Cardiovascular Significance of Endothelium-Derived Vasoactive Factors

Edited by

Gabor M. Rubanyi, M.D., Ph.D.

Professor of Pharmacology
New York University Medical Center
New York, New York;

Director of Institute of Pharmacology
Research Center, Schering AG,
Berlin, Germany

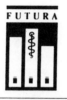

FUTURA

**Futura Publishing
Company, Inc.**
Mount Kisco, NY
1991

Library of Congress Cataloging-in-Publication Data

Cardiovascular significance of endothelium-derived vasoactive factors
 / editor, Gabor M. Rubanyi.
      p.   cm.
    Includes bibliographical references.
    Includes index.
    ISBN 0-87993-359-3
    1. Endothelium-derived contracting factors.   2. Endothelium-
derived relaxing factors.   3. Blood—Circulation—Regulation.
4. Cardiovascular system—Diseases—Pathophysiology.   I. Rubanyi,
Gabor M., 1947–
    [DNLM: 1. Cardiovascular Diseases—physiopathology.
2. Endothelium-Derived Relaxing Factor—physiology.   3. Endothelium,
Vascular—physiology.   4. Hemodynamics—physiology.
5. Prostaglandins X—physiology.   QV 150 C2754]
QP88.45.C37   1991
616.1'07—dc20
DNLM/DLC
for Library of Congress   90-14132
                                                   CIP

Copyright 1991
Futura Publishing Company, Inc.

Published by
 Futura Publishing Company, Inc.
 2 Bedford Ridge Road
 Mount Kisco, New York 10549

LC #: 90-14132
ISBN #: 0-87993-359-3

Every effort has been made to ensure that the information in this
book is as up to date and as accurate as possible at the time of
publication. However, due to the constant developments in
medicine, neither the author, nor the editor, nor the publisher
can accept any legal or any other responsibility for any errors
or omissions that may occur.

Printed in the United States of America.

To my wife,
Edith,
and my children,
Thomas and Dora

Contributors

Regina M. Botting
The William Harvey Research Institute, St. Bartholomew's Hospital Medical College, Charterhouse Square, London, England

Chantal Boulanger, Ph.D.
Department of Research. Laboratory of Vascular Research, University Hospital, Basel, Switzerland

Fritz R. Buhler, M.D.
Laboratory of Hypertension, University Hospital, Basel, Switzerland

Geoffrey Burnstock, M.D.
Department of Anatomy and Developmental Biology and Centre for Neuroscience, University College of London, London, England

Sidney Cassin, Ph.D.
Department of Physiology, College of Medicine, University of Florida, Gainesville, Florida

John P. Cooke, M.D., Ph.D.
Division of Vascular Medicine and Atherosclerosis, Brigham and Women's Hospital, Boston, Massachusetts

Mark A. Creager, M.D.
Division of Vascular Medicine and Atherosclerosis, Brigham and Women's Hospital, Boston, Massachusetts

Yasuaki Dohi, M.D., Ph.D.
Department of Research, Laboratory of Vascular Research, University Hospital, Basel, Switzerland

John A. Dormandy, M.D.
Department of Vascular Surgery, St. George's Hospital and Medical School, London, England

Victor J. Dzau, M.D.
Division of Cardiovascular Medicine, Falk Cardiovascular Research Center, Stanford University School of Medicine, Stanford, California, formerly at Division of Vascular Medicine and Atherosclerosis, Brigham and Women's Hospital, Boston, Massachusetts

Peter Ganz, M.D.
Brigham and Women's Hospital and Harvard Medical School, Boston, Massachusetts

Gary H. Gibbons, M.D.
Molecular and Cellular Research Laboratory, Brigham and Women's Hospital, Harvard Medical School, Boston, Massachusetts

Katsutoshi Goto, Ph.D.
Institute of Basic Medical Sciences, University of Tsukuba, Tsukuba, Iberaki, Japan

Garrett J. Gross, Ph.D.
Department of Pharmacology and Toxicology, The Medical College of Wisconsin, Milwaukee, Wisconsin

Richard J. Gryglewski, M.D.
Department of Pharmacology, Copernicus Academy of Medicine, Grzegorzecka, Cracow, Poland

Ricardo Guerra, M.D.
Department of Medicine, The University of Iowa, Iowa City, Iowa

David G. Harrison, Ph.D., M.D.
Department of Medicine, Emory University, Atlanta, Georgia

Philip J. Kadowitz, Ph.D.
Department of Pharmacology, Tulane University School of Medicine, New Orleans, Louisiana

Gabor Kaley, Ph.D.
Department of Physiology, New York Medical College, Valhalla, New York

Sadao Kimura, Ph.D.
Institute of Basic Medical Sciences, University of Tsukuba, Tsukuba, Iberaki, Japan

Akos Koller, M.D.
Department of Physiology, New York Medical College, Valhalla, New York

Hermes A. Kontos, M.D., Ph.D.
Division of Cardiology, Department of Internal Medicine, Medical College of Virginia, Richmond, Virginia

Malcolm J. Lewis, M.B., Ph.D.
Department of Cardiology, University of Wales College of Medicine, Cardiff, Wales

Jill Lincoln, Ph.D.
Department of Anatomy and Developmental Biology and Centre for Neuroscience, University College of London, London, England

Thomas F. Lüscher, M.D.
Department of Medicine, Division of Cardiology, and Department of Research, Laboratory of Vascular Research, University Hospital, Basel, Switzerland

J. Jeffrey Marshall, M.D.
Department of Medicine, Medical College of Virginia, Richmond, Virginia

Tomoh Masaki, M.D., Ph.D.
Institute of Basic Medical Sciences, University of Tsukuba, Tsukuba, Iberaki, Japan

Fiona M. McDonald, M.D.
Research Laboratories of Schering AG, Berlin, Germany

James M. McLenachan, M.D.
Brigham and Women's Hospital and Harvard Medical School, Boston, Massachusetts

Dennis B. McNamara, Ph.D.
Department of Pharmacology, Tulane University School of Medicine, New Orleans, Louisiana

Edward J. Messina, Ph.D.
Department of Physiology, New York Medical College, Valhalla, New York

Robert K. Minkes, Ph.D.
Department of Pharmacology, Tulane University School of Medicine, New Orleans, Louisiana

Robert L. Minor, M.D.
Department of Medicine, The University of Iowa, Iowa City, Iowa

B. Müller, D.V.M.
Research Laboratories of Schering AG, Berlin, Germany

Galen M. Pieper, M.D.
Department of Pharmacology and Toxicology, The Medical College of Wisconsin, Milwaukee, Wisconsin

James E. Quillen, M.D.
Department of Medicine, The University of Iowa, Iowa City, Iowa

V. Ralevic
Department of Anatomy and Developmental Biology and Centre for Neuroscience, University College of London, London, England

Gabor M. Rubanyi, M.D., Ph.D.
Professor of Pharmacology, New York University Medical Center, New York, New York; Director of Institute of Pharmacology, Research Center, Schering AG, Berlin, Germany

Thomas J. Ryan, Jr., M.D.
Brigham and Women's Hospital and Harvard Medical School, Boston, Massachusetts

Frank W. Sellke, M.D.
Department of Medicine, The University of Iowa, Iowa City, Iowa

Andrew P. Selwyn, M.D.
Brigham and Women's Hospital and Harvard Medical School, Boston, Massachusetts

John T. Shepherd, M.D., D.Sc.
Department of Physiology and Biophysics, Mayo Clinic and Foundation, Rochester, Minnesota

Jerry A. Smith, B.Sc., Ph.D.
Department of Pharmacology and Therapeutics, University of Wales College of Medicine, Cardiff, Wales

Yoh Takuwa, Ph.D.
Institute of Basic Medical Sciences, University of Tsukuba, Tsukuba, Iberaki, Japan

Charles B. Treasure, M.D.
Brigham and Women's Hospital and Harvard Medical School, Boston, Massachusetts

Julie I. Tucker, B.S.
Division of Vascular Medicine and Atherosclerosis, Brigham and Women's Hospital, Boston, Massachusetts

Sir John R. Vane, Ph.D., D.Sc.
The William Harvey Research Institute, St. Bartholomew's Hospital Medical College, Charterhouse Square, London, England

Paul M. Vanhoutte, M.D., Ph.D.
Department of Medicine, Center for Experimental Therapeutics, Baylor College of Medicine, Houston, Texas

Vladimir I. Vekshtein, M.D.
Brigham and Women's Hospital and Harvard Medical School, Boston, Massachusetts

Joseph A. Vita, M.D.
Brigham and Women's Hospital and Harvard Medical School, Boston, Massachusetts

Franz F. Weidinger, M.D.
Brigham and Women's Hospital and Harvard Medical School, Boston, Massachusetts

Werner Witt
Research Laboratories of Schering AG, Berlin, Germany

Michael S. Wolin, Ph.D.
Department of Physiology, New York Medical College, Valhalla, New York

Masashi Yanagisawa, M.D., Ph.D.
Institute of Basic Medical Sciences, University of Tsukuba, Tsukuba, Iberaki, Japan

Alan C. Yeung, M.D.
Brigham and Women's Hospital and Harvard Medical School, Boston, Massachusetts

Preface

It has long been recognized that endothelial cells play an important role in essentially all aspects of normal animal biology and that most major diseases are associated with pathophysiological alterations in endothelial cell structure and function. In addition to its other important functions (which include, among others, capillary transport of water and solutes, regulation of plasma lipids, participation in inflammatory and immune responses, in cell growth and proliferation and tumor angiogenesis and metastasis), the endothelial cell contributes to cardiovascular homeostasis by maintaining the fluidity of the blood and by adjusting the caliber of blood vessels to the ever-changing hemodynamic and hormonal environment.

The vascular endothelium performs these functions primarily by the production of a host of biologically active substances including pro- and anticoagulant molecules, proliferative and antiproliferative substances and factors which modulate the tone of underlying vascular smooth muscle. The latter, termed endothelium-derived vasoactive factors, is the focus of this monograph.

Due to the tremendous progress in the past decade, we have a better understanding not only of the chemical nature of these factors but also of their diverse biological activities in health and disease. For example, under physiological conditions, by virtue of their vasodilator, antiplatelet, and cytoprotective properties, endothelium-derived relaxing factors (EDRFs) and prostacyclin act synergistically to maintain the fluidity of blood and adequate tissue perfusion. Endothelial dysfunction, characterized by decreased synthesis/release of these relaxing substances and maintained or facilitated synthesis/release of contracting factors (EDCFs), can lead to various pathological consequences such as thrombosis, vasospasm, and hypertension. These pathophysiological results of endothelial dysfunction have been observed not only in intact animals but also in patients with various cardiovascular diseases.

Historically, researchers have approached the study of the endothelium and endothelium-derived vasoactive factors from many different fields including molecular biology, cell biology, biochemistry, pharmacology, physiology, pathology, and clinical sciences. Technical reports are dispersed across many scientific journals that often do not share a common audience. Although several excellent reviews, monographs, and books on endothelium-derived vasoactive factors have been published in recent years, they dealt with one or more of the specific features of this exponentially growing field. It was imperative, therefore, to try to summarize the existing knowledge from a different perspective. The editor and participating authors with their excellent contributions have recognized this need and have attempted to create a book that unites these diverse interests and that provides a concise introduction and review to major conceptual issues, theoretical questions, and practical (clinical) considerations. By so doing, this volume will provide the reader with a sense of not only what these novel factors represent today, but where this field may be headed in the future. This monograph is, therefore, different from its predecessors in many ways.

First, its major goal is not only to give a comprehensive summary of the state-of-the-art of present knowledge about these factors, but to also put this knowledge into perspective as to what may be the potential significance of these factors in the control of the cardiovascular system. Second, it is consciously organized to give an in-depth summary, not only about the chemical nature and biological action of these factors, but also to focus on their potential role in different vascular beds, in different cardiovascular diseases, and also in novel therapeutic concepts which are emerging from the key discoveries of the past decade.

In line with these goals, the book is divided into four parts: Part I gives comprehensive reviews (written by the pioneers of each field) on the key endothelium-derived vasoactive factors: prostacyclin, EDRF, EDCF, and endothelin. The last chapter in this part of the book introduces a novel concept that the endothelium is the site of synthesis and storage of several known neurohumoral mediators (e.g., acetylcholine, histamine, serotonin, angiotensin II, substance P, vasopressin, etc.) which can act in an autocrine fashion to release the vasoactive factors from endothelial cells. Part II discusses the significance of endothelium-derived vasoactive factors in the control of blood flow through special vascular beds under normal and pathological conditions including the coronary, the cerebral, and the pulmonary circulation and the peripheral microcirculation. Part III gives an in-depth analysis of the potential pathophysiological significance of endothelial dysfunction in hypertension, in diabetes, in hyperlipidemia, in atherosclerosis, and in thrombosis. Part IV focuses on novel therapeutic potentials represented by the stable prostacyclin analogue, iloprost.

This book is a valuable source of integrated information and also raises novel ideas and potential directions for future research in this exciting field of cardiovascular sciences. It is therefore recommended for basic scientists and clinicians alike from a variety of disciplines including, for the basic scientist, cell biology, biochemistry, physiology, pharmacology, and pathology and for the clinical sciences, angiology, vascular surgery, organ transplantation, cardiology, lipid disorders, atherosclerosis, diabetes, coagulopathies, etc.

It is our hope that this book will be not only a useful source of information providing a pleasant and exciting reading experience but will also stimulate further thoughts and research ideas to the readers, whether they are actively involved in the field or just watching its glorious progress.

I wish to thank the leading scholars for their excellent contributions that made this book possible, and the staff of Futura Publishing Co. for their very efficient handling and timely publication of this volume.

Gabor M. Rubanyi, M.D., Ph.D.

Introduction

Endothelium-Derived Vasoactive Factors in Health and Disease

Gabor M. Rubanyi

Key discoveries in the past 15 years have proved that the vascular endothelium is more than just a lining for blood vessels and have led to many important new concepts in vascular biology and pathophysiology. Because of its key localization in the circulation, its ability to *sense* changes in the mechanical (hemodynamic forces such as shear stress or pressure) (Rubanyi et al., 1986; Harder, 1987; Rubanyi, 1988d) chemical (pO_2) (Rubanyi and Vanhoutte, 1985) and humoral environment (circulating or locally produced amines, peptides, proteins, nucleotides, and arachidonic acid and its metabolites) and to *transduce* these changes into compensatory adjustments of vascular tone (short-term adjustment) (Vanhoutte et al., 1986; Vanhoutte, 1987) or structure (long-term adjustment) (Langille and O'Donell, 1986; Dzau et al., 1989) by the production of biologically active substances (Fig. 1), the vascular endothelium plays a significant role in cardiovascular homeostasis.

The series of key discoveries in the field of endothelium-derived vasoactive factors started in 1976 when Vane and his colleagues demonstrated that the vascular endothelium synthesizes and releases prostacyclin, a potent antiplatelet, vasodilator, profibrinolytic, and cytoprotective metabolite of arachidonic acid (Moncada et al., 1976), which contributes to the thrombo-resistant and vasodilator properties of the endothelium (Fig. 2) (see Chapter 1). This was followed in 1980 by the cornerstone observation of Furchgott and Zawadzki showing that the presence of endothelium is obligatory for acetylcholine to evoke relaxation in isolated rings of rabbit aorta (Furchgott and Zawadzki, 1980). Endothelium-dependent vascular relaxation is mediated by a nonprostanoid substance(s), which was termed endothelium-derived relaxing factor or EDRF (see Chapter 2). In the following 6 years, bioassay studies revealed that (1) EDRF is a diffusible substance with a very short biological half-life (Griffith et al., 1984; Rubanyi et al., 1985); (2) similar to nitrovasodilators, it activates soluble guanylate cyclase and increases cyclic GMP levels (Rapoport and Murad, 1983); (3) it can be inhibited by hemoglobin (Martin et al., 1985); and (4) it is destroyed by superoxide anion and protected by superoxide dismutase (SOD) (Rubanyi and Vanhoutte, 1986; Gryglewski et al., 1986; Rubanyi, 1988b). The nature of EDRF remained unknown until 1986 when, based on their striking similarities, Furchgott and Ignarro independently proposed that it is identical with nitric oxide (NO) (Furchgott et al., 1987; Ignarro et al., 1987). In 1987, Moncada and his colleagues demonstrated the presence of NO in the effluent of cultured endothelial cells (Palmer et al., 1987), and later discovered that it is derived from L-arginine (Palmer et al., 1988). Recent findings suggest that EDRF may be identical with

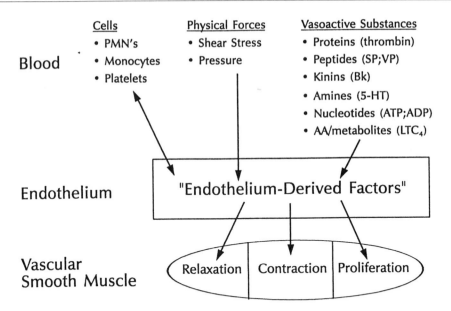

Figure 1: *Modulation of the tone and structure of vascular smooth muscle by the vascular endothelium.* The endothelial cell has the ability to "sense" changes in hemodynamic (physical) forces, and respond to vasoactive substances (circulating or locally produced), and mediators released from blood cells (e.g., polymorphonuclear neutrophils, PMNs) and platelets. These stimuli then trigger the synthesis/release of biologically active substances from the endothelium ("Endothelium-Derived [Vasoactive] Factors") which modulate the tone (relaxation or contraction) of underlying vascular smooth muscle. By virtue of these recently discovered properties, the vascular endothelium contributes to cardiovascular homeostasis in a significant way. SP = substance P; VP = vasopressin; BK = bradykinin; 5-HT = serotonin; ATP, ADP = adenosine, tri- and diphosphate; LTC_4 = leukotriene C_4.

a labile nitroso compound (e.g., S-nitroso-L-cysteine) rather than free NO (Myers et al., 1989; Rubanyi et al., 1989, 1990). It has been recognized that not all endothelium-dependent vascular responses can be explained by the classic EDRF(NO) (Rubanyi and Vanhoutte, 1987). The existence of an endothelium-derived hyperpolarizing factor (EDHF) was postulated, which mediates endothelium-dependent smooth muscle hyperpolarization (Komori and Suzuki, 1987; Vanhoutte, 1987) (Fig. 2).

In the early 1980s, Vanhoutte and colleagues made pioneering observations that introduced concepts about the potential cardiovascular significance of endothelium-derived vasoactive factors (see Chapter 2). They discovered, for example, that thrombin and aggregating platelets stimulate the release of EDRF, which in turn will dilate blood vessels, increase blood flow, and inhibit platelet aggregation, thereby preventing the formation of occlusive thrombi (Fig. 3) (DeMey and Vanhoutte, 1982; Cohen et al., 1983). By virtue of its vasodilator and antiplatelet effects, EDRF(NO) acts synergistically with prostacyclin, but via a different signal transduction pathway. While prostacyclin elevates cyclic AMP, EDRF(NO) (similar to organic nitrovasodilators) stimulates soluble guanylate cyclase and elevates cellular cyclic GMP levels (Fig. 3). Recently it was proposed that cytoprotection (by virtue of eliminating toxic free radicals) may be an important additional biological function of EDRF(NO) (Fig. 4) (Feigl 1988; Rubanyi, 1988a). Endothelium-dependent relaxation was shown to be a ubiquitous phenomenon

Thrombo-Resistance

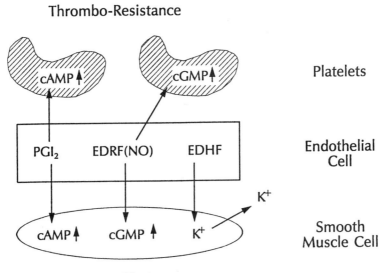

Figure 2: *Endothelium-derived relaxing factors (EDRFs).* Prostacyclin (PGI$_2$) and EDRF [identical with nitric oxide (NO) or a labile nitroso compound] relax vascular smooth muscle and inhibit platelet aggregation by elevating tissue levels of cyclic AMP (cAMP) and cyclic GMP (cGMP), respectively. Endothelium-derived hyperpolarizing factor (EDHF) relaxes vascular smooth muscle by membrane hyperpolarization presumably via activating K$^+$ channels. These factors contribute to the "thrombo-resistant" and "vasodilator function" of the endothelium.

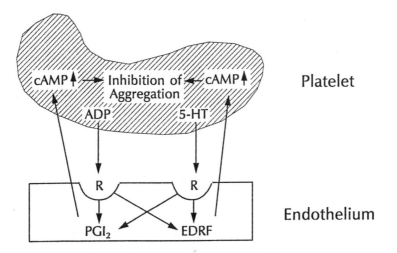

Figure 3: *Antithrombogenic function of the endothelium.* Aggregating platelets release adenosine diphosphate (ADP) and 5-hydroxytryptamine (5-HT; serotonin) which activate specific receptors (R) on the endothelium and stimulate the synthesis/release of PGI$_2$ and EDRF. These endothelium-derived vasoactive factors will inhibit platelet aggregation and trigger vasodilation (see Fig. 2), which will prevent the development of occlusive thrombi.

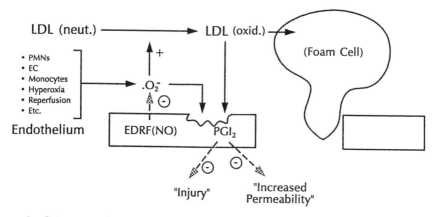

Figure 4: *Cytoprotective function of the endothelium.* By virtue of its interaction with superoxide anion radicals ($.O_2^-$), EDRF(NO) can be regarded as an extracellular scavenger of this toxic radical species produced by activated leukocytes (PMNs) and by several cell types under various pathological conditions (e.g., hypoxia, reoxygenation/reperfusion, etc.) (Rubanyi, 1988a,b; Feigl, 1988). Prostacyclin (PGI$_2$) on the other hand, "protects" endothelial cells from injury caused by various noxious stimuli (including free radicals) and also decreases endothelial permeability. The synergistic cytoprotective actions of EDRF(NO) and PGI$_2$ may hypothetically play an important role in preventing or delaying the development of atherosclerosis by virtue of protecting LDL from oxidative modification by $.O_2^-$ (EDRF) and by maintaining endothelial cell integrity (PGI$_2$).

present in various species (from bony fishes to humans) (Miller and Vanhoutte, 1986). EDRF(NO) is produced by a variety of cells and tissues (e.g., leukocytes, monocytes, and neurons) other than the endothelium, suggesting that it is a widely distributed mediator which may modulate a variety of bodily functions.

Soon after the discovery of EDRF, Vanhoutte and his co-workers demonstrated that the endothelium can mediate not only vasorelaxation, but also vasoconstriction (Fig. 5) (DeMey and Vanhoutte, 1982). Similar to EDRF(s), bioassay studies revealed that endothelium-dependent vasoconstriction is mediated by diffusible substance(s) termed endothelium-derived contracting factors (EDCFs) (Rubanyi and Vanhoutte, 1985; Rubanyi, 1988c) (Fig. 5). The exact nature of EDCFs has not been established, but cyclooxygenase products (or free radicals) of the arachidonic acid metabolic cascade (EDCF$_1$) may be responsible for several of the endothelium-mediated contractions described (Fig. 5). In contrast to the widespread *popularity* of EDRF, the phenomenon of endothelium-mediated contraction and EDCFs remained the interest of only a few laboratories. As a consequence, knowledge regarding the nature and cardiovascular significance of EDCFs is relatively limited. Nonetheless, endothelium-dependent vasoconstriction evoked by hypoxia (Rubanyi and Vanhoutte, 1985) or increases in transmural pressure (Harder, 1987; Rubanyi, 1988d) have been postulated to contribute to *physiological* responses such as exclusion of poorly ventilated alveoli from the pulmonary circulation (hypoxic pulmonary vasoconstriction) or autoregulation of blood flow in the cerebral and renal vascular beds. Discovery of a peptidergic vasoconstrictor produced by cultured endothelial cells (Hickey et al., 1985) and its isolation, purification, and identification as a 21-amino acid unique peptide, endothelin (Yanagisawa et al., 1988) further emphasized the potential importance of the endothelium in modulating vascular tone. Although endothelin is not likely to be the EDCF that mediates rapid

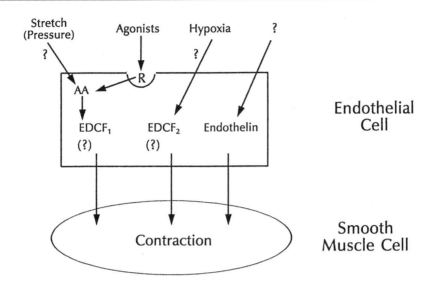

Figure 5: *Endothelium-derived contracting factors (EDCFs).* Bioassay studies showed that similar to EDRFs, endothelium-dependent contraction of vascular preparations in response to (1) stretch or increased transmural pressure, (2) various agonists (e.g., arachidonic acid and thrombin in canine veins; acetylcholine, ADP, and 5-HT in the aorta of SHR, etc.), and (3) hypoxia are mediated by diffusible vasoactive substances released from the endothelium (EDCF). Endothelium-dependent contractions evoked by stretch and agonists can be prevented by inhibition of cyclooxygenase, suggesting that the mediator is probably a vasoconstrictor metabolite of arachidonic acid (TXA$_2$, endoperoxide) or a free radical (e.g., .O$_2^-$) (EDCF$_1$). The nature of the bioassayable mediator released by hypoxia is still unknown (?) (EDCF$_2$). The recently discovered potent vasoconstrictor polypeptide endothelin can also be regarded as an endothelium-derived contracting factor; however, the stimuli which trigger its synthesis/release under physiological or pathological conditions are still unknown (?).

changes in vascular tone, its wide distribution in the body and intriguing diverse biological activity make it a potential candidate to play a role in many physiological and pathological processes (Rubanyi, 1989) (see Chapter 3). Using histochemical, biochemical, and biological techniques, Burnstock and his colleagues found that the endothelium can store and probably synthesize a variety of known neurohumoral mediators which are released under various conditions and may act in an autocrine fashion to stimulate the release of endothelium-derived vasoactive factors (see Chapter 4).

It is believed that under physiological conditions, a balance between endothelium-derived relaxing (EDRF, EDHF, PGI$_2$) and contracting (TXA$_2$, free radicals, EDCFs, endothelin) substances contribute to the maintenance of optimal vessel caliber and adequate tissue perfusion (Fig. 6). The discovery of endothelium-dependent regulation of vascular smooth muscle growth/proliferation (Langille and O'Donell, 1986) added a new dimension to the potential significance of endothelium-derived vasoactive factors. They may be involved not only in short-term modulation of vascular tone, but also in long-term adjustment of vascular structure (remodeling) (Dzau et al., 1989).

In certain diseases the endothelium cannot perform its physiological function. Dysfunction of the endothelium can be defined as an imbalance between relaxing and

Balance Between Contracting and Relaxing Factors

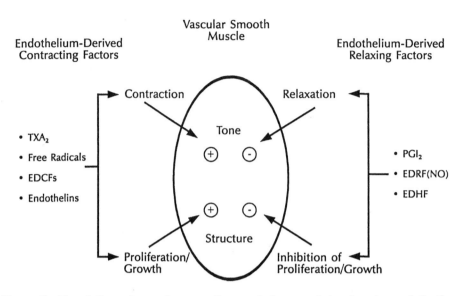

Figure 6: *Regulation of vascular smooth muscle tone and structure by endothelium-derived vasoactive factors.* Under physiological conditions, a delicate balance exists between relaxing (right) and contracting (left) factors produced by the endothelium. These factors (in concert with a wide variety of other growth-promoting and inhibiting substances, which are not mentioned here) can also influence the growth and proliferation of cellular elements (e.g., smooth muscle) in the blood vessel wall. When the endothelial cell functions normally, the physiological balance between EDRFs and EDCFs contributes to short-term (tone) and long-term (structure) adjustment of vessel caliber to the ever-changing demands of the hemodynamic and humoral environment. However, after endothelial injury (not denudation!) these cells become dysfunctional [i.e., loss of protective function by EDRFs (see Figs. 2, 3, and 4), with maintained or augmented synthesis/release of EDCFs]. This imbalance (or endothelial dysfunction) can lead to various pathological conditions (e.g., thrombosis, vasospasm, hypertension, etc.) (see Fig. 7).

contracting factors, between anti- and procoagulant mediators or growth-inhibiting and growth-promoting factors (Fig. 6). This imbalance can develop by reduced synthesis/release of *protective* factors (EDRF, PGI_2) or augmented synthesis/release of contracting/growth-promoting substances, or both. This imbalance can lead to serious pathophysiological consequences, including localized (vasospasm) or generalized (hypertension) increase in vascular tone or proliferation (e.g., hypertension, atherosclerosis) and thrombosis. Endothelial dysfunction (either as a cause or consequence) has been identified for numerous cardiovascular diseases, including thrombosis (see Chapter 14), hyperlipidemia (see Chapter 11), atherosclerosis (see Chapter 12), hypertension (see Chapter 9), diabetes (see Chapter 10), coronary (see Chapter 5) and cerebral vasospasm (see Chapter 6), and peripheral arterial occlusive diseases (see Chapters 8 and 16) (Fig. 7). The more we learn about these factors (their nature, the cellular mechanism(s) of their synthesis/release and action) in health and

Endothelial Dysfunction
and Cardiovascular Diseases

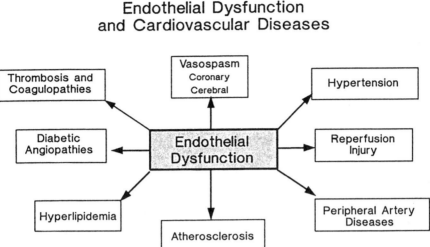

Figure 7: *Cardiovascular diseases where the existence of endothelial dysfunction (see Fig. 6) has been demonstrated.* Endothelial dysfunction can develop as the consequence of the pathological process (e.g., diabetes, reperfusion after myocardial ischemia [MI], hyperlipidemia) or may play a pathogenetic role contributing to certain diseases (e.g., thrombosis, vasospasm, hypertension, peripheral artery disease, atherosclerosis). Better understanding of the exact nature of endothelial dysfunction (including the role played by endothelium-derived vasoactive factors) may provide a basis for novel therapies in these vasculopathies.

disease, the more focused our attempts will be to investigate their contribution to cardiovascular diseases and to seek appropriate novel therapies to prevent or treat such diseases. As an example, only a few years after its discovery, stable analogues of prostacyclin (e.g., iloprost) have already been used with significant clinical success for the treatment of various vascular diseases (see Chapters 15 and 16). It is our hope that similar progress can (and will) be made with other endothelium-derived vasoactive factors as well. By summarizing the present knowledge on the cardiovascular significance of PGI_2, EDRFs, EDCFs, and endothelin, this book may contribute to this cause in a significant way.

References

1. DeMey J.G., Vanhoutte P.M.: Heterogenous behavior of the canine arterial and venous wall. Circ. Res. 51:439–447, 1982.
2. Cohen R.A., Shepherd J.T., Vanhoutte P.M.: Inhibitory role of the endothelium in the response of isolated coronary arteries to platelets. Science 221:273–274, 1983.
3. Dzau V.J., Cooke J.P., Rubanyi G.M.: Significance of endothelial derived vasoactive substances. J. Vasc. Med. Biol. 1:43–45, 1989.
4. Feigl E.O.: EDRF: a protective factor? Nature 331:490–491, 1988.
5. Furchgott R.F., Zawadzki J.V.: The obligatory role of endothelial cells in the relaxation of arterial smooth muscle by acetylcholine. Nature 288:373–376, 1980.

6. Furchgott R.F., Khan M.T., Jothianandan D.: Comparison of endothelium dependent relaxation and nitric oxide induced relaxation in rabbit aorta. Fed. Proc. (Abstract) 46:385, 1987.
7. Griffith T.M., Edwards D.H., Lewis M.J., Newby A.C., Henderson A.H.: The nature of endothelium-derived vascular relaxant factor. Nature 308:645–647, 1984.
8. Gryglewski R.F., Palmer R.M.F., Moncada S.: Superoxide anion plays a role in the breakdown of EDRF. Nature 320:454–456, 1986.
9. Harder D.R.: Pressure-induced myogenic activation of cat cerebral arteries is dependent on intact endothelium. Circ. Res. 60:102–107, 1987.
10. Hickey K.A., Rubanyi G., Paul R.J., Highsmith R.F.: Characterization of a coronary vasoconstrictor produced by cultured endothelial cells. Am. J. Physiol. 248 (Cell. Physiol. 17):C550–C556, 1985.
11. Ignarro L.J., Byrns R.E., Buga G.M., Wood K.S.: Endothelium-derived relaxing factor from pulmonary artery and vein possess pharmacologic and chemical properties identical to those of nitric oxide radical. Circ. Res. 61:866–879, 1987.
12. Komori K., Suzuki H.: Heterogeneous distribution of muscarinic receptors in the rabbit saphenous artery. Br. J. Pharmacol. 92:657–664, 1987.
13. Langille B.L., O'Donell F.: Reductions in arterial diameter produced by chronic decreases in blood flow are endothelium-dependent. Science 231:405–407, 1986.
14. Martin W., Villani G.M., Jothianandan D., Furchgott R.F.: Selective blockade of endothelium-dependent and glyceryl trinitrate-induced relaxation by hemoglobin and by methylene blue in the rabbit aorta. J. Pharmacol. Exp. Ther. 232:708–716, 1985.
15. Miller V.M., Vanhoutte P.M.: Endothelium-dependent responses in isolated blood vessels of lower vertebrates. Blood Vessels 23:225–235, 1986.
16. Moncada S., Gryglewski R., Bunting S., Vane J.R.: An enzyme isolated from arteries transforms prostaglandin endoperoxidase to an unstable substance that inhibits platelet aggregation. Nature 263:663–665, 1976.
17. Palmer R.M.J., Ferrige A.G., Moncada S.: Nitric oxide release accounts for the biological activity of endothelium-derived relaxing factor. Nature 327:524–526, 1987.
18. Palmer R.M.J., Ashton D.S., Moncada S.: Vascular endothelial cells synthesize nitric oxide from L-arginine. Nature 333:664–666, 1988.
19. Rapoport R.M., Murad F.: Agonist-induced endothelium-dependent relaxation in rat thoracic aorta may be mediated through cGMP. Circ. Res. 52:352–357, 1983.
20. Rubanyi G.M., Vanhoutte P.M.: Hypoxia releases a vasoconstrictor substance from canine vascular endothelium. J. Physiol. (Lond) 364:24–56, 1985.
21. Rubanyi G.M., Lorenz R.R., Vanhoutte P.M.: Bioassay of endothelium-derived relaxing factor(s). Inactivation by catecholamines. Am. J. Physiol. 249:H95–H101, 1985.
22. Rubanyi G.M., Vanhoutte P.M.: Superoxide anions and hypoxia inactivate endothelium-derived relaxing factor. Am. J. Physiol. 250:H822–H827, 1986.
23. Rubanyi G.M., Romero J.C., Vanhoutte P.M.: Flow-induced release of endothelium-derived relaxing factor. Am. J. Physiol. 250:H1145–H1149, 1986.
24. Rubanyi G.M., Vanhoutte P.M.: Nature of endothelium-derived relaxing factor: Are there two relaxing mediators? Circ. Res. (Suppl II) 61:II61–II67, 1987.
25. Rubanyi G.M.: Potential role of endothelium-derived relaxing factor in the protection against free radical injury. J. Mol. Cell. Cardiol. 20 (suppl V):2S56, 1988a.
26. Rubanyi G.M.: Vascular effects of oxygen-derived free radicals. Free Radical Biol. Med. 4:107–120, 1988b.
27. Rubanyi, G.M.: Endothelium-derived vasoconstrictor factors. In: Endothelial Cell, edited by Una S. Ryan, Cleveland, OH: CRC, Vol. III:61–74, 1988c.
28. Rubanyi G.M.: Endothelium-dependent pressure-induced contraction of isolated canine carotid arteries. Am. J. Physiol. 255:H783–H788, 1988d.
29. Rubanyi G.M., Johns A., Harrison D.G., Wilcox D.: Evidence that EDRF may be identical with an S-nitrosothiol and not with free nitric oxide. Circulation 80 (Suppl II):II-281, 1989.
30. Rubanyi G.M.: Maintenance of "basal" vascular tone may represent a physiologic role for endothelin. J. Vasc. Med. Biol. 1:315–316, 1989.
31. Rubanyi G.M., Greenberg S.S., Wilcox D.E.: Endothelium-derived relaxing factor cannot be identified as free nitric oxide by electron paramagnetic resonance spectroscopy. In: Endothelium-Derived Relaxing Factors. Eds. G.M. Rubanyi and P.M. Vanhoutte, Karger, Basel, pp. 32–38, 1990.

32. Vanhoutte P.M., Rubanyi G.M., Miller V.M., Houston, D.S.: Modulation of vascular smooth muscle contraction by the endothelium. Annu. Rev. Physiol. 48:307–320, 1986.
33. Vanhoutte P.M.: Endothelium and the control of vascular tissue. News Physiol. Sci. 2:18–22, 1987.
34. Yanagisawa M., Kurihara H., Kimura A., Tomobe Y., Kabayashi M., Mitsui Y., Yazaki Y., Goto K., Masaki T.: A novel potent vasoconstrictor peptide produced by vascular endothelial cells. Nature 332:411–415, 1988.

Contents

Part I
Endothelium-Derived Vasoactive Factors

Part II
Endothelial Control of Special Vascular Beds
in Health and Disease

Part III
Endothelial Dysfunction and Cardiovascular Diseases

Part IV
Therapeutic Considerations

Abbreviations Used in This Book

AA = arachidonic acid, eicosatetraenoic acid
ACAT = acyl-CoA/cholesterol o-acyltransferase
ACE = angiotensin I converting enzyme
ACEH = acid cholesterol ester hydrolase
ADP = adenosine diphosphate
cAMP = cyclic adenosine monophostate
Apo A-I = apolipoprotein A-I, a major Apo of HDL
Apo B = apolipoprotein B, a major Apo of LDL
ATP = adenosine-5'-triphosphate
CAT = catalase
CoQ_{10} = coenzyme Q_{10}, ubiquinone
DAG = 1,2-diacylglycerol
EDCF = endothelium-derived contracting factor
EDRF = endothelium-derived relaxing factor
EGF = epidermal growth factor
EPA = eicosapentaenoic acid
GC/MS = gas chromatography/mass spectrometry
cGMP = cyclic guanosine monophostate
GSH = reduced glutathione
GTP = guanosine-5'-phosphate
HDL = high density lipoprotein
HETE = hydroxyeicosatetraenoic acid
HHT = 12-hydroxyheptadecatrienoic acid
HPETE = hydroperoxyeicosatetraenoic acid
5-HT = 5-hydroxytryptamine
IP_3 = inositol 1,4,5-triphosphate
Kd = dissociation constant
kDa = kilodalton
LDL = low density lipoprotein
LT = leukotriene
MDA = malondialdehyde
t-PA = tissue plasminogen activator
PAD = peripheral arterial disease
PAI-1 = specific t-PA inhibitor
PDGF = platelet-derived growth factor
PG = stable prostaglandin
PGG_2 and PGH_2 = prostaglandin endoperoxides
PGI_2 or PGX = prostacyclin
PIP_2 = phosphatidylinositol 4,5-biphosphate
PLA_2 = phospholipase A_2
PLC = phospholipase C
PUFA = polyunsaturated fatty acids
RIA = radioimmunoassay
mRNA = messenger ribonucleic acid
SHR = spontaneously (genetically) hypertensive rats
SOD = superoxide dismutase
SRS-A = slow reacting substance of anaphylaxis
TX = thromboxane
TXSI = thromboxane synthase inhibitors

Part 1

Endothelium-Derived Vasoactive Factors

1

Prostacyclin: From Discovery to Clinical Application

Richard J. Gryglewski, Regina M. Botting, John R. Vane

Discovery of PGX

Prostaglandin X (PGX), the name of which was later changed to prostacyclin (prostaglandin I_2, PGI_2) was discovered as a product of the biotransformation of prostaglandin endoperoxides (PGG_2 or PGH_2) by an enzyme from arterial walls.[26,90,195,196] This discovery was deeply rooted in the principles of bioassay which had been founded by Dale, Burn, and Gaddum and which were developed into a philosophy for making discoveries by Vane.[305-307]

In 1969 Piper and Vane[230] had shown that immunologically challenged guinea pig lungs released in addition to histamine, SRS-A (slow reacting substance of anaphylaxis), and prostaglandins, another unstable "rabbit aorta contracting substance" (RCS), the generation of which was inhibited by aspirin. In 1972 Gryglewski and Vane[98] demonstrated that RCS from dog spleen had a half-life of 2–4 minutes, its generation was boosted by

arachidonic acid (AA) and hindered by nonsteroidal anti-inflammatory drugs. Therefore, it was proposed that RCS represented the biological activity of an unstable intermediate in the biosynthesis of prostaglandins from AA.

In 1967 Samuelsson and colleagues[253] postulated the existence of such an unstable intermediate—a cyclic prostaglandin endoperoxide. Indeed, in 1973 two cyclic prostaglandin (PG) endoperoxides (PGG_2 and PGH_2) were isolated, their chemical structures elucidated and their biological RCS-like activity confirmed.[108,213] In addition, Samuelsson and colleagues discovered that PG endoperoxides aggregated blood platelets, and then their RCS-like potency was augmented and their half-life substantially shortened to 30 seconds.[110,282] This change in the profile of the RCS-like activity of PG endoperoxides by platelets led to the discovery of their enzymatic conversion to thromboxane A_2 (TXA_2) which is a platelet activator, vasoconstrictor, and cytotoxic agent with a half-life of 30 seconds.[109] The corresponding

Rubanyi G.M.: Cardiovascular Significance of Endothelium-Derived Vasoactive Factors, Futura Publishing Co., Inc., Mount Kisco, NY, © 1991.

enzyme, TXA_2 synthase, was soon indentified in platelet microsomes.[207]

An urgent question emerged at that stage of research: do microsomes from other cells or organs convert PG endoperoxides to TXA_2? We employed the Vane bioassay system composed of smooth muscle detectors which were superfused in cascade[305] in such a way that they could differentiate between stable prostaglandins (PGE_2, $PGF_{2\alpha}$) prostaglandin endoperoxides (PGH_2 $PGG_{2\alpha}$) and thromboxane A_2 (TXA_2).

When incubated with PG endoperoxides, microsomes from kidney, lung, liver, brain, skin, and spleen of laboratory animals generated mainly stable PGs at the expense of the disappearing PG endoperoxides. Some of the microsomal preparations generated traces of TXA_2. However, only microsomes from porcine aorta avidly consumed PG endoperoxides without a concomitant generation of stable PGs or TXA_2.

The first and false assumption was that aortic microsomes had catalyzed breakdown of PG endoperoxides to malondialdehyde (MDA) and a 12-hydroxyheptadecatrienoic acid (HHT) thus scavenging substrates for the generation of PGs and TXA_2. In fact, aortic microsomes were making from PGH_2 an unstable (half-life of 3–5 minutes at 37°C, pH 7.4) vasodilator and platelet-suppressant agent which we named "prostaglandin X" – PGX. PGX was more stable when generated on ice. The biological activity of PGX could then be extracted into ethyl acetate and stayed there for hours, although in aqueous solutions PGX decomposed within a few minutes to a stable and biologically inactive prostaglandin. When $1\text{-}^{14}C$ AA was incubated with a coupled system of ram seminal vesicle and porcine aortic microsomes, radiochromatograms showed a peak located between standard peaks of PGE_2 and $PGF2_\alpha$. However, that novel peak had no biological activity at all.

Johnson et al.[136] elucidated the chem-ical structure of the product of decomposition of PGX as 6-keto-prostaglandin $F_{1\alpha}$ (6-keto-$PGF_{1\alpha}$ or 6-oxo-$PGF_{1\alpha}$) whereas PGX itself was 9-deoxy-6, 9α-epoxy-$^{\Delta5}$-$PGF_{1\alpha}$. The name given to PGX was prostacyclin,[136] although the abbreviation introduced subsequently—PGI_2—is a misleading one. Prostacyclin is a nonprostaglandin, unstable enol-ether system which is easily hydrolyzed (especially at low pH and high temperature) to a stable and inactive prostaglandin. Tribute should be paid to Pace-Asciak and Wolfe[222] who as early as 1971 recognized the potential of 6(9)-oxo products as intermediates in the formation of a novel stable prostaglandin by rat stomach homogenates, which turned out to be 6-keto-$PGF_{1\alpha}$.[220] The elegant biochemical studies of Pace-Asciak[221] gave an important clue to the biosynthetic pathway of prostacyclin and, consequently, to its chemical structure.

At the time of the discovery of prostacyclin[26,90,195,196] four additional observations were made.

(1) A high yield from the conversion of PG endoperoxides to prostacyclin was found in porcine aortic and rat stomach microsomes. However, microsomes obtained from other sources, except for platelets, also generated small amounts of prostacyclin. Thus, the principal product of cyclooxygenation of AA in arterial walls can also be generated by other tissues.

(2) Prostacyclin synthase from aortic microsomes was inhibited by micromolar concentrations of lipid peroxides, eg by 15-HPETE (15-hydroperoxyeicosatetraenoic acid). The significance of this finding for etiopathogenesis of thrombosis and atherosclerosis was recognized in the very same series of papers which dealt with the discovery of PGX.

(3) Aggregation of blood platelets in platelet-rich plasma by adenosine diphosphate (ADP) was not only prevented by PGX but preformed platelet aggregates were also dissipated. Thus, not only the antiaggregatory but also the disaggrega-

tory action of prostacyclin on platelet clumps was discovered.

(4) Blood platelets could feed indomethacin-treated arterial rings with their PG endoperoxides. In consequence, vascular PGX was generated at the expense of platelet PG endoperoxides. Teleologically speaking, this appeared to be an attractive arrangement since aortic microsomes converted AA to PGX at a very low rate (<1%) in contrast to their high conversion rate of PGH_2 to PGX (>30%). At that point we formulated the idea of collaboration between platelets and vascular wall in generating prostacyclin, an idea confirmed by others.[2,224,255,292] The core of this concept was later developed and made more general by Marcus[176] in a hypothesis on "transcellular metabolism of eicosanoids."

At the end of 1976, it was already obvious that prostaglandin endoperoxides, apart from being transformed to stable prostaglandins, were also the substrates for the biosynthesis of a pair of chemically unstable substances with opposing activities—thromboxane A_2 and prostacyclin.

Actions of Prostacyclin

Prostacyclin is a vasodilator, platelet-suppressant, fibrinolytic and cytoprotective agent which is considered to be an endogenous antithrombotic and antiatherogenic principle. The platelet-suppressant action of prostacyclin is associated with activation of platelet adenylate cyclase and a rise in cAMP levels.[18,85,293] Platelet receptors for prostacyclin are the same as those for PGE_1 and 6-keto-PGE_1 but different from those for PGD_2.[172,192,236,320] These receptors have been recently purified as a protein of molecular weight 190 kilodaltons (kDa) and high affinity binding sites for PGE_1 of kDa = 9.8 nM.[60] The surface expression of these receptors on human platelets is down-regulated by cholesterol.[81] The introduction of the radioligand

(^{3}H) iloprost, a chemically stable analogue of prostacyclin, allowed the study of prostacyclin receptors in several types of cells including neoplastic ones.[310]

The rise in platelet cAMP stimulated by prostacyclin inhibits mobilization of fibrinogen binding sites on thrombin and ADP-treated platelets.[114] A similar prostacyclin-induced rise in cAMP in vascular smooth muscle[130] and in endothelial cells[254] may well be responsible for vasodilatation and maintenance of endothelial integrity, although vasodilatation by prostacyclin has also been attributed to membrane hyperpolarization which is induced by the opening of K^+ channels.[264]

Prostacyclin activates adenylate cyclase in lungs.[171] Unlike PGE_2, prostacyclin is not removed on passage through the pulmonary circulation.[3] In contrast, when the lung receives blood containing activated platelets, this organ enriches the arterial blood with endogenous prostacyclin from the pulmonary endothelium.[92] Not only platelet-derived nucleotides but also endothelin and other vasoactive peptides release prostacyclin from perfused isolated lungs.[54,88] Prostacyclin dilates the pulmonary vascular bed,[128] although it has weak effects on bronchial tone.[111]

Fluctuations in the biosynthesis of prostacyclin do not seem to play a role in the pathogenesis of hypertension. Hypertensive, salt-sensitive Dahl rats[301] or patients with essential hypertension[280] have abnormally high rates of prostacyclin synthesis, whereas spontaneously (genetically) hypertensive rats (SHR) rats either have low prostacyclin levels[272] or show no difference from normal.[169] Vascular prostacyclin synthesis can be low at the time immediately preceding development of hypertension[194] and this may contribute to its progression.[71] The enhanced synthesis of prostacyclin by vascular smooth muscle that parallels raised blood pressure may therefore be a compensatory adaptive mechanism in response to the hypertensive state. It is just as difficult to reconcile the renal effects of prostacyclin—stimulation of intravascular renin release and urinary kallikrein excretion—with a possible role in the pathogenesis of hypertension.[262]

In vascular smooth muscle, prostacyclin (via cAMP) enhances the activity of acid cholesterol ester hydrolase (ACEH), though it does not influence the activity of acyl-CoA/cholesterol O-acyl-transferase (ACAT). The latter is inhibited by PGE_2. Thus, the concerted actions of prostacyclin and PGE_2 will trigger an outflow of free cholesterol from the vascular wall. This process is facilitated by the extracellular presence of HDL apoproteins that serve as cholesterol carriers.[101] It could well be that, in vivo, the prostacyclin and PGE_2 generating system is responsible for clearing cholesterol esters off the vascular wall, whereas an inhibition of this system by lipid peroxides[90,154] brings about an accumulation of cholesterol esters in the vascular wall, followed by formation of foam cells and atherogenesis. In this respect there is good news for moderate drinkers, in whose arteries acetaldehyde is a potent stimulant for the production of prostacyclin,[81] possibly through the induction of cytochrome-P 450-dependent prostacyclin synthase[113,302,303] and in whose blood HDL goes up after an intake of alcohol. However, this has only been shown so far in rats!

Willis and colleagues[321–323] found that prostacyclin and its analogues suppress the accumulation of cholesterol esters by macrophages and also suppress the release of growth factors from endothelial cells, macrophages and platelets. The latter effect is seen at concentrations that are one-tenth of those required to inhibit platelet aggregation. Prostacyclin inhibits the release of platelet-derived growth factor (PDGF) from α-granules in preference to β-thromboglobulin and platelet factor 4. In addition, a decrease in the lipid content of vascular walls has been seen in humans after prostacyclin infusion, in this way supporting the in vitro data of Hajjar[101] of an enhanced removal of cholesterol from vascular smooth muscle cells under the influence of prostacyclin.

The first observation on the thrombolytic action of prostacyclin in dogs with pulmonary thromboembolism[304] was followed by reports on shortening of euglobulin clot lysis time in patients who had been treated with prostacyclin for peripheral vascular disease[50,286] or central retinal vein occlusion.[336] The inhibitory effect of aspirin on fibrinolysis in human volunteers is prevented by replacing endogenous prostacyclin with its stable analogue iloprost.[17] The release of t-PA (tissue plasminogen activator) from the vascular wall[203,274,286] or inhibition of PAI-1 secretion from platelets, endothelial cells and hepatocytes[16] have been claimed and denied[17] as mechanisms of the fibrinolytic action of prostacyclin. Indeed, prostacyclin exhibits fibrinolytic action only in vivo and ex vivo but it has no activity on lysis time of euglobulin clots in vitro.[88] However, in whole coagulating human blood, prostacyclin stimulates thrombolysis at concentrations that have no effect on hemostasis.[86] Even though the thrombolytic effect of prostacyclin in humans is weaker and less general than that of streptokinase,[203,286] prostacyclin potentiates streptokinase-induced thrombolysis in vivo.[259] Moreover, streptokinase alone activates platelets and thus it evokes a generalized increase in the production of endogenous prostacyclin in patients with myocardial infarction.[69] It is likely that the fibrinolytic effect of streptokinase is supported by the fibrinolytic action of endogenously released prostacyclin.

André Robert[245] introduced the term *cytoprotection* to describe the ability of several prostaglandins (including prostacyclin)[199] to protect the gastric mucosa from damage by ethanol or other noxious agents. This term has been borrowed to describe the phenomenon of protection by prostacyclin of other cells, tissues and organs against multifactorial injury. Attempts to replace this term by *cellular protection, metabolic protection,* or *histoprotection* have not been successful. The term *cytoprotection* is still used to describe protection by prostacyclin of platelets against aging,[191] cardiac myocytes against hypoxic damage,[63] glial cells and neurons against anoxia[242] and hepatocytes against chemical injury.[28] Prostacyclin also protects against postischemic reperfusion damage to animal brains[102,103] and hearts.[138,160,189] In the heart, prostacyclin reduces the frequency of arrhythmias and limits the size of myocardial infarction.[137]

Among possible mechanisms underlying the cytoprotective action of prostacyclin, the most interesting explanation is that prostacyclin combats oxygen free radicals that are generated during tissue injury, for instance in the ischemic area after reperfusion.[185] In ischemic myocardium, free radicals may arise from infiltrating leukocytes,[260,318] from the ischemic tissue itself subsequent to intercoversion of xanthine dehydrogenase to xanthine oxidase[185] or as a result of the depletion of ubiquinone (CoQ_{10}) from cardiac mitochondria.[219] Indeed, free radical scavengers such as superoxide dismutase (SOD),[318] CoQ_{10},[215,219] nitric oxide donors[80] and others[204] are cardioprotective in a similar fashion to prostacyclin,[137,138,189] prostacyclin analogues[257,291] and prostacyclin activators.[36,209,219]

Biosynthesis of Prostacyclin

Metabolism of Arachidonic Acid in the Vascular Wall

The rate-limiting step in the biosynthesis of prostacyclin by the vascular wall is the availability of substrate. Arachidonic acid (eicosatetraenoic acid, 20:4n6, AA) is released in endothelial cells and in the smooth muscle of the vascular wall by a variety of agents that stimulate either phospholipase A_2 (PLA_2) or phospholipase C (PLC).[124,153,155] Prostacyclin is the major metabolite of AA produced by the vascular endothelium of large blood vessels while the underlying vascular smooth muscle cells are less efficient generators of prostacyclin unless they undergo transformation to neointima. Formation of PGE_2 and PGD_2 takes precedence over generation of prostacyclin in isolated[83] and cultured[198] endothelial cells of brain microvessels. The PGI_2/PGE_2 production ratio is lower in microvascular than in macrovascular endothelial cells.[84,294]

Vascular tissue may generate small amounts of TXA_2 along with prostacyclin.[188] A variety of monohydroxy-, dihydroxy-, and epoxy derivatives of AA are also formed as products of lipoxygenation, cyclooxygenation, and cytochrome P-450-dependent monooxygenation of AA[184,229,233,243] (Fig. 1). There is a variety of species-dependent, age-dependent, region-dependent, diet-dependent, and culture-medium-dependent profiles of oxidative metabolism of AA in blood vessels.[1,39,233,294]

Powell and Funk[233] have recently demonstrated that vascular tissue from fetal calves is particularly active in metabolizing free AA to prostacyclin and other eicosanoids. In fetal aorta the conversion rate of AA to prostacyclin is >10%, whereas in most arteries of adult laboratory animals it remains in the range of 0.5–1% and in human colic and gastric arteries and veins it does not exceed 0.01%.[197] Thus, fetal calf arteries are especially suitable for studies of AA metabolism.

The enzyme that initiates the metabolism of AA is named PGH synthase or PGG/H synthase. It is a heme-containing glycoprotein and catalyzes two reactions—bis-dioxygenation of AA to the hydroperoxy endoperoxide PGG_2 (cyclooxygenation activity) and reduction of PGG_2 to the

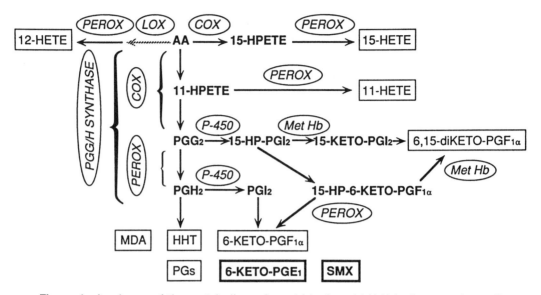

Figure 1: A scheme of the metabolism of arachidonic acid (AA) in the vascular wall as modified after Powell and Funk.[233] Stable products that have been isolated and identified are surrounded by square frames. Enzymes (COX = cyclooxygenase; LOX = lipoxygenase; PEROX = peroxidase; P-450 = P-450-dependent PGI$_2$ synthase); and cofactors (Met Hb = methemoglobin) that catalyze the conversion reactions are surrounded by circles. HP = hydroperoxide; SMX = a stable metabolite X (for structure, see text); for others, same abbreviations as used in text.

hydroxy endoperoxide PGH$_2$ (peroxidase activity). The cyclooxygenase and peroxidase activities cannot be separated by physical methods. At present, the enzymic homodimer composed of two 70 kDa subunits is being studied for localization of active sites of dioxygenase and peroxidase.[181] PGG/H synthase has been cloned.[56] Adrenaline, hydroquinone, and other polyphenols such as flavonols activate the peroxidase function of PGH synthase.[233] Kuehl and colleagues[148] were the first to point out the biological significance of the peroxidase function of PGG/PGH synthase. According to them, weakening of that function leads to accumulation of the pro-inflammatory lipid peroxide, PGG$_2$. Phenolic derivatives activate peroxidase and thus act as anti- inflammatory agents, which are alternatives to aspirin-like inhibitors of cyclooyganase.[307]

In the vascular wall, PGH$_2$ undergoes a rearrangement consisting of the activa-tion of the 9-oxygen atom for a new oxygen-carbon (9, 6) bond is formed during the biosynthesis of bicyclic prostacyclin. This is brought about by PGI$_2$ synthase which is a cytochrome P-450-dependent enzyme like TXA$_2$ synthase.[113,302,303] Incidentally, liver microsomal cytochrome P-450-dependent monooxygenases do not catalyze TXA$_2$ or PGI$_2$ formation. Therefore, PGI$_2$ and TXA$_2$ synthases constitute a new class of cytochrome P-450 enzymes in which the heme iron does not undergo a redox cycle between ferrous and ferric forms. Thereby, the term *cytochrome* is not appropriate for these hemoproteins.[303] "Regular" cytochrome P-450-dependent and NADPH-dependent enzymes monooxidize AA to a number of epoxy- and hydroxy-trienoic and tetraenoic acids (the third pathway of AA metabolism), some of which may replace AA as substrates for cyclooxygenase and, subsequently, for PGI$_2$ synthase.[261]

It is possible that instead of PGH_2, small amounts of PGG_2 are used as substrate for PGI_2 synthase. In that case, instead of PGI_2, 15-hydroperoxy PGI_2 (15-HP-PGI_2) is formed. Both of these are spontaneously hydrolyzed to inactive 6-keto-$PGF_{1\alpha}$ and to its 15-hydroperoxy derivative, which in turn is rapidly converted to 6-keto-$PGF_{1\alpha}$ by peroxidases or in the presence of heme compounds (e.g., methemoglobin) nonenzymatically dehydrated to 6,15-diketo-$PGF_{1\alpha}$[233] (Fig. 1). It was claimed that platelet 9-hydroxy-PG-dehydrogenase may convert prostacyclin to its stable and biologically active mebolite, 6-keto-PGE_1.[326] We consider 6-keto-PGE_1 as a minor product (conversion rate ~0.1%) of nonenzymatic hydrolysis of prostacyclin. 6-keto-PGE_1 is formed along with biologically inactive 6-keto-$PGF_{1\alpha}$ and 7-[3-(hydroxy-1-octenyl)-4-hydroxy-tetrahydro-pyranel-6-oxo-heptanoic acid (SMX) with conversion rates ~96% and 4%, respectively.[174]

In a series of elegant papers, Fitzgerald,[73,74] Patrono[37,226] and their colleagues have shown that in humans the secretion rate of prostacyclin amounts to 0.08–0.1 ng/kg/min and the maximal estimate of its circulating concentration is 3.4 pg/mL with a half-life of 3 minutes. After an intravenous infusion of prostacyclin into volunteers, 6-keto-$PGF_{1\alpha}$ and 13,14-dihydro-6,15-diketo-$PGF_{1\alpha}$ accumulate in plasma to similar levels. However, the latter enzymic metabolite of prostacyclin is cleared at a considerably lower rate than 6-keto-$PGF_{1\alpha}$. In turn, 2,3-dinor-6-keto-$PGF_{1\alpha}$ is the major urinary metabolite of systemically infused prostacyclin, whereas urinary 6-keto-$PGF_{1\alpha}$ represents the renal capacity to generate prostacyclin. The corresponding "low turnover" major metabolites of TXA_2 in plasma and urine are 11-dehydro-TXB_2 and 2,3-dinor-TXB_2. These findings suggest caution in assessing data on plasma levels of 6-keto-$PGF_{1\alpha}$ and TXB_2 as an index of PGI_2/TXA_2 balance in vivo, since these "high turnover" products may be formed during blood sampling.

Microsomes from fetal calf aorta also convert AA to 11-, 12-, and 15-hydroxyeicosatetraenoic acids (HETEs).[233] As expected, adrenaline (a peroxidase cofactor) stimulates the generation of HETEs. Surprisingly, indomethacin inhibits the formation not only of 6-keto-$PGF_{1\alpha}$ and 11-HETE but also of 15-HETE whereas it stimulates the generation of 12-HETE. Consequently, 11-HETE and 15-HETE must be considered as products of cyclooxygenation and 12-HETE as a product of lipoxygenation of AA (Fig. 1). In other vascular beds and in other species the profile of cyclooxygenation and lipoxygenation products may differ considerably.[233]

Lipid Peroxides, Oxygen Free Radicals, and Prostacyclin

Lands[154] has shown that hydroperoxides of fatty acids at low concentrations (10 pM-100 nM) are required to initiate cyclooxygenation of PA. Activation of PGG/H synthase may be initiated from inside the cell by PGG_2, 15-hydroperoxy-PGI_2 (15-HP-PGI_2), or HPETEs (Fig. 1) or from outside through a transcellular regulating mechanism[176] which consists of a transfer of 5-HPETE and H_2O_2 from leukocytes or 12-HPETE from platelets. For instance, human and guinea pig neutrophils and macrophages produce sufficiently low amounts (60 nM) of lipid peroxides to activate PGG/H synthase in co-incubated cultured U937 cells,[182] possibly in concert with other neutrophil-derived stimulators of prostacyclin synthesis.[193] Peroxides or free radicals produce arteriolar vasodilatation in dog brain,[144] rat cremaster muscle[325] and bovine lungs.[324] The complex mechanism of this response includes activation of the prostacyclin release from endothelial cells[325] and an indirect activation of guanylate cyclase by peroxides in vascular smooth muscle.[324]

It may appear unusual that the peroxidase subunit of PGG/H synthase removes an intermediate (PGG_2) which triggers the activity of its cyclooxygenase subunit. This apparent paradox has two possible explanations. First, "peroxide tone," which regulates cyclooxygenase activity, is maintained not only by PGG_2 but also by linear lipid peroxides (e.g., HPETEs) which are decomposed by gluthathione peroxidases.[179] Second, hydroperoxides at concentrations >1 μM inhibit cyclooxygenation of AA. The peroxidase subunit within PGG/H synthase might be considered an intrinsic mechanism regulating enzymic activity of the whole complex including a possible irreversible self-deactivation in the presence of an excess of substrate.[61] In that case, because of a difference in kinetics between cyclooxygenase and peroxidase, lipid peroxides (11-HPETE, 15-HPETE, or PGG_2) will accumulate and destroy PGG/H and PGI_2 synthases.[329] This destruction can be prevented by a group of antioxidants which includes flavonols,[93] ascorbic acid,[91] α-tocopherol,[216,284] nafazatrom,[21,47] nordihydroguaiaretic acid,[329] BW 755C, or dipyridamole[9] which may protect the prostacyclin-generating capacity of blood vessels from being inhibited by lipid peroxides.

A further enzymic step, i.e., that mediated by PGI_2 synthase, is also susceptible to inhibition by lipid peroxides.[90] Lipid peroxides at concentrations >1 μM inhibit both PGG/H and PGI_2 synthases. The inhibitory potency of 15-HPETE on PGI_2 synthase in porcine aortic microsomes (IC_{50} = 1.5 μM)[90,250] is much weaker than in A23187-stimulated cultured endothelial cells from bovine coronary artery (IC_{50} <<0.1 μM).[243] This may point to a high susceptibility of coronary arteries to biochemical damage by lipid peroxides although species differences cannot be excluded.

It is possible that the inhibitory action of peroxides on PGI_2 synthase is mediated by oxygen free radicals which are formed during peroxidase-dependent reduction of lipid hydroperoxides.[106] Hydroxyl radicals are the most likely to be involved.[249] In contrast to PGI_2 synthase, TXA_2 synthase is resistant to destruction by oxygen free radicals,[106] while endothelium-derived relaxing factor (EDRF, nitric oxide) is selectively destroyed by superoxide anions[96] rather than by hydroxyl radicals. The differential action of superoxide anions and hydroxyl radicals has also recently been described in platelets, the aggregation and adhesiveness of which are increased by superoxide anions but not by hydroxyl radicals.[252] Nonetheless, superoxide anions can serve as an alternative source of hydroxyl radicals[104,271] which in turn would be capable of affecting the activity of PGG/H and PGI_2 synthases. Low intracellular concentrations of lipid peroxide and oxygen free radicals are likely to stimulate cyclooxygenation of AA, but they do not affect PGI_2 synthase: the resultant effect would be to stimulate prostacyclin formation. However, high concentrations of free radicals inhibit both enzymes,[154] reduce prostacyclin synthesis, and cause damage to many cells and tissues[65] including endothelial cells.[125]

Superoxide anions are generated not only by activated neutrophils, macrophages, and platelets[177] but also by cultured endothelial cells exposed to calcium ionophore, phorbol esters,[183] or menadione.[246] In rats, guinea pigs, and dogs, but not in humans, endothelial cells contain xanthine dehydrogenase/oxidase.[276] Any potential hazard from intracellular generation of oxygen free radicals or their transfer from the extracellular space is reduced by endothelial superoxide dismutase, catalase, and the glutathione redox cycle,[29,125,281] as well as by antioxidant molecules of tocopherols, carotenes, ascorbic acid, and reduced glutathione

(GSH) which scavenge free upaired electrons from radical molecules.[276]

Interestingly, hyperoxia (95% O_2:5% CO_2) applied to cultured bovine pulmonary artery endothelial cells for 72 hours increases rather than diminishes the generation of prostacyclin, although the production of superoxide anions is markedly enhanced.[131] Hyperoxia (50% O_2:5% CO_2:45% N_2) applied to cultured rat fetal lung endothelial cells for 72 hours does not change the generation of prostacyclin, although hypoxia (1% O_2:5% CO_2:94% N_2) suppresses the AA- and A23187 ionophore-stimulated release of prostacyclin.[217] In vivo, hyperoxia is responsible for acute and chronic lung injury which is paradoxically prevented by pretreatment with endotoxin,[77] possibly because endotoxin increases the activity of superoxide dismutase in cultured bovine pulmonary endothelial cells.[263] On the other hand, a short exposure (10 min) of cultured endothelial cells to hydrogen peroxide (100 μM) irreversibly inactivates cyclooxygenase. The generation of prostacyclin becomes re-established only after new enzyme has been synthesized.[61]

The inactivation of superoxide anions by endothelial cells is potentiated by the mere act of adhesion of neutrophils to the endothelial surface.[125] On the other hand, this enzymic defense system is overcome by the topical application of AA or bradykinin to the brain surface of anesthetized cats, a procedure that produces cerebral arteriolar vasodilatation[144] and increased blood-brain barrier permeability to proteins.[314] These vascular effects are mediated by superoxide anions and hydrogen peroxide since they are prevented by exogenously applied superoxide dismutase and catalase. Anticancer antibiotics adriamycin, mitomycin, or bleomycin also destroy the endothelial antioxidant barrier since they cause injury to the endothelium,[158] generate superoxide anions in biological systems, and are cardiotoxic for

humans.[139] A substantial body of literature connects the PGG/H synthase embedded peroxidase activity with the formation of potential carcinogens by a mechanism which involves co-oxygenation of xenobiotics.[24,180]

The most prolific producers of superoxide anions, hydrogen peroxide, hydroxyl radicals, and lipid peroxides in the circulation are neutrophils activated with opsonized zymosan, N-formyl-L-methionyl-L-leucyl-L-phenylalanine (f-MLP), calcium ionophores, phorbol esters, and other agents.[64] In neutrophils stimulated with f-MLP or zymosan, prostacyclin is a weak superoxide suppressant and much less effective than PGE_1, 6-keto-PGE_1, PGE_2, PGD_2, or the stable prostacyclin analogues iloprost, taprostene, or naxaprostene in inhibiting generation of superoxide anions.[64,256,275,333] The efficacy of prostaglandins to suppress superoxide anions parallels their potency in stimulating adenylate cyclase in leukocytes. However, this is not the case with prostacyclin analogues which only marginally raise cAMP levels in leukocytes.[275] The concept of Kuehl and colleagues[107,147,148] seems to be valid: in neutrophils PGE_2 acts as a stimulator of adenylate cyclase whereas in platelets a similar function is performed by PGI_2.

Along with superoxide anions, neutrophils generate a "nitric oxide-like factor."[251] This factor stimulates cystosol-soluble guanylate cyclase[251] in a manner similar to EDRF[82,87,240] and lipid or hydrogen peroxides.[219] Synthetic nitric oxide donors (e.g., a metabolite of molsidomine, SIN-1) synergize with iloprost in its protective action against aging of neutrophils and activation of platelets.[145] Studies of the interactions between a biochemical triangle—eicosanoids:oxygen free radicals: nitric oxide radical—and a biological triangle — endothelial cells : leukocytes : platelets—present a challenging field for new research.

Physiology, Pathology, and Pharmacology of Prostacyclin Release

Substances that Release Prostacyclin

The recognized intracellular signal for the biosynthesis of prostacyclin is a rise in free calcium concentration $[Ca^{++}]_i$ in the cytoplasm of endothelial cells. Most of the substances that release prostacyclin increase $[Ca^{++}]_i$ by stimulation of cell membrane receptors which are linked through a pertussis-toxin-sensitive guanosine monophostate- (GTP) binding protein (protein G) to phospholipase C (PLC). Thus, activated PLC digests membrane phosphoinositides (PIP$_2$) and generates two second messengers—diacylglycerol (DAG) and inositol triphosphate (IP$_3$). Both of these influence $[Ca^{++}]_i$: DAG by activation of protein kinase C and IP$_3$ by a direct effect on the endoplasmic reticulum.[15]

In cultured bovine aortic endothelial cells, the receptor-mediated release of prostacyclin is coupled to the release of EDRF, and both are associated with activation of the PLC-phosphoinositide system,[53] although differently influenced by extra- and intracellular calcium.[167] The vascular release of prostacyclin by adrenaline and sodium fluoride is not mediated by cAMP, as might be expected, but through activation of either α-adrenergic receptors linked to PLC[134] or G protein linked to protein kinase C.[135] The same intracellular endothelial signaling system is linked to the activation of purinergic P$_2$ receptors by ADP and ATP[22,116,227,231] and kinin B$_2$ receptors by bradykinin and its analogues.[53,167] A similar linkage may exist between thrombin,[316] substance P,[11] muscarinic,[25,212] 5-HT$_2$,[143] endothelin-3,[164] and PDGF[41] receptors, and the biochemical machinery that releases prostacyclin from the vascular wall.

Receptor-mediated activation of PLC is an attractive hypothesis explaining the initiation of the biosynthesis of prostacyclin in endothelial cells. According to this concept, DAG may serve not only as a messenger for activation of protein kinase C but also as a source of AA. On the other hand, by mobilizing $[Ca^{++}]_i$, IP$_3$ may activate PLA$_2$[155] and again additional free AA would appear in the vicinity of PGG/H synthase. However, it has also been claimed that in cultured porcine aortic endothelial cells, bradykinin-induced activation of PLA$_2$ is independent of the activation of PIP$_2$ by PLC.[140] Nonreceptor-mediated mechanisms of prostacyclin release include direct activation of PLA$_2$, entry of extracellular calcium into endothelial cells or feeding endothelial cells with exogenous AA.[316] Interestingly, in cultured porcine[95] and bovine[53] aortic endothelial cells, most receptor agonists are ineffective as prostacyclin releasers and these cells lack voltage-sensitive calcium channels.[40] It may be that in these nonphysiological cells, bradykinin releases prostacyclin by a nonreceptor-mediated mechanism, that of direct stimulation of PLA$_2$.

The endogenous mechanisms for controlling the release of prostacyclin are not known. Studies with vasoactive peptides such as angiotensin or bradykinin reveal a complex picture. Bradykinin but not angiotensin releases prostacyclin from cultured porcine or bovine aortic endothelial cells and from perfused guinea pig lungs.[44,55,95] In perfused lungs, but not in cultured cells, this effect of bradykinin is potentiated by captopril, an ACE inhibitor.[55] However, angiotensin I and angiotensin II release prostacyclin from isolated perfused lungs, kidneys, and the mesenteric vascular bed of rabbits, and from blood vessels of anesthetized cats.[88] This release of prostacyclin by angiotensin I is blocked by captopril. On the other hand, captopril elevates plasma levels of 6-keto-PGF$_{1\alpha}$ in man[273] and increases the urinary excretion of 6-keto-PGF$_{1\alpha}$ in dogs.[313] Both prostacyclin and captopril potentiate left ventricular reflexes to veratridine in dogs,[223] which in the case of captopril can be inhibited by indomethacin. These findings are in line with the assumption that in humans and dogs inhibition of ACE prevents the breakdown of bradykinin, which is a potent generator of prostacyclin in man.[115] Thus, in humans the kinin system overrides the angiotensin system in promoting the generation of prostacyclin. However, the blood pressure lowering effects of captopril in hypertensive subjects[235] lead to the opposite conclusion.

Acetylcholine is another example of the ambiguous behavior of an endogenous mediator of prostacyclin release. Acetylcholine was used as an agonist to stimulate the release of EDRF from the endothelium of fresh arterial tissues.[82] In these preparations agonists at muscarinic receptors released prostacyclin along with EDRF[76] (Fig. 2), although they failed to do so in cultured porcine[95] and bovine[53] aortic endothelial cells, in perfused rabbit lungs, and in anesthetized dogs.[201] However, in anesthetized cats, acetylcholine and methacholine are among the most potent triggers which release an unstable, aspirin-ablated disaggregatory principle into arterial blood, and in volunteers carbachol releases from the lungs prostacyclin metabolites that can be detected by gas chromatography/mass spectrometry) (GC/MS).[25,212]

Platelet-derived PG endoperoxides are the best candidates for the role of endogenous modulators of the biosynthesis of vascular prostacyclin, as we originally proposed at the time of the discovery of prostacyclin.[26,90,196] This shunt for feeding arteries with platelet PG endoperoxides was later renamed the "steal" phenomenon, and its existence was confirmed in experiments with a mixture of platelets and cultured endothelial cells[178,255] or with rabbit de-endothelialized aorta which interacted with platelets in vivo.[224] When TX synthase inhibitors—TXSI (dazoxiben,

OKY-046, CGS 13080, and others) became available, there appeared reports on the promotion by TXSI of a transfer of PGH_2 from platelets to aortic microsomes in vitro[151] or from anticoagulated blood to aortic rings.[244] Prostacyclin-like effects of TXSI in vivo have also been described, e.g., potentiation by TXSI of an increase in coronary blood flow induced by local intra-arterial administration of AA[260] or the prevention by TXSI of the recurrent obstruction of coronary arteries in dogs, a phenomenon that was reversed by a cyclooxygenase inhibitor.[2] However, the definitive experiment was performed in rabbits with a nylon thread inserted into one of the jugular veins.[47] In these animals administration of dazoxiben resulted in a distinct rise in 6-keto-$PGF_{1\alpha}$ at the thread site but a smaller rise at a control site in the contralateral vein. Thus, platelets in which TXA_2 synthase is blocked have to be activated (by a nylon thread!) in order to supply PG endoperoxides to the vascular endothelium. It is a local transfer of PG endoperoxides to a well-defined group of endothelial cells that makes prostacyclin locally and not a general process. Thus, TXSI can amplify the generation of prostacyclin in patients whose platelets are activated, as happens in atherosclerosis.

Fitzgerald et al.[73] detected a two- to threefold increase in the urinary excretion of 2,3-dinor-6-keto-$PGF_{1\alpha}$ following the administration of two out of three TXSI tested, while others[68] found both plasma 6-keto-$PGF_{1\alpha}$ and urinary 2,3-dinor-6-keto-$PGF_{1\alpha}$ unchanged after treatment with a TXSI, UK-38485. These and similar studies in man (for review see reference 73), although interesting, may not reflect the local generation of prostacyclin by the vascular wall at the particular site of its interaction with activated platelets. Should generalized activation of platelets occur in a subject who has a sufficiently large area of healthy endothelium to metabolize PG endoperoxides from activated platelets, then measurement of urinary 2,3-dinor-6-keto-

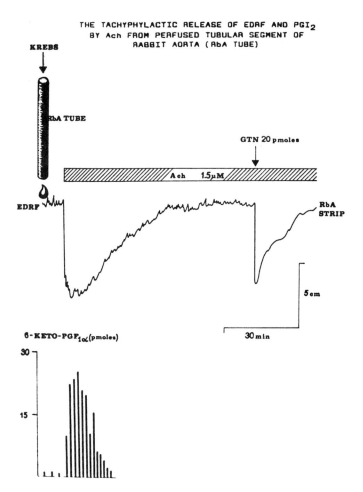

Figure 2: The acetylcholine-induced coupled tachyphylactic release of EDRF (assayed by relaxation of a precontracted rabbit aortic strip and compared to a standard relaxation with glyceryl trinitrate, GTN) and prostacyclin (measured by radioimmunoassay of 6-keto-PGF$_{1\alpha}$) as measured in the effluent from a tubular segment of rabbit aorta perfused with Krebs' buffer containing acetylcholine hydrochloride (Ach) at a concentration of 1.5 μM.

PG$_{1\alpha}$ would assess an enhancement of total prostacyclin turnover in the body. This situation occurs in patients with acute myocardial infarction who have been treated with streptokinase[69] or in patients with severe atherosclerosis.[75]

Two serum factors influence prostacyclin turnover: PGI$_2$ synthesis stimulating factor[173,244] and PGI$_2$ stabilizing factor.[332] The first has not yet been chemically characterized and is deficient in patients with

thrombotic microangiopathy.[241] The second was thought to be serum albumin[328] until its recent characterization as Apo A-I, the major apolipoprotein of HDL.[332] Thus Apo A-I not only serves as a carrier for cholesterol from the vascular wall to the liver[101,321] but also lengthens the half-life of prostacyclin. Apo A-I makes prostacyclin available for its anti-atherosclerotic action.[321,332]

There are many physiological and

pharmacological agents that modify the release of prostacyclin by little known mechanisms. For instance, γ-interferon,[62] interleukin-1,[175,247] and interleukin-2[327] induce prostacyclin formation in endothelial and smooth muscle cells following an incubation period longer than 6 hours, possibly through de novo synthesis of PGG/H synthase. Epidermal growth factor (EGF) stimulates phosphorylation of lipocortin and thus removes the lipocortin blockade of m-RNA (messenger ribonucleic acid) which is responsible for the formation of PGG/H synthase.[4,5] Platelet-derived growth factor (PDGF), a mitogen and vasoconstrictor,[131] enhances the vascular release of prostacyclin, and in turn prostacyclin inhibits PDGF release from platelets. Atherosclerotic vascular tissue is less responsive to PDGF-stimulation.[269] The vasodilator and fibrinolytic actions of nicotinic acid derivatives in humans and in cats are mediated through the release into the blood of a prostacyclin-like substance.[49] Low molecular weight serum factor,[241,244] a new kallikrein-induced peptide,[202] endotoxin,[312] and nitroglycerine[187] are all claimed to stimulate the formation of prostacyclin in vitro. Before accepting a substance as a potentially important stimulator of prostacyclin synthesis, it is prudent to confirm its activity in more than one experimental system and to demonstrate that its pharmacological actions supposedly mediated through prostacyclin release are abolished by pretreatment with a cyclooxygenase inhibitor. Many so-called "PGI$_2$ releasers" do not fulfill these criteria.[21]

Inhibitors of Prostacyclin Release

Since aspirin and other nonsteroidal anti-inflammatory drugs inhibit AA cyclooxygenase[307] it is not surprising that they impair the generation of prostacyclin in various vascular preparations in vitro.[21] Aspirin also inhibits the spontaneous generation of prostacyclin by human arterial and venous tissues ex vivo.[317] In volunteers, the bradykinin-induced rise of plasma 6-keto-PGF$_{1\alpha}$ is inhibited by 90% after administration of 600 mg of aspirin. However, this inhibitory effect disappears within 6 hours.[115] Aspirin, in a dose of 1 g, suppresses the urinary excretion of 2,3-dinor-6-keto-PGF$_{1\alpha}$ for only 3 hours.[309] This short-lasting inhibitory effect of aspirin on the biosynthesis of prostacyclin in vivo may be explained by the de novo synthesis of cyclooxygenase enzyme in the vascular wall. The inhibition disappears more rapidly from endothelial cells compared to vascular smooth muscle.[78] Platelets lack the capacity to resynthesize cyclooxygenase, and after a high dose of aspirin, the full reappearance of the enzymic activity in platelets requires the total exchange of "aspirinized" platelets for new ones from bone marrow. This process requires 6–8 days.[279]

The preferential inhibition by aspirin (following its oral administration) of the platelet rather than vascular cyclooxygenase is of therapeutic value when coupled to the reduced bioavailability of aspirin for the vascular wall in the systemic circulation because of its avid deacetylation in the liver. Platelets, however, are exposed in the portal circulation to higher than systemic concentrations of aspirin and therefore their cyclooxygenase is preferentially inhibited by the drug.[31,228] This hypothesis is confirmed by findings that aspirin at low doses (20–40 mg daily) hardly inhibits the generation of prostacyclin by vascular tissues from patients[317] and does not affect the urinary excretion of either 6-keto-PGF$_{1\alpha}$[255] or 2,3-dinor-6-keto-PGF$_{1\alpha}$[72] while inhibiting the generation of thromboxane by platelets.[226] Aspirin at low doses is almost as selective for TX synthase as TXSI might be; the major difference is that, unlike TXSI,[73] aspirin does not increase the endogenous generation of prostacyclin. These findings correlate with the moderate beneficial effect of aspirin in the prevention of ischemic heart disease.

Steroidal anti-inflammatory drugs such as hydrocortisone and dexamethasone reduce the histamine- and bradykinin-induced biosynthesis of prostacyclin in cultured endothelial cells from human umbilical vein[163] and bovine pulmonary artery.[43] This inhibitory action of glucocorticosteroids develops following a latent period of at least 18 hours; it is receptor-mediated; it depends on the capacity of endothelial cells to synthesize proteins and it can be overcome by exogenous AA. In other words, it seems to be a lipocortin-mediated phenomenon. The classic explanation is that lipocortin, the synthesis of which is induced by steroids, serves as an inhibitory subunit for PLA_2. Recent studies[4] point to the fact that epidermal growth factor (EGF)-dependent synthesis of cyclooxygenase is blocked by glucocorticosteroids. Lipocortin appears to be an inhibitor of the transformation of inactive m-RNA to its active form which is reponsible for the synthesis of cyclooxygenase. EGF induces protein kinase-dependent phosphorylation of lipocortin and removes the blockade of m-RNA, while glucocorticosteroids provide cells with new molecules of lipocortin. Much less is known about the in vivo action of glucocorticosteroids on the release of prostacyclin. In rabbits, dexamethasone does not inhibit the urinary excretion of prostaglandin metabolites.[206] In cultured rat aortic smooth muscle cells, testosterone inhibits[205] and estradiol stimulates[33] the production of prostacyclin. These findings fit the concept of a delay in the biological aging of females as compared to males.

Other in vitro inhibitors of the biosynthesis of prostacyclin include lipid peroxides and other organic peroxides,[295] a monoamine oxidase inhibitor tranylcypromine,[90] vitamin K_1,[211] a hair growth-promoting agent minoxidil,[152] and cyclosporin A.[208] Heparin neutralizes the antiaggregatory action of prostacyclin by binding into a complex with it.[248] The relevance of these in vitro findings to the in vivo situation is not fully understood.

Prostacyclin and Atherosclerosis

The discovery of prostacyclin and of the inhibitory effect of lipid peroxides on PGI_2 synthase promoted the concept that the peroxide-induced deficiency of prostacyclin could trigger the development of atherogenesis and thrombogenesis.[90] Indeed, a diminished capacity of the vascular wall to generate prostacyclin has been reported in the aortae, coronary, and mesenteric arteries of rabbits fed an atherogenic diet,[48,91,94] in blood vessels of patients with atherosclerosis[45,266,267] and in cultured smooth muscle cells from atherosclerotic rabbit aortae.[156,157] At the same time, high plasma levels of lipid hydroperoxides in patients with hyperlipoproteinemias,[58] an enhanced formation of 15-HPETE[120] and increased SOD activity[118] in atherosclerotic arteries of rabbits point to an increased generation of lipid peroxides and oxygen free radicals in atherosclerosis. A similar decrease in prostacyclin synthesizing capacity and an increase in lipid peroxide formation by arterial walls have been reported in infants of diabetic mothers,[329] in vitamin E deficiency,[32,216] and during aging.[190] Atherosclerosis also impairs endothelium-dependent vascular relaxation in rabbits[34,99,199,132,133,308] primates,[79] and humans.[14,168] This defect could be reversed by treatment with an anti-atherosclerotic diet[112] or with a calcium channel blocker.[99] Although the above data are rightly interpreted as a suppression of the release of EDRF or of its relaxant effect on smooth muscle, in humans and in primates prostacyclin deficiency in the endothelium cannot, however, be excluded.

In contrast to the above findings, in atheromatous human or rabbit[186] arteries, the biosynthesis of prostacyclin is either unchanged or increased while the generation of TXA_2 is enhanced. Also, urinary metabolites of prostacyclin are elevated in patients with severe atherosclerosis.[75] We believe that this last finding may reflect the overproduction of prostacyclin by those areas of the vascular wall that are not affected by atheromatous changes. The mechanism of this compensatory phenomenon may consist of the activation of platelets over prostacyclin-deficient[45] and EDRF-deficient[168] atheromatous plaques. Subsequently, activated platelets may supply PG endoperoxides to those areas of the intima that have preserved their PGI_2 synthesizing ability.

An interaction between oxidized lipoproteins, endothelial cells, smooth muscle cells, and monocytes is crucial for atherogenesis. Oxidation of LDL can occur either during the isolation procedure of LDL[97] or during their interaction with endothelial cells, smooth muscle cells, monocytes, or neutrophils. Superoxide anions or other free radicals participate in this process.[123] During the extensive oxidation of LDL, products of the decomposition of lipid peroxides and denaturation processes of the protein core of LDL[277] cause changes in the lysine residues of apo B. These changes in apo B enhance the uptake of the modified LDL by the scavenger receptor on monocytes/macrophages or smooth muscle cells and promote their transformation to foam cells. In addition, oxidatively modified LDLs recruit circulating monocytes into the subendothelial space and prevent the resident monocytes/macrophages from leaving the vascular wall.[237] Another deleterious effect of oxidatively modified LDLs is the biochemical and morphological damage to the endothelial lining. This may be the determining factor for the development of fatty streaks—the first macroscopic signs of atherosclerosis.

Oxidized LDLs produce injury to cultured endothelial cells[117] in a concentration-dependent manner. They also inhibit the generation of prostacyclin following a 3-minute preincubation with fresh rat aortic slices or during superfusion of a strip of bovine coronary artery with oxidized LDL.[97,283] Nonoxidized LDLs have hardly any effect on the biosynthesis of prostacyclin in the above system.[97] This observation indicates that LDL may serve as a carrier for lipid peroxides which subsequently inactivate vascular PGG/H and/or PGI_2 synthases. Nonoxidized LDLs stimulate formation of prostacyclin in cultured human endothelial cells. This stimulation occurs after 60 minutes' exposure to LDL and lasts up to 12 days.[191] It indicates either activation of PGG/H synthase[154] by a trace of lipid peroxides which might be present in nonoxidized LDL or promotion of a shuttle of AA from LDL to endothelial membrane phospholipids, as it has been proposed for HDL.[232] Interestingly, spontaneous oxidation of HDL hardly ever occurs, and HDLs have been consistently reported to stimulate biosynthesis of prostacyclin in endothelial cells.[97,191]

Apart from triggering other atherogenic mechanisms, a low HDL/LDL ratio and a high rate of LDL peroxidation hampers the vascular biosynthesis of prostacyclin and EDRF which exert a synergistic suppressant effect on platelets[239] and leukocytes[145] and thus prevent damage to endothelial cells by adhering platelets, rolling neutrophils, and infiltrating monocytes.

Prostacyclin exerts a wide range of potentially anti-atherosclerotic and anti-thrombotic effects. Platelet adhesion and aggregation in arteries correlates negatively with their capacity to produce prostacyclin,[297] while prostacyclin itself inhibits the formation of thrombi in medium-sized arteries,[299] in arterioles and venules,[122] on the subendothelium,[315] on collagen surfaces in extracorporeal circulations[88,92] and it protects against an immune complex-induced vasculitis.[149] In blood of patients with atherosclerosis, prostacyclin prolongs the life span of platelets and decreases the number of circulating endothelial cells[265] as well as short-ening the euglobulin clot lysis time.[50,88] The above findings are best explained by the platelet-suppressant, fibrinolytic, and cytoprotective properties of prostacyclin which maintain the thromboresistance of the endothelial surface and protect against injury by oxygen free radicals (see section on "Actions of Prostacyclin"). Prostacyclin is a powerful inhibitor of the release of mi-togens from platelets, endothelial cells, and macrophages[322,323] and therefore it is a possible suppressant of smooth muscle proliferation in atherosclerotic plaques. Prostacyclin inhibits accumulation of cho-lesterol in macrophages[322] and in vascular smooth muscle cells,[101] in this way being a possible suppressant of the formation of foam cells. This last effect is accomplished in conjunction with PGE_2 and HDL. PGE_2 inhibits ACAT and prostacyclin stimulates ACEH whereas HDL serves as a choles-terol carrier.[101]

Prostacyclin or its stable analogues have been suggested as the drugs for "re-placement therapy" to restore the lost en-dogenous prostacyclin defense mechanism in patients with atherosclerosis.[88,285,287] However, it appears that atherosclerosis needs to be treated with more than one drug (see next section). Possible co-drugs for anti-atherosclerotic therapy with pros-tacyclin are those which neutralize cyto-toxic eicosanoids (TXA$_2$, LTs), e.g., TXSI,[73] TXA$_2$/PGH$_2$ receptor antagonists,[105] or low doses of cyclooxygenase inhibitors and other antiplatelet drugs.[226] Drugs that act through the release of nitric oxide and thus stimulate guanylate cyclase synergize with prostacyclin in its suppressant action on platelets and leukocytes but not as vaso-relaxants.[145] Inhibitors of cyclic nucleotide phosphodiesterases potentiate cAMP- and cGMP-mediated responses to prostacyclin and EDRF.[46] Scavengers of oxygen free radicals such as SOD[318] or flavonols[93] and lipid-lowering drugs quench LDL oxida-tion.[129] Repeatedly, for many good—though changing—reasons, treatment

with eicosapentaenoic acid (EPA) and other polyunsaturated fatty acids (PUFA) is proposed as a preventive measure against atherosclerosis.[23,321]

Clinical Applications

A year after the pharmacological ac-tions of prostacyclin had been studied in healthy volunteers,[285] prostacyclin was given to five patients with peripheral ar-terial disease (PAD). In these patients a sustained relief of rest pain and healing of ischemic ulcers were noticed.[287] Patients with arteriosclerosis of the lower limbs were chosen for the first clinical trial with prostacyclin since Carlson and his col-leagues successfully treated patients with a similar disease with intra-arterial[29] and intravenous[30] infusions of PGE$_1$ which shares platelet receptors with prostacy-clin.[172] During the last 10 years, patients with critical ischemia resulting from ath-erosclerosis or other vascular diseases have been treated with prostacyclin or its stable analogues[59] (see Chapter 12).

Peripheral Arterial Disease (PAD)

For the treatment of patients with PAD we introduced a continuous IV in-fusion of Na-PGI$_2$, epoprostenol or Flolan from Wellcome Research Labs, UK, dis-solved in a glycine buffer of pH 10.5, in a dose of 2–10 ng/kg/min for 72 to 84 hours.[89] Sinzinger's group[278] has reported the down-regulation of platelet receptors by a long-term infusion of prostacyclin with a subsequent desensitization of platelets to prostacyclin[170,268] and their paradoxical ac-tivation.[52] Intermittent infusions of the drug, e.g., 6-hour courses daily for a month, are recommended to avoid this "rebound" phenomenon. In the Depart-ment of Clinical Pharmacology of Copernicus Academy of Medicine in Cracow, we have continued to use prostacyclin in preselected PAD patients, excluding those with severe diabetes, Leriche syndrome, or black gangrene. At present we have records of 176 PAD patients (156 with arteriosclerosis and 20 with thrombangiitis obliterans), who have been treated with prostacyclin. Long-term (>3 months) improvement occurred in 61% of 102 patients with intermittent claudication and in 52% of 74 patients with rest pain. In the last group, 19 patients suffered from ischemic ulcers that healed or improved significantly in 31% of patients. Similar results were obtained in another open trial in PAD patients[89] as well as in small randomized controlled trials.[11,210]

The placebo-controlled, 13-center study performed in inoperable patients with arteriosclerosis obliterans who suffered from ischemic ulcers showed that an IV infusion of a stable analogue of prostacyclin, iloprost, at a dose of 2 ng/kg/min for 6 hours daily for 28 days led to complete or partial healing of the major ulcer in 62% of patients by the 28th day compared with 17% of patients treated with placebo. This improvement was maintained in most patients in an uncontrolled follow-up after 9–12 months.[57,59] The greater beneficial effect of iloprost than that of prostacyclin[210] on the healing of ischemic ulcers could be due to the improved dosing schedule which was used for the administration of iloprost[57] or to a greater intrinsic therapeutic action of iloprost compared to that of prostacyclin.

In placebo-controlled studies, prostacyclin[10] and iloprost[330] were shown to be particularly effective in reducing pain and promoting the healing of ischemic ulcers in patients with Raynaud's syndrome. In arteriosclerosis obliterans, thrombangiitis obliterans (Buerger's disease) and Raynaud's syndrome, a common symptom is the critical ischemia which appears peripherally to the occluded blood vessels. Prostacyclin and its analogues seem to exert their therapeutic effect at the level of the microcirculation where they repair damage done by activated platelets and leukocytes as well as preventing these cells from being further activated.[59]

Ischemic Stroke

Huczynski and colleagues[126,127] have reported the results of two randomized, controlled studies in 56 patients after ischemic stroke who were assigned at random to IV infusion of prostacylcin (2–5 ng/kg/min) or placebo in 6-hour courses for 4 days (26 patients in the first trial) or a 14-day treatment (30 patients in the second trial). Two weeks after prostacyclin had been administered to the patients, their neurological deficit (mainly hemiparesis and aphasia) improved compared to the placebo group. However, this difference did not reach statistical significance in either of two controlled trials. Prostacyclin produced a brief improvement in the neurological status[94] only during the initial 54 hours of treatment.

Experimental postischemic brain injury is associated with lipid peroxidation[331] while indomethacin and heparin in conjunction with prostacyclin protect against postischemic impairment of reperfused brain in dogs.[102,103] In humans, a high dose of 1.3 g daily of aspirin reduced the risk of stroke in patients with transient ischemic attacks (TIA).[7,67] Lack of a therapeutic effect of prostacyclin alone should not discourage trials of the treatment of ischemic stroke with prostacyclin plus SOD or other oxygen free radical scavengers, and cyclooxygenase, lipoxygenase, or TXA_2 synthase inhibitors or heparin.

Myocardial Ischemia

In several experimental models, prostacyclin has protected the myocardium from (post)ischemic injury.[137,138,160,189] In thrombotic occlusion of canine coronary arteries, the activation of TXA_2/PGH_2 receptors plays a major role,[70] although prostacyclin is a weak antagonist of coronary vasospasm induced by TXA_2 and 5-HT.[258] Myocardial contactility is also not influenced by prostacyclin.[42]

Abnormal metabolism of AA has been reported in patients with acute myocardial infarction or active unstable angina. In these patients, AA in serum[270] and platelets[234] is elevated and the generation of TXA_2[121,234] and prostacyclin[121] is enhanced, although the ratio of 6-keto-$PGF_{1\alpha}/TXB_2$ in the systemic circulation is decreased.[150,200] Their platelets are also less susceptible to inhibition by prostacyclin.[200]

Intracoronary infusion of prostacyclin has been reported to recanalize the obstructed arteries[300] in patients with acute myocardial infarction. However, systemic administration of prostacyclin to these patients produced a mild improvement[119] or none at all[142] in the course of the disease. Unlike glyceryl trinitrate, prostacyclin has hardly any effect in patients with stable angina,[290] nor is it of any significant therapeutic value in patients with variant angina[37,38] except for patients with a subtype of unstable angina that is characterized by nocturnal attacks and ST-segment suppression.[288] In conclusion, prostacyclin seems to be of limited therapeutic benefit for patients with ischemic heart disease.

Pulmonary Hypertension

Together with PGE_1, sodium nitroprusside, hydralazine, and some calcium channel blockers, prostacyclin belongs to the group of vasodilators that are active in the pulmonary vascular bed. Prostacyclin lowers pulmonary wedge resistance and total pulmonary resistance. Infusions of prostacyclin into patients with mitral ste-

nosis reduce the risks involved in subsequent cardiac surgery and may prove to be life-saving if pulmonary hypertension occurs in the postoperative period. Prostacyclin is also used in children with idiopathic pulmonary artery stenosis or vasoconstriction. Long and Rubin[165] have recently reviewed 26 reports on the therapeutic use of prostacyclin in 134 patients with primary and secondary pulmonary hypertension. Prostacyclin and PGE_1 are equally promising therapeutic agents. Chronic infusions of prostacyclin may prove to be particularly useful in patients with primary pulmonary hypertension awaiting heart-lung transplants. Stable, orally active prostacyclin analogues will be highly valued when available for the treatment of patients with pulmonary hypertension.[165]

Thrombotic Microangiopathy (TMA)

Thrombotic microangiopathy (TMA) includes thrombotic thrombocytopenic purpura (TTP), hemolytic uremic syndrome (HUS), systemic lupus erythematosus (SLE), and complications in preeclampsia. Immunosuppressive treatment with cyclosporin A or mitomycin may promote the development of HUS. Prostacyclin deficiency is a common biochemical feature of these clinical disturbances.[241] TMA patients lack "prostacyclin stimulating plasma factor," which is a stable, polar molecule of 300–400 daltons molecular weight, capable of reactivating the production of prostacyclin from exhausted rat aortic rings in vitro. Remuzzi and colleagues[241] have recently reviewed the therapeutic approaches to TMA which include the administration of steroids, heparin, dipyridamole, aspirin, streptokinase, vitamin E, plasma exchange, and last but not least infusions of prostacyclin. The results of these therapeutic strategies are difficult to interpret because very few controlled prospective and comparative studies have been made. Prostacyclin therapy has been successful in some patients but equivocal or disappointing in others.[241]

Extracorporeal Circulation

A series of early clinical trials with infusions of prostacyclin during cardiopulmonary bypass surgery[12,27,35,141,166,238,311] has shown that prostacyclin preserves platelet count and function as well as potentiating the anticoagulant action of heparin when extracorporeal circulation is being maintained. Thus, in these patients, infusions of prostacyclin make it possible to decrease the dose of heparin and reduce postoperative blood loss, thrombocytopenia, and microembolization of brain blood vessels. The hypotensive properties of prostacyclin are useful in controlling intrabypass hypertension.[141] The heparin-sparing properties of prostacyclin were exploited to the utmost when 15 patients were hemodialyzed in two clinical studies[298,334] using prostacyclin as the sole antithrombotic agent. Prostacyclin has a well-established position in preserving platelets in extracorporeal circulations.[89]

Central Retinal Vein Occlusion (CRVO)

CRVO shows up as a hemorrhage or ischemic unilateral retinopathy that causes a sudden unilateral loss of vision in half of the affected patients. The disturbing acute phase of CRVO usually subsides within 2 weeks following conventional therapy with anti-inflammatory drugs, hydergine, or vitamins C and P. In open trials, prostacyclin therapy (2–5 ng/kg/min for 72 hours by IV infusion) accelerated the recovery of the visual acuity in the initial stages of CRVO.[89,335,336] However, in a

controlled trial, this difference was not statistically significant. The prevention by prostacyclin of the appearance of late complications of CRVO (6–12 months after the start of the disease) such as neovascularization, glaucoma, and atrophy of the optic nerve disc[94] was statistically significant.

Miscellaneous

Therapy with prostacyclin has been tried in small groups of patients suffering from a variety of other diseases. Sudden unilateral deafness (SUD) is a severe sensorineuronal loss of hearing of thrombovascular or viral origin. Thirty SUD patients were entered for a placebo-controlled trial with an end-point of 2 weeks. Therapy with prostacyclin resulted in statistically significant improvement in audiometric parameters[94] similar to that seen in an open trial.[218] Beneficial effects of treatment with prostacyclin have also been reported in patients with peptic gastric ulcers,[51] kidney grafts,[162] acute renal failure associated with septicemia,[159] and preeclamptic toxemia.[66] Beneficial effects of prostacyclin in experimental endotoxemia have also been reported.[146,161]

Side Effects of Prostacyclin Therapy

The most common side effect of prostacyclin therapy is headache. It usually appears at doses higher than 5 ng/kg/min and disappears when the infusion rate is reduced. Occasionally, patients tolerate a dose of 10 ng/kg/min prostacyclin without headache. The most consistent but less serious side effect is facial flush. Flushing of palms and feet and a feeling of warmth are also quite common. Restlessness, uneasiness, and drowsiness are experienced by some patients. Typical cardiovascular side effects that occur during intravenous infusions of prostacyclin consist of moderate hypotension and blunted tachycardia. An overdose of prostacyclin (50 ng/kg/min) may result in a sudden drop of arterial blood pressure, bradycardia, and fainting. Therapeutic doses of prostacyclin usually range from 2.5 to 7.5 ng/kg/min given IV and the dose has to be adjusted for individual patients depending on their susceptibility to side effects. Based on our experience with 240 patients treated with prostacyclin, other side effects that can occur are the following: a paradoxical rise in blood pressure (7 patients, mostly with a history of hypertension), chest pain and ectopic heart beats (11 patients, mainly with a history of myocardial ischemia), and articular jaw pain during chewing (27 patients, usually with a history of rheumatoid arthritis). The hyperglycemic effect of prostacyclin[289] disappears after termination of the infusion of prostacyclin but should be monitored and corrected with an increased dose of insulin in patients with diabetes. Unlike others,[214] we hardly observed in our patients any gastrointestinal disturbances during the administration of prostacyclin apart from the rare occurrence of nausea. Side effects of therapy with prostacyclin do not constitute serious clinical problems, although highly qualified staff are required for running these trials.[89]

Conclusion

Prostacyclin is an important regulating mediator in the cardiovascular system. It is a vasorelaxant, antithrombotic, and cytoprotective agent, the actions of which oppose those of TXA_2. Its release coupled to that of EDRF by a PLC signaling system, and its generation are regulated by free radicals. Its biological actions are mediated by adenylate cyclase, and like EDRF, endothelin-1, and t-PA, it originates in the vascular endothelium. Its biochemical actions are linked to those of EDRF since there is synergism between compounds which increase cAMP and cGMP in target cells. Clinical trials with prostacyclin have shown that its therapeutic action for the treatment of some cardiovascular disorders needs to be supplemented by other drugs such as cyclooxygenase, lipoxygenase, or thromboxane synthase inhibitors, TXA_2/PGH_2 receptor antagonists, nitric oxide donors, superoxide dismutase or other free radical scavengers, heparin, or streptokinase. The development of new stable, orally active analogues of prostacyclin constitutes another promising approach to exploiting the therapeutic potential of prostacyclin.

Acknowledgment: The William Harvey Research Institute is supported by a grant from Glaxo Group Research Limited.

References

1. Ager A., Gordon J.L., Moncada S., Pearson J.D., Salmon J.A., Trevethick M.A.: Effects of isolation and culture on prostaglandin synthesis by porcine aortic endothelial and smooth muscle cells. J. Cell. Physiol. 110:9–16, 1982.
2. Aiken J.W., Shebuski R.J., Miller O.V., Gorman R.: Endogenous prostacyclin contributes to the efficacy of a thromboxane synthetase inhibitor for preventing coronary artery thrombosis. J. Pharmacol. Exp. Ther. 219:299–308, 1981.
3. Armstrong J.M., Dusting G.J., Moncada S., Vane J.R.: Cardiovascular actions of

prostacyclin (PGI$_2$), a metabolite of arachidonic acid which is synthesized by blood vessels. Circ. Res. 43:I-112–I-119, 1978.

4. Bailey J.M.: Regulation of cyclooxygenase synthesis by EGF and corticosteroids. Adv. Prostaglandin Thromboxane Leukotriene Res. 19:450–453, 1989.

5. Bailey J.M., Muza B., Hla T., Salata K.: Restoration of prostacyclin synthase in vascular smooth muscle cells after aspirin treatment: regulation by epidermal growth factor. J. Lipid Res. 26:54–61, 1985.

6. Barchowsky A., Kent R.S., Whorton A.R.: Recovery of porcine endothelial prostacyclin synthesis following inhibition of sublethal concentrations of hydrogen peroxide. Biochim. Biophys. Acta 927:372–381, 1987.

7. Barnett H.J.M., Gent M., Sackett D.L., Taylor D.W., Blakeley J.A., Hitsh J., Mustard J.F., Stuart R.K.: A randomized trial of aspirin and sulfinpyrazone in threatened stroke. The Canadian Cooperative Study Group. N. Engl. J. Med. 299:53–59, 1978.

8. Barona E., Guivernau M., Lieber C.S.: Relationship between ethanol, HDL and vascular prostacyclin production. Trans. Assoc. Am. Physicians C:70–79, 1987.

9. Beetens J.R., Herman A.G.: Vitamin C increases the formation of prostacyclin by aortic rings from various species and neutralizes the inhibitory effect of 15-hydroperoxy arachidonic acid. Br. J. Pharmacol. 80:249–254, 1983.

10. Belch J.J.F., Drury J.K., Capell H., Forbes C.D., Newman P., McKenzie F., Liebeman P., Prentice C.R.M.: Intermittent epoprostenol (prostacyclin) infusions in patients with Raynaud's syndrome. Lancet 1:313–315, 1983.

11. Belch J.J.F., McArdle B., Pollock J.G., Forbes C.D., McKay A., Liebeman P., Lowe G.D.O., Prentice C.R.M.: Epoprostenol (prostacyclin) and severe arterial disease: a double blind trial. Lancet 1:315–317, 1983.

12. Bennett J.G., Longmore D.B., O'Grady J.: Use of prostacyclin in cardiopulmonary bypass in man. In: Clinical Pharmacology of Prostacyclin, Lewis P.J., O'Grady J. (eds.). Raven Press, New York, pp 201–208, 1981.

13. Berk B.C., Alexander R.W., Brock F.A., Gimbrone M.A., Webb R.C.: Vasoconstriction: a new activity for platelet-derived growth factor. Science 232:87–90, 1986.

14. Berkenboom G., Depierreux M., Fontaine J.: The influence of atherosclerosis on the mechanical responses of human isolated coronary arteries to substance P, isoprenaline and noradrenaline. Br. J. Pharmacol. 92:113–120, 1987.

15. Berridge M.J.: Inositol triphosphate and diacylglycerol, two interacting second messengers. Annu. Rev. Biochem. 56:159–193, 1987.

16. Bertele V., Mussoni L., del Rosso G., Pintucci G., Carriero M.R., Merati M.G., Liberti A., de Gaetano G.: Defective fibrinolytic response in atherosclerotic patients: Effect of iloprost and its possible mechanism of action. Thromb. Haemostas. 60:141–144, 1988.

17. Bertele V., Mussoni L., Pintucci G., del Rosso G., Romano G., de Gaetano G., Libertti A.: The inhibitory effect of aspirin on fibrinolysis is reversed by iloprost, a prostacyclin analogue. Thromb. Haemostasis 61:286–288, 1989.

18. Best L.C., Martin T.J., Russell R.G.G., Preston F.E.: Prostacyclin increases cyclic AMP levels and adenylate cyclase activity in platelets. Nature 267:850–852, 1977.

19. Blackwell G.J., Radomski M., Vargas J.R., Moncada S.: Prostacyclin prolongs viability of washed human platelets. Biochim. Biophys. Acta 718:60–65, 1982.

20. Block E.R., Patel J.M., Sheridan N.P.: The effect of oxygen and endotoxin on lactate dehydrogenase release, 5-hydroxytryptamine uptake and antioxidant enzyme activities in endothelial cells. J. Cell. Physiol. 122:240–248, 1985.

21. Boeynaems J.M.: Drugs influencing the vascular production of prostacyclin. Prostaglandins, Leukotrienes and Essential Fatty Acids—Reviews 34:197–204, 1988.

22. Boeynaems J.M., Galand N.: Stimulation of vascular prostacyclin synthesis by extracellular ADP and ATP. Biochem. Biophys. Res. Commun. 112:290–296, 1983.

23. Böttinger L.E., Dyerberg J., Nordoy A.: n-3 Fish oils in clinical medicine. J. Intern. Med. 225(Suppl 731):1–238, 1989.

24. Boyd J.A., Eling T.E.: Metabolism of aromatic amines by prostaglandin H synthase. Environ. Health Perspect. 64:45–52, 1985.

25. Brandt R., Dembińska-Kieć A., Korbut R., Gryglewski R.J., Nowak J.: Release of prostacyclin from the human pulmonary vascular bed in response to cholinergic stimulation. Naunyn-Schmiedeberg's Arch. Pharmacol. 325:69–75, 1984.

26. Bunting S., Gryglewski R.J., Moncada S., Vane J.R.: Arterial walls generate from prostaglandin endoperoxides a substance (prostaglandin X) which relaxes strips of mesenteric and coeliac arteries and inhibits platelet aggregation. Prostaglandins 12:897–913, 1976.

27. Bunting S., O'Grady J., Fabiani J.N., Terrier E., Moncada S., Vane J.R., Dubost C.: Cardiopulmonary bypass in man: effects of prostacyclin. In: Clinical Pharmacology of Prostacyclin, Lewis P.J., O'Grady J. (eds.). Raven Press, New York, p 181, 1981.

28. Bursch W., Schulte-Hermann R.: Cytoprotective effect of iloprost against liver cell death induced by carbon tetrachloride (CCl_4) or bromobenzene. In: Prostacyclin and Its Stable Analogue Iloprost, Gryglewski R.J., Stock G. (eds.). Springer Verlag, Berlin, pp 257–268, 1987.

29. Carlson L.A., Eriksson J.: Femoral artery infusion of PGE_1 in severe peripheral vascular disease. Lancet 1:155, 1973.

30. Carlson L.A., Olsson A.: Intravenous PGE_1 in severe peripheral vascular disease. Lancet 2:810, 1976.

31. Cerletti C., Gambino M.C., Garettini S., de Gaetano G.: Biochemical selectivity of oral versus intravenous aspirin in rats. J. Clin. Invest. 78:323–326, 1986.

32. Chan A.C., Leith M.K.: Decreased prostacyclin synthesis in vitamin E-deficient rabbit aorta. Am. J. Clin. Nutr. 34:2341–2347, 1981.

33. Chang-Chang W., Nakao J., Orimo H., Murota S.J.: Stimulation of prostaglandin cyclooxygenase and prostacyclin synthase activities by estradiol in rat aortic smooth muscle cells. Biochim. Biophys. Acta 620:472–476, 1980.

34. Chappell S.P., Lewis M.J., Henderson A.H.: Effect of lipid feeding on endothelium dependent relaxation in rabbit aortic preparations. Cardiovasc. Res. 21:34–38, 1987.

35. Chelly J., Tricot C., Garcia A., Boucherie J.C., Fabiani J.N., Passalecq J., Dubost C.: Haemodynamic effects of prostacyclin infusion after coronary bypass surgery. In: Clinical Pharmacology of Prostacyclin, Lewis P.J., O'Grady J. (eds.). Raven Press, New York, pp 209–218, 1981.

36. Chen X., Pi X.J., Li D.Y., Li Y.J., Deng H.W.: Prostacyclin-mediated cardioprotection of captopril and ramiprilate against lipid peroxidation in rat. In: Prostaglandins in Clinical Res. Cardiovasc. System,

Schrör K., Sinzinger H. (eds.) A.R. Liss Inc., New York, pp. 167–173, 1989.

37. Chierchia S., Patrono C.: Role of platelet and vascular eicosanoids in pathophysiology of ischaemic heart disease. Fed. Proc. 46:81–88, 1987.

38. Chierchia S., Patrono C., Crea F., Ciabattoni G., Da Caterina R., Cinotti G.A., Distante A., Maseri A.: Effects of intravenous prostacyclin in variant angina. Circulation 65:470–477, 1982.

39. Chung-Welch N., Shepro D., Dunham B., Hechtman H.B.: Prostacyclin and prostaglandin E_2 secretions by bovine pulmonary microvessel endothelial cells are altered by change in culture conditions. J. Cell. Physiol. 135:224–234, 1988.

40. Colden-Stanfield M., Schilling W.P., Richie A.K., Eskin S.G., Navarro L.T., Kunze D.L.: Bradykinin-induced increases in cytosolic calcium and ionic currents in cultured bovine aortic endothelial cells. Circ. Res. 61:632–640, 1987.

41. Coughlins S.R., Moskowitz M.A., Zetter B.R., Antoniades H.N., Levine L.: Platelet-dependent stimulation of prostacyclin synthesis by platelet-derived growth factor. Nature 288:600–602, 1980.

42. Couttenye M.M., De Cerck N.M., Herman A.G., Brutsaert D.L.: Effect of prostacyclin on contractile properties of isolated mammalian cardiac muscle. J. Cardiovasc. Pharmacol. 7:971–976, 1985.

43. Crutchley D.J., Ryan V.S., Ryan J.M.: Glucocorticoid modulation of prostacyclin production in cultured bovine pulmonary endothelial cells. J. Pharmacol. Exp. Ther. 233:650–655, 1985.

44. Crutchley D.J., Ryan J.W., Ryan U.S., Fisher G.H.: Bradykinin-induced release of prostacyclin and thromboxanes from bovine pulmonary artery endothelial cells. Biochim. Biophys. Acta 751:99–107, 1983.

45. D'Angelo V., Myśliwiec M., Donati M.B., De Gaetano G.: Defective fibrinolytic and prostacyclin-like activity in human atheromatous plaque. Thromb. Haemostas. 39:535–536, 1978.

46. Darius H., Lefer A.M., Lepran I., Smith J.B.: In vivo interaction of prostacyclin with an inhibitor of cyclic nucleotide phosphodiesterase, HL 725. Br. J. Pharmacol. 84:735–741, 1985.

47. Deckmyn H., Van Houtte E., Verstraete M., Vermylen J.: Manipulation of the local thromboxane and prostacyclin balance in vivo by the antithrombotic compounds dazoxiben, acetylsalicylic acid and nafaza-

trom. Biochem. Pharmacol 32:2757–2762, 1983.

48. Dembińska-Kieć A., Gryglewska T., Żmuda A., Gryglewski R.J.: The generation of prostacyclin by arteries and by coronary vascular bed is reduced in experimental atherosclerosis in rabbits. Prostaglandins 14:1025–1035, 1977.

49. Dembińska-Kieć A., Korbut R., Bieroń K., Kostka-Trąbka E., Gryglewski R.J.: Betapyridyl-carbinol (Ronicol) releases a prostacyclin-like substance into arterial blood of patients with arteriosclerosis obliterans. Pharmacol. Res. Commun. 15:377–385, 1983.

50. Dembińska-Kieć A., Kostka-Trąbka E., Gryglewski R.J.: Effect of prostacyclin on fibrinolytic activity in patients with arterioslerosis obliterans. Thromb. Haemostas. 47:190, 1982.

51. Dembińska-Kieć A., Kostka-Trąbka E., Kosiniak-Kamysz A., et al.: Prostacyclin in patients with peptic gastric ulcers—a placebo controlled study. Hepato-Gastroenterol. 33:262–266, 1986.

52. Dembińska-Kieć A., Żmuda A., Grodzińska L., Bieroń K., Basista M., Kędzior A., Kostka-Trąbka E., Żelazny T.: Increased platelet activity after termination of prostacyclin infusion into man. Prostaglandins. 21:827–832, 1981.

53. De Nucci G., Gryglewski R.J., Warner T.D., Vane J.R.: Receptor-mediated release of endothelium-derived relaxing factor (EDRF) and prostacyclin from bovine aortic endothelial cells is coupled. Proc. Natl. Acad. Sci. U.S.A. 85:2334–2338, 1988.

54. De Nucci G., Thomas R., D'Orleans-Juste P., Antunes E., Walder C., Warner T.D., Vane J.R.: Pressor effects of circulating endothelin are limited by its removal in the pulmonary circulation and by the release of prostacyclin and endothelium-derived relaxing factor. Proc. Natl. Acad. Sci. U.S.A. 85:9797–9800, 1988.

55. De Nucci G., Warner T., Vane J.R.: Effect of captopril on the bradykinin-induced release of prostacyclin from guinea pig lungs and bovine aortic endothelial cells. Br. J. Pharmacol. 95:783–788, 1988.

56. De Witt D.L., El-Harith E.A., Smith W.L.: Molecular cloning of prostaglandin G/H synthase. Adv. Prostaglandin Thromboxane Leukotriene Res. 19:454–457, 1989.

57. Diehm C.: Placebo-Kontrollierte Doppelblinde 13-Center-Studie zum Nachweis der Therapeutischen Wirksamkeit von Il-oprost bei Patienten mit Arterieller Verschlusskrankheit (Stad. IV). Vein Woschr. 65:38–39, 1987.

58. Domagała B., Hartwich J., Szczeklik A.: Incidence of lipid peroxidation in patients with hypercholesterolemia and hypertriglicerydemia. Wiener Klin. Wochenschr. 101:425–428, 1989.

59. Dormandy J.A. (ed.): The pathophysiology of critical limb ischaemia and pharmacological intervention with a stable prostacyclin analogue, iloprost. Royal Soc. Med. Services, London, 1–54, 1989.

60. Dutta-Roy A.K., Sinha A.K.: Purification and properties of prostaglandin E_1/prostacyclin receptor of human blood platelets. J. Biol. Chem. 262:12685–12691, 1987.

61. Egan R.W., Paxton J., Kuehl F.A. Jr.: Mechanism for irreversible self-deactivation of prostaglandin synthetase. J. Biol. Chem. 251:7329–7335, 1976.

62. Eldor A., Friedman R., Vlodavsky I., Hy-Am E., Fuks Z., Panet A.: Interferon enhances prostacyclin production by cultured vascular endothelial cells. J. Clin. Invest. 73:251–257, 1984.

63. Escoubet B., Griffaton G., Samuel J.L., Lechat P.: Calcium antagonists stimulate prostaglandin synthesis by cultured rat cardiac myocytes and prevent the effects of hypoxia. Biochem. Pharmacol. 35:4401–4408, 1986.

64. Fantone J.C., Kinnes D.A.: Prostaglandin E_1 and prostaglandin I_2 modulation of superoxide production by human neutrophils. Biochim. Biophys. Res. Commun. 113:506–512, 1983.

65. Fantone A.U., Ward P.A.: Polymorphonuclear leukocyte-mediated cell and tissue injury: oxygen metabolites and their relation to human disease. Hum. Pathol. 16:973–978, 1985.

66. Fidler J., Ellis C., Bennett M.J., de Swiet M., Lewis P.J.: PGI_2 in pre-eclactic toxaemia. In: Clinical Pharmacology of Prostacyclin, Lewis P.J., O'Grady J. (eds.). Raven Press, New York, pp 141–143, 1981.

67. Fields W.S., Lemak N.A., Frankowski R.F., Hady R.J.: Controlled trial of aspirin in cerebral ischaemia. Stroke 8:301–316, 1977.

68. Fischer S., Struppler M., Böhling B., Bermutz C., Wober W., Weber P.: The influence of selective thromboxane synthase inhibition with a novel imidazole derivative UK 38 485 on prostanoid formation in man. Circulation 68:821–826, 1983.

69. Fitzgerald D.J., Catella F., Roy L., Fitzgerald G.A.: Marked platelet activation in vivo after intravenous streptokinase in patients with acute myocardial infarction. Circulation 77:142–150, 1988.

70. Fitzgerald D.J., Doran J., Jackson E., Fitzgerald J.A.: Coronary vascular occlusion mediated via thromboxane A_2-prostaglandin endoperoxide receptor activation in vivo. J. Clin. Invest. 77:496–502, 1986.

71. Fitzgerald D.J., Entman S.S., Mulloy K., Fitzgerald G.A.: Decreased prostacyclin biosynthesis preceding the clinical manifestation of pregnancy-induced hypertension. Circulation 75:956–963, 1987.

72. Fitzgerald G.A., Oates J.A., Hawiger J., Maas R.L., Roberts L.J., Lawson J.A., Brash A.R.: Endogenous biosynthesis of prostacyclin and thromboxane and platelet functioning during chronic administration of aspirin in man. J. Clin. Invest. 71:676–688, 1983.

73. Fitzgerald G.A., Reilly J.A.G., Pedersen A.K.: The biochemical pharmacology of thromboxane synthase inhibition in man. Circulation 72:1194–1201, 1985.

74. Fitzgerald D.J., Roy L., Fitzgerald G.A.: Enhanced prostacyclin and thromboxane A_2 synthesis in vivo in ischaemic heart disease: noninvasive evidence of sporadic platelet activation in unstable angina. Circulation 72:111–113, 1985.

75. Fitzgerald G.A., Smith B., Pedersen A.K., Brash A.R.: Increased prostacyclin biosynthesis in patients with severe atherosclerosis and platelet activation. New Engl. J. Med. 310:1060–1065, 1984.

76. Förstermann U., Hertting G., Neufang B.: The role of endothelial and nonendothelial prostaglandins in the relaxation of isolated blood vessels of the rabbit induced by acetylcholine and bradykinin. Br. J. Pharmacol. 87:521–532, 1986.

77. Frank L., Roberts R.J.: Endotoxin protection against oxygen-induced acute and chronic lung injury. J. Appl. Physiol. 47:577–581, 1979.

78. Frazer C.E., Ritter J.M.: Recovery of prostacyclin synthesis by rabbit aortic endothelium and other tissues after inhibition by aspirin. Br. J. Pharmacol. 91:251–256, 1987.

79. Freiman P.C., Mitchell G.G., Heistad D.D., Armstrong M.L., Harrison D.G.: Atherosclerosis impairs endothelium-dependent vascular relaxation to acetylcholine and thrombin in primates. Circ. Res. 58:783–789, 1986.

80. Fuchs J., Freisleben H.J., Mainka L., Zimmer G.: Mitochondrial sulfhydryl groups under oligomycin-inhibited, ageing and uncoupling conditions: beneficial influence of cardioprotective drugs. Arch. Biochem. Biophys. 266:83–88, 1988.

81. Funck M., Muller C.P., Jaschonek K.: Modulation of surface expression of human platelet prostacyclin receptors by cholesterol, dibucaine and pentoxiphilline. Thromb. Res. 52:343–347, 1988.

82. Furchgott R.F., Zawadzki J.: The obligatory role of endothelial cells in the relaxation of smooth muscle by acetylcholine. Nature 288:373–376, 1980.

83. Gecse A., Ottlecz A., Mezei Z., Telegdy G., Ioo F., Dux E., Karnushina J.: Prostacyclin and prostaglandin synthesis in isolated brain capillaries. Prostaglandins 234:287–297, 1982.

84. Gerritsen M.E.: Functional heterogeneity of vascular endothelial cells. Biochem. Pharmacol. 36:2701–2711, 1987.

85. Gorman R.R., Bunting S., Miller O.V.: Modulation of human platelet adenylate cyclase by prostacyclin (PGX). Prostaglandins 13:377–388, 1977.

86. Görög P., Kovacs J.B.: Prostacyclin is a more potent stimulator of thrombolysis than inhibitor of haemostasis. Haemostasis 16:337–345, 1986.

87. Griffith T.M., Edwards D.H., Lewis M.J., Henderson A.H.: Evidence that cyclic guanosine monophosphate (cGMP) mediates endothelium-dependent relaxation. Eur. J. Pharmacol. 112:195–202, 1985.

88. Gryglewski R.J.: Prostaglandins, platelets and atherosclerosis. In: CRC Critical Review on Biochemistry, vol. 7. Fasman J.D. (ed.). CRC Press Inc., New York, pp 291–338, 1980.

89. Gryglewski R.J.: Prostacyclin in vascular disease. In: Biological Protection with Prostaglandins, vol. 1, Cohen M.M. (ed.). CRC Press Inc., Boca Raton, Florida, pp 145–168, 1985.

90. Gryglewski R.J., Bunting S., Moncada S., Flower R.J., Vane J.R.: Arterial walls are protected against deposition of platelet thrombi by a substance (prostaglandin X) which they make from prostaglandin endoperoxides. Prostaglandins 12:685–713, 1976.

91. Gryglewski R.J., Dembińska-Kieć A., Żmuda A., Gryglewska T.: Prostacyclin and thromboxane A_2 biosynthesis capacities of heart, arteries and platelets at various stages of experimental atherosclerosis

in rabbits. Atherosclerosis 31:385–394, 1978.

92. Gryglewski R.J., Korbut R., Ocetkiewicz A.: Generation of prostacyclin by lungs in vivo and its release into the arterial circulation. Nature 273:765–767, 1978.

93. Gryglewski R.J., Korbut R., Robak J., Święs J.: On the mechanism of antithrombotic action of flavonoids. Biochem. Pharmacol. 36:317–322, 1987.

94. Gryglewski R.J., Kostka-Trąbka E., Dembińska-Kieć A., Korbut R.: Prostacyclin and atherosclerosis—experimental and clinical approaches. In: Eicosanoids, Apoproteins, Lipoproteins, Particles and Atherosclerosis, Malmendier C.L., Alaupovic P (eds.). Plenum Press, New York, pp 21–29, 1988.

95. Gryglewski R.J., Moncada S., Palmer R.M.J.: Bioassay of prostacyclin and endothelium-derived relaxing factor (EDRF) from porcine aortic endothelial cells. Br. J. Pharmacol. 87:685–694, 1986.

96. Gryglewski R.J., Palmer R.M.J., Moncada S.: Superoxide anion is involved in the breakdown of endothelium-derived vascular relaxing factor. Nature 320:454–456, 1986.

97. Gryglewski R.J., Szczeklik A.: Prostaglandins and atherosclerosis. In: Prostaglandins in Clinical Medicine: Cardiovascular and Thrombotic Disorders. Wu K.K., Rossi E.C. (eds.). Year Book Med. Publ. Inc., Chicago, pp 177–190, 1982.

98. Gryglewski R., Vane J.R.: The release of prostaglandins and rabbit aorta contracting substance (RCS) from rabbit spleen and its antagonism by anti-inflammatory drugs. Br. J. Pharmacol. 45:37–47, 1972.

99. Habib J.B., Bossaller C., Wells S., Williams C., Morrisett J.D., Henry P.D.: Preservation of endothelium-dependent vascular relaxation in cholesterol-fed rabbit by treatment with the calcium blocker PN 200110. Circ. Res. 58:305–309, 1986.

100. Habib J.B., Wells S.L., Williams C.L., Henry P.D.: Atherosclerosis impairs endothelium-dependent arterial relaxation. Circulation 70(Suppl. II): 123, 1984.

101. Hajjar D.P.: Prostaglandins and cyclic nucleotides: modulators of arterial cholesterol metabolism. Biochem. Pharmacol. 34:295–300, 1985.

102. Hallenbeck J.M.: Effect of prostacyclin, indomethacin and heparin on postischaemic nerve cell function. In: Prostacyclin: Clinical Trials, Gryglewski R.J., Szczeklik A., McGiff J.C. (eds.). Raven Press, New York, pp 83–93, 1985.

103. Hallenbeck J.M., Furlow T.W. Jr.: Prostaglandin I₂ and indomethacin prevent impairment of postischaemic brain reperfusion in the dog. Stroke 10:629–637, 1979.

104. Halliwell B., Gutteridge J.M.C.: The importance of free radicals and catalytic metal ions in human disease. Mol. Aspects Med. 8:89–193, 1985.

105. Halushka P.V., Mais D.E., Saussy D.L.: Platelet and vascular smooth muscle thromboxane A₂/prostaglandin H₂ receptors. Fed. Proc. 46:149–153, 1987.

106. Ham E.A., Egan R.W., Soderman P.D., Gale P.H., Kuehl F.A. Jr.: Peroxidase-dependent deactivation of prostacyclin synthetase. J. Biol. Chem. 254:2191–2194, 1979.

107. Ham E.A., Soderman D.D., Zanetti M.E., Dougherty H.W., McCauley E., Kuehl F.A., Jr.: Inhibition by prostaglandins of leukotriene B₄ release from activated neutrophils. Proc. Natl. Acad. Sci. U.S.A. 80:4349–4353, 1983.

108. Hamberg M., Samuelsson B.: Detection and isolation of an endoperoxide intermediate in prostaglandin biosynthesis. Proc. Natl. Acad. Sci. U.S.A. 70:899–903, 1973.

109. Hamberg M., Svensson J., Samuelsson B.: Thromboxanes: A new group of biologically active compounds derived from prostaglandin endoperoxides. Proc. Natl. Acad. Sci. U.S.A. 72:2994–2998, 1975.

110. Hamberg M., Svensson J., Wakabayashi T., Samuelsson B.: Isolation and structure of two prostaglandin endoperoxides that cause platelet aggregation. Proc. Natl. Acad. Sci. U.S.A. 71:345–349, 1974.

111. Hardy C.C., Bradding P., Robinson C., Holgate S.T.: Bronchoconstrictor and antibronchoconstrictor properties of inhaled prostacyclin in asthma. J. Appl. Physiol. 64:1567–1574, 1988.

112. Harrison D.G., Armstrong M.L., Freiman P.C., Heistad D.D.: Restoration of endothelium-dependent relaxation by dietary treatment of atherosclerosis. J. Clin. Invest. 80:1808–1811, 1987.

113. Haurand M., Ullrich V.: Isolation and characterization of thromboxane synthase from human platelets as a cytochrome P-450 enzyme. J. Biol. Chem. 260:15059–15067, 1985.

114. Hawiger J., Parkinson S., Timmons S.: Prostacyclin inhibits mobilisation of fibrinogen binding sites on human ADP and thrombin-treated platelets. Nature 283:195–198, 1980.

115. Heavey D., Barrow S.E., Hickling N.E., Ritter J.M.: Aspirin causes short lived inhibition of bradykinin-stimulated prostacyclin production in man. Nature 318:186–187, 1985.

116. Hellewell P.G., Pearson J.D.: Purinoceptor mediated stimulation of prostacyclin release in the porcine pulmonary vasculature. Br. J. Pharmacol. 83:457–462, 1984.

117. Henriksen T., Evensen S.A., Carlander B.: Injury to cultured endothelial cells induced by low density lipoproteins. Scand. J. Clin. Lab. Invest. 39:369–375, 1979.

118. Henriksson P., Bergström K., Edhag O.: Experimental atherosclerosis and a possible generation of free radicals. Thromb. Res. 38:195–198, 1985.

119. Henriksson P., Edhag O., Wennmalm A.: Prostacyclin infusion in patients with myocardial infarction. Br. Heart J. 53:173–179, 1985.

120. Henriksson P., Hamberg M., Diczfalusy U.: Formation of 15-HETE as a major hydroxyeicosatetraenoic acid in the atherosclerotic vessel wall. Biophys. Acta 834:272–274, 1985.

121. Henriksson P., Wennmalm A., Edhag O., Vesterquist O., Green K.: In vivo production of prostacyclin and thromboxane in patients with acute myocardial infarction. Br. Heart J. 55:543–548, 1986.

122. Higgs E.A., Higgs, G.A., Moncada S., Vane J.R.: Prostacyclin (PGI$_2$) inhibits the formation of platelet thrombi in arterioles and venules of the hamster cheek pouch. Br. J. Pharmacol. 63:535–539, 1978.

123. Hiramatsu K., Rosen H., Heinecke J.W., Wolfbaur G., Chait A.: Superoxide initiates oxidation of low density lipoprotein by human monocytes. Atherosclerosis 7:55–60, 1987.

124. Hong S.L., Deykin D.: Activation of phospholipases A$_2$ and C in pig aortic endothelial cells synthesizing prostacyclin. J. Biol. Chem. 257:7151–7154, 1982.

125. Hoover R.L., Robinson J.M., Karnovsky M.J.: Adhesion of polymorphonuclear leukocytes to endothelium enhances the efficiency of detoxification of oxygen free radicals. Am. J. Pathol. 126:258–268, 1987.

126. Huczyński J., Kostka-Trąbka E., Sotowska W., Bieron K., Grodzińska L., Dembinska-Kiec A., Pykosz-Mazur E., Peczak E., Gryglewski R.J.: Double-blind controlled trial on the therapeutic effects of prostacyclin in patients with completed ischaemic stroke. Stroke 16:810–814, 1985.

127. Huczyński J., Gryglewski R.J., Kostka-Trąbka E., Dembinska-Kiec A., Pykosz-Mazur E., Sotowska W., Grodzinska L., Peczak E., Bieron K., Kedziov A., et al.: Prostacyclin in patients with ischaemic stroke—double blind trial II. Neuro. Neurochir. Pol. 22:299–304, 1988.

128. Hyman A.L., Kadowitz P.J.: Vasodilator actions of prostaglandin 6-keto-PGE$_1$ in the pulmonary vascular bed. J. Pharmacol. Exp. Ther. 213:468–472, 1980.

129. Illingworth D.R.: Lipid-lowering drugs: an overview of indications and optimum therapeutic use. Drugs 33:259–279, 1987.

130. Ito T.T., Ogawa K., Enomoto J., Hashimoto H., Kai J., Satake T.: Comparison of effects of PGI$_2$ and PGE$_1$ on coronary and systemic hemodynamics and on coronary cyclic nucleotide levels in dogs. In: Advances in Prostaglandin Thromboxane Leukotriene Research, vol. 7. Samuelsson B., Ramwell P., Paoletti R. (eds.). Raven Press, New York, pp 641–646, 1980.

131. Jackson R.M., Chandler D.B., Fulmer J.D.: Production of arachidonic acid metabolites by endothelial cells in hyperoxia. J. Appl. Physiol. 61:584–591, 1986.

132. Jayakody L., Kappagoda T., Senarante M.P.Y., Thomson A.B.R.: Impairment of endothelium-dependent relaxation: an early marker for atherosclerosis in rabbits. Br. J. Pharmacol. 94:335–346, 1988.

133. Jayakody R.L., Senartane M.P.J., Thomson A.B.R., Kappagoda C.T.: Cholesterol feeding impairs endothelium-dependent relaxation of rabbit aorta. Can. J. Physiol. Pharmacol. 63:1206–1209, 1985.

134. Jeremy J.Y., Dandone P.: The role of the diacylglycerol-protein kinase C system in mediating adrenoceptor-prostacyclin synthesis coupling in the rat aorta. Eur. J. Pharmacol. 136:311–316, 1987.

135. Jeremy J.Y., Dandone P.: Fluoride stimulates in vitro vascular prostacyclin synthesis: interrelationship of G proteins and protein kinase C. Eur. J. Pharmacol. 146:179–284, 1988.

136. Whittaker N., Bunting S., Salmon J., Moncada S., Vane J.R., Johnson R.A., Morton D.R., Kinner J.H., Gorman R.R., McGuire J.C., Sun F.F.: The chemical structure of prostaglandin X (prostacyclin). Prostaglandins 12:915–928, 1976.

137. Jouve R., Puddu E.: Prostacyclin and protection of the ischaemic myocardium. Cardiologia 33:339–341, 1988.

138. Jugdutt B.J., Hutchins G.M., Bulkley B.H., Becker L.C.: Dissimilar effects of prostacyclin, prostaglandin E$_1$ and protag-

landin E_2 on myocardial infarct size after coronary occlusion in conscious dogs. Circ. Res. 49:685–700, 1981.

139. Kappus H.: Overview of enzyme systems involved in bioreduction of drugs and in redox cycling. Biochem. Pharmacol. 35:1–6, 1986.

140. Kaya H., Hong S.L.: Bradykinin-induced activation of phospholipase A_2 is independent of the activation of polyphosphoinositide-hydrolyzing phospholipase C. Advances in Prostaglandin Thromboxane Leukotriene Research, vol. 19, Samuelsson B., Wong P.Y.K., Sun F.F. (eds.). Raven Press, New York, pp 580–583, 1989.

141. Kaye M.P., Peterson K.A., Noback C.R., Dewanjee M.K.: Hemodynamic and platelet-preserving effects of prostacyclin during cardiopulmonary bypass. In: Prostaglandins in Clinical Medicine, Wu K.K., Rossi E.C. (eds.). Year Book Medical Publishers, Chicago, p 371, 1982.

142. Kiernan F.J., Kluger J., Regnier J.C., Rutkowski M., Fieldman A.: Epoprostenol sodium (prostacyclin) infusion in acute myocardial infarction. Br. Heart J. 56:428–432, 1986.

143. Kokkas B., Boeynaems J.M.: Release of prostacyclin from the dog saphenous vein by 5-hydroxytryptamine. Eur. J. Pharmacol. 147:473–476, 1988.

144. Kontos H.A., Wei E.P., Povlishok T., Christman C.W.: Oxygen radicals mediate cerebral arteriolar dilatation from arachidonate and bradykinin in cats. Circ. Res. 55:295–303, 1984.

145. Korbut R., Trąbka-Janik E., Gryglewski R.J.: Cytoprotection of human polymorphonuclear leukocytes by stimulators of adenylate and guanylate cyclases. Eur. J. Pharmacol. 165:171–172, 1989.

146. Krausz M.M., Utsunomiya T., Feurstein G., Shepro D., Hechtman H.B.: Reversal of lethal endotoxemia with prostacyclin. Surg. Forum 31:37–39, 1980.

147. Kuehl F.A., Dougherty H.W., Ham E.A.: Interactions between prostaglandins and leukotrienes. Biochem. Pharmacol. 33:1–5, 1984.

148. Kuehl F.A., Humes J.L., Egan R.W., Ham E.A., Beveridge G.C., Arman C.G.: Role of prostaglandin endoperoxide G_2 in inflammatory processes. Nature 265:170–173, 1977.

149. Kunkel S.L., Thrall R.S., Kunkel C.K., McCromick J.R., Ward P.A., Zurier R.B.: Suppression of immune complex vasculitis in rats by prostaglandin. J. Clin. Invest. 64:1525–1529, 1979.

150. Kurita A., Takase B., Vehata A. et al.: The role of prostacyclin during exercise in patients with chronic angina pectoris. Jap. Heart J. 29:401–413, 1988.

151. Kuzuya T. et al.: Effect of OKY-046, a thromboxane synthase inhibitor on arachidonate-induced platelet aggregation: possible role of "prostaglandin H_2 steal" mechanism. Jap. Circ. J. 50:1071–1078, 1986.

152. Kvedar J.C., Baden H.P., Levine L.: Selective inhibition by minoxidil of prostacyclin production by cells in culture. Biochem. Pharmacol. 37:867–874, 1988.

153. Lambert T.L., Kent R.S., Whorton A.P.: Bradykinin stimulation of inositol polyphosphate production in porcine aortic endothelial cells. J. Biol. Chem. 262:15288–15293, 1986.

154. Lands W.E.M.: Interaction of lipid hydroperoxides with eicosanoid biosynthesis. J. Free Radicals Biol. Med. 1:97–101, 1985.

155. Lapetina E.G., Crouch M.F.: Relationship of inositol phospholipid metabolism to phospholipase A_2. In: Advances in Prostaglandin and Thromboxane Leukotriene Res., vol. 19, Samuelsson B., Wong P.Y.K., Sun F.F. (eds.). Raven Press, New York, pp 568–573, 1989.

156. Larrue J., Leroux C., Daret D., Bricaud H.: Decreased prostacyclin production in cultured smooth muscle cells from atherosclerotic rabbit aorta. Biochim. Biophys. Acta 710:257–263, 1982.

157. Larrue J., Rigaud M., Daret D., Demond J., Durand J., Bricaud H.: Prostacyclin production by cultured smooth muscle cells from atherosclerotic rabbit aorta. Nature 285:480–482, 1980.

158. Lazo J.S.: Endothelial injury caused by antineoplastic agents. Biochem. Pharmacol. 35:1919–1923, 1986.

159. Leaker B., Miller R., Cohen S.: Treatment of acute renal failure, symmetrical peripheral gangrene and septicaemia with plasma exchange and epoprostenol. Lancet 1:156, 1987.

160. Lefer A.M., Ogletree M.L., Smith J.B., Silver M.J., Nicolau K.C., Barnette W.E., Gasic G.P.: Prostacyclin: a potentially valuable agent for preserving myocardial tissue in acute myocardial ischaemia. Science 200:52–54, 1978.

161. Lefer A.M., Tabas J., Smith E.F.: Salutary effects of prostacyclin in endotoxic shock. Pharmacology 21:206–212, 1980.

162. Leithner C., Sinzinger H., Schwartz H.: Treatment of chronic kidney transplant re-

jection with prostacyclin-reduction of platelet deposition in the transplant: prolongation of platelet survival and improvement of transplant function. Prostaglandins 22:783–788, 1981.

163. Lewis G.D., Campbell W.B., Johnson A.R.: Inhibition of prostaglandin synthesis by glucocorticosteroids in human endothelial cells. Endocrinology 119:62–69, 1986.

164. Lidbury P.S., Thiemermann C., Thomas G.R., Vane J.R.: Endothelin-3: selectivity as an anti-aggregatory peptide in vivo. Eur. J. Pharmacol. 166:335–338, 1989.

165. Long W.A., Rubin L.J.: Prostacyclin and PGE$_1$ treatment of pulmonary hypertension. Am. Rev. Respir. Dis. 136:773–776, 1987.

166. Longmore D.B., Bennett J.G., Hoyle P.M., Smith M.A., Gregory A., Osivand T., Jones W.A.: Prostacyclin administered during cardiopulmonary bypass in man. Lancet 1:800–804, 1981.

167. Luckhoff A.: Release of prostacyclin and EDRF from endothelial cells is differentially controlled by extra- and intracellular calcium. Eicosanoids 1:5–11, 1988.

168. Ludmer P.L., Selwyn A.P., Shook T.L., Wayne R.R., Mudge G.H., Alexander R.W., Ganz P.: Paradoxical vasoconstriction induced by acetylecholine in atherosclerotic coronary arteries. New Engl. J. Med 315:1046–1051, 1986.

169. Lukacsko P.: Effect of arachidonic acid on the basal release of prostaglandins E$_2$ and I$_1$ by rat arteries during the development of hypertension. Clin. Exp. Hypertens. [A] 5:1471–1473, 1983.

170. MacDermot J.: Desensitization of prostacyclin responsiveness in platelets: Apparent differences in the mechanism in vitro and in vivo. Biochem. Pharmacol. 35:2645–2649, 1986.

171. MacDermot J., Barnes P.J.: Activation of guinea pig pulmonary adenylate cyclase by prostacyclin. Eur. J. Pharmacol 67:419–425, 1980.

172. MacIntyre D.E., Gordon J.L.: Discrimination between platelet prostaglandin receptors with a specific antagonist of bisenoic prostaglandins. Thromb. Res. 11:705–713, 1977.

173. MacIntyre D.E., Pearson J.D., Gordon J.L.: Localisation and stimulation of prostacyclin production in vascular cells. Nature 271:549–551, 1978.

174. Madej J.: Identification of novel products of prostacyclin hydrolysis. PhD Thesis,

Copernicus Academy of Medicine in Cracow, 1990.

175. Mantovani A., Dejana E.: Modulation of endothelial function by interleukin-1. Biochem. Pharmacol. 36:301–305, 1987.

176. Marcus A.J.: Transcellular metabolism of eicosanoids. Progr. Hemostasis Thromb. 8:127–142, 1986.

177. Marcus A.J., Silk S.T., Safier L.B., Ullman H.L.: Superoxide production and reducing activity in human platelets. J. Clin. Invest. 59:149–158, 1977.

178. Marcus A.J., Weksler B.B., Jaffe E.A., Broekman M.J.: Synthesis of prostacyclin from platelet-derived endoperoxides by cultured human endothelial cells. J. Clin. Invest. 66:979–986, 1980.

179. Markey C.M., Alward A., Weller P.E., Marnett L.J.: Quantitative studies of hydroperoxide reduction by prostaglandin H synthase. J. Biol. Chem. 262:6266–6279, 1987.

180. Marnett L.J.: Peroxyl free radicals potential mediators of tumor initiation and promotion. Carcinogenesis (London) 8:1365–1374, 1987.

181. Marnett L.J., Chen Y-N.P., Madipati K.R., Labeque R., Ple R.: Localisation of the peroxidase active site of PGH synthase. In: Advances in Prostaglandin and Thromboxane Leukotriene Research. vol. 19. Samuelsson B., Wong P.Y.K., Sun F.F. (eds.). Raven Press, New York, pp 458–461, 1989.

182. Marshall P.Y., Lands W.E.M.: In vitro formation of activators for prostaglandin synthesis by neutrophils and macrophages from humans and guinea pigs. J. Lab. Clin. Med. 108:525–534, 1986.

183. Matsubara T., Ziff M.: Superoxide anion release by human endothelial cells: synergism between a phorbol ester and a calcium ionophore. J. Cell Physiol. 127:207–210, 1986.

184. Mayer B., Moser R., Gleispagh H., Kukovetz W.R.: Possible inhibitory function of endogenous 15-hydroxyeicosatetraenoic acid on prostacyclin formation in bovine aortic endothelial cell. Biochem. Biophys. Acta 875:641–653, 1986.

185. McCord J.M.: Oxygen-derived free radicals in postischaemic tissue injury. N. Engl. J. Med. 312:159–163, 1985.

186. Mehta J.L., Lawson D., Mehta P., Sladeen T.: Increased prostacyclin and thromboxane A$_2$ biosynthesis in atherosclerosis. Proc. Natl. Acad. Sci. U.S.A. 85:4511–4515, 1988.

187. Mehta J, Mehta P., Ostrowski N.: Effects of nitroglycerin on human vascular prostacyclin and thromboxane A_2 generation. J. Lab. Clin. Med. 102:106–125, 1983.

188. Mehta J., Roberts A.: Human vascular tissue produces thromboxane as well as prostacyclin. Am. J. Physiol. 244:R839–R844, 1983.

189. Melin J.A., Becker L.C.: Salvage of ischaemic myocardium by prostacyclin during experimental myocardial infarction. J. Am. Col. Cardiol. 2:279–286, 1983.

190. Menconi M., Taylor L., Martin B., Polgar P.: A review: prostaglandins, ageing and blood vessels. J. Am. Geriatrics Soc. 35:239–247, 1987.

191. Miano J.M., Holland J.A., Pritchard K.A. Jr., Rogers N.Y., Stemerman M.B.: Low-density lipoprotein-mediated endothelial cell perturbation: effects on endothelial cell eicosanoid metabolism. In: Advances in Prostaglandin Thromboxane Leukotriene Research, Samuelsson B., Wong P.Y.K., Sun F.F. (eds.). Raven Press, New York, pp 248–254, 1989.

192. Miller O.V., Gorman R.R.: Evidence for distinct PGI_2 and PGD_2 receptors in human platelets. J. Pharmacol. Exp. Ther. 210:134–140, 1979.

193. Miller D.K., Sadowski S., Soderman D.D., Kuehl F.A. Jr.: Endothelial cell prostacyclin production induced by activated neutrophils. J. Biol. Chem. 260:1006–1014, 1985.

194. Miyamori J., Yasuhara S., Ikeda M., Koshida H., Takeda Y., Morse T., Nagai K., Okamoto S., Takeda R.: Participation of vascular prostacyclin for the pathogenesis of experimental glucocorticoid hypertension in rats. Clin. Exp. Hypertens. [A] 7:513–524, 1985.

195. Moncada S., Gryglewski R., Bunting S., Vane J.R.: An enzyme isolated from arteries transforms prostaglandin endoperoxides to an unstable substance that inhibits platelet aggregation. Nature 263:663–665, 1976.

196. Moncada S., Gryglewski R.J., Bunting S., Vane J.R.: A lipid peroxide inhibits the enzyme in blood vessel microsomes that generates from prostaglandin endoperoxides the substance (prostaglandin X) which prevents platelet aggregation. Prostaglandins 12:715–737, 1976.

197. Moncada S., Higgs E.A., Vane J.R.: Human arterial and venous tissues generate prostacyclin (prostaglandin X), a potent inhibitor of platelet aggregation. Lancet 1:18–20, 1977.

198. Moore S.A., Spector A.A., Hart M.N.: Eicosanoid metabolism in cerebrovascular endothelium. Am. J. Physiol. 254:C37–C44, 1988.

199. Mozsik G., Moron F., Javor T.: Cellular mechanism of the development of gastric mucosal damage and gastrocytoprotection induced by prostacyclin in rats: a pharmacological study. Prostaglandins Leukotrienes Med. 9:71–84, 1982.

200. Mueller H.S., Rao P.S., Greenberg M.A., et al.: Systemic and transcardiac platelet activity in acute myocardial infarction in man: resistance to prostacyclin. Circulation 72:1336–1345, 1985.

201. Mullane K.M., Moncada S.: Prostacyclin release and the modulation of some vasoactive hormones. Prostaglandins 20:25–49, 1980.

202. Murata S., Morita I., Kanayasu T.: A kallikrein induced new peptide stimulating prostacyclin production by vascular endothelial cells. In: Advances in Prostaglandin Thromboxane Leukotriene Research, vol. 19, Samuelsson B., Wong P.Y.K., Sun F.F. (eds.). Raven Press, New York, pp 244–247, 1989.

203. Musial J., Wilczyńska M., Sladek K., Cierniawski C.S., Niżankowski R., Szczeklik A.: Fibrinolytic activity of prostacyclin and iloprost in patients with peripheral arterial disease. Prostaglandins 31:61–70, 1986.

204. Myers M.L., Bolli R., Lekich R.F., Hartley C.J., Roberts R.: Enhancement of recovery of myocardial function by oxygen free radical scavengers after reversible regional ischaemia. Circulation 72:915–921, 1985.

205. Nakano J., Chang W.C., Murata S., Orimo H.: Testosterone inhibits prostacyclin production by rat aortic smooth muscle cells in culture. Atherosclerosis 39:203–209, 1981.

206. Naray-Fejes-Toth A., Fejes-Toth G., Fischer C., Fröhlich J.C.: Effect of dexamethasone on in vivo prostanoid production in the rabbit. J. Clin. Invest. 74:120–123, 1984.

207. Needleman P., Moncada S., Bunting S., Vane J.R., Hamberg M., Samuelsson B.: Identification of an enzyme in platelet microsomes which generates thromboxane A_2 from prostaglandin endoperoxides. Nature 26:558–560, 1976.

208. Neild G.H., Rocchi I., Imberti L., Fumagalli F., Brown Z., Remuzzi G., Williams D.G.: Effect of cyclosporin A on prostacyclin synthesis by vascular tissue. Thromb. Res. 32:373–379, 1983.

209. Niada R., Porta R., Pescador R., Mantovani M., Prino G.: Cardioprotective effect of defibrotide in acute myocardial ischaemia in cat. Thromb. Res. 38:71–81, 1985.

210. Niżankowski R., Królikowski W., Bielatowicz J., Schaller J., Szczeklik A.: Prostacyclin for ischemic ulcers in peripheral arterial disease: a random assignment placebo-controlled study. In: Prostacyclin: Clinical Trials, Gryglewski R.J., Szczeklik A., McGiff J.C. (eds.). Raven Press, New York, pp 15–22, 1985.

211. Nolan R.D., Eling T.E.: Inhibition of prostacyclin synthesis in cultured bovine aortic endothelial cells by vitamin K_1. Biochem. Pharmacol. 35:4273–4281, 1986.

212. Nowak J., Brandt R., Dembińska-Kieć A., Gryglewski R.J., Korbut R.: Carbaminoylcholine stimulates release of prostacyclin from the human pulmonary vascular bed. In: Prostacyclin: Clinical Trials, Gryglewski R.J., Szczeklik A., McGiff J.C. (eds.). Raven Press, New York, pp 95–106, 1985.

213. Nugteren D.H., Hazelhof E.: Isolation and properties of intermediates in prostaglandin biosynthesis. Biochim. Biophys. Acta 326:448–461, 1973.

214. O'Grady J., Warrington S., Moti J., Bunting S., Flower R., Fowle A.S.E., Higgs E.A., Moncada S.: Effects of intravenous infusion of prostacyclin (PGI_2) in man. Prostaglandins 19:319–332, 1980.

215. Ohara H., Kanaide H., Yoshimura R., Okada M., Nakamura M.: A protective effect of coenzyme Q_{10} on ischaemia and reperfusion of the isolated perfused rabbit heart. J. Mol. Cell Cardiol. 13:65–74, 1981.

216. Okuma M., Takayama H., Uchino H.: Generation of prostacyclin-like substance and lipid peroxidation in vitamin E-deficient rats. Prostaglandins 19:527–536, 1980.

217. Olson D.M., Tanswell A.K.: Effects of oxygen, calcium ionophore and arachidonic acid on prostaglandin production by monolayer cultures of mixed cells and endothelial cells from rat fetal lungs. Exp. Lung Res. 12:207–221, 1987.

218. Olszewski E., Sekula J., Kostka-Trąbka E., Grodzińska L., et al.: Prostacyclin in the treatment of sudden deafness. In: Prostacyclin: Clinical Trials, Gryglewski R.J., Szczeklik A., McGiff J.C. (eds.). Raven Press, New York, pp 77–82, 1985.

219. Otani H., Tanaka H., Inoue T., Umemeto M., Omoto K., Tanaka K., Sato T., Osako T., Masuda A., Nonoyama A., Kagawa T.: In vitro study on contribution of oxidative metabolism of isolated rabbit heart mitochondria to myocardial reperfusion injury. Circ. Res. 55:168–175, 1984.

220. Pace-Asciak C.: A new prostaglandin metabolite of arachidonic acid. Formation of 6-keto-$PGF_{1\alpha}$ by the rat stomach. Experientia 32:291–292, 1976.

221. Pace-Asciak C., Nashat M., Menon N.K.: Transformation of prostaglandin G_2 into 6(9)-11,15-dihydroxy-prosta-7,13-dienoic acid by the rat stomach fundus. Biochim. Biophys. Acta 424:323–325, 1976.

222. Pace-Asciak C., Wolfe L.S.: A novel prostaglandin derivative formed from arachidonic acid by rat stomach homogenates. Biochemistry 10:3657–3664, 1971.

223. Panzenbeck M.J., Tan W., Hajdu M.A., Zucker I.H.: Prostaglandins mediate the increased sensitivity of left ventricular reflexes after captopril treatment in conscious dogs. J. Pharmacol. 244:384–390, 1988.

224. Papp A.C., Crowe L., Pettigrew L.C., Wu K.K.: Production of eicosanoids by de-endothelialized rabbit aorta: interaction between platelets and vascular wall in the synthesis of prostacyclin. Thromb. Res. 42:549–556, 1986.

225. Patrigniani P., Filabozzi P., Patrono C.: Selective cumulative inhibition of platelet thromboxane production by low-dose aspirin in healthy subjects. J. Clin. Invest. 69:1366–1372, 1982.

226. Patrono C., Ciabattoni G., Patrigniani P., Pugliese F., Filabozzi P., Catella F., Davi G., Forni L.: Clinical pharmacology of platelet cyclooxygenase. Circulation 75:1177–1184, 1985.

227. Pearson J.D., Slakey L.L., Gordon J.L.: Stimulation of prostaglandin production through purinoceptors on cultured porcine endothelial cells. Biochem. J. 214:273–276, 1983.

228. Pedersen A.K., Fitzgerald G.A.: Dose-related kinetics of aspirin: presystemic acetylation of platelet cyclooxygenase. New Engl. J. Med. 311:1206–1211, 1984.

229. Pinto A., Abraham N.G., Mullane K.M.: Cytochrome P-450-dependent monooxygenase activity and endothelial-dependent relaxations induced by arachidonic acid. J. Pharmacol. Ther. 236:445–451, 1986.

230. Piper P.J., Vane J.R.: Release of additional factors in anaphylaxis and its antagonism by anti-inflammatory drugs. Nature 223:29–35, 1969.

231. Pirrotton S., Erneux G., Boeynaems J.M.: Dual role of GTP-binding proteins in the control of endothelial prostacyclin. Biochem. Biophys. Res. Commun. 147:1113–1120, 1987.

232. Pomerantz K.B., Fleisher L.N., Tall A.R., Cannon P.J.: Enrichment of endothelial cell arachidonic acid by lipid transfer from high density lipoproteins: relationship to prostaglandin I_2 synthesis. J. Lipid Res. 26:1269–1276, 1985.

233. Powell W.S., Funk C.D.: Metabolism of arachidonic acid and other polyunsaturated fatty acids by blood vessels. Prog. Lipid Res. 26:183–210, 1987.

234. Prisco D., Rogasi P.G., Matuci M., Abbate R., Gensini F.G., Neri Serneri G.G.: Increased thromboxane A_2 generation and altered membrane fatty acid composition in platelets from patients with active angina pectoris. Thromb. Res. 44:101–112, 1986.

235. Quilley J., Duchin K.L., Hudes E.M., McGiff J.C.: The antihypertensive effect of captopril in essential hypertension: relationship to prostaglandins and the kallikrein-kinin system. J. Hypertension 5:121–128, 1987.

236. Quilley C.P., McGiff J.C., Lee W.H., Sun F.F., Wong P.Y.K.: 6-keto-PGE_1: a possible metabolite of prostacyclin having platelet antiaggregatory effects. Hypertension 2:524–528, 1980.

237. Quinn M.T., Parthasarathy S., Fong L., Steinberg D.: Oxidatively modified low density lipoproteins: a potential role in recruitment and retention of monocyte/macrophages during atherogenesis. Proc. Natl. Acad. Sci. U.S.A. 84:2995–2998, 1987.

238. Radegran K., Aren C., Egberg N., Papaconstantinou C., Teger-Nilsson A.C.: Experiences with use of prostacyclin in open heart surgery. In: Prostaglandins in Clinical Medicine, Wu K.K., Rossi C.E. (eds.). Year Book Med. Publisher, Chicago, p 379, 1982.

239. Radomski M.W., Palmer R.M.J., Moncada S.: The antiaggregating properties of vascular endothelium: interactions between prostacyclin and nitric oxide. Br. J. Pharmacol. 92:639–646, 1987.

240. Rapoport R.M., Murad F.: Agonist-induced endothelium-dependent relaxation in rat thoracic aorta may be mediated through cGMP. Circ. Res. 52:352–357, 1983.

241. Remuzzi G., Zoja C., Rossi E.C.: Prosta-cyclin thrombotic microangiopathy. Semin. Hematol. 24:110–118, 1987.

242. Renkawek K., Herbaczyńska-Cedro K., Mossakowski M.J.: The effect of prostacyclin on morphological and enzymatic properties of CNS cultures exposed to anoxia. Acta Neurol. Scand. 73:111–118, 1986.

243. Revtyak G.E., Johnson A.R., Campbell H.B.: Cultured bovine coronary arterial endothelial cells synthesize HETEs and prostacyclin. Am. J. Physiol. 23:254(C8–C19), 1988.

244. Ritter J.M.: Prostanoid synthesis by aortic rings in human blood: selective increase of prostacyclin mediated by a serum factor. Br. J. Pharmacol. 83:409–418, 1984.

245. Robert A.: On the mechanism of cytoprotection by prostaglandins. Am. Clin. Res. 16:335–338, 1984.

246. Rosen G.M., Freeman B.A.: Detection of superoxide generated by endothelial cells. Proc. Natl. Acad. Sci. U.S.A. 81:7269–7273, 1984.

247. Rossi V., Breviario F., Ghezzi P., Dejana E., Mantovani A.: Prostacyclin synthesis induced in vascular cells by interleukin-1. Science 229:174–176, 1985.

248. Saba S.R., Saba H.J.: Heparin-mediated neutralisation of platelet antiaggregatory activity of prostacyclin (PGI_2): studies on mechanism. Am. J Hematol. 20:97–105, 1985.

249. Sagone A.L., Wells R.M., De Mocko C.: Evidence that OH production by human PMNs is related to prostaglandin metabolism. Inflammation 4:65–71, 1980.

250. Salmon J.A., Smith D.R., Flower R.J., Moncada S., Vane J.R.: Further studies on the enzymatic conversion of prostaglandin endoperoxide into prostacyclin by porcine aortic microsomes. Biochim. Biophys. Acta 523:250–262, 1978.

251. Salvemini D., de Nucci G., Gryglewski R.J., Vane J.R.: Human neutrophils and mononuclear cells inhibit platelet aggregation by releasing a nitric oxide-like factor. Proc. Natl. Acad. Sci. 86:6328–6332, 1989.

252. Salvemini D., de Nucci G., Sneddon J.M., Vane J.R.: Superoxide anions enhance platelet adhesion and aggregation. Br. J. Pharmacol. 97:1145–1150, 1989.

253. Samuelsson B., Granström E., Hamberg M.: On the mechanism of biosynthesis of prostaglandins. In: Proceedings of 2nd Nobel Symposium, Bergström S., Samuelsson B., Interscience Publishers, London pp 31–44, 1967.

254. Schafer A.I., Gimbrone M.A., Jr., Hadin R.J.: Endothelial cell adenyl cyclase: activation by catecholamines and prostaglandin I_2. Biochem. Biophys. Res. Commun. 96:1640–1647, 1980.

255. Schafer A.I., Crawford D.D., Gimbrone M.A.: Unidirectional transfer of prostaglandin endoperoxides between platelets and endothelial cells. J. Clin. Invest. 73:1105–1108, 1984.

256. Schrör K., Hecker G.: Potent inhibition of superoxide anion generation by PGE_1 analogue OP-1206 in human PMNs: unrelated to its antiplatelet PGI_2-like activity. Vasa Suppl. 17:11–16, 1987.

257. Schrör K., Ohlendorf R., Darius H.: Beneficial effects of new carbacyclin derivative ZK 36374 in acute myocardial ischaemia. J. Pharmacol. Exp. Ther. 219:243–249, 1981.

258. Schrör K., Verheggen R.: Prostacyclins are only weak antagonists of coronary vasospasm induced by authentic thromboxane A_2 and serotonin. J. Cardiovasc. Pharmacol. 8:607–613, 1986.

259. Schumacher W.A., Lee E.C., Lucchesi B.R.: Augmentation of streptokinase thrombolysis by heparin and prostacyclin. J. Cardiovasc. Pharmacol. 7:739–766, 1985.

260. Schumacher W.A., Lucchesi B.R.: Effect of thromboxane synthetase inhibitor UK-37248 (Dazoxiben) upon platelet aggregation, coronary artery thrombosis and vascular reactivity. J. Pharmacol. Exp. Ther. 227:790–796, 1983.

261. Schwartzmann M.L., Falck J.R., Yadagiri P., Escalante B.: Metabolism of 20-hydroxyeicosatetraenoic acid by cyclooxygenase. J. Biol. Chem. 264:11658–11662, 1989.

262. Schwertschlag U., Stahl T., Hackenthal E.: Comparison of the effects of prostacyclin and 6-keto-PGE_1 on renin release in the isolated rat and rabbit kidney. Prostaglandins 23:129–138, 1982.

263. Shiki Y., Meyriek B.O., Brigham K.L., Burr J.M.: Endotoxin increases superoxide dismutase in cultured bovine pulmonary endothelial cells. Am. J. Physiol. 1987 (Cell Physiol. 21) 252:C436–C440.

264. Siegel G., Schnalke F., Stock G., Grote J.: Prostacyclin, endothelium-derived relaxing factor and vasodilatation. In: Advances in Prostaglandin Thromboxane Leukotriene Res., vol. 19, Samuelsson B., Wong P.Y.K., Sun F.F. (eds.). Raven Press, New York, pp 267–270, 1989.

265. Sinzinger H., Rauscha F., Fitscha P., Kaliman J.: Beneficial effect of PGI_2 on circulatory endothelial cells. Basic Res. Cardiol. 83:597–601, 1988.

266. Sinzinger H., Silberbauer K., Feigl W.: Diminished PGI_2 function by human atherosclerotic arteries. Lancet 1:469–470, 1979.

267. Sinzinger H., Silberbauer K., Feige W., Wagner W., Witner M., Auerswald A.: Prostacyclin activity is diminished in differential types of morphologically controlled human atherosclerotic lesions. Thromb. Haemostas. 42:803–805, 1979.

268. Sinzinger H., Silberbauer K., Harsch A.K., Gall A.: Decreased sensitivity of human platelets to PGI_2 during long-term intra-arterial prostacyclin infusion in patients with peripheral vascular disease: a rebound phenomenon. Prostaglandins 21:49–51, 1981.

269. Sinzinger H., Zidek T., Fitscha P., Kaliman J., Steuer G.: Platelet derived growth factor (PDGF) and prostacyclin (PGI_1, PGI_2) as modulators of the atherogenic process. Folia Haematol. 115:439–442, 1988.

270. Skuladottir G., Hardarson T., Sigfusson N., Oddson G., Gudbjarnason S.: Arachidonic acid levels in serum phospholipids of patients with angina pectoris or fatal myocardial infarction. Acta Med. Scand. 218:55–58, 1985.

271. Slater T.F., Cheeseman K.H., Davies M.J., Proudfort D.K., Xin W.: Free radical mechanisms in relation to tissue injury. Proc. Nutrition Soc. 46:1–12, 1987.

272. Soma M., Manku M.S., Jenkins D.K., Horrobin D.F.: Prostaglandins and thromboxane outflow from the perfused mesenteric vascular bed in spontaneously hypertensive rats. Prostaglandins 29:323–333, 1985.

273. Someya N., Kodama K., Tanaka K.: Effects of captopril on plasma prostacyclin concentration in essential hypertensive patients. Prostaglandins Leukotrienes Med. 20:187–195, 1985.

274. Sprengers E.D.: A sensitive assay, specific for endothelial cell type plasminogen activator in blood plasma. Thromb. Haemostas. 55:74–77, 1986.

275. Stahlberg H.J., Loschen G., Flohe L.: Effects of prostacyclin analogs in cyclic adenosine monophosphate and superoxide formation in human polymorphonuclear leukocytes stimulated by formyl-methionyl-leucyl-phenylalanine. Biol. Chem. Hoppe-Seyler 369:329–336, 1988.

276. Stam H., Hülsmann W.C., Jongkind J.F.,

van der Kraaij A.M.M., Koster J.F.: Endothelial lesions, dietary composition and lipid peroxidation. Eicosanoids 2:1–14, 1989.

277. Steinbrecher U.P.: Oxidation of human low density lipoprotein results in derivatization of lysine residues of apoprotein B by lipid peroxide decomposition products. J. Biol. Chem. 262:3603–3608, 1987.

278. Steuer P., Fitscha P., Sinzinger H.: The platelet rebound phenomenon during PGI_2-infusion occurs at receptor level. Folia Haematol. 115:435–438, 1988.

279. Stuart M.J., Murphy S., Oski F.A.: A simple non-radioiosope technic for the determination of platelet life-span. New Engl. J. Med. 292:1310–1313, 1975.

280. Sundar S.: Prostacyclin in (extracted) plasma of essential hypertensives. Acta Cardiol. 42:135–139, 1987.

281. Suttorp N., Toepfer W., Roka L.: Antioxidant defense mechanism of endothelial cells: glutathione redox cycle versus catalase. Am. J. Physiol. 252:C671–C680, 1986.

282. Svensson J., Hamberg M., Samuelsson B.: Prostaglandin endoperoxides IX. Characterization of rabbit aorta contracting substance (RCS) from guinea pig lungs and human platelets. Acta Physiol. Scand. 94:222–228, 1975.

283. Szczeklik A., Gryglewski R.J.: Low density lipoproteins (LDL) are carriers for lipid peroxides and invalidate prostacyclin (PGI_2) biosynthesis in arteries. Artery 7:489–491, 1980.

284. Szczeklik A., Gryglewski R.J., Domagala B., Dworski R., Basista M.: Dietary supplementation with vitamin E in hyperlipoproteinemias: effects on plasma lipid peroxides, antioxidant activity, prostacyclin generation and platelet aggregability. Thromb. Haemostas. 54:1–6, 1985.

285. Szczeklik A., Gryglewski R.J., Niżankowski R., Musial J., Pietoń R., Mruk J.: Circulatory and anti-platelet effects of intravenous prostacyclin in healthy men. Pharmacol. Res. Commun. 10:545–556, 1978.

286. Szczeklik A., Kopeć M., Sładek K.: Prostacyclin and the fibrinolytic system in ischaemic vascular disease. Thromb. Res. 29:655–660, 1983.

287. Szczeklik A., Niżankowski R., Skawiński S., Gluszko P., Gryglewski R.J.: Successful therapy of advanced arteriosclerosis obliterans with prostacyclin. Lancet 1:1111–1114, 1979.

288. Szczeklik A., Niżankowski R., Szczeklik J., Tabeau J., Królikowski W.: Treatment with prostacyclin of various forms of spontaneous angina pectoris not responding to placebo. Pharmacol. Res. Commun. 16:1117–1130, 1984.

289. Szczeklik A., Piętoń R., Sieradzki J., Niżankowski R.: The effects of prostacyclin on glycemia and insulin release in man. Prostaglandins 19:959–968, 1980.

290. Szczeklik J., Szczeklik A., Niżankowski R.: Prostacyclin, nitroglycerin and effort angina (letter). Lancet 1:1006, 1981.

291. Szekeres L., Balint Z., Karcsus S., Tosaki A., Udvary E.: On the 7-oxo-PGI_2 induced late appearing long-lasting cytoprotective effect. In: Prostaglandins in Clinical Research: Cardiovascular System, Schrör K., Sinzinger H., (eds.). Alan R. Liss, New York, pp 143–147, 1989.

292. Tansik R.L., Namm D.H., White H.L.: Synthesis of prostaglandin 6-keto-$F_{1\alpha}$ by cultured aortic smooth muscle cells and stimulation of its formation in a coupled system with platelet lysates. Prostaglandins 15:399–408, 1978.

293. Tateson J.E., Moncada S., and Vane J.R.: Effects of prostaglandin X (PGI_2) on cyclic AMP concentration in human platelets. Prostaglandins 13:389–397, 1977.

294. Taylor L., Foxall T., Auger K., Heinsohn C., Polgar P.: Comparison of prostaglandin synthesis by endothelial cells from blood vessels originating in the rat, baboon, calf and human. Atherosclerosis 65:227–236, 1987.

295. Terashita Z., Nishikawa K., Terao S., Nakagawa M., Hino T.: A specific prostaglandin I_2 synthetase inhibitor 3-hydroperoxy-3-methyl-Z-phenyl-^{3}H-indole. Biochem. Biophys. Res. Commun. 91:72–78, 1979.

296. Thiemermann G., Löbl P., Schrör K.: Usefulness of defibrotide in protecting ischemic myocardium from early reperfusion damage. Am. J. Cardiol. 56:978–982, 1985.

297. Tschapp T.B., Baumgartner H.R.: Platelet adhesion and aggregation in arteries of rats, rabbits and guinea pigs in vivo and vitro correlates negatively with their prostacyclin (PGI_2) production. Agents and Actions (Suppl.) 4:156–159, 1979.

298. Turney J.H., Dodd N.J., Weston M.J.: Prostacyclin in extracorporeal circulation. Lancet 1:1101, 1981.

299. Ubatuba F.B., Moncada S., Vane J.R.: The effect of prostacyclin (PGI_2) on platelet behaviour, thrombus formation in vivo and bleeding time. Thromb. Diath. Haemorrh. 41:425–434, 1979.

300. Uchida Y., Hanai T., Hasegawa K., Kawamura K., Oshima T.: Recanalisation of obstructed coronary artery by intracoronary administration of prostacyclin in patients with acute myocardial infarction. Adv. Prostagl. Thromb. Leukotr. Res. 11:377–383, 1983.

301. Uehara Y., Tobian L., Iwai J., Ishii M., Sugimoto T.: Alterations of vascular prostacyclin and thromboxane A_2 in Dahl genetic strain susceptible to salt-induced hypertension. Prostaglandins 33:727–738, 1987.

302. Ullrich V., Castle L., Weber P.: Spectral evidence for the cytochrome P-450 nature of prostacyclin synthetase. Biochem. Pharmacol. 30:2033–2037, 1981.

303. Ullrich V., Graf H.: Prostacyclin and thromboxane synthase as P-450 enzymes. TIPS 5:352–355, 1984.

304. Utsunomiya T., Krausz M.M., Valeri C.R., Shepro D., Hechtman H.B.: Treatment of pulmonary embolism with prostacyclin. Surgery 88:25–30, 1980.

305. Vane J.R.: The use of isolated organs for detecting active substances in the circulatory blood. Br. J. Pharmacol. Chemother. 23:360–373, 1964.

306. Vane J.R.: The release and fate of vasoactive hormones in the circulation. Br. J. Pharmacol 35:209–242, 1969.

307. Vane J.R.: Inhibition of prostaglandins as a mechanism of action for aspirin-like drugs. Nature (New Biol.) 231:232–235, 1971.

308. Verbeuren T.J., Jordaens F.A., Zonnekeyn L.L., Van Hove C.E., Coene M.C., Herman A.G.: Effect of hypercholesterolemia on vascular reactivity in the rabbit. I. Endothelium-independent and endothelium-dependent contractions and relaxations in isolated arteries of control and hyperchlesterolemic rabbits. Circ. Res. 58:552–564, 1986.

309. Vesterquist O.: Rapid recovery of in vivo prostacyclin formation after inhibition by aspirin. Eur. J. Clin. Pharmacol. 30:69–73, 1986.

310. Virgolini I., Herman M., Sinzinger H.: Decrease of prostaglandin I_2 binding sites in thyroid cancer. Br. J. Cancer 58:584–588, 1988.

311. Walker J.D., Davidson J.F., Faichney A., Wheatley D., Davidson K.: Prostacyclin in cardiopulmonary bypass surgery. In: Clinical Pharmacology of Prostacyclin, Lewis P.J., O'Grady J. (eds.). Raven Press, New York, pp 195–200, 1981.

312. Watanabe K., McCaffrey T.M., Weksler B.B., Jaffe E.A.: Endotoxin stimulates the production of prostacyclin by cultured human endothelial cells. Advances in Prostaglandin Thromboxane Leukotriene Research, vol. 19. Samuelsson B., Wong P.Y.K., Sun F.F. (eds.). Raven Press, New York, pp 242–243, 1989.

313. Jones R.L., Watson M.L.: The contribution of PGI_2 to the effect of captopril in conscious dogs in differing states of sodium balance. Clin. Sci. 71:527–532, 1986.

314. Wei E.P., Ellison M.D., Kontos H.A., Povlishok J.T.: O_2 radicals in arachidonate-induced increased blood-brain barrier permeability to proteins. Am. J. Physiol. 251(Heart Circ. Physiol. 20):H693–H699, 1986.

315. Weiss H.J., Turitto V.T.: Prostacyclin (prostacyclin I_2, PGI_2) inhibits platelet adhesion and thrombus formation on subendothelium. Blood 53:244–250, 1979.

316. Weksler B.B., Ley C.W., Jaffe E.A.: Stimulation of endothelial cell prostacyclin production by thrombin, trypsin and the ionophore A 23187. J. Clin. Invest. 62:923–930, 1978.

317. Weksler B.B., Pett S.B., Alonso D., Richter R.C., Sfelzer P., Subramanian V., Tack-Goldman K., Gay W.A.: Differential inhibition by aspirin of vascular and prostaglandin synthesis in atherosclerotic patients. New Engl. J. Med. 308:800–805, 1983.

318. Warns S.W., Shea M.J., Driscoll E.M., Cohen C., Abrams G.D., Pitt B., Lucchesi B.R.: The independent effects of oxygen radical scavengers on canine infarct size. Reduction by superoxide dismutase and not catalase. Circ. Res. 56:895–898, 1985.

319. White A.A., Karr D.B., Patt C.S.: Role of lipoxygenase in O_2-dependent activation of soluble guanylate cyclase from rat lungs. Biochem. J. 204:383–392, 1982.

320. Whittle B.J.R., Moncada S., Vane J.R.: Comparison of the effects of prostacyclin (PGI_2), prostaglandin E_1 and D_2 on platelet aggregation in different species. Prostaglandins 16:373–388, 1978.

321. Willis A.L., Smith D.L.: Therapeutical impact of eicosanoids in atherosclerotic disease. Eicosanoids 2:69–99, 1989.

322. Willis A.L., Smith D.L., Vigo C.: Suppression of principal atherosclerotic mechanisms by prostacyclins and other eicosanoids. Prog. Lipid Res. 25:645–666, 1986.

323. Willis A.L., Smith D.L., Vigo C., Kluge A.F.: Effects of prostacyclin and orally sta-

ble nimetic agent RS-93427-007 on basic mechanisms of atherogenesis. Lancet 2:682–683, 1987.

324. Wolin M.S., Burke-Wolin T., Cohn L.A., Cherry P.D.: Potential mechanism of pulmonary arterial relaxation and guanylate cyclase activation by 15-hydroperoxy eicosatetraenoic acid. In: Advances in Prostaglandin Thromboxane Leukotriene Research, vol. 19, Samuelsson B., Wong P.Y.K., Sun F.F. (eds.). Raven Press, New York, pp 285–288, 1989.

325. Wolin M.S., Messina E.J., Kaley G.: Involvement of prostaglandins in arteriolar vasodilatation to peroxides. In: Advances in Prostaglandin Thromboxane Leukotriene Research, vol. 19, Samuelsson B., Wong P.Y.K., Sun F.F. (eds.). Raven Press, New York, pp 281–284, 1989.

326. Wong P.Y.K., Lee W.H., Chao P.H.W., Reiss R.F., McGiff J.C.: Metabolism of prostacyclin by 9-hydroxyprostaglandin dehydrogenase in human platelets. J. Biol. Chem. 255:9021–9024, 1980.

327. Wu K.K., Lo S.S., Papp A.C., Vijjeswarapu H.N.: Stimulation of de novo synthesis of prostaglandin G/H synthase in endothelial cells. In: Advances in Prostaglandin Thromboxane Leukotriene Research, vol. 19, Samuelsson B., Wong P.Y.K., Sun F.F. (eds.). Raven Press, New York, pp 237–241, 1989.

328. Wynalda M.A., Fitzpatrick F.A.: Albumins stabilize prostaglandin I_2. Prostaglandins 20:853–861, 1980.

329. Yamaja Setty B.N., Stuart M.J.: 15-hydroxy-5,8,11,13-eicosatetraenoic acid inhibits human vascular cyclooxygenase. Potential role in diabetic vascular disease. J. Clin. Invest. 77:202–211, 1986.

330. Yarduman D.A., Isenberg D.A., Rustin M., Belcher G., Snaith M.L., Dowd P., Machin S.J.: Successful treatment of Raynaud's syndrome with Iloprost, a chemically stable prostacyclin analogue. Br. J. Rheumatol. 27:220–226, 1988.

331. Yoshida S., Inoh S., Asano T., Sano K., Kubota M., Shimazoki H., Ueta N.: Lipid peroxidation as a cause of postischaemic brain injury. In: Pathology and Pharmacotherapy of Cerebrovascular Disorders, Betz E., et al., (eds.). Verlag-Witzstrock, Baden-Baden, pp 85–89, 1980.

332. Yui Y., Aoyama T., Morishita H., Takahashi M., Takatsu Y., Kawai C.: Serum prostacyclin stabilizing factor is identical to apolipoprotein A-I(Apo AI). A novel function of Apo A-I. J. Clin. Invest. 82:803–807, 1988.

333. Zimmerman J.J.: Pharmacologic modulation by prostaglandin E_1 of superoxide anion production by human polymorphonuclear leukocytes. Crit. Care Med. 14:761–767, 1986.

334. Zusman R.M., Rubin R.H., Cato A.E., Cocchetto D.M., Crow J.W., Tolkoff-Rubin N.: Hemodialysis using prostacyclin instead of heparin as the sole antithrombotic agent. N. Engl. J. Med. 304:934, 1981.

335. Zygulska-Mach H., Kostka-Trąbka E., Nitoń A., Gryglewski R.J.: Prostacyclin in central retinal vein occlusion. Lancet 1:1075, 1980.

336. Zygulska-Mach H., Kostka-Trąbka E., Grodzińska L., Bieroń K., Telesz E., Gryglewski R.J.: Prostacyclin in the therapy of central retinal vein occlusion. In: Prostacyclin: Clinical Trials, Gryglewski R.J., Szczeklik A., McGiff J.C. (eds.). Raven Press, New York, pp 67–75, 1985.

2

Endothelium-Derived Relaxing (EDRF) and Contracting Factors (EDCF) in the Control of Cardiovascular Homeostasis: The Pioneering Observations

John T. Shepherd, Paul M. Vanhoutte

Introduction

It has long been recognized that the fluidity of the blood depends on interactions between the cells of the blood and the endothelium. Examples of the complex factors involved are the ability of the endothelial cells to synthesize key factors,[50] such as mucopolysaccharides,[10] von Willebrand factor,[66] tissue plasminogen activator,[20] platelet activating factor,[131] growth-promoting factor,[103] and antioxidant enzymes.[5]

Endothelial cells also can metabolize 5-hydroxytryptamine (serotonin) and norepinephrine, mainly by the enzyme monoamine oxidase, and convert angiotensin I to angiotensin II and degrade bradykinin (Fig. 1). In addition they synthesize a series of autocrine and paracrine substances including prostacyclin,[89] a nonprostanoid

endothelium-derived relaxing factor (EDRF),[37] a hyperpolarizing factor,[30,120] and an enzyme that is capable of activating prorenin. This enzyme, in conjunction with angiotensin converting enzyme and other angiotensinases might, by amplifying the generation of angiotensin, affect local vascular tone.[28] Endothelial cells can also form constrictor substances, among which are the oxygen-derived free radical superoxide anion and the peptide endothelin.[69–72,124,129]

In 1976, Moncada et al.[89] showed that an enzyme isolated from arteries transforms prostaglandin endoperoxides to an unstable substance that inhibits platelet aggregation. The substance can be found both in the vascular smooth muscle cells and in the endothelium. This protects the vessels from deposition of platelet thrombi.[11,50] Later, it was shown that the substance generated was the endoperox-

Rubanyi G.M.: Cardiovascular Significance of Endothelium-Derived Vasoactive Factors, Futura Publishing Co., Inc., Mount Kisco, NY, © 1991.

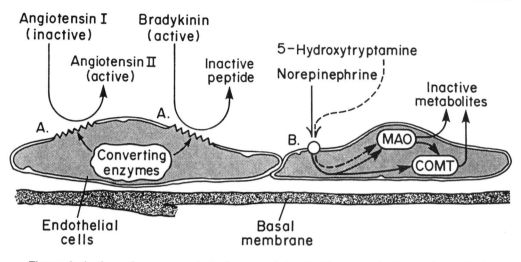

Figure 1: In the pulmonary endothelium, angiotensin I is converted to angiotensin II, bradykinin is inactivated, serotonin (5-hydroxytryptamine) is degraded by the enzyme monoamine oxidase (MAO), as is norepinephrine by catechol-O-methyltransferase (COMT). Prostaglandins are also metabolically degraded (from Lüscher and Vanhoutte, 1990, by permission).

ide, prostacyclin, which, in addition to inhibiting platelet adhesion and aggregation, can evoke vasodilatation. Cultured cells from human umbilical veins, when stimulated by thrombin, trypsin, or calcium ionophores, synthesized prostacyclin.[128] The effects of prostacyclin are mediated by the stimulation of adenylate cyclase in vascular smooth muscle and in platelets.[51]

Turning to the events leading to the demonstration that acetylcholine can release an endothelium-derived relaxing factor, it was long known that spiral strips of blood vessels contract to acetylcholine. It was also known that injection of acetylcholine into the arterial system caused a vasodilatation. For example, when injected into the brachial artery at increasing doses, flows as large as those obtained during severe exercise of those muscles could be obtained.[27] Part of this dilatation was later explained by the presence of muscarinic receptors on the sympathetic nerve terminals, which, when activated, reduced the output of norepinephrine.[123] How-

ever, since blocking the sympathetic nerve causes about a threefold increase in blood flow, this could not explain the much larger dilatation seen with intra-arterial infusions. What was not thought of at this time was that in the preparation of the spiral strips, the endothelium is accidentally removed. Thus, it remained for Furchgott and Zawadzki to reconcile the different findings.[37] They demonstrated that acetylcholine causes an endothelium-dependent relaxation of mammalian arteries. Using an isolated preparation of the descending thoracic aorta of the rabbit, they concluded that this relaxation was initiated by the action of acetylcholine on a muscarinic receptor on the endothelial cells. This in turn stimulated these cells to release some factor or factors which diffuses to the smooth muscle cells and causes them to relax.[39] This they called "endothelium-derived relaxing factor" (EDRF). It was not prostacyclin or another prostaglandin since none of the many prostaglandins tested cause relaxation of the rabbit aorta and inhibitors of cyclooxygenase did not prevent the acetylcholine-induced relaxation.[37] Thus, by definition, the term EDRF refers to a nonprostanoid relaxing factor. The quest for its identity led to the discovery that it may be nothing else but nitric oxide.[40,63,64,96]

In 1982, while exploring differences in endothelium-dependent responsiveness between canine arteries and veins, DeMey and Vanhoutte found that stimuli such as arachidonic acid and thrombin could evoke endothelium-dependent contractions rather than relaxations in the veins. They also demonstrated that profound anoxia could evoke endothelium-dependent contractions in some but not all arteries and veins of the same species.[22] Subsequent work demonstrated that the response to anoxia was due to a diffusible substance that was not a metabolite of arachidonic acid,[105] while the endothelium-dependent contractions evoked by arachidonic acid could be prevented by inhibitors of cyclooxygenase.[22,86] Thus the concept emerged that endothelial cells could release several endothelium-derived contracting factors (EDCF). These initial observations were corroborated by the demonstration that cultured endothelial cells produce a potent vasoconstrictor peptide, which has been characterized as endothelin.[129]

The pioneering studies on prostacyclin, EDRF, and endothelium-dependent contractions have led to increased understanding of vascular physiology and pathology.

In this chapter, we will concentrate on the important normal heterogeneity of endothelium-mediated vasomotor responses, the factors involved in the release of EDRF, its nature, the existence of other relaxing and constricting factors (EDCFs, apart from endothelin) that operate in physiological and pathological circumstances, and how these can participate in normal regulation of the vascular system.

Heterogeneity of Endothelium-Mediated Vascular Responses

Species Differences

Endothelium-mediated responses are present in all vertebrates that have been examined, including bony fishes and amphibia.[87] However, there are species differences in responses to various agonists. For example, acetylcholine causes an endothelium-dependent relaxation of isolated coronary arteries of the dog but not the pig,[46] whereas 5-hydroxytryptamine (serotonin) causes an endothelium-dependent relaxation in both.[17,18,111]

Differences Within Species

Acetylcholine causes endothelium-dependent relaxation of isolated canine arteries from different vascular beds, except for the basilar artery where it induces an endothelium-dependent contraction.[22,68,69] Isolated segments from the porcine aorta relax to acetylcholine, but not those from the coronary arteries.[45,46,115] Another example is the responses to serotonin, which causes endothelium-dependent relaxation of isolated segments of coronary but not of femoral or renal arteries.[18,19,59] In humans, adenosine diphosphate and thrombin evoke endothelium-dependent relaxations in isolated segments of coronary, internal mammary and renal arteries, but not in peripheral arteries.[82,83] The responses to vasopressin are another example of heterogeneity within species. In the dog, vasopressin causes marked endothelium-dependent relaxation of the basilar artery without any direct effect on the smooth muscle; coronary artery segments also relax and this is me-

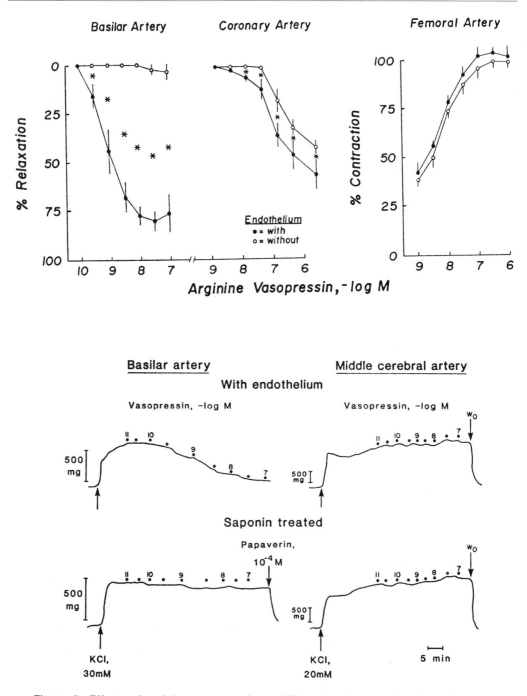

Figure 2: Effects of arginine vasopressin on different canine arteries. Top: It causes endothelium-dependent relaxation of the cerebral basilar artery, relaxation of the coronary arteries by an endothelium-dependent mechanism as well as a direct relaxing action on the smooth muscle, and endothelium-independent constriction of the smooth muscle of the femoral artery (from Katusic et al., 1984, by permission of the American Heart Association). Bottom: While vasopressin causes endothelium-dependent relaxation of the basilar artery, it causes an endothelium-independent contraction of the middle cerebral artery (Katusic, unpublished data).

diated both by an endothelium-dependent mechanism and a direct effect on the smooth muscle, whereas in the femoral artery an endothelium-independent contraction of the smooth muscle occurs. All of these actions are mediated through V_1-vasopressinergic receptors.[69,70] Also, while the canine basilar arteries relax as mentioned above, more distal canine cerebral arteries contract (Fig. 2) (Katusic, unpublished observations).

Responses of Arteries and Veins of the Same Species

Examination of isolated segments of canine arteries and veins showed that while the former demonstrated endothelium-dependent relaxation to both arachidonic acid and thrombin, the veins showed endothelium-dependent contractions (Fig. 3). Also, acetylcholine, which evokes potent endothelium-dependent relaxations of most arterial segments, has little effect on venous segments.[22,83]

Causes of Heterogeneity

No specific information is available to explain the heterogeneity in endothelium-dependent responsiveness. Obviously, differences in receptor population on en-

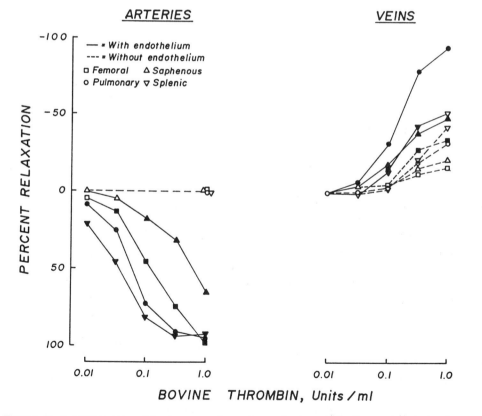

Figure 3: Arachidonic acid causes a dose-dependent endothelium-mediated relaxation of arteries, but an endothelium-dependent contraction of the corresponding veins (from DeMey and Vanhoutte, 1982, by permission of the American Heart Association).

dothelial cells, differences in the relaxing or contracting factors released, or in the sensitivity of the smooth muscle to the factors released could be key factors.[107a] For example, in examining endothelium-dependent responses to aggregating platelets, species and regional differences are found in the receptors involved. Also, there could be differences in the cellular mechanisms leading to release, for example, in the guanine nucleotide regulatory proteins.

Whatever the mechanism(s) of these different responses, they have important clinical implications. For example, a differing response to vasopressin may serve to redistribute blood flow and conserve arterial blood pressure during hemorrhage. The vasodilator response to thrombin in arteries will help to disperse an incipient clot, whereas the vasoconstrictor response in the veins will help to retain it and so prevent pulmonary embolization.

Physiological Responses

Changes in Blood Flow

It has been known for many years that a dilatation of the conduit arteries occurs when the blood flow through the artery is increased. For example, in cats, a dilatation of the femoral artery occurs in response to a contraction of the hindlimb muscles or by opening an arteriovenous fistula in that leg.[24] Similar findings have been noted in the epicardial coronary arteries of the dog[42] and in the human brachial and coronary arteries.[1,26,92]

In the canine femoral artery in situ, removal of the endothelium by a balloon catheter prevents the flow-induced dilatation, demonstrating that it depends on the presence of endothelial cells.[97,98] The explanation lies in the release of relaxing factor by the endothelium of the conduit vessels. In bioassay experiments using the

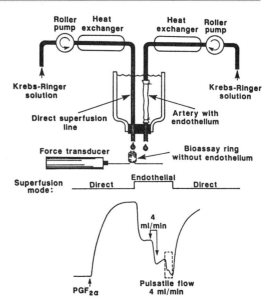

Figure 4: Bioassay technique to assess release of vasoactive factors by the endothelium. In this study, the bioassay ring without endothelium was contracted with prostaglandin $F_{2\alpha}$ (PGF$_{2\alpha}$). On changing the steady flow (02 mL/min) from the direct superfusion line to an artery with intact endothelium, relaxation of the bioassay ring occurs. On increasing the steady flow to 4 mL/min, a further relaxation occurs and when the flow is made pulsatile, there is an additional relaxation (data from Rubanyi et al., unpublished).

canine femoral artery perfused with oxygenated physiological salt solution, increases in laminar or pulsatile flow from 2 to 4 mL per minute augments the release of endothelium-derived relaxing factor (Fig. 4) and prostacyclin.[106] Since the dilatation is not blocked by inhibitors of cyclooxygenase, it can be attributed to the release of EDRF. This endothelium-mediated dilatation of the conduit artery when the distal resistance vessels dilate helps to optimize the flow to metabolically active vascular beds. An increase in the viscosity of the perfusate augments the response, indicating that changes in local shear stress are likely to be the initiating factor.[19,73,121] In cultured human endothelial cells, flow increases the production of prostacyclin and that of tissue plasmino-gen activator.[4,25,36] In the intact vascular system, the endothelial cells are continu-ously exposed to shear forces. It is evident that these cells recognize these forces, since normally they are elongated in the direction of the flow.[78]

Endothelial cells have mechanotrans-ducing ion channels which are cation se-lective and permeable to Ca^{2+}.[79] Ca^{2+} ions are necessary for the release of EDRF. An increased shear stress activates a potas-sium-ion current across the membrane of endothelial cells.[94] The resultant hyper-polarization of the endothelium could help explain the local release of a relaxing factor and the consequential relaxation of the un-derlying smooth muscle. Chronic in-creases in flow also increase the endothe-lium-dependent vasodilator responses to acetylcholine.[88,130] Shear stress can influ-ence many endothelial cell functions in-cluding permeability[23] and the synthesis of prostacyclin and endothelium-derived re-laxing factor.[97,98]

Endothelium-dependent, flow-in-duced vasodilatation also has been ob-served in isolated resistance vessels of the cat and rabbit, when contracted with nor-epinephrine or prostaglandin $F_{2\alpha}$. After re-moval of the endothelium by rubbing, the flow-induced relaxation was reduced from a mean of 70% to 37%, indicating that it originates both in the endothelium and in the smooth muscle. The mechanism of the relaxation in the absence of the endothe-lium is unknown.

Transmural Pressure

In vascular beds in vivo, the trans-mural pressure dictates the length of the contractile components of the circular mus-cle and hence the force generated by the muscle in response to a given stimulus. An increase in transmural pressure can cause resistance vessels to contract to less than

their initial diameter and to dilate when the pressure is decreased.[67] These adjust-ments in resistance serve to maintain a fairly constant flow and tend to hold cap-illary hydrostatic pressure constant over a wide range of arterial pressures. It has been suggested that this autoregulation either is the result of a myogenic mecha-nism or that the change in contractile force was secondary to a difference in the met-abolic levels around the resistance blood vessels during the initial flow changes that follow the changes in transmural pres-sure.[67]

Another possibility is that the endo-thelium senses changes in transmural pressure. A quick stretch of an isolated ring of canine basilar artery is followed at once by an active increase in tension if the endothelium is present, but not if it is ab-sent.[71] The contraction is prevented by in-hibiting the enzyme cyclooxygenase by in-domethacin, but not by diethylcarbama-zine, a lipoxygenase inhibitor. This indicates that a product of the cyclooxy-genase pathway is involved (Fig. 5).

In the cat cerebral artery, an increase in transmural pressure also causes endo-thelium-dependent contraction accompa-nied by depolarization of the smooth mus-cle.[54] Stretch-activated ion channels are present in endothelial cells,[79] and these are permeable to Ca^{2+}. Their opening fre-quency increases with stretching of the cell membrane. The stretch-induced contrac-tions, in response to a sudden change in transmural pressure, such as the autore-gulatory responses in the intact circulation, are characterized by a rapid onset followed by a sustained contraction. Further studies are needed in other arteries and vascular beds to see if a stretch-induced release of an endothelium-dependent contracting factor(s) is the key mediator of autoregu-lation. In the canine basilar artery, in-creases in the extracellular concentrations of potassium induce endothelium-depen-dent rhythmic activity.[72] These depend on the activity of cyclooxygenase and are in-

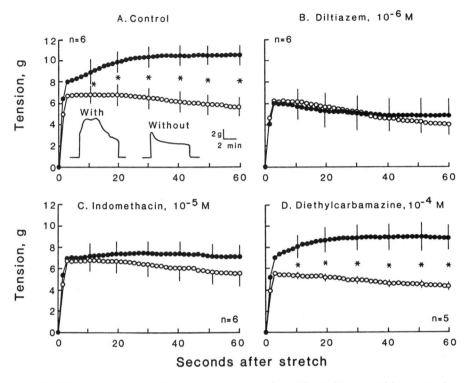

Figure 5: When a ring of canine cerebral artery is subjected to a sudden stretch, a further and persistent increase in tension occurs if the endothelium is present, but not if it is absent. The increase in tension is prevented by the calcium antagonist diltiazem, by the cyclooxygenase inhibitor indomethacin, but not by the beta-lipoxygenase inhibitor diethylcarbamazine (from Katusic et al., 1987, by permission).

hibited by Ca^{2+} antagonists. This suggests that they are mediated by an endothelium-derived contracting factor which is released or acts intermittently.[108] In isolated perfused carotid arteries of the dog, increases in transmural pressure trigger endothelium-dependent contraction, which is mediated by a decrease in basal release of EDRF, rather than an increased release of an EDCF.[109a]

Endothelium and Platelets

When platelets are made to aggregate in the vicinity of unstimulated isolated seg-ments of arteries without endothelium, this causes their contraction. However, the contraction is prevented, or considerably reduced, by the presence of the endothelium. When segments of canine, porcine, or human coronary arteries are contracted, aggregating platelets cause endothelium-dependent relaxations (Fig. 6).[12,15,16,34,59,60,111,115] If platelets were to aggregate in an artery in situ, and this enhanced the release of EDRF from endothelial cells at the site, this, by opposing further aggregation[99,119] and by relaxing the smooth muscle,[15,16,59] would operate to inhibit progression of the coagulation process. Thus, in normal blood vessels, EDRF, together with the release of prostacyclin

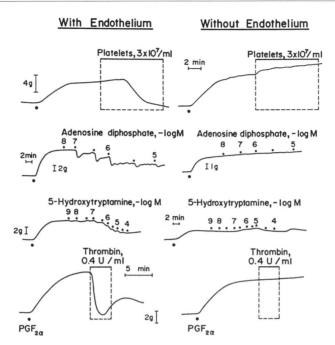

Figure 6: Studies on isolated segments of canine coronary arteries contracted with prostaglandin $F_{2\alpha}$ (PGF$_{2\alpha}$). Aggregating platelets, adenosine diphosphate, serotonin (5-hydroxytryptamine) and thrombin cause endothelium-dependent relaxation (from Shepherd JT: The Management of the Acute Coronary Attack, Academic Press, Inc., London, 1986; chapter 2).

may act to relax the blood vessels and at the same time work synergistically to inhibit platelet adhesion and aggregation (Fig. 7).[62,90,125]

Mediators of Platelet-Induced Release of EDRF

Adenine Nucleotides

In the coronary arteries of the dog, the adenine nucleotides are the prime mediators of endothelium-mediated relaxation (Fig. 6), since the enzyme apyrase, which catalyzes the breakdown of adenosine triphosphate, prevents most of the relaxa-

tion.[59,60] This is true also in human coronary and internal mammary arteries and the porcine basilar artery.[34,83,114] In the canine coronary artery and porcine basilar arteries, the adenine nucleotides act on endothelial purinergic receptors of the P_{2y}-purinergic subtype.[53,58,114] In cultured porcine endothelial cells, adenosine diphosphate causes the release of another relaxing factor which is not nitric oxide.[6,7]

Serotonin (5-Hydroxytryptamine)

In various animal and human quiescent arterial segments, the contractions caused by serotonin are greater in the absence of the endothelium.[17,41,44] In the por-

PROSTACYCLIN AND ENDOTHELIUM-DERIVED RELAXING FACTOR(S)

Thrombin

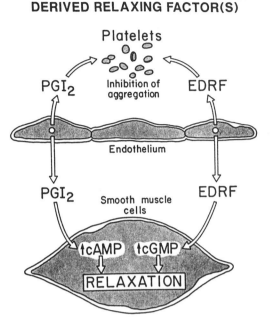

Figure 7: Both prostacyclin (PGI_2) formed in vascular endothelial cells and in the smooth muscle, as well as endothelium-derived relaxing factor (EDRF) formed in endothelial cells cause relaxation of the underlying smooth muscle. They also inhibit platelet adhesion and aggregation. Prostacyclin acts by increasing cyclic adenosine 3',5'-monophosphate (cAMP) while endothelium-derived relaxing factor increases cyclic guanosine 3',5'-monophosphate (cGMP).

The role of the platelet products in preventing obstruction to blood flow by causing release of EDRF is reinforced if

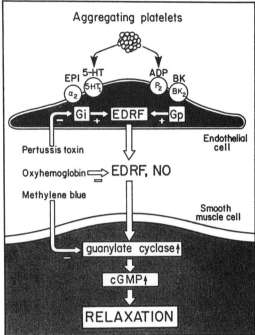

Figure 8: Guanine nucleotide-binding proteins (G-proteins) function as intermediaries in transmembrane signaling pathways that consist of three proteins: receptors, G-proteins, and effectors (from Gilman: Annu. Rev. Biochem. 56:615–619, 1987). The G-proteins act to signal transducers from the activated membrane receptors by various agonists to the effector enzymes and channels, including adenylate cyclase and phospholipase C. The release of endothelium-derived relaxing factor involves at least two G-proteins, one of which, G_i but not Gp, is inhibited by pertussis toxin. Epi = epinephrine; 5-HT = 5-hydroxytryptamine (serotonin); ADP = adenosine diphosphate; BK = bradykinin; cGMP = cyclic guanosine 3',5'-monophosphate; NO = nitric oxide; EDRF = endothelium-derived relaxing factor; P_2 = P_{2y}—purinergic receptor; α_2-alpha$_2$-adrenoceptor; BK_2-bradykinin receptor; $5HT_1$ = serotonin receptor (from Vanhoutte PM, 1989, by permission).

cine coronary artery, after blockade of $5HT_2$-serotonergic receptors on the vascular smooth muscle, serotonin is the key mediator of the endothelium-dependent relaxations to aggregating platelets.[112,113] The receptors on the endothelium are of the $5HT_1$-like subtype.[61] The transducer of the signal from these receptors to the release of the relaxing factor involves a pertussin toxin-sensitive G-protein.[32,112,113] By contrast, the coupling between the activation of the endothelial purinergic receptors and the subsequent increase in cyclic GMP does not involve this G-protein (Fig. 8).[112,113]

thrombin is formed, since the latter can cause a potent endothelium-dependent relaxation of arterial vessels which can be blocked by heparin (Fig. 6).

Platelet-Activating Factor

While platelet-activating factor can cause endothelium-dependent relaxation in certain vessels, this requires much greater concentrations than are necessary for its other biological effects, including platelet aggregation.[59,62]

Release of Renin from Juxtaglomerular Cells

In the afferent glomerular arterioles the endothelial cells are in close proximity to the juxtaglomerular cells (Fig. 9). Since endothelial cells respond to an increase in flow by releasing EDRF, the latter could modulate renin release. This is suggested by the demonstration that EDRF released from isolated canine blood vessels or from cultured porcine endothelial cells can decrease the production of renin from slices of dog kidneys (Fig. 10).[9,127]

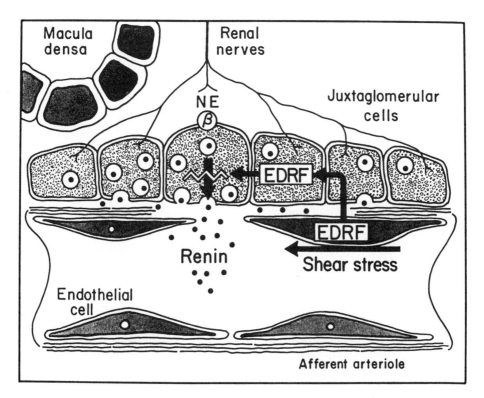

Figure 9: The relation of the juxtaglomerular cells to the afferent arteriole and the macula densa. In addition to regulation of renin release from these juxtaglomerular cells, changes in sodium load to the macula densa and by activation of the renal sympathetic nerves, the endothelial cells of the afferent arterioles may release endothelium-derived relaxing factor in response to an increase in shear stress. This factor, by acting on juxtaglomerular cells, can inhibit renin release. β = beta-adrenoceptor; NE = norepinephrine (from Lüscher and Vanhoutte, 1990, by permission).

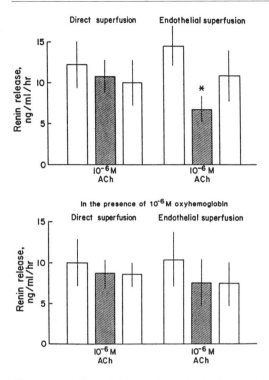

Figure 10: Superfusion of cortical slices of dog kidney. When these are superfused directly, there is no change in the amount of renin they release. If, however, the superfusate passes through an artery with intact endothelium, and the endothelium is stimulated by acetylcholine, inhibition of renin release occurs. This inhibition is prevented by oxyhemoglobin, which indicates that it is caused by endothelium-derived relaxing factor (from Vidal-Ragout et al., 1988, by permission).

Arterial Mechanoreceptors

These receptors respond to changes in transmural pressure. Studies of afferent nerve traffic from the isolated carotid mechanoreceptors in the dog, from which the endothelial cells were removed, have demonstrated that the threshold pressure for activating these receptors is elevated when cultured endothelial cells, stimulated by either bradykinin or a calcium ionophore, are added. During stepwise increases in pressure in the sinus, the affer-

ent activity was lower after infusion of the cells.[13]

Atrial Natriuretic Peptide

Atrial natriuretic peptide(s) is released from the atria in response to changes in transmural pressure.[29] To examine the influence of the endocardium on the release, the endocardium of the rat atrium was removed by saponin. This augmented the basal release of the atrial natriuretic peptide, as did inhibition of EDRF by agents such as methylene blue, hydroquinone, and oxyhemoglobin.[80]

Alpha$_2$-Adrenoceptors

The endothelial cells of some blood vessels have alpha$_2$-adrenoceptors. When activated by norepinephrine, they cause a release of EDRF.[14,32,86] This could contribute to the vasodilator effect that circulating catecholamines have in the coronary and splanchnic vascular beds. Augmentation of endothelium-dependent vasodilator effects of catecholamines may contribute to the vasodilator properties of beta-adrenergic blocking agents.

Nature of Endothelium-Derived Vasoactive Factors

Endothelium-Derived Relaxing Factor(s)

After the discovery of EDRF by Furchgott and Zawadzki,[37] subsequent studies demonstrated that this had a half-life of about 6 seconds, was released continuously, and could be stimulated by many substances and physical factors. The release was demonstrated originally using a "sandwich" preparation of the rabbit aorta.[37,38] In this procedure, the response to acetylcholine of a transverse strip freed of endothelial cells was tested when mounted separately and also tested when mounted, intimal surface against intimal surface, with a longitudinal strip of the same width and length with the endothelial cells present. This was confirmed by other bioassay procedures in which isolated arteries, with and without endothelium, are perfused and the EDRF released is bioassayed by an endothelium-free preparation of artery downstream attached to a force transducer.[33,34,47–49,104] Another approach is to use cultured endothelial cells on the surface of microcarrier beads contained in a superfused column, again with a downstream superfused ring or strip of artery attached to a force transducer as the detector.[7,14,43,47,81,103] The scavenger of superoxide anions, superoxide dismutase, prolongs the half-life of EDRF, indicating that the oxygen-derived free radical superoxide anion rapidly inactivates it.[52,105,107] The finding that the calcium ionophore A23187 is a potent endothelium-dependent relaxing agent suggested that an increase in calcium ions in the region of some key Ca^{2+} activating enzyme could be a step in the reactions mediating release of EDRF.[38] It was later shown that the production of EDRF depends on extracellular calcium, although the activation of voltage-operated Ca^{2+} channels is not involved.[39,48,118] In the rabbit aorta, agents that inhibit mitochondrial electron transport or uncouple oxidative phosphorylation interfere with either the synthesis or the release of EDRF.[48]

In porcine coronary arteries, the inhibitor of certain guanine nucleotide regulatory proteins attenuates the endothelium-dependent relaxations to serotonin and the selective α_2-adrenergic agonist UK14304, but not those to adenosine diphosphate, bradykinin, or the calcium ionophore A23187.[32] This toxin does not inhibit the relaxing action of nitric oxide on the smooth muscle. These studies suggest that there are at least two mechanisms leading to the production of EDRF, one of which involves a pertussis toxin-sensitive G-protein, probably G_i (Fig. 8).

Knowing that EDRF is an unstable nonprostanoid substance that can be inactivated by superoxide anions, that EDRF stimulates an increase in soluble guanylate cyclase in vascular smooth muscle (Fig. 11), and that this increase precedes the relaxation, Furchgott[40] and Ignarro et al.[63,64] proposed that EDRF might be nitric oxide. Using chemiluminescence, Palmer et al.[96] demonstrated that cultured endothelial cells exposed to bradykinin release nitric oxide, which is synthesized from the terminal guanidine nitrogen atom(s) of the amino acid L-arginine in the vascular endothelial cells.[95] The nitric oxide released from the endothelial cells is indistinguishable from EDRF in terms of its biological activity and stability and its action was inhibited similarly by hemoglobin (Fig. 11). The latter inhibits endothelium-dependent relaxation by reacting with EDRF before the factor gains access to the soluble guanylate cyclase of the smooth muscle.[85,96]

The L-arginine analogue N-omega monomethyl arginine (L-NMMA) but not its dextro-isomer inhibits the generation of nitric oxide by endothelial cells.[102] It is still uncertain whether nitric oxide is secreted by the endothelial cells or is bound to a carrier molecule (R-NO) that dissociates at the cell membrane of the vascular smooth muscle.[91,109]

The cyclic nucleotide, cyclic GMP, formed following the activation of soluble guanylate cyclase and leading to cyclic GMP-dependent protein phosphorylation, most likely mediates the vasodilator action of EDRF (Fig. 11).[33,57,63,64,76,85,100,101]

The EDRF-evoked increase in cyclic

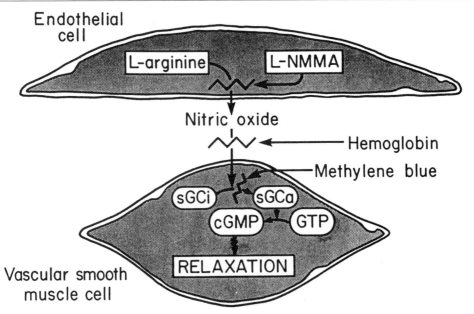

Figure 11: The production of endothelium-derived nitric oxide from L-arginine and the inhibitory effect of L-N^G-monomethyl arginine (L-NMMA). The nitric oxide derived from L-arginine activates the soluble guanylate cyclase (sGC) in the smooth muscle leading to the accumulation of cyclic guanosine monophosphate (cGMP). Hemoglobin inactivates nitric oxide, while methylene blue prevents the activation of soluble guanylate cyclase. i = inactive; a = active; GTP = guanosine triphosphate.

GMP inhibits the release of Ca^{2+} from intracellular stores and its entry through receptor-operated Ca^{2+} channels.[21] The increase in cyclic AMP caused by prostacyclin stimulates the phosphorylation of myosin light chain kinase. Thus their different mechanisms of causing relaxation of the underlying smooth muscle permits their synergistic action, not only in enhancing the relaxation but also in inhibiting platelet adhesion and aggregation. Subthreshold concentrations of EDRF and prostacyclin together markedly inhibit platelet aggregation, thus contributing to the antiaggregation properties of the endothelial surface.[99]

In the anesthetized rabbit, intravenous administration of L-NMMA induced a dose-dependent enantiomer-specific hypertension. This suggests that there is a continuous utilization of L-arginine for the enzymatic formation of nitric oxide by resistance blood vessels and indicates that formation of nitric oxide contributes to the regulation of blood pressure.[102]

Endothelium-Derived Hyperpolarizing Factor

In response to acetylcholine applied to isolated arteries with intact endothelium, the cell membrane of the smooth muscle becomes hyperpolarized. After removal of the endothelium, no hyperpolarization is observed. The hyperpolarization is mediated by a diffusible substance since it can be transferred from femoral arteries with endothelium to coronary arteries without endothelium (Fig. 12).[30] Exogenous nitric

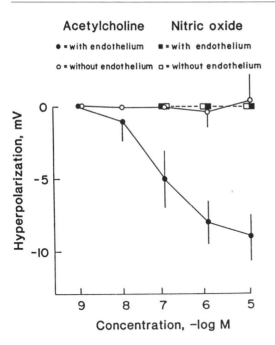

Acetylcholine   **Nitric oxide**

● = with endothelium   ■ = with endothelium

○ = without endothelium   □ = without endothelium

Figure 12: Acetylcholine causes a dose-dependent and endothelium-dependent hyperpolarization of the underlying smooth muscle, whereas nitric oxide does not. This indicates that there are at least two nonprostanoid relaxing factors, one of which acts by hyperpolarizing the muscle (endothelium-derived hyperpolarizing factor) (from Komori et al., 1988, by permission).

oxide does not affect the membrane potential in vascular smooth muscle, and methylene blue or hemoglobin do not prevent the endothelium-dependent hyperpolarization.[30,120] Thus, the endothelium-derived hyperpolarizing factor (EDHF) is not nitric oxide.[74] Ouabain applied only to the smooth muscle of the bioassay tissue prevents the hyperpolarization, but not the sustained relaxation to acetylcholine. Also, the hyperpolarization is transient while the relaxation to acetylcholine is sustained.[30] The receptors involved also differ, with an M_1-muscarinic receptor responsible for the release of the hyperpolarizing factor but an M_2-receptor responsible for the release of nitric oxide (Fig. 13).[75]

Other evidence for more than one en-

dothelium-derived relaxing substance includes the finding that under bioassay conditions (Fig. 4) pretreatment of the bioassay tissue with ouabain prevents the effect of the substance released from the endothelium of the canine coronary artery by acetylcholine and by shear stress, but not that released by bradykinin.[55] Similar conclusions have been reached using cultured porcine endothelial cells, where ouabain applied to the bioassay tissue inhibits the effects on this tissue of the EDRF released by adenosine diphosphate and by shear stress but not by the relaxing substance released by bradykinin or the calcium ionophore A23187 (Fig. 14).[6] The relaxation of the bioassay tissue caused by the latter two substances is inhibited by hemoglobin and by methylene blue, suggesting that it is nitric oxide.[6] In addition, treatment of the endothelial cells with ouabain reduces bradykinin and A23187-induced release of EDRF, but not that induced by ADP or shear stress.[6,35]

Endothelium-Derived Contracting Factors

In 1982, DeMey and Vanhoutte demonstrated that in canine systemic and pulmonary veins, arachidonic acid augmented the contractions evoked by norepinephrine. This augmentation did not occur after removal of the endothelium. This was the first demonstration of an endothelium-dependent vasoconstrictor substance(s) (EDCF). Since the contractions were prevented by inhibitors of the enzyme cyclooxygenase, but not by those of prostacyclin synthetase, venous endothelial cells can metabolize arachidonic acid into a vasoconstrictor prostanoid, which is not prostacyclin or thromboxane A_2.[86]

In the dog basilar artery, the fatty acid arachidonic acid causes endothelium-dependent contractions, which also are pre-

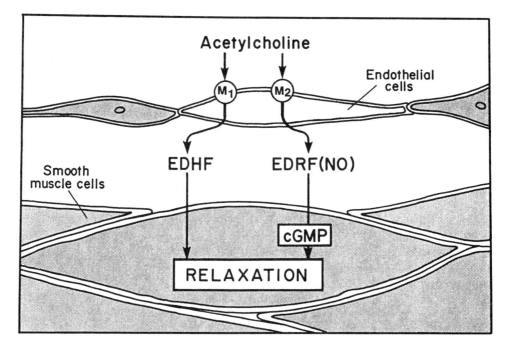

Figure 13: Acetylcholine activates an M_2-muscarinic receptor on the endothelial cells which causes them to release a relaxing substance (EDRF) which is probably nitric oxide (NO). Acetylcholine also acts on an M_1-muscarinic receptor of the endothelium to release another relaxing factor which hyperpolarizes the smooth muscle and thus initiates relaxation (endothelium-derived hyperpolarizing factor; EDHF). Nitric oxide sustains the relaxation by entering the smooth muscle and activating soluble guanylate cyclase which leads to the accumulation of cyclic GMP (cGMP) (from Lüscher and Vanhoutte, 1990, by permission).

vented by inhibition of cyclooxygenase.[70,110] The contractions can be prevented by inhibitors of thromboxane synthetase and thromboxane receptors. This suggests that thromboxane A_2 has an important role in the response. Since the calcium ionophore A23187 also causes contraction which is inhibited similarly, this indicates that an increase in cytosolic Ca^{2+} concentration activates the production of arachidonic acid by the endothelial cells which in turn is metabolized to thromboxane A_2. Since these contractions are prevented by superoxide dismutase, a scavenger of superoxide anion, it is likely that the radical generated during the metabolism of arachidonic acid, rather than thromboxane A_2, results in the activation of the vascular smooth muscle.[70]

Anoxia causes endothelium-dependent contractions in a variety of isolated blood vessels.[22,70,107] The contractions are due to the release of a diffusible substance, which does not require the activity of cyclooxygenase, and is not likely to be endothelin.[105,126] The EDCF released by anoxia causes contraction of vascular smooth muscle by activating the entry of extracellular Ca^{2+}.[70]

Pathophysiological Responses

Hypercholesteremia

In the pig, a high cholesterol diet (2%) reduces the endothelium-dependent relax-

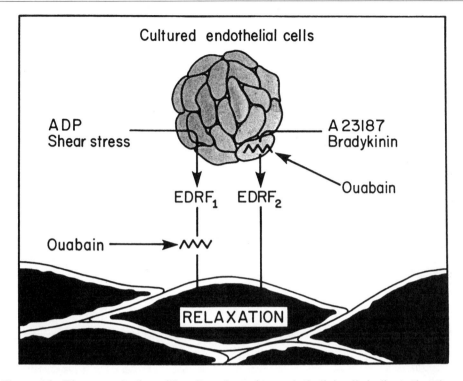

Figure 14: Bioassay studies with cultured porcine endothelial cells indicate that these cells release at least two relaxing factors (EDRF). One is most likely nitric oxide (NO); its release, stimulated by bradykinin or the Ca^{2+} ionophore A23187, but not its action, can be prevented by ouabain. The other factor is of unknown nature; it is released under basal conditions or when the endothelial cells are exposed to adenosine diphosphate (ADP) or to a shear stress; its action, but not its release, can be prevented by ouabain (from Lüscher and Vanhoutte, 1990, by permission).

ations to adenosine diphosphate, aggregating platelets, and serotonin in the coronary, basilar, and other arteries (Fig. 15).[19,116,117] In the rabbit aorta, contracted with either norepinephrine or serotonin, low-density lipoproteins inhibit endothelium-dependent relaxation to acetylcholine at a concentration seen in the plasma of patients with severe hyperlipidemia. The inhibition persists after washing out the lipoproteins.[2] Similar findings have been seen in porcine coronary arteries.[122] High density lipoproteins are without effect on the relaxation. In isolated porcine endothelial cells, native LDL inhibits the basal release and the receptor-operated release of EDRF.[6] Primary cultures of endothelial cells from human umbilical veins have a spontaneous inhibitory effect on adenosine diphosphate and collagen-induced platelet aggregation. This inhibitory effect is reduced by incubation of the cells with LDL prepared from normolipemic subjects.[93]

Fish Oil

In the pig, dietary supplementation with fish oil enhances endothelium-dependent relaxation of the coronary artery to aggregating platelets, and to adenosine diphosphate, bradykinin, and serotonin

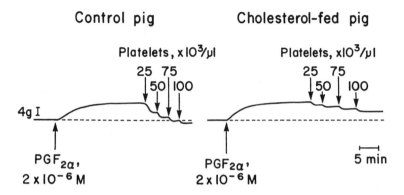

Figure 15: A diet rich in cholesterol inhibits the release of endothelium-derived re-laxing factor(s) by the coronary artery endothelial cells of the pig. In this study, the arterial segments were contracted by prostaglandin $F_{2\alpha}$ (PGF$_{2\alpha}$) and aggregating platelets were used to release the relaxing factor(s).

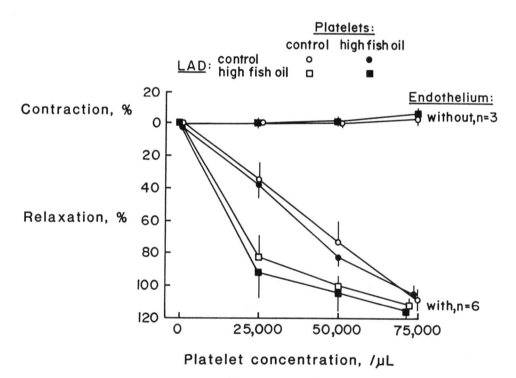

Figure 16: A diet rich in fish oil enhances the release of endothelium-derived relaxing factor(s) from the coronary arteries of the pig. In these studies the arterial segments were precontracted with prostaglandin $F_{2\alpha}$ and aggregating platelets were used to release the relaxing factor(s). It made no difference to the response whether or not the platelets came from a control pig or a pig on a high fish oil diet (from Shimokawa et al., 1987, by permission of the American Heart Association).

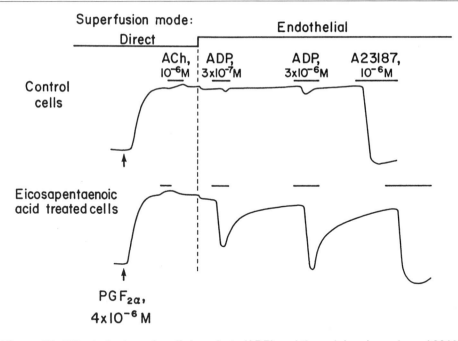

Figure 17: Effect of adenosine diphosphate (ADP) and the calcium ionophore A23187 on the release of relaxing factor(s) by porcine aortic endothelial cells cultured on microcarrier beads. As compared to control cells, cells incubated with the active principle of fish oil, eicosapentaenoic acid, cause a potent relaxation to ADP (bioassayed with a segment of porcine coronary artery without endothelium attached to a force transducer). Acetylcholine (ACh) was given at the beginning of the study to confirm the absence of endothelial cells in the bioassay segment. The response to the calcium ionophore was unchanged by the eicosapentaenoic acid (from Boulanger et al., 1990, by permission).

(Fig. 16). However, the relaxation to the Ca^{2+} ionophore A23187 is unchanged.[115] Bioassay studies show that the fish oil diet augments the release of EDRF. When cultured endothelial cells are grown in a medium containing eicosapentaenoic acid (EPA), the active component of fish oil, the amount of EDRF on stimulation by adenosine diphosphate is increased, whereas that released by the Ca^{2+} ionophore is unchanged (Fig. 17), suggesting that the EPA may augment the release of the endothelial factor that differs from nitric oxide.[7] Fish oil in the diet not only enhances the production of EDRF in atherosclerotic porcine coronary arteries but also helps to suppress the atherosclerotic process.[114]

Regenerated Endothelium

If the endothelium of pig coronary arteries is removed, it regenerates rapidly. In 8 days there are normal endothelium-mediated relaxations to platelets. However, at 4 weeks, the relaxations are impaired (Fig. 18). This is due to a specific lack of responsiveness to serotonin which is still seen at 5 months, since the relaxations to adenosine diphosphate, bradykinin, and thrombin are preserved. The lack of response to serotonin appears to be due to the loss of the pertussis toxin-sensitive component of the response, indicative of a deficient G-protein-mediated mechanism.[112,113]

PLATELETS AND REGENERATED ENDOTHELIUM IN ISOLATED PORCINE CORONARY ARTERIES
(Contracted with PGF$_{2\alpha}$ in the presence of ketanserin)

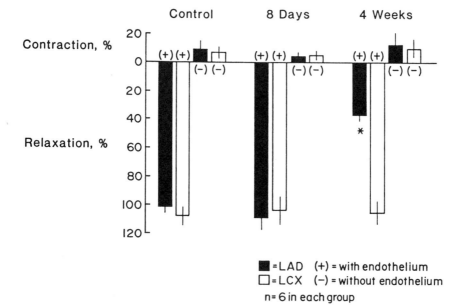

Figure 18: After balloon denudation of the left circumflex coronary artery of the pig, the regenerated endothelium shows a normal release of relaxing factor(s) in response to aggregating platelets (70,000/µL) at 8 days but the response is diminished at 4 weeks. LAD = segment of left anterior descending coronary artery (control) ; LCX = segment of left circumflex coronary artery. The arterial segments were precontracted with prostaglandin F$_{2\alpha}$ (PGF$_{2\alpha}$) and the S$_1$-serotonergic receptors on the smooth muscle were blocked by ketanserin. The segments were treated with indomethacin for 40 minutes prior to inducing contraction with prostaglandin F$_{2\alpha}$ to prevent the synthesis of vasoactive prostanoids. Since endothelium-derived relaxing factor is not a product of cyclooxygenase, its release is not affected by indomethacin (from Shimokawa et al., 1987, by permission of the American Heart Association).

References

1. Anderson E.A., Mark A.L.: Flow-mediated and reflex changes in large peripheral artery tone in humans. Circulation 79:93–100, 1989.
2. Andrews H.E., Bruckdorfer K.R., Dunn R.C., Jacobs M.: Low-density lipoproteins inhibit endothelium-dependent relaxation in rabbit aorta. Nature 327:237–239, 1987.
3. Bevan J.A., Joyce E.H., Wellman G.C.: Flow-dependent dilation in a resistance artery still occurs after endothelium removal. Circ. Res. 63:980–985, 1988.
4. Bhagyalakshmi A., Frangos J.A.: Mechanism of shear-induced prostacyclin production in endothelial cells. Biochem. Biophys. Res. Commun. 158:31–37, 1989.

5. Block E.R., Patel J.M., Sheridan N.P.: The effect of oxygen and endotoxin on acetate dehyrogenase release, 5-hydroxytryptamine uptake and antioxidant enzyme activity in endothelial cells. J. Cell. Physiol. 122:240–248, 1985.

6. Boulanger C., Bühler F.R., Lüscher T.F.: Low density lipoproteins impair the release of endothelium-derived relaxing factor from cultured porcine endothelial cells (Abstract). Eur. Heart J. 10:331, 1989.

7. Boulanger C., Hendrickson H., Lorenz R.R., Vanhoutte P.M.: Release of different relaxing factors by cultured porcine cells. Circ. Res. 64:1070–1078, 1989.

8. Boulanger C., Schini V.B., Hendrickson H., Vanhoutte P.M.: Chronic exposure of cultured endothelial cells to eicosapentaenoic acid potentiates the release of endothelium-derived relaxing factor(s). Br. J. Pharmacol. 99(1):176–180, 1990.

9. Boulanger C., Vidal-Ragout M., Fiksen-Olsen M., Romero J.C., Vanhoutte P.M.: Cultured endothelial cells release a nonprostanoid inhibitor of renin release (Abstract). Clin. Res. 36:539, 1988.

10. Buonassisi V.: Sulphated mucopolysaccharide synthesis and modulation in endothelial cell cultures. Exp. Cell. Res. 76:363–368, 1973.

11. Bunting S., Gryglewski R., Moncada S., Vane J.R.: Arterial walls generate from prostaglandin endoperoxides and substance (prostaglandin X) which relaxes strips of mesenteric and coeliac arteries and inhibits platelet aggregation. Prostaglandins 12:897–913, 1976.

12. Busse R., Ogilvie A., Pohl U.: Vasomotor activity of diadenosine triphosphate and diadenosine tetraphosphate in isolated arteries. Am. J. Physiol. 254:H828–H832, 1988.

13. Chapleau M.W., Hajduczok G., Shasby D.M., Abboud F.M.: Activated endothelial cells in culture suppress baroreceptors in the carotid sinus of dog. Hypertension 11:586–590, 1988.

14. Cocks T.M., Angus J.A., Campbell J.H., Campbell G.R.: Release and properties of endothelium-derived relaxing factor (EDRF) from endothelial cells in culture. J. Cell Physiol. 123:310–320, 1985.

15. Cohen R.A., Shepherd J.T., Vanhoutte P.M.: Inhibitory role of the endothelium in the response of isolated coronary arteries to platelets. Science 221:273–274, 1983.

16. Cohen R.A., Shepherd J.T., Vanhoutte P.M.: 5-Hydroxytryptamine can mediate endothelium-dependent relaxations of coronary arteries. Am. J. Physiol. 245:H1077–H1080, 1983.

17. Cohen R.A., Shepherd J.T., Vanhoutte P.M.: Inhibitory role of the endothelium in response of isolated coronary arteries to platelets. Blood Vessels 20:188–189, 1983.

18. Cohen R.A., Shepherd J.T., Vanhoutte P.M.: Endothelium and asymmetrical responses of the coronary arterial wall. Am. J. Physiol. 247:H403–H408, 1984.

19. Cohen R.A., Zitnay K.M., Haudenschild C.C., Cunningham L.D.: Loss of selective endothelial cell vasoactive functions caused by hypercholesterolemia in pig coronary arteries. Circ. Res. 63:903–910, 1988.

20. Collen D., Lijnen H.R.: Tissue-type plasminogen activator-mechanism of action and thrombolytic properties. Haemostasis 16 (Suppl 3):25–32, 1986.

21. Collins P., Lewis M.J., Henderson A.H.: Endothelium-derived factor relaxes vascular smooth muscle by cyclic GMP-mediated effects on calcium movements. In: Relaxing and Contracting Factors: Biological and Clinical Research. P.M. Vanhoutte (ed.). Humana Press, Clifton, NJ, pp. 267–283, 1988.

22. DeMey J.G., Vanhoutte P.M.: Heterogeneous behavior of the canine arterial and venous wall: importance of the endothelium. Circ. Res. 51:439–447, 1982.

23. Dewey C.F. Jr., Bussolari S.R., Gimbrone M.A. Jr., Davies P.F.: The dynamic response of vascular endothelial cells to fluid shear stress. J. Biomech. Eng. 103:177–185, 1981.

24. D'Silva J., Fouché R.F.: The effect of changes in blood flow on the calibre of large arteries. J. Physiol. (Lond.) 150:23P–24P, 1960.

25. Diamond S.L., Eskin S.G., McIntire L.V.: Fluid flow stimulates tissue plasminogen activator secretion by cultured human endothelial cells. Science 243:1483–1485, 1989.

26. Drexler H., Zeiher A.M., Wollschläger H., Meinertz T., Just H., Bonzel T.: Flow-dependent coronary artery dilatation in humans. Circ. 80:466–474, 1989.

27. Duff F., Greenfield A.D.M., Shepherd J.T., Thompson I.D.: A quantitative study of the response to acetylcholine and histamine of the blood vessels of the human hand and forearm. J. Physiol. Lond. 120:160–170, 1953.

28. Dzau V.J., Roth T., Gonzales D.: Endothelium-derived prorenin-activating enzyme. J. Vasc. Med. Biol. 1:13–17, 1989.

29. Edwards B.S., Schwab T.R., Zimmerman R.S., Burnett J.C. Jr.: Increased transmural but not intra-atrial pressure stimulates atrial natriuretic peptide (ANP) release. Circulation 74:II 462, 1986.

30. Feletou M., Vanhoutte P.M.: Endothelium-dependent hyperpolarization of canine coronary smooth muscle. Br. J. Pharmacol. 93:515–524, 1988.

31. Feletou M., Hoeffner U., Vanhoutte P.M.: Endothelium-dependent relaxing factors do not affect the smooth muscle of portal-mesenteric veins. Blood Vessels 26:21–32, 1989.

32. Flavahan N.A., Shimokawa H., Vanhoutte P.M.: Pertussis toxin inhibits endothelium-dependent relaxations to certain agonists in porcine coronary arteries. J. Physiol. 408:549–560, 1989.

33. Förstermann U., Mülsch A., Böhme E., Busse R.: Stimulation of soluble guanylate cyclase by an acetylcholine-induced endothelium-derived factor from rabbit and canine arteries. Circ. Res. 58:531–538, 1986.

34. Förstermann U., Mügge A., Bode S.M., Frölich J.C.: Response of human coronary arteries to aggregating platelets: importance of endothelium-derived relaxing factor and prostanoids. Circ. Res. 63:306–312, 1988.

35. Freismuth M., Nees S., Böck M., Schutz W.: Binding of oubain to endothelial cells derived from various beds. Basic Res. Cardiol. 82:544–550, 1987.

36. Frangos J.A., Eskin S.G., McIntire L.V., Ives L.V.: Flow effects on prostacyclin production by cultured human endothelial cells. Science 227:1477–1479, 1985.

37. Furchgott R.F., Zawadzki J.V.: The obligatory role of endothelial cells in the relaxation of arterial smooth muscle by acetylcholine. Nature 299:373–376, 1980.

38. Furchgott R.F., Zawadzki J.V., Cherry P.P.: Role of endothelium in the vasodilator response to acetylcholine. In: Vasodilation. P.M. Vanhoutte, I. Leusen (eds.). Raven Press, New York, pp 59–66, 1981.

39. Furchgott R.F.: Role of endothelium in responses of vascular smooth muscle. Circ. Res. 53:557–573, 1983.

40. Furchgott R.F.: Studies on relaxation of rabbit aorta by sodium nitrite: the basis for the proposal that the acid-activatable inhibitory factor from bovine retractor penis is inorganic nitrite and the endothelium-derived relaxing factor is nitric oxide. In: Vanhoutte P.M. (ed.). Vasodilatation. Raven Press, New York, pp 401–414, 1988.

41. Garland C.J.: Endothelial cells and the electrical and mechanical responses of the rabbit coronary artery to 5-hydroxytryptamine. J. Pharmacol. Exp. Ther. 233:158–162, 1985.

42. Gerova M., Smiesko V., Gero J., Barta E.: Dilatation of conduit coronary artery induced by high blood flow. Physiol. Bohemoslov. 32:55–63, 1983.

43. Glover W.E., Marks R.M., Petrenas G.G.: Evidence for the release of a vascular relaxing factor from cultured human endothelial cells. In: Vasodilatation: Vascular Smooth Muscle, Peptides, Autonomic Nerves and Endothelium. P.M. Vanhoutte (ed.). Raven Press, New York, pp 421–426, 1988.

44. Glusa E., Markwardt F.: Influence of endothelium on the vasoconstrictor effect of dihydroergotamine in the isolated rat aorta. Arch. Int. Pharmacol. 296:66–75, 1988.

45. Gordon J.L., Martin W.: Endothelium-dependent relaxation of the pig aorta: relationship to stimulation of ^{86}Rb efflux from isolated endothelial cells. Br. J. Pharmacol. 79:531–541, 1983.

46. Gräser T., Leisner H., Tiedt N.: Absence of role of endothelium in the response of isolated porcine coronary arteries to acetylcholine. Cardiovasc. Res. 20:299–302, 1986.

47. Griffith T.M., Henderson A.H., Edwards D.H., Lewis M.J.: Isolated perfused rabbit coronary artery and aortic strip preparations: the role of endothelium-derived relaxant factor. J. Physiol. 351:13–24, 1984.

48. Griffith T.M., Edwards D.H., Lewis M.J., Newby A.C., Henderson A.H.: Production of endothelium-derived relaxant factor is dependent on oxidative phosphorylation and extracellular calcium. Cardiovasc. Res. 20:7–12, 1986.

49. Griffith T.M., Henderson A.H.: The nature of endothelium-derived relaxing factor. In: Relaxing and Contracting Factors: Biological and Clinical Research. P.M. Vanhoutte (ed.). Humana Press, Clifton, NJ, pp 41–64, 1988.

50. Gryglewski R.J., Bunting S., Moncada S., Flower R.J., Vane J.R.: Arterial walls are protected against deposition of platelet thrombosis by a substance (prostaglandin X), which they make from prostaglandin

endoperoxides. Prostaglandins 12:685–713, 1976.

51. Gryglewski R.J., Botting R.M., Vane J.R.: Mediators produced by the endothelial cell. Hypertension 12:503–548, 1988.

52. Gryglewski R.J., Palmer R.M.J., Moncada S.: Superoxide anion is involved in the breakdown of endothelium-derived vascular relaxing factor. Nature 320:454–456, 1986.

53. Hardebo J.E., Kahrström J., Owman C.: P_1- and P_2-purine receptors in brain circulation. Eur. J. Pharmacol. 144:343–352, 1987.

54. Harder D.R.: Pressure-induced myogenic activation of cat cerebral arteries is dependent on intact endothelium. Circ. Res. 60:102–107, 1987.

55. Hoeffner U., Feletou M., Flavahan N.A., Vanhoutte P.M.: Canine arteries release different endothelium-derived relaxing factors. Am. J. Physiol. 257:H330–H333, 1989.

56. Holtz J., Foerstermann U., Pohl U., Giesler M., Bassenge E.: Flow-dependent, endothelium-mediated dilatation of epicardial coronary arteries in conscious dogs: effects of cyclooxygenase inhibition. J. Cardiovasc. Pharmacol. 6:1161–1169, 1984.

57. Holzmann S.: Endothelium-induced relaxation by acetylcholine associated with larger rises in cyclic GMP in coronary arterial strips. J. Cyclic Nucl. Res. 8:409–419, 1982.

58. Houston D.S., Burnstock G., Vanhoutte P.M.: Different P_2-purinergic receptor subtypes on endothelium and smooth muscle in canine blood vessels. J. Pharmacol. Exp. Ther. 241:501–506, 1987.

59. Houston D.S., Shepherd J.T., Vanhoutte P.M.: Adenine nucleotides, serotonin and endothelium-dependent relaxations to platelets. Am. J. Physiol. 248:H389–H395, 1985.

60. Houston D.S., Shepherd J.T., Vanhoutte P.M.: Aggregating human platelets cause direct contraction and endothelium-dependent relaxation in isolated canine coronary arteries. J. Clin. Invest. 78:539–544, 1986.

61. Houston D.S., Vanhoutte P.M.: Comparison of serotonergic receptor subtypes on the smooth muscle and endothelium of the canine coronary artery. J. Pharmacol. Exp. Ther. 244:1–10, 1988.

62. Houston D.S., Vanhoutte P.M.: Platelets, endothelium and vasospasm. Circulation 72:728–734, 1985.

63. Ignarro L.J., Byrns R.E., Wood K.S.: Endothelium-dependent regulation of resting levels of cyclic GMP and cyclic AMP and tension in pulmonary arteries and veins. In: Relaxing and Contracting Factors: Biological and Clinical Research. P.M. Vanhoutte (ed.). Humana Press, Clifton, NJ, pp 309–332, 1988.

64. Ignarro L.J., Byrns R.E., Wood K.S.: Biochemical and pharmacological properties of endothelium-derived relaxing factor and its similarity to nitric oxide radical. In: Vasodilatation: Vascular Smooth Muscle, Peptides, Autonomic Nerves and Endothelium. P.M. Vanhoutte (ed.). Raven Press, New York, pp 427–436, 1988.

65. Inoue T., Tomoike H., Hisano K., Nakamura M.: Endothelium determines flow-dependent dilation of the epicardial coronary artery in dogs. J. Am. Coll. Cardiol. 11:187–191, 1988.

66. Jaffe E.A.: Endothelial cells and the biology of factor VIII. N. Engl. J. Med. 196:377–386, 1977.

67. Johnson P.C.: The myogenic response. In: Handbook of Physiology: The Cardiovascular System. Vascular Smooth Muscle, D.F. Bohr, A.P. Somlyo, H.V. Sparks, Jr., (eds.). American Physiological Society, Bethesda, MD, Sect. 2, Vol. II, Chapter 15, pp 409–442, 1980.

68. Kanamaru K., Waga S., Kojima T., Fujimoto K., Itoh H.: Endothelium-dependent relaxation of canine basilar arteries. Part 1: Difference between acetylcholine- and A23187-induced relaxation and involvement of lipoxygenase metabolite(s). Stroke 18:932–937, 1987.

69. Katusic Z.S., Shepherd J.T., Vanhoutte P.M.: Vasopressin causes endothelium-dependent relaxations of the canine basilar artery. Circ. Res. 55:575–579, 1984.

70. Katusic Z.S., Shepherd J.T., Vanhoutte P.M.: Oxytocin causes endothelium-dependent relaxations of canine basilar arteries by activating V_1-vasopressinergic receptors. J. Pharmacol. Exp. Ther. 236:166–170, 1986.

71. Katusic Z.S., Shepherd J.T., Vanhoutte P.M.: Endothelium-dependent contractions to stretch in canine basilar arteries. Am. J. Physiol. 252:H671–H673, 1987.

72. Katusic Z.S., Shepherd J.T., Vanhoutte P.M.: Potassium-induced endothelium-dependent rhythmic activity in the canine basilar artery. J. Cardiovasc. Pharmacol. 12:37–41, 1988.

73. Khayutin V.M., Melkumyants A.M., Ro-

goza A.N., Veselova E.S., Balashov, S.A., Nikolsky V.P.: Flow-induced control of arterial lumen. Acta Physiol. Hung. 68:241–251, 1986.

74. Komori K., Lorenz R.R., Vanhoutte P.M.: Nitric oxide, acetylcholine, and electrical and mechanical properties of arterial smooth muscle. Am. J. Physiol. 255:H207–H212, 1988.

75. Komori K., Suzuki H.: Heterogeneous distribution of muscarinic receptors in the rabbit saphenous artery. Br. J. Pharmacol. 92:657–664, 1987.

76. Kukovetz W.R., Holzmann S.: Cyclic GMP in endothelium-dependent relaxation of coronary smooth muscle by acetylcholine. In: Vascular Neuroeffector Mechanisms. J.A. Bevan, T. Godfraind, R.A. Maxwell, J.C. Stoclet, M. Worcel (eds.). Elsevier Science Publishers, Amsterdam, pp 115–121, 1985.

77. Kuriyama H., Suzuki H.: The effects of acetylcholine on the membrane and contractile properties of smooth muscle cells of the rabbit superior mesenteric artery. Br. J. Pharmacol. 64:493–501, 1978.

78. Langille B.L., Adamson S.L.: Relationship between blood flow direction and endothelial cell orientation at arterial branch sites in rabbits and mice. Circ. Res. 48:481–488, 1981.

79. Lansman J.B., Hallam T.J., Rink T.J.: Single stretch-activated ion channels in vascular endothelial cells as mechanotransducers? Nature 325:811–813, 1987.

80. Lorenz R.R., Sanchez-Ferrer C.F., Burnett J.C., Vanhoutte P.M.: Influence of endocardial-derived factor(s) on the release of atrial natriuretic factor (Abstract). FASEB Journal 2:1293, 1988.

81. Lückhoff A., Busse R., Winter I., Bassenge E.: Characterization of vascular relaxant factor released from cultured endothelial cells. Hypertension 9:295–303, 1987.

82. Lüscher T.F., Cooke J.P., Houston D.S., Neves R., Vanhoutte P.M.: Endothelium-dependent relaxations in human peripheral and renal arteries. Mayo Clin. Proc. 62:601–606, 1987.

83. Lüscher T.F., Diederich D., Siebenmann R., Lehmann K., Stulz P., von Segesser L., Yang Z., Turina M., Grädel E., Weber E., Bühler F.R.: Difference between endothelium-dependent relaxations in arterial and in venous coronary bypass grafts. N. Engl. J. Med. 319:462–467, 1988.

84. Lüscher T.F., Vanhoutte P.M.: The endothelium: Modulator of cardiovascular function. CRC Press, Inc., Boca Raton, FL, 1990.

85. Martin W., Villani G.M., Jothianandan D., Furchgott R.F.: Selective blockade of endothelium-dependent and glyceryl trinitrate-induced relaxation by hemoglobin and by methylene blue in the rabbit aorta. J. Pharmacol. Exp. Ther. 232:708–716, 1985.

86. Miller V.M., Vanhoutte P.M.: Endothelial alpha$_2$-adrenoceptors in canine pulmonary and systemic blood vessels. Eur. J. Pharmacol. 118:123–129, 1985.

87. Miller V.M., Vanhoutte P.M.: Endothelium-dependent responses in isolated blood vessels of lower vertebrates. Blood Vessels 23:225–235, 1986.

88. Miller V.M., Vanhoutte P.M.: Enhanced release of endothelium-derived factor(s) by chronic increases in blood flow. Am. J. Physiol. 255:H446–H451, 1988.

89. Moncada S., Gryglewski R., Bunting S., Vane J.R.: An enzyme-isolated from arteries transforms prostaglandin endoperoxidase to an unstable substance that inhibits platelet aggregation. Nature 263:663–665, 1976.

90. Moncada S., Vane J.R.: Pharmacology and endogenous roles of prostaglandin endoperoxides, thromboxane A$_2$, and prostacyclin. Pharmacol. Rev. 30:293–331, 1979.

91. Myers P.R., Guerra R., Bates J.N., Harrison D.G.: Comparitive studies on nitrosothiols: Similarities between EDRF and S-nitroso-1-cysteine (cysNO). FASEB J. (Abstract) 3:5336, 1989.

92. Nabel E.G., Ganz P., Selwyn A.P.: Atherosclerosis impairs flow-mediated dilatation in human coronary arteries. Circulation 78 (Suppl. II):474, 1988.

93. Nordoy A., Svensson B., Wiebe D., Hoak J.C.: Lipoprotein and the inhibitory effect of human endothelial cells on platelet function. Circ. Res. 43:527–534, 1978.

94. Olesen S.-P., Clapham D.E., Davies P.F.: Haemodynamic shear stress activates a K$^+$ current in vascular endothelial cells. Nature 331:168–170, 1988.

95. Palmer R.M.J., Ashton D.S., Moncada S.: Vascular endothelial cells synthesize nitric oxide from L-arginine. Nature 333:664–666, 1988.

96. Palmer R.M.J., Ferrige A.G., Moncada S.: Nitric oxide release accounts for the biological activity of endothelium-derived relaxing factor. Nature 327:524–526, 1987.

97. Pohl U., Holtz J., Busse R., Bassenge E.: Crucial role of endothelium in the vaso-

dilator response to increased flow in vivo. Hypertension 8:37–44, 1986a.

98. Pohl V., Busse R., Juan E., Bassenge E.: Pulsatile perfusion stimulates the release of endothelial autocoids. J. Appl. Cardiol. 1:215–235, 1986b.

99. Radomski M.W., Palmer R.M.J., Moncada S.: Endogenous nitric oxide inhibits human platelet adhesion to vascular endothelium. Lancet 2:1057–1058, 1987.

100. Rapoport R.M., Murad F.: Agonist-induced endothelium-dependent relaxation in rat thoracic aorta may be mediated through cGMP. Circ. Res. 52:352–357, 1983.

101. Rapoport R.M., Murad F.: Role of cyclic GMP in endothelium-dependent relaxation of vascular smooth muscle. In: Relaxing and Contracting Factors: Biological and Clinical Research. P.M. Vanhoutte (ed.). The Humana Press, Clifton, NJ, pp 219–239, 1988.

102. Rees D.D., Palmer R.M.J., Moncada S.: Role of endothelium-derived nitric oxide in the regulation of blood pressure. Proc. Natl. Acad. Sci. USA 86:3375–3378, 1989.

103. Ross R., Raines E.W., Bowen-Pope D.F.: The biology of platelet derived growth factor. Cell 46:155–169, 1986.

104. Rubanyi G.M., Lorenz R.R., Vanhoutte P.M.: Bioassay of endothelium-derived relaxing factor(s): inactivation by catecholamines. Am. J. Physiol. 249:H95–H101, 1985.

105. Rubanyi G.M., Vanhoutte P.M.: Hypoxia releases vasoconstrictor mediator(s) from the vascular endothelium. J. Physiol. (Lond.) 249:H95–H101, 1985.

106. Rubanyi G.M., Romero J.C., Vanhoutte P.M.: Flow-induced release of endothelium-derived relaxing factor. Am. J. Physiol. 250:H1145–H1149, 1986.

107. Rubanyi G.M., Vanhoutte P.M.: Superoxide anions and hyperoxia inactivate endothelium-derived relaxing factor. Am. J. Physiol. 250:H822–H827, 1986.

107a. Rubanyi G.M., Vanhoutte P.M.: Heterogeneity of endothelium-dependent responses to acetylcholine in canine blood vessels. Blood Vessels 25:75–81, 1988.

108. Rubanyi G.M., Harder D.R., Sanchez-Ferrer C., Kauser K., Stekiel W.J.: Pressure releases a transferable endothelial contractile factor in cat cerebral arteries. Circ. Res. 65:193–198, 1989.

109. Rubanyi G.M., Johns A., Harrison D.G., Wilcox D.: Evidence that EDRF may be identical with an S-nitrosothiol and not with free nitric oxide. Circulation 80 (Suppl II):II-281, 1989.

109a. Rubanyi G.M.: Pressure-induced endothelium-mediated contraction of canine carotid arteries. Am. J. Physiol. 255:H783–H788, 1988.

110. Shirahase H., Usui H., Fujiwara M.: Possible role endothelial thromboxane A_2 in the resting tone and contractile responses to acetylcholine and arachidonic acid in canine cerebral arteries. Cardiovasc. Pharmacol. 10:517–522, 1987.

111. Shimokawa H., Aarhus L.L., Vanhoutte P.M.: Porcine coronary arteries with regenerated endothelium have a reduced endothelium-dependent responsiveness to aggregating platelets and serotonin. Circ. Res. 61:256–270, 1987.

112. Shimokawa H., Aarhus L.L., Vanhoutte P.M.: Dietary Ω_3 polyunsaturated fatty acids augment endothelium-dependent relaxation to bradykinin in porcine coronary microvessels. Br. J. Pharmacol. 95:1191–1196, 1989.

113. Shimokawa H., Flavahan N.A., Vanhoutte P.M.: Natural course of the impairment of endothelium-dependent relaxations after balloon endothelium-removal in porcine coronary arteries. Circ. Res. 65:740–753, 1989.

114. Shimokawa H., Kim P., Vanhoutte P.M.: Endothelium-dependent relaxation to aggregating platelets in isolated basilar arteries of control and hypercholesterolemic pigs. Circ. Res. 63:604–612, 1988.

115. Shimokawa H., Lam J.Y.T., Chesebro J.H., Bowie E.J.W., Vanhoutte P.M.: Effects of dietary supplementation with cod-liver oil on endothelium-dependent responses in porcine coronary arteries. Circulation 76:898–905, 1987.

116. Shimokawa H., Vanhoutte P.M.: Impaired endothelium-dependent relaxation to aggregating platelets and related vasoactive substances in porcine coronary arteries in hypercholesterolemia and atherosclerosis. Circ. Res. 64:900–914, 1989.

117. Shimokawa H., Vanhoutte P.M.: Hypercholesterolemia causes generalized impairment of endothelium-dependent relaxation to aggregating platelets in porcine arteries. J. Am. Coll. Cardiol. 13(6):1402–1408, 1989.

118. Singer H.A., Peach M.J.: Calcium and endothelial-mediated vascular smooth muscle relaxation in rabbit aorta. Hypertension 4 (Suppl. II):19–25, 1982.

119. Sneddon J.M., Vane J.R.: Endothelium-

derived relaxing factor reduces platelet adhesion to bovine endothelial cells. Proc. Natl. Acad. Sci. USA 85:2800–2804, 1988.

120. Taylor S.G., Weston A.H.: Endothelium-derived hyperpolarizing factor: a new endogenous inhibitor from the vascular endothelium. Tr. Pharm. Sci. 9:272–274, 1988.

121. Tesfamariam B., Cohen R.A.: Inhibition of adrenergic vasoconstriction by endothelial cell shear stress. Circ. Res. 63:720–725, 1988.

122. Tomita T., Ezaki M., Miwa M., Nakamura K., Inoue Y.: Rapid and reversible inhibition by low density lipoprotein of the endothelium-dependent relaxation to hemostatic substances in porcine coronary arteries. Circ. Res. 66:18–27, 1990.

123. Vanhoutte P.M.: Inhibition by acetylcholine of adrenergic neurotransmission in vascular smooth muscle. Circ. Res. 34:317–326, 1974.

124. Vanhoutte P.M.: Endothelium and the control of vascular tissue. News Physiol. Sci. 2:18–22, 1987.

125. Vanhoutte P.M., Shimokawa H.: Endothelium-derived relaxing factor and coronary vasospasm. Circulation 80:1–9, 1989.

126. Vanhoutte P.M.: Endothelium and control of cardiovascular function. State of the art lecture. Hypertension 13:658–667, 1989.

127. Vidal-Ragout M.J., Romero J.C., Vanhoutte P.M.: Endothelium-derived relaxing factor inhibits renin release. Eur. J. Pharmacol. 149:401–402, 1988.

128. Weksler B.B., Ley C.W., Jaffe E.A.: Stimulation of endothelial cell prostacyclin production by thrombin, trypsin and the ionophore A 28187. J. Clin. Invest. 62:923–930, 1978.

129. Yanagisawa M., Kurihara H., Kimuri S., Mitsui Y., Kobayashi M., Watanabe T.X., Masaki T.: A novel potent vasoconstrictor peptide produced by vascular endothelial cells. Nature 332:411–415, 1988.

130. Young M.A., Vatner S.F.: Blood flow- and endothelium-mediated vasomotion of iliac arteries in conscious dogs. Circ. Res. 61 (Suppl. II):88–93, 1987.

131. Zimmerman G.A., McIntyre T.M., Prescott S.M.: Production of platelet-activating factor by human vascular endothelium cells: evidence for a requirement for specific agonists and modulation by prostacyclin. Circ. 72:718–727, 1985.

3

Cardiovascular Significance of Endothelin

Tomoh Masaki, Masashi Yanagisawa,
Katsutoshi Goto, Sadao Kimura, Yoh Takuwa

Introduction

It is generally accepted that the vascular endothelial cell plays an important role in regulation of vascular functions. Historically, the first report on the regulatory function of the endothelium on vascular tone was the discovery of the production of prostacyclin by the vascular wall by Moncada et al.[68] This was followed by the discovery of endothelium-derived relaxing factor (EDRF) by Furchgott and Zawadski.[20] The latter finding triggered tremendous research activities in this field. Several investigators have become aware that the endothelium produces not only vasodilator mediators, but a peptidic vasoconstrictor as well.[26,74] This substance had remained unknown until recently when endothelin was isolated and purified from the conditioned medium of cultured porcine aortic endothelial cells.[105]

Endothelin is the most potent vasoconstrictor peptide known in isolated vascular preparations and in intact animals.

Endothelin causes vasodilation at relatively low doses as well as vasoconstriction. Endothelin may affect blood pressure not only through vasoconstriction and vasodilation, but also through regulation of body fluid balance by its endocrinological or neurohumoral actions. Although more evidence will be necessary, endothelin is likely to play some role in the maintenance of basal vascular tone in cooperation with other vasoactive factors, for instance, EDRF or atrial natriuretic peptide (ANP). Impediment of this system is supposed to cause hypertensive state or vasospasm.

Analysis of human endothelin gene revealed the existence of three distinct isoforms of endothelin.[34] These three endothelins and closely related polypeptides of a snake venom, sarafotoxin S6b, S6a1, S6a2, and S6c reported subsequently,[96] constitute a family of evolutionarily related peptides (Fig. 1).

Recent progress in endothelin-research revealed that the actions of endothelins include not only the cardiovascular system, but also the central nervous sys-

Rubanyi G.M.: Cardiovascular Significance of Endothelium-Derived Vasoactive Factors, Futura Publishing Co., Inc., Mount Kisco, NY, © 1991.

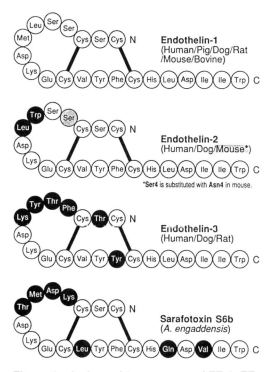

Figure 1: Amino acid sequences of ET-1, ET-2, ET-3, and sarafotoxin S6b.

tem, kidney, lung, and cell growth. In this chapter, we will summarize the cardiovascular functions of endothelin.

Chemistry and Structure-Activity Relation

Endothelin comprises 21 amino acid residues with free amino- and carboxyl-termini, including four cysteine residues at positions 1, 3, 11, 15. The native form of endothelin has two disulfide bonds, 1–15 and 3–11. The molecular weight of endothelin is estimated to be 2492 from the amino acid sequence.[105] It consists of a hydrophilic amino terminal half and a strongly hydrophobic C-terminal half. It includes two turns. Residues 1 through 4 constitute the first turn, while residues 8 through 11 constitute the second. The C-

terminal half of endothelin forms β-sheets.[100] Nuclear magnetic resonance analysis of the endothelin molecule reveals a snail-like structure with a helical tail.[72]

The nucleotide sequences of the three distinct endothelin-related genes[34] are highly conserved within the regions encoding the 21-residue endothelin, one of which matches exactly the sequence of endothelin initially isolated from the conditioned medium of cultured porcine aortic endothelial cells. This was named ET-1. The other two were designated as ET-2 and ET-3 (Fig. 1). Comparison of the biological activities among these three forms revealed that all of these forms were bioactive, but considerable differences exist in their pharmacological potency and profile. ET-2, with the replacement of Leu6 and Met7 in ET-1 by Trp6 and Leu7, is the most potent vasoconstrictor and pressor agent. ET-3, in which 6-amino-acid residues in the amino terminal side of ET-1 were replaced, was the least active as a vasoconstrictor/pressor agent. ET-1 is common at least in human, pig, dog, and rat, and probably all mammals. ET-3 is common in human and rat. Interestingly, the highly homologous sequence of endothelin was found in the sequence of sarafotoxin S6b, which is a constituent of the venom of the burrowing asp, *Atractaspis engaddensis*.[96]

Endothelial cells produce exclusively ET-1. ET-1 was isolated not only from the conditioned medium of cultured vascular endothelial cells, but also from porcine brain and spinal cord.[87,88] ET-3 was also isolated from porcine brain, but the relative amount of ET-3 to that of ET-1 was small.[87] In situ hybridization and immunocytochemical studies detected the ET-1 mRNA and ET-like immunoreactivity in the spinal cord, dorsal root ganglia, as well as the endothelial layer of some blood vessels.[21] Two distinct mRNAs of endothelins, probably corresponding to ET-1 and ET-3, were demonstrated in various tissues of rats.[50] Northern blot analysis demonstrated the existence of abundant ET-3 in the porcine hypophysis and intestine.[54]

The characteristic biological activities of these peptides are dependent on both the cyclic portion of the amino-terminal side of the peptide and hydrophobic residues of the carboxyl terminal tail.[40] Thus, opening the cysteine disulfide bonds of ET-1 in which a 1–15 disulfide bond existed and Cys3 and Cys11 were protected with acetamidomethyl groups, had no significant pressor response.[61] Two analogous peptides of ET-1 which comprised two disulfide bonds, other than native 1–15 and 3–11 bonds, also revealed far less biological activity than the native peptide.[46] According to the results of the vasoconstrictive activities of endothelin and endothelin analogues, potency of the vasoconstrictor and pressor response is likely to be regulated by the sequence heterogeneity at the amino terminal portion, especially at positions 4 through 7 which show the unordered secondary structure.[72,90] In addition, importance of the terminal amino group was also pointed out.[71]

On the other hand, the sequence of several amino acid residues at the carboxyl-terminus is essential for the characteristic features of the vasoconstriction.[40] Removal of the amino acid residues from the carboxyl-terminus attenuated the activity. Trp21 is especially essential. Progressive deletion of amino acid residues from the carboxyl terminal further decreased the activity. Both native ET-1 and the modified ET-1 in which D-Trp or Phe replaced Trp21 of ET-1 induced slowly developing and sustained vasoconstriction, while the truncated peptide ET-1,[1–20] carboxyamidomethylated ET-1 and Lys9-nicked ET-1 elicited a much more rapid contraction. Asp8, Glu10, and Phe14 are also essential for vasoconstriction. Replacement of Asp8 by Asn, Glu10 by Gln or Phe14 by Ala elicited significant decrease in the biological activity, indicating the importance of the carboxyl group of Asp8, Glu10, and Phe14 in the vasoconstrictor activity.[72] Additionally, the carboxyl-terminal hexapeptide ET-1[16–21] showed no contraction in rat aorta, but elicited constriction in guinea pig bronchus.[52] Receptor replacement experiments also demonstrated that ET-1[16–21] did not replace ET-1 bound to its receptor in cultured rat vascular smooth muscle cells.[31] These results suggest that the rigid conformation of the middle part of endothelin molecule is necessary for the binding of the peptide to the receptor of vascular smooth muscle, and carboxyl-terminal hydrophobic residues are important in exerting the characteristic (slowly developing) vascular contraction.

Synthesis and Secretion

Porcine prepro ET-1 contains 203 amino acids.[105] The sequence comprises a characteristic signal peptide sequence which is probably cleaved intracellularly. The resulting pro ET-1 must cross the internal membrane before secretion. Pre ET-1 is initially cleaved by endopeptidases specific for the paired dibasic residues to form an intermediate, 39 amino acid peptide, designated as big ET-1, by a putative endothelin converting enzyme. The big ET-1 is a vasocontrictor but about 140-fold less active than ET-1 in terms of molar potency in denuded porcine coronary arteries,[40] suggesting the significance of the conversion from big ET-1 to ET-1 in regulation of vascular tone. Chymotrypsin-treated big ET-1 produced endothelin-like contraction when applied to isolated rat aortic rings and a characteristic endothelin-like effect on blood pressure in vivo.[55] Big ET-1, the carboxyl terminal fragment of big ET-1 and ET-1 were secreted concomitantly into the medium from cultured bovine endothelial cells.[16,85] The same molar concentrations of big ET-1 and ET-1 were detected in human plasma.[66] These results corroborate the concept of conversion of big ET-1 to ET-1.

Expression of prepro ET-1 mRNA in

porcine endothelial cells is enhanced by various factors, including thrombin, phorbol ester, ionomycin, and TGF-β.[47,105] ET-1 is released from endothelial cells by TGF-β, TPA, ionomycin, angiotensin II, or arginine vasopressin.[17,47,105] Increased shear stress was also able to induce the prepro form of mRNA in cultured endothelial cells.[107] However, the mechanism of controlling the synthesis and release of endothelin remains to be determined.

Physiological and Pharmacological Properties

The primary action of endothelin administered exogenously to isolated vascular preparations is vasoconstriction. Relatively higher concentrations of endothelin are required to elicit vasoconstriction during intraluminal infusion into perfused blood vessel segments. At lower concentrations, endothelin elicits vasodilation in some (but not all) blood vessels. However, this response varies in the blood vessel employed. In contrast, in isolated vascular strips, endothelin causes only contraction. Exogenous endothelin injected intravenously into animals evokes significant changes in blood pressure. The response of blood pressure is complicated because of the multifunction of endothelin on the cardiovascular system. Although the function of endogenous endothelin still remains to be solved, evidence for the physiological role of endothelin in the maintenance of vascular tone has been accumulated.[83]

Contraction of Isolated Blood Vessels

Endothelin elicits concentration-dependent increases in tension in isolated vascular tissue. A characteristic feature of this contraction is that it develops slowly and it lasts long after endothelin has been removed. The estimated concentration at which ET-1 was 50% effective (EC_{50}) was around 10^{-9} M and 10^{-8} M in canine femoral vein and artery,[58] and about 10^{-10} M in porcine coronary artery.[105] The sensitivity varies according to the blood vessel and species employed. Veins are more sensitive to the peptide than arteries. Lymphatic vessels are also sensitive to endothelin, although they are not sensitive to norepinephrine.

The vasoconstrictor action of endothelin is potentiated by removal of the endothelium in some (but not all) vascular preparations. The maximum tension developed by endothelin is not affected by removal of the endothelium. This potentiation mechanism still remains unclear. However, it may be postulated that the inhibitory role of the endothelium results from the basal release of EDRF. In fact, EDRF was released from endothelium by endothelin itself in the rat mesenteric vascular bed.[13] Response of the endothelial cell to endothelin in releasing EDRF also depends on the blood vessel, but it seems to be weaker in arteries than in veins. For instance, the ability of the endothelium to release EDRF in response to endothelin is greater in canine saphenous vein than in the mesenteric artery, because removal of the endothelium enhanced the sensitivity only of venous smooth muscle to endothelin.[58]

Endothelin-induced vasodilation is not always ascribed to the release of EDRF from endothelial cells. EDRF was not released by endothelin in rabbit aorta despite the occurrence of potentiation of vasoconstriction by endothelin after removal of the endothelium.[75]

Vascular endothelial cells also release prostacyclin and thromboxane in response to endothelin.[15] Armstead et al. observed that vasodilation of cranial pial arterioles of piglets induced by endothelin was blocked by either indomethacin or aspirin in situ.[2] Endothelin produced concentration-dependent increases in cortical periarachnoid cerebrospinal fluid level of 6-keto prostaglandin $F_{1\alpha}$, prostaglandin E_2, prostaglandin $F_{2\alpha}$, and thromboxane B_2. The contraction of isolated rat aorta by endothelin was also reduced in the presence of either the cyclooxygenase inhibitor, indomethacin, or a thromboxane receptor antagonist.[15] These results imply that endothelin stimulates the arachidonic acid metabolic cascade as well. However, endothelin-induced vasoconstriction could not be ascribed solely to these prostanoids because endothelin was able to elicit constriction even in the presence of indomethacin.

Anoxia elicits endothelium-dependent vasoconstriction,[82] but endothelin is probably not the mediator of this phenomenon.[58]

Endothelin-induced vasoconstriction is not abolished by antagonists of known neurotransmitters or autoacoids. However, the sustained contraction of porcine coronary artery strips by endothelin was abolished by a dihydropyridine calcium antagonist or removal of calcium ion from the bathing medium. The dose-response curve for ET-1 was shifted to the right in a competitive manner in the presence of increasing concentrations of a dihydropyridine calcium antagonist.[38] The maximal responses in the presence and absence of the calcium antagonist were unaltered. Further, ET-1 markedly enhanced high-threshold calcium channel current on whole cell patches of porcine coronary artery. This inward calcium current was inhibited by nicardipine.[24] These results strongly suggested that endothelin stimulated the L-type calcium channel, causing sustained and long-lasting vasoconstriction. However, the results reported later by many investigators are not in agreement with the above hypothesis because responses of endothelin-induced vasoconstriction to dihydropyridine calcium antagonists varied depending on the blood ves-

sel and species.[53] In confirmation of the above results, calcium antagonists do not displace endothelin from its binding sites. Nicardipine, diltiazem, and verapamil did not displace iodine-labeled endothelin from the binding sites in membranes from chicken cardiac and cultured rat aortic smooth muscles.[67] Conversely, endothelin did not displace bound PN210–100 or ω-conotoxin.

Cellular Mechanism of Endothelin-Induced Vasoconstriction

Endothelin Receptor

It appears that endothelin acts on a specific receptor(s). Autoradiographic experiments with iodine-labeled endothelin demonstrated wide distribution of endothelin-receptors including the blood vessel wall, cardiac muscle, central nervous system, kidney cortex, lung, adrenal medulla, spleen, corneal endothelium and intestine.[45]

Expression of ET-1 receptor in vascular smooth muscle is regulated not only by ET-1 itself,[32] but also by angiotensin II. Either ET-1 or angiotensin II selectively down-regulated the number of ET-1 binding sites. This fact suggests interaction of these two agents on vascular smooth muscle.[32,81]

Multiple subtypes of endothelin-receptor were shown by several investigators. Receptor subtypes reported so far are able to be classified into two types; i.e., the "large type" which has higher affinity for ET-1 and ET-2 than for ET-3, and the "small type" which has higher affinity for ET-3 than for ET-1 or ET-2.[103] The former type may include a 53 kDa species in chicken cardiac membrane, 44 kDa species in rat lung membrane and probably a 70 kDa protein detected in rat aortic vascular smooth muscle A-10 cells have a single class of affinity site for ET-1.[98] A 58 kDa species in rat mesangial cells, and a 40 kDa protein in human placenta may also be included in this class.[91,102] The latter class comprises a 43 kDa or 34 kDa species in chicken cardiac membrane, 32 kDa in rat lung and a 34 kDa protein in rat mesangial cells.[92]

Intracellular Signaling System

Endothelin evokes an immediate and transient increase followed by sustained elevation in intracellular free calcium ion ($[Ca^{2+}]_i$) in cultured and isolated smooth muscles.[24,28] Rapid transient increase in intracellular free calcium by ET-1 is due to the release of calcium ion from a caffeine-sensitive calcium store probably via phosphatidyl inositol trisphosphate[57,97] (Fig. 2). Endothelin stimulates a concentration-de-pendent increase in calcium efflux, which is not blocked by calcium antagonists.[5,57] The increase in $[Ca^{2+}]_i$ is partially dependent on the presence of extracellular calcium. When cells were exposed to endothelin in calcium-free buffer, the initial transient increase was still observed, but no sustained increase could be detected. Nickel or lanthanum ions, or removal of external calcium completely blocked the sustained increase in intracellular free calcium but did not interfere with the mobilization of intracellular calcium.[98]

In isolated porcine coronary artery, the sustained increase of intracellular calcium in the presence of endothelin is blocked by a dihydropyridine calcium antagonist at a relatively high concentration.[24] However, in rat vascular smooth muscle, dihydropyridine calcium antagonists did not interfere with the increase in $[Ca^{2+}]_i$. These data strongly suggest the existence of a calcium channel which is ac-

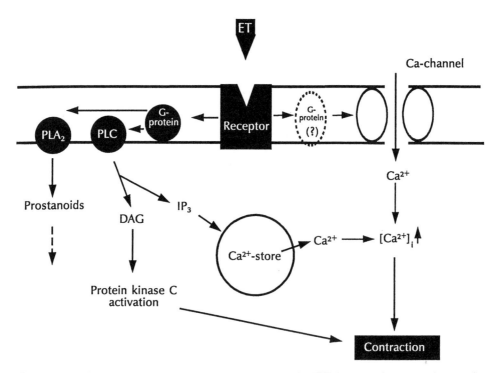

Figure 2: Cellular mechanism of action of endothelin (ET) in vascular smooth muscle.

tivated by endothelin, but not sensitive to the classical calcium channel antagonists (Fig. 2). Since two distinct types of calcium channels in their sensitivity to dihydropyridines have been identified in various vascular smooth muscles, the sustained increase in $[Ca^{2+}]_i$ may be mediated by at least two types of calcium channels. In A10 cells, oscillations in $[Ca^{2+}]_i$ were superimposed on the plateau phase. The oscillations in $[Ca^{2+}]_i$ could be inhibited by the addition of nifedipine or by the removal of extracellular Ca^{2+},[89] suggesting that calcium influx is partly due to the activation of L-type calcium channel.

It has been demonstrated by many investigators that endothelin activates phospholipase C which leads to the production of inositol-triphosphate and 1,2-diacylglycerol in vascular smooth muscle and other types of cells.[1,39,79] In rat aortic smooth muscle cell membrane, the endothelin-receptor is coupled to phospholipase C via a guanine nucleotide binding regulatory protein (G-protein) which is not the substrate of pertussis toxin[98] (Fig. 2). Analysis of the time course of increase in calcium and phosphatidyl inositol in isolated smooth muscle cell from porcine coronary artery[39] or in rings of canine coronary artery[77] revealed that this signalling system contributed to the initiation of vasoconstriction. The rapid production of inositol-1,4,5-trisphosphate is consistent with the time course for mobilization of intracellular free calcium ion from the caffeine-sensitive store in both isolated and cultured vascular smooth muscle cells. However, even after the complete depletion of calcium ion from caffeine-sensitive and histamine-sensitive intracellular calcium stores in calcium-free solution, a slow rising tonic contraction with no increase in intracellular free calcium ion was elicited by endothelin.[39,43] This apparent calcium-independent component was largely inhibited by the protein kinase C inhibitor H-7, but not by W-7, a calmodulin antagonist.[43] Indeed, sustained increase in ac-

tivation of protein kinase C by endothelin has been demonstrated.[48]

Although a G-protein which is sensitive to pertussis toxin was not involved in the activation of phospholipase C by endothelin, ADP-ribosylation of a 41 kDa protein of the membrane was observed in the presence of the toxin in rat aortic smooth muscle cell.[99] This protein may be responsible for the activation of phospholipase A_2 by endothelin (shown in cultured smooth muscle) because the endothelin-induced response of phospholipase A_2 was partially inhibited by pretreatment with pertussis toxin.[80] This response was independent of the activation of phospholipase C by endothelin, because pretreatment with phorbol ester inhibited endothelin-induced inositol phosphate formation, but potentiated endothelin-stimulated arachidonic acid release (80) (Fig. 2).

The mechanism of the opening of calcium channels by endothelin is unclear. Van Tentergham et al. have reported that endothelin opens a nonspecific cation channel permeable to Ca^{2+} and Mg^2, and the resulting membrane depolarization opens L-type Ca^{2+} channels.[100] However, membrane depolarization induced by endothelin in porcine coronary artery did not exceed 8.4 mV in the presence of the maximum concentration of the peptide.[38] The depolarization may not be the cause of activation of voltage-dependent calcium channels in this case. Depolarization can also be elicited by an increase in sodium conductance. However, it is unlikely that a sodium-channel is involved in the mechanism of endothelin-induced vasoconstriction, because the contractile responses to endothelin were unaffected by tetrodotoxin or by the removal of sodium chloride from the bathing solution.[7] Additionally, endothelin evoked intracellular alkalinization which was blocked by pretreatment with amiloride, suggesting a potential role of the sodium/proton antiport system.[56] Thus the mechanism by which endothelin evokes a sustained increase in cytosolic calcium ion concentration is still unclear.

Pressor and Depressor Actions in Intact Animals

Endothelin is by far the most powerful pressor agent. After a single intravenous bolus injection of a moderate dose of endothelin, systemic blood pressure first decreases transiently and subsequently rises rapidly in anesthetized, chemically denervated, as well as conscious, rats.[14,65] When the peptide is infused continuously, blood pressure is maintained at an elevated level for a long time.

The initial transient depressor response observed after intravenous bolus injection is probably due to the release of vasodilators (e.g., prostacyclin and EDRF).[103] ET-3 was more potent than ET-1 or ET-2 as a vasodilator.[103] This response to ET is dependent on the dose and vascular bed.[25,49,61-64] For instance, in squirrel monkey, the blood flow to the brain and stomach was not decreased by endothelin.[11]

The pressor response is chiefly attributable to direct vasoconstrictor actions. Threshold pressor dose of endothelin in intact rat or dog is between 10 and 100 ng/kg/min. At higher doses, mean blood pressure increases, cardiac output decreases and total peripheral resistance increases.[23,27,30,41,59] An apparently more potent effect of endothelin has been reported with bolus injections in conscious rats. However, these doses of the exogenously administered peptide are much higher than the normal plasma levels of endothelin (1–2 pg/mL)[66] observed in humans and in dogs.

A marked decrease in blood flow to the splanchnic organs was observed after endothelin administration. Decreases in vascular conductance of the pulmonary, renal, and mesenteric vascular beds were usually prominent. Vasoconstrictor responses to endothelin of isolated renal, pulmonary, and mesenteric arteries were also reported. Since microvessels, especially venules, are very sensitive to endothelin, exogenously administered endothelin was able to abolish blood flow in the microcirculation of the mesenteric vascular bed.

Endothelin has a profound effect on the kidney. Continuous intravenous infusion of endothelin into rats caused a marked reduction of renal blood flow, glomerular filtration rate (GFR), and sodium excretion. Additional infusion of atrial natriuretic peptide completely reversed the change in blood pressure and renal hemodynamics caused by endothelin, resulting in marked natriuresis.[30] Similar results were obtained in the isolated perfused kidney of the rabbit. In response to bolus injection of a relatively low dose of endothelin, renal plasma flow fell more than GFR, resulting in an increase in filtration fraction.[41] On the other hand, endothelin contracted mesangial cells[4] which can contribute to the fall in filtration coefficient and consequently GFR. Micropuncture experiments demonstrated elevation of hydrostatic pressure in glomerular capillaries because of greater elevation of efferent than afferent arteriolar resistance.[41] However, a renal vascular casting study revealed that endothelin primarily constricted the arcuate and interlobular arteries, as well as afferent arterioles.[30] Thus, the reason for the fall in GFR is still obscure. Endothelin also directly inhibits tubular sodium reabsorption.[18] Thus endothelin can influence blood pressure not only through vasoconstriction but also by controlling the water and electrolyte balance in the kidney (Fig. 3).

The possible involvement of additional factors other than vasoconstriction in cardiovascular responses to endothelin was suggested (Fig. 3). Although endothelin inhibits release of renin from juxtaglomerular cells,[78,95] it activates the renin-

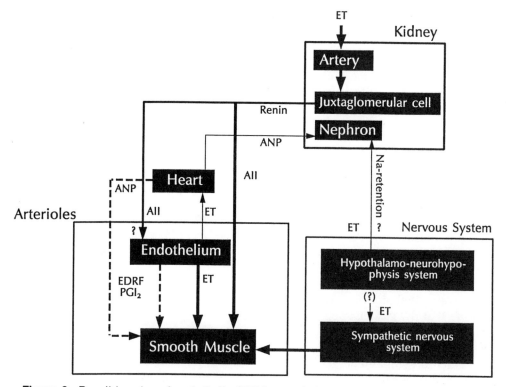

Figure 3: Possible roles of endothelin (ET) in regulation of blood pressure (vascular smooth muscle tone in arterioles).

angiotensin system in vivo, producing an increase in plasma renin activity.[59] Endothelin stimulates aldosterone production by zona glomerulose cells[70] and, in addition, endothelin acts at picomolar concentrations as a potent secretagogue of atrial natriuretic peptide (ANP) from cultured neonatal rat atrial cardiocytes[19] (Fig. 3). Intravenous infusion of endothelin caused significant and progressive increases in plasma levels of ANP.[30] Since synthetic rat ANP exerted a potent vasorelaxant activity in rabbit vascular preparations precontracted by synthetic porcine ET-1,[6] ANP release by endothelin may influence the basal tone of blood vessels and the balance of the body fluids (Fig. 3). These findings suggest that endothelin may act as a circulating hormone, although endothelin introduced into the blood stream was removed rapidly.[86] It was re-

cently demonstrated that endothelin is present in paraventricular and supraoptic nuclear neurons and their terminals in the neurohypophysis of the rat. Water deprivation depleted endothelin from these neurons. This result strongly suggests that endothelin may play some role in the hypothalamo-neurohypophysial system, and therefore may contribute to the central regulation of water balance and blood pressure (Fig. 3).

In this context, another important finding is that endothelin enhanced the responsiveness of α-adrenergic receptors to norepinephrine.[94] Interestingly, this enhancement was attenuated by nicardipine. Threshold concentration of endothelin also enhanced the contractile responses of aortic rings to clonidine.[22]

Endothelin-induced vasoconstriction was potentiated by hypoxia and hypercapnia in pithed rats.[51] The pressor effect was due to the combination of an increase in gastrointestinal vasoconstriction and an increase in cardiac output. In rats with moderate hypoxia, hypercapnia, and acidosis, endothelin-induced vasoconstriction of the mesenteric bed and an increase in cardiac contractility were potentiated.

Endothelin can influence blood pressure through the central nervous system. Cerebroventricularly administrated endothelin elicited an increase in mean arterial blood pressure in a dose-dependent manner.[77] Pretreatment with phenoxybenzamine significantly suppressed this pressor response. Recently, Knuepfer et al. demonstrated that the increase in rat hindquarter vascular resistance induced by endothelin was attenuated by pentolinium, suggesting that the vascular actions of endothelin are at least partly dependent on a mechanism involving nicotinic cholinergic receptors in sympathetic ganglia.[42] In addition, endothelin-induced bradycardia was also attenuated by pentolinum. These results show that endothelin-induced pressor responses may involve (at least in part) the sympathetic nervous system (Fig. 3).

Cardiac Actions: Positive Inotropic and Chronotropic Effects

Autoradiographic and biochemical experiments revealed the existence of high affinity endothelin binding sites in cardiac muscles.[45,104] Indeed, endothelin exerted positive inotropic effects in the electrically driven left atria of guinea pig and rat.[36,69,101] The endothelin-induced positive inotropic response was slowly developing and long-lasting. In spontaneously beating rat right atria, endothelin induced a positive inotropic effect but no chronotropic effects were observed.[101] However, Ishikawa et al. demonstrated positive

chrontropic response in the isolated right atria of the guinea pig.[37]

Endothelin-induced positive chronotropic response is due to direct effects of endothelin on cardiac muscle because it could not be antagonized by adrenergic, histaminergic, or serotonergic antagonists. It was antagonized by dihydropyridine calcium antagonists and low external calcium concentration. However, infusion of endothelin decreased cardiac output in conscious rats.[27,30] This decrease in cardiac output was not observed in chemically denervated rats,[27] indicating that the decrease in cardiac output may be due to some indirect neuroendocrine mechanism(s).

Endothelin evokes bradycardia in vivo, following the initial transient depressor response. Atropine reversed this bradycardiac response and caused a concomitant increase in arterial pressure, suggesting that the bradycardia was not mediated via baroreflex mechanisms.

Clinical Implications

Because of the characteristic biological properties of endothelin, it is hypothesized that this peptide family may play some role in the pathomechanism of hypertension and vasospasm.

Hypertension

The concentration of endothelin in human plasma is 1–2 pg/mL,[93] but higher values (around 5 pg/mL)[84] were also reported. Plasma levels of endothelin increase with age in healthy subjects, and they are significantly lower in females than in males (Miyauchi, unpublished data). Release of other endothelium-derived contractile factors (thromboxane A_2 and other prostanoids) also increase with age in rats.[44] These results strongly suggest that vascular tone is maintained and increases with age by these endothelium-derived contractile factors, especially by endothelin because of its long-lasting action. However, the plasma ET-1 level of normal subjects is not significantly lower than that of patients with essential hypertension. Circulating ET-1 may be the result of aging of endothelium. Locally secreted ET-1 may be involved in increases in vascular tone with age and may contribute to the development of hypertension. In addition, endothelin is produced in peripheral resistance vessels which are important in maintenance of blood pressure.

Vasospasm

Coronary vasospasm frequently occurs in patients with angina pectoris and myocardial infarction. In the presence of thrombus or plaque rupture especially, endothelin is likely to be released from the injured arterial wall. Although the dysfunction of endothelium in releasing EDRF was demonstrated as a potential cause of coronary vasospasm in dogs, production of endothelin may also contribute to the phenomenon, because coronary arteries (especially subepicardial branches) are very sensitive to endothelin.[10]

The mechanism of slowly developing *cerebral vasospasm* after subarachnoid hemorrhage is still unknown. When endothelin was administered intracisternally, a characteristic long-lasting vasoconstriction of cat and dog basilar arteries developed. However, the basilar arteries did not respond to endothelin when it was applied intra-arterially.[3,33,60] These observations suggest that endothelin cannot penetrate the blood-brain barrier, and that endothelin acts on intracerebral vessels from the adventitial side but not from the luminal side. Canine basilar arteries are very sensitive to endothelin when administrated

intracisternally. Therefore, endothelin may be a potential candidate to play a role in cerebral vasospasm after subarachnoid hemorrhage.

The plasma concentration of ET-1 in patients with acute myocardial infarction increased 24 hours after the onset of chest pain and then gradually declined over the next 4–6 days.[66] Similarly, the concentration of ET-1 increased significantly immediately after surgical operations and then returned to the preoperative levels within the next day.[29] In the state of cardiogenic shock, the plasma ET-1 level also increases.[9]

Analysis of the sequence of the ET-1 gene revealed the existence of the sequence for the acute phase of regulatory elements in the 5'-flanking region.[35] This fact implies that ET-1 production may be the consequence of acute phase reactions, at least in acute myocardial infarction, cardiogenic shock, or surgical interventions.

Recently, Coceani et al. demonstrated that endothelin induced long-lasting constriction of isolated *ductus arteriosus* from mature fetal lamb at low oxygen concentration at relatively low doses, suggesting a potential role of endothelin in the closure of the ductus arteriosus at birth.[12]

Conclusions

Endothelin is a potent vasoconstrictor peptide produced by vascular endothelial cells. Evidence accumulating thus far suggests an important role of endothelin in the cardiovascular system. We speculate that endothelin is produced in peripheral vascular beds and acts on the neighboring vascular smooth muscle. Production and release of endothelin may be regulated by other vasoactive factors. Endothelial dysfunction such as during atherosclerosis or aging can lead to augmented production and release of endothelin. Thus basal tone of peripheral resistance vessels is maintained and endothelial dysfunction can lead to the hypertensive state or vasospasm of the endothelin-sensitive vessels. Endothelin can affect blood pressure via a central mechanism including influence of water balance, renin-angiotensin system, or the autonomic nervous system. Recent progress in endothelin research revealed that endothelin may influence several bodily functions other than the cardiovascular system.

References

1. Araki S., Kawahara Y., Kariya K., Sunako M., Fukuzaki H., Takai Y.: Stimulation of phospholipase C-mediated hydrolysis of phosphoinositide by endothelin in cultured rabbit aortic smooth muscle cells. Biochem. Biophys. Res. Commun. 159:1072–1079, 1989.

2. Armstead W.M., Mirro R., Leffler C.V., Busija D.W.: Influence of endothelin on piglet cerebral microcirculation. Am. J. Physiol. 257:H707-H710, 1989.

3. Asano T., Ikezaki T., Suzuki Y., Satoh S., Shibuya M.: Endothelin and a production of cerebral vasospasm in dogs. Biochem. Biophys. Res. Commun. 59:1345–1351, 1989.

4. Bader K.F., Murray J.L., Breyer M.D., Takahashi K., Inagami T., Harris R.C.: Mesangial cells, glomerular and renal vascular responses to endothelin in rat kidney. J. Clin. Invest. 83:336–342, 1989.

5. Bialecki R.A., Izzo N.J.J., Colucci W.S.: Endothelin-1 increases intracellular calcium mobilization but not calcium uptake in rabbit vascular smooth muscle cells. Biochem. Biophys. Res. Commun. 164:474–479, 1989.

6. Bonhomme M.C., Cantin M., Garcia R.: Relaxing effect of atrial natriuretic factor on endothelin-precontracted vascular strips. Exp. Biol. Med. 191:309–315, 1989.

7. Bolges R., Carter D.V., von Grafenstein H., Halliday J., Knight D.E.: Ionic requirements of the endothelin response in aorta and portal vein. Circ. Res. 65:265–271, 1989.

8. Cairns H.S., Rogerson M.E., Fairbanks L.D., Neild G.H., Westwick J.: Endothelin induces an increase in renal vascular resistance and a fall in glomerular filtration rate in the rabbit isolated perfused kidney. Br. J. Pharmacol. 98:155–160, 1989.

9. Cernacek P., Stewart D.J.: Immunoreactive endothelin in human plasma: marked elevations in patients in cardiogenic shock. Biochem. Biophys. Res. Commun. 161:562–567, 1989.

10. Clozel J.P., Clozel M.: Effect of endothelin on the coronary vascular bed in open-chest dogs. Circ. Res. 65:1193–1200, 1989.

11. Clozel M., Clozel J.P.: Effects of endothelin on regional flows in squirrel monkeys. J. Pharmacol. Exp. Ther. 250:1125–1131, 1989.

12. Coceani F., Armstrong C., Kelsey L.: Endothelin is a potent constrictor of the lamb ductus arteriosus. Can. J. Physiol. Pharmacol. 67:902–904, 1989.

13. D'Orleans-Juste P., Finet M., DeNucci G., Vane J.R.: Pharmacology of endothelin-1 in isolated vessels: effect of nicardipine, methylene blue, hemoglobin, and gossypol. J. Cardiovasc. Pharmacol. 13 (Suppl. 5):S19-S22, 1989.

14. DeNucci G., Thomas R., D'Orleans-Juste P., Autunes E., Walder C., Warner T.D., Vane J.R.: Pressor effects of circulating endothelin are limited by its removal in the pulmonary circulation and by the release of prostacyclin and endothelium-derived relaxing factor. Proc. Natl. Acad. Sci. USA 85:9797–9800, 1988.

15. Eglen R.M., Michel A.D., Sharif N.A., Swank S.R., Whiting R.L.: The pharmacological properties of the peptide, endothelin. Br. J. Pharmacol. 97:1297–1307, 1989.

16. Emori T., Hirata Y., Ohta K., Shichiri M., Marumo F.: Secretory mechanism of immunoreactive endothelin in cultured bovine endothelial cells. Biochem. Biophys. Res. Commun. 160:93–100, 1989.

17. Emori T., Hirata Y., Ohta K., Shichiri M., Shimokado K., Marumo F.: Concomitant secretion of big endothelin and its C-terminal fragment from human and bovine

endothelial cells. Biochem. Biophys. Res. Commun. 162:217–223, 1989.

18. Ferrario R.G., Foulkes R., Salvati P., Patrons C.: Hemodynamic and tubular effects of endothelin and thromboxane in the isolated perfused rat kidney. Eur. J. Pharmacol. 171:127–134, 1989.

19. Fukuda Y., Hirata Y., Yoshimi H., Kojima T., Kobayashi Y., Yanagisawa M., Masaki T.: Endothelin is a potent secretagogue for atrial natriuretic peptide in cultured rat atriai myocytes. Biochem. Biophys. Res. Commun. 155:167–172, 1988.

20. Furchgott R.F., Zawadzki J.V.: The obligatory role of endothelial cells in the relaxation of arterial smooth muscle by acetylcholine. Nature (Lond) 288:373–376, 1980.

21. Giaid A., Gibson S.J., Ibrahim N.B.N., Legon S., Bloom S.R., Yanagisawa M., Masaki T., Varndell I.M., Polak J.M.: Endothelin-1, an endothelium-derived peptide is expressed in to neurons of the human spinal cord and dorsal root ganglia. Proc. Natl. Acad. Sci. USA 86:1989.

22. Godfraind T., Mennig D., Morel N., Wobo M.: Effect of endothelin-1 on calcium channel gating by agonists in vascular smooth muscle. J. Cardiovasc. Pharmacol. 13 (Suppl. 5):S112-S117, 1989.

23. Goetz K.L., Wang B.C., Madwed J.B., Zhu J.L., Leadley R.J. Jr.: Cardiovascular, renal, and endocrine responses to intravenous endothelin in conscious dogs. Am. J. Physiol. 255:R1064-R1068, 1988.

24. Goto K., Kasuya Y., Matsuki N., Takuwa Y., Kurihara H., Ishikawa T., Kimura S., Yanagisawa M., Masaki T.: Endothelin activates the dihydropyridine-sensitive, voltage-dependent Ca channel in vascular smooth muscle. Proc. Natl. Acad. Sci. USA 86:3915–3918, 1989.

25. Han S.P., Trapani A.J., Fok K.F., Westfall T.C., Knuepfer M.M.: Effects of endothelin on regional hemodynamics in conscious rats. Eur. J. Pharmacol. 159:303–305, 1989.

26. Hickey K.A., Rubanyi G., Paul R.F., Highsmith R.F: Characterization of a coronary vasoconstrictor produced by cultured endothelial cells. 248:C550-C556, 1985.

27. Hinojosa-Laborde C., Osborn J.W. Jr., Cowley A.W. Jr.: Hemodynamic effects of endothelin in conscious rats. Am. J. Physiol. 256:H1742-H1746, 1989.

28. Hirata Y., Fukuda Y., Yoshimi H., Emori T., Schichiri M., Marumo F.: Specific receptor for endothelin in cultured rat car-

diocytes. Biochem. Biophys. Res. Commun. 160(3):1438–1444, 1989.

29. Hirata Y., Itoh K., Ando K., Endo M., Marumo F.: Plasma endothelin levels during surgery. N. Engl. J. Med. 321:1686, 1989.

30. Hirata Y., Matsuoka H., Kimura K., Fukui K., Hayakawa H., Suzuki E., Sugimoto T., Sugimoto T., Yanagisawa M., Masaki T.: Renal vasoconstriction by the endothelial cell-derived peptide endothelin in spontaneously hypertensive rats. Circ. Res. 65:1370–1379, 1989.

31. Hirata Y., Yoshimi H., Emori T., Shichiri M., Marumo F., Watanabe T.X., Kumagae S., Naskajima K., Kimura T., Sakakibara S.: Receptor binding activity and cytosolic free calcium response by synthetic endothelin analogues in cultured rat vascular smooth muscle cells. Biochem. Biophys. Res. Commun. 160:228–234, 1989.

32. Hirata Y., Yoshimi H., Takaichi S., Yanagisawa M., Masaki T.: Binding and receptor down-regulation of a novel vasoconstrictor endothelin in cultured rat vascular smooth muscle cells. FEBS Lett. 239:13–17, 1988.

33. Ide K., Yamakawa K., Nakagomi T., Sasaki T., et al.: The role of endothelin in the pathogenesis of vasospasm following subarachnoid hemorrhage. Neurol. Res. 11(2):101–104, 1989.

34. Inoue A., Yanagisawa M., Kimura S., Kasuya Y., Miyauchi T., Goto K., Masaki T.: The human endothelin family: three structurally and pharmacological distinct isopeptides predicted by three separate genes. Proc. Natl. Acad. Sci. USA 86:2863–2867, 1989.

35. Inoue A., Yanagisawa M., Takuwa Y., Mitsui Y., Kobayashi M., Masaki T.: The human preproendothelin-1 gene: complete nucleotide sequence and regulation of expression. J. Biol. Chem. 264:14954–14959, 1989.

36. Ishikawa T., Yanagisawa M., Kimura S., Goto K., Masaki T.: Positive inotropic action of novel vasoconstrictor peptide endothelin on guinea pig atria. Am. J. Physiol. 255:H970-H973, 1988.

37. Ishikawa T., Yanagisawa M., Kimura S., Goto K., Masaki T.: Positive chronotropic effects of endothelin, a novel endothelium-derived vasoconstrictor peptide. Pflügers Arch. 413:108-11O, 1988.

38. Kasuya Y., Ishikawa T., Yanagisawa M., Kimura S., Goto K., Masaki T.: Mechanism of contraction to endothelin in the

isolated porcine coronary artery. Am. J. Physiol. 257(6, Pt. 2):H1828–H1835, 1989.

39. Kasuya Y., Takuwa Y., Yanagisawa M., Kimura S., Goto K., Masaki T.: Endothelin-1 induces vasoconstriction through two functionally distinct pathways in porcine coronary artery: contribution of phosphoinositide turnover. Biochem. Biophys. Res. Commun. 161:1049–1055, 1989.

40. Kimura S., Kasuya Y., Sawamura T., Shinmi 0., Sugita Y., Yanagisawa M., Goto K., Masaki T.: Structure-activity relationships of endothelin: importance of the C-terminal moiety. Biochem. Biophys. Res. Commun. 156:1182–1186, 1988.

41. King A.J., Brenner B.M., Anderson S.: Endothelin: a potent renal and systemic vasoconstrictor peptide. Am. J. Physiol 256:F1051-F1058, 1989.

42. Knuepfer M.M., Han S.P., Trapani A.J., Fok K.F., Westfall T.C.: Regional hemodynamic and baroreflex effects of endothelin in rats. Am. J. Physiol. 257:H918-H926, 1989.

43. Kodama M., Kanaide H., Abe S., Hirano K., Kai H., Nakamura M.: Endothelin-induced CA-independent contraction of the porcine coronary artery. Biochem. Biophys. Res. Commun. 160:1302–1308, 1989.

44. Koga T., Takata Y., Kobayashi K., Takishita S., Yamashita Y., Fujishima M.: Age and hypertension promote endothelium-dependent contractions to acetylcholine in the aorta of the rat. Hypertension 14:542–548, 1989.

45. Koseki C., Imai M., Hirata Y., Yanagisawa M., Masaki T.: Autoradiographic distribution in rat tissues of binding sites ior endothelin: a neuropeptide? Am. J. Physiol. 256:R858-R866, 1989.

46. Kumagaye S., Kuroda H., Nakajima K., Watanabe T.X., Kimura T., Masaki T., Sakakibara S.: Synthesis and disulfide structure determination of porcine endothelin: an endothelium-derived vasoconstricting peptide. Int. J. Pept. Protein Res. 32:519–526, 1988.

47. Kurihara H., Yoshizumi M., Sugiyama T., Takaku F., Yanagisawa M., Masaki T., Hamaoki M., Kato H., Yazaki Y.: Transforming growth factor-beta stimulates the expression of endothelin mRNA by vascular endothelial cells. Biochem. Biophys. Res. Commun. 159:1435–1440, 1989.

48. Lee T.S., Chao T., Hu K.Q., King G.L.: Endothelin stimulates a sustained 1,2-diacylglycerol increase and protein kinase C activation in bovine aortic smooth muscle

cells. Biochem. Biophys. Res. Commun. 162:381–386, 1989.

49. Lippton H., Goff J., Hyman A.: Effect of endothelin in the systemic and renal vascular beds in vivo. Eur. J. Pharmacol. 155:197–199, 1988.

50. MacCumber M.W., Ross C.A., Glaser B.M., Snyder S.H.: Endothelin: visualization of mENAs by in situ hybridization provides evidence for local action. Proc. Natl. Acad. Sci. USA 86:7285–7289, 1989.

51. MacLean M.R., Randall M.D., Hiley C.R.: Effect of moderate hypoxia, hypercapnea and acidosis on haemodynamic changes induced by endothelin-1 in the pithed rat. Br. J. Pharmacol. 98:1055–1065, 1989.

52. Maggi C.A., Giuliani S., Patacchini R., Santicioli P., Roberto P., Giachetti A., Meli A.: The C-terminal hexapeptide, endothelin-(16–21), discriminates between different endothelin receptors. Eur. J. Pharmacol. 166:121–122, 1989.

53. Masaki T., Yanagisawa M., Kimura S., Goto K.: Diversity of pharmacological responses of endothelin. Exp. Biol. Med., in press.

54. Matsumoto H., Syzyki N., Onda H., Fujino M.: Abundance of endothelin-3 in rat intestine, pituitary gland and brain. Biochem. Biophys. Res. Commun. 164:74–80, 1989.

55. McMahon E.G., Fok K.F., Moore W.M., Smith C.E., Siegel N.R., Trapani A.J.: In vitro and in vivo activity of chymotrypsin-activated big endothelin (porcine 1–40). Biochem. Biophys. Res. Commun. 161:406–413, 1989.

56. Meyer-Lehnert H., Wanning C., Pledel H.G., Backer A., Stelkens H., Krammer H.J.: Effects of endothelin on sodium transport mechanisms: potential role in cellular Ca^{2+} mobilization. Biochem. Biophys. Res. Commun. 163:458–465, 1989.

57. Miasiro N., Yamamoto H., Kanaide H., Nakamura M.: Does endothelin mobilize calcium from intracellular store sites in rat aortic vascular smooth muscle cells in primary culture? Biochem. Biophys. Res. Commun. 156:312–317, 1988.

58. Miller V.M., Komori K., Burnett J.C.J., Vanhoutte P.M.: Differential sensitivity to endothelin in canine arteries and veins. Am. J. Physiol. 257:H1127-H1131, 1989.

59. Miller W.L., Redfield M.M., Burnett J.C. Jr.: Integrated cardiac, renal and endocrine actions of endothelin. J. Clin. Invest. 83:317–320, 1989.

60. Mima T., Takakura K., Shigeno T., Yan-

agisawa M., Saito A., Goto K., Masaki T.: Endothelin induces sustained constriction of feline andcanine basilar arteries in vivo, when administrated cisternally but not intraarterially. Stroke, in press.

61. Minkes R.K., Coy D.H., Murphy W.A., McNamara D.B., Kadowitz P.J.: Effect of porcine and rat endothelin and an analog on blood pressure in the anesthetized cat. Eur. J. Pharmacol 164:571–575, 1989.

62. Minkes R.K., Kadowitz P.J.: Differential effects of rat endothelinon regional blood flow in the cat. Eur. J. Pharmacol. 165:161–164, 1989.

63. Minkes R.K., Kadowitz P.J.: Influence of endothelin on systemic arterial pressure and regional blood flow in the cats. Eur. J. Pharmacol. 163:163–166, 1989.

64. Minkes R.K., MacMillan L.A., Bellan J.A., Kerstein M.D., McNamara D.B., Kadowitz P.J.: Analysis of regional responses to endothelin in hindquarters vascular bed of cats. Am. J. Physiol. 256:H598-H602, 1989.

65. Miyauchi T., Ishikawa T., Tomobe Y., Yanagisawa M., Kimura S., Sugishita Y., Ito I., Goto K., Masaki T.: Characteristics of pressor response to endothelin in spontaneously hypertensive and Wistar Kyoto rats. Hypertension 14:427–434, 1989.

66. Miyauchi T., Yanagisawa M., Tomizawa T., Sugishita Y., Suzuki N., Fujino M., Ajisasaka R., Goto K., Masaki T.: Increased plasma concentrations of endothelin-1 and big endothelin-1 in acute myocardial infarction. Lancet ii:53–54, 1989.

67. Miyazaki H., Kondoh M., Watanabe H., Masuda Y., Murakami K., Takahashi M., Yanagisawa M., Kimura S., Goto K., Masaki T.: Affinity labelling of endothelin receptor and characterization of solubilized endothelin-endothelin receptor complex. Eur. J. Biochem. 187(1):125–129, 1990.

68. Moncada S., Gryglewski R., Bunting S., Vane J.R.: An enzyme isolated from arteries transforms prostaglandin endoperoxidase to an unstable substance that inhibits platelet aggregation. Nature (London) 263:663–665, 1976.

69. Moravec C.S., Reynolds E.E., Stewart R.W., Bond M.: Endothelin is a positive inotropic agent in human and rat heart in vitro. Biochem. Biophys. Res. Commun. 159:14–18, 1989.

70. Morishita R., Higaki J., Ogihara T.: Endothelin stimulates aldosterone biosynthesis by dispersed rabbit adreno-capsular cells. Biochem. Biophys. Res. Commun. 160:628–632, 1989.

71. Nakajima K., Kubo S., Kumagae S., Nishio H., Tsunemi M., Inui T., Kuroda H., Chino N., Watanabe T.X., Kimura T., Sakakibara S.: Structure-activity relationship of endothelin: importance of charged groups. Biochem. Biophys. Res. Commun. 163:424–429, 1989.

72. Nakajima K., Kumagae S., Nishio H., Kuroda H., Watanabe T.X., Kobayashi Y., Tamaoki H., Kimura T., Sakakibara S.: Synthesis of endothelin-1 analogues, endothelin-3, and sarafotoxin S6b: Structure-activity relationships. J. Cardiovasc. Pharmacol. 13 (Suppl. 5):S8-S12, 1989.

73. Nakio S., Sugiura M., Snajdar R. M., Boehm F. H., Inagami T.: Solubilization and identification of human placental endothelin receptor. Biochem. Biophys. Res. Commun. 164:205–211, 1989.

74. O'Brien R., Robbins R.J., McMurtry I.F.: Endothelial cells inculture produce a vasoconstrictor substance. J. Cell Physiol. 135:263–270, 1987.

75. Ohlstein E.H., Horohonich S., Hay D.W.P.: Cellular mechanisms of endothelin in rabbit aorta. J. Pharmacol. Exp. Ther. 250:548–555, 1989.

76. Ouchi Y., Kim S., Souza A.C., Iijima S., Hattori A., Orimo H., Yoshizumi M., Kurihara H., Yazaki Y.: Central effect of endothelin on blood pressure in conscious rats. Am. J. Physiol. 256:H1747–1751, 1989.

77. Pang D.C., Johns A., Patterson K., Parker-Botelho L.H., Rubanyi G.M.: Endothelin stimulates phosphatidylinositol hydrolysis and calcium uptake in isolated canine coronary arteries. J. Cardiovasc. Pharmacol. 13 (Suppl. 5):S75-S79, 1989.

78. Rakugi H., Nakamura M., Tabuchi Y., Nagano M., Mikami H., Ogihara T.: Endothelin stimulates the release of prostacyclin from rat mesenteric arteries. Biochem. Biophys. Res. Commun. 160:924–928, 1989.

79. Resink T.J., Scott-Burden T., Buhler F.R.: Activation of phospholipase A_2 by endothelin in cultured vascular smooth muscle cells. Biochem. Biophys. Res. Commun. 158:279–286, 1989.

80. Reynolds E.E., Mok L.L.S., Kurosawa S.: Phorbol ester dissociates endothelin-stimulated phosphoinositide hydrolysis and arachidonic acid release in vascular smooth muscle cells. Biochem. Biophys. Res. Commun. 160:868–873, 1989.

81. Roubert P., Gillard V., Plas P., Guillon J.M., Chabrier P.E., Braquet P.: Angiotensin II and phorbol-esters potently down-

regulate endothelin (ET-1) binding sites in vascular smooth muscle cells. Biochem. Biophys. Res. Commun. 164:809–815, 1989.

82. Rubanyi G.M., Vanhoutte P.M.: Hypoxia releases vasoconstrictor mediator(s) from the vascular endothelium. J. Physiol. (Lond.) 364:431–434, 1984.

83. Rubanyi G.M. Maintenance of "basal" vascular tone may represent a physiological role for endothelin (Editorial). J. Vasc. Med. Biol. 1:315–316, 1989.

84. Saito Y., Nakao K., Itoh H., Yamada T., Mukoyama M., Arai H., Hosoda K., Shirakami G., Suga S., Jougasaki M., Morichika S., Imura H.: Endothelin in human plasma and culture medium of aortic endothelial cells-detection and characterization with radioimmunoassay using monoclonal antibody. Biochem. Biophys. Res. Commun. 161:320–326, 1989.

85. Sawamura T., Kimura S., Shinmi 0., Sugita Y., Yanagisawa M., Masaki T.: Analysis of endothelin related peptides in cultured supernatant of pocine aortic endothelial cells: evidence for biosynthetic pathway of endothelin-1. Biochem. Biophys. Res. Commun. 162:1287–1294, 1989.

86. Shiba R., Yanagisawa M., Miyauchi T., Ishii Y., Kimura S., Uchiyama Y., Masaki T., Goto K.: Elimination of intravenously injected endothelin-1 irom the circulation of the rat. J. Cardiovasc. Pharmacol. 13 (Suppl. 5):S98-SlOl, 1989.

87. Shinmi O., Kimura S., Sawamura T., Sugita Y., Yoshizawa T., Uchiyama Y., Yanagisa A.W., Goto K., Masaki T., Kanazawa I.: Endothelin-3 is a novel neuropeptide: Isolation and sequence determination of endothelin-1 and endothelin-3 in porcine brains. Biochem. Biophys. Res. Commun. 164:587–593, 1989.

88. Shinmi O., Kimura S., Yoshizawa T., Sawamura T., Uchiyama Y., Sugita Y., Kanazawa I., Yanagisawa M., Goto K., Masaki T.: Presence of endothelin-1 in porcine spinal cord: isolation and sequence determination. Biochem. Biophys. Res. Commun. 340–346, 1989.

89. Simpson A.W.M., Ashley C.C.: Endothelin evoked Ca^{2+} transients and oscillations in A10 vascular smooth muscle cells. Biochem. Biophys. Res. Commun. 163:1223–1229, 1989.

90. Spinella M.J., Krystek S.R.J., Peapus D.H., Wallace P.A., Bruner C., Andersen T.T.: A proposed structural method of endothelin. Pept. Res. 2:286–291, 1989.

91. Sugiura M., Inagami T., Hare G.M.T., Johns J.A.: Endothelin action: inhibition by a protein kinase C inhibitor and involvement of phosphoinositols. Biochem. Biophys. Res. Commun. 158:170–176, 1989.

92. Sugiura M., Snajdar R.M., Schwartzberg M., Badr K.F., Inagami T.: Identification of two types of specific endothelin receptors in rat mesangial cell. Biochem. Biophys. Res. Commun. 162:1396–1401, 1989.

93. Suzuki N., Matsumoto H., Kitada C., Masaki T., Fujino M.: A sensitive sandwichenzyme immunoassay for human endothelin. J. Immunol. Meth. 118:245–250, 1989.

94. Tabuchi Y., Nakamura M., Rakugi H., Nagano M., Ogihara T.: Endothelin enhances adrenergic vasoconstriction in perfused rat mesenteric arteries. Biochem. Biophys. Res. Commun. 159:1304–1308, 1989.

95. Takagi M., Matsuoka H., Atarashi K., Yagi S.: Endothelin: a new inhibitor of renin release. Biochem. Biophys. Res. Commun. 157:1164–1168, 1988.

96. Takasaki C., Tamiya N., Bdolah A., Wolleberg Z., Kochva E.: Sarafotoxins S6: several isotoxins from *Atractaspis engaddensis* (burrowing asp) venom that affect the heart. Toxicon 26:543–548, 1988.

97. Takuwa N., Takuwa Y., Yanagisawa M., Yamashita K., Masaki T.: A novel vasoactive peptide endothelin stimulates mitogenesis through inositol lipid turnover in Swiss 3T3 iibroblasts. J. Biol. Chem. 264:7856–7861, 1989.

98. Takuwa Y., Kasuya Y., Takuwa N., Kudo M., Yanagisawa M., Goto K., Masaki T., Yamashita K.: Endothelin receptor is coupled to phospholipase C via a pertussis toxin-insensitive guanine nucleotide binding regulatory protein in vascular smooth muscle cells. J. Clin. Invest. 85(3):653–658, 1990.

99. Takuwa Y., Yanagisawa M., Takuwa N., Masaki T.: Endothelin, its diverse biological activities and mechanism of action. Prog. Growth Factor Res. in press.

100. Van Renterghem C., Vigne P., Barhanin J., Schmid-Alliana A., Frelin C., Lazdunski M.: Molecular mechanism of action of the vasoconstrictor peptide endothelin. Biochem. Biophys. Res. Commun. 157:977–985, 1988.

101. Vigne P., Lazdunski M., Frelin C.: The inotropic effect of endothelin-1 on rat atria involves hydrolysis of phosphatidylinositol. FEBS Lett. 249:143–146, 1989.

102. Wada K., Tabuchi H. Ohbe, R. Satoh M.,

Tachibana Y., Akiyama N., Hiraoka O. Asakura A., Miyamoto C., Fruichi Y.: Purification of an endothelin receptor from human placenta. Biochem. Biophys. Res. Commun. 167(1):251–257, 1990.

103. Warner T.D., Mitchell J.A., DeNucci G., Vane J.R.: Endothelin-1 and endothelin-3 release EDRF from isolated perfused arterial vessels of the rat and rabbit. J. Cardiovasc. Pharmacol. 13 (Suppl. 5):S85-S88, 1989.

104. Watanabe H., Miyazaki H., Kondoh M., Masuda Y., Kimura S., Yanagisawa M., Masaki T., Murakami K.: Two distinct types of endothelin receptors are present on chick cardiac membranes. Biochem. Biophys. Res. Commun. 161:1252–1259, 1989.

105. Yanagisawa M., Kurihara H., Kimura S., Tomobe Y., Kobayashi M., Mitsui Y., Yazaki Y., Goto K., Masaki T.: A novel potent vasoconstrictor peptide produced by vascular endothelial cells. Nature 332:411–415, 1988.

106. Yoshizawa T., Shinmi O., Giaid A., Yanagisawa M., Gibson J., Kimura S., Ochiyama Y., Polak J.M., Masaki T., Kanazawa I.: Endothelin is a novel peptide in the posterior pituitary system. Science, in press.

107. Yoshizumi M., Kurihara H., Sugiyama T., Takaku F., Yanagisawa M., Masaki T., Yazaki Y.: Hemodynamic shear stress stimulates endothelin production by cultured endothelial cells. Biochem. Biophys. Res. Commun. 161:859–864, 1989.

4

Neurohumoral Substances and the Endothelium

Jill Lincoln, V. Ralevic, Geoffrey Burnstock

Introduction

Since the first demonstration that acetylcholine (ACh) is able to cause vascular relaxation via the endothelium,[65] many other established and putative neurotransmitters have been shown to elicit effects on vascular tone through specific receptors located on endothelial cells. The growing list of substances for which a neurotransmitter role has been described has been matched and even superseded by the list of substances shown to have endothelium-dependent actions. These include adenosine 5'-triphosphate (ATP), adenosine diphosphate (ADP), substance P (SP), bradykinin (BK), serotonin (5-HT), vasopressin (VP), angiotensin II (AgII) and histamine.[2,63,99,146,186] For some of these substances, evidence of a pharmacological action has been complemented by autoradiographic demonstration of specific receptors on the endothelium.[181]

A change in vascular tone is the culmination of a chain of events initiated by endothelial receptor activation with subsequent release of endothelium-derived relaxing factors (EDRFs), constrictor factors (EDCFs), or prostaglandins. Many of the substances having receptors on the endothelium also have different subtypes of receptors on the underlying smooth muscle. Hence, the same vasoactive substance may produce opposite effects on vascular tone depending on the presence or absence of the endothelium, with a corresponding exposure of endothelial or smooth muscle receptors, respectively. An example of the opposite effects of ATP on the rat femoral artery, with and without endothelium, is shown in Figure 1. This emphasizes the importance of endothelial function and integrity and is likely to explain some of the abnormalities in vascular reactivity seen in various pathophysiological conditions.

Endothelium-dependent responses to many substances in a number of different vessels have been extensively documented, and progress in the characterization of EDRF favors its identity as nitric oxide.[64,90,144] Advances have also been made as to the origin of the neurohumoral substances acting via endothelial mechanisms, and several lines of evidence suggest that, at least for some of these, a

Rubanyi G.M.: Cardiovascular Significance of Endothelium-Derived Vasoactive Factors, Futura Publishing Co., Inc., Mount Kisco, NY, © 1991.

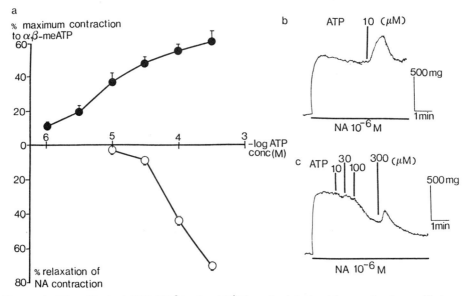

Figure 1: The effect of ATP (10^{-6} to 3×10^{-4}M) on isolated rat femoral artery with tone raised by 10^{-6}M NA (a) when endothelium is intact (open circles) or removed (closed circles) (n = 4). Vertical bars show SEM. Upper curve shows ATP-induced contractions in the absence of endothelium. Lower curve shows ATP-induced relaxations in the presence of endothelium. (b) Endothelium removed. Contraction to 10^{-5}M ATP. (c) Endothelium intact. Relaxations to ATP (10^{-5}M to 3×10^{-4}M). Used with permission from Kennedy C., Delbro D., Burnstock G.: Eur. J. Pharmacol. 107:161–168, 1985.

source is the endothelial cells themselves. The vascular geometry of blood vessels (except for capillaries and possibly precapillary arterioles) makes it unlikely that perivascular nerves are the source of substances acting on the endothelium, since these are located at the adventitial-medial border, posing several diffusion barriers between neurotransmitters and the luminal surface. Aggregating platelets in the vicinity of endothelial cells may be important in vascular pathophysiology as a readily releasable source of 5-HT and ATP. These are not, however, a source of substances such as ACh and SP, for which endothelium-dependent relaxations have also been demonstrated, since rapid breakdown processes keep the plasma concentrations of ACh and SP low.

In this chapter, we present evidence for the storage and release of neurohumoral substances from endothelial cells. This is drawn from electron microscopic immunocytochemical localization, with complementary release studies on isolated vascular beds and columns of cultured endothelial cells. The implications of endothelial cells as a source of releasable neurohumoral substances are considered in relation to changes occurring in endothelial integrity and local environment under different physiological and pathophysiological conditions.

Localization and Synthesis of Neurohumoral Substances in Endothelial Cells

In order to establish that endothelial cells themselves are a source in the intact organism of vasoactive substances that regulate vascular tone via endothelium-dependent responses, it is necessary to demonstrate that such substances are synthesized and/or localized in the endothelial cells. In the past, the metabolic activities of the endothelium in relation to vasoactive agents has been considered largely in terms of inactivation of those agents present in the circulation. Thus, it has been known for some time that endothelial cells, particularly in the pulmonary vascular bed, have a marked capacity to degrade and/or take up vasoactive substances such as 5-HT, NA, BK, and adenine nucleotides.[29,50,93,94,148,150,158,167,179] Less attention has been paid to the fate of vasoactive substances once they have been taken up or to whether endothelial cells have the ability to synthesize their own stores of vasoactive substances. The following section will summarize some of the evidence that has accumulated for the presence of stores of vasoactive substances and/or their synthesis in endothelial cells.

Neurohumoral Substances

Acetylcholine (ACh)

Since circulating levels of ACh and SP are low due to their rapid breakdown, it has often been assumed that the source of ACh and SP, which act on endothelial receptors to produce endothelium-dependent vasodilatation, is the perivascular nerves. However, in the case of ACh, it has been demonstrated that ACh released from perivascular nerves does not reach the endothelial cells.[37] This has brought into question whether the endothelium-dependent effect of ACh can contribute to the local regulation of blood flow via the endothelium in the intact organism.[194] The first evidence that ACh may be localized in endothelial cells in situ was provided in 1985 when Parnavelas et al. demonstrated that choline acetyltransferase (ChAT), the enzyme responsible for the synthesis of ACh, was present in the endothelial cells of small vessels and capillaries in the rat cortex.[145] Immunocytochemical staining combined with electron microscopy revealed immunoreactivity for ChAT within the cytoplasm of endothelial cells. Since this time ChAT has also been demonstrated in endothelial cells of the coronary artery.[125] In both coronary and brain vessels, not all the endothelial cells were immunoreactive for ChAT; positive staining was observed only in approximately 10% of the cells. This indicates that, even within the same vascular bed, endothelial cells may not be a homogeneous population. This was a finding observed repeatedly with immunocytochemical studies of other vasoactive agents in a variety of blood vessels (see the following sections entitled *Neurosecretory and Locally Produced Hormones* and *Biogenic Amines*). Endothelial cells in pial vessels have been shown to be able to take up choline.[76] In addition, by use of a combination of ultrastructural and neurochemical techniques, the ability of endothelial cells in microvessels of the rat cortex to synthesize ACh has been demonstrated.[3,70] Thus there is mounting evidence that endothelial cells can synthesize their own stores of ACh. By implication, the endothelium is likely to be the source of the ACh that acts on the endothelial receptors to produce local vasodilatation.

Substance P (SP)

The fact that there is a non-neuronal source of SP in intracranial and extracranial feline cephalic arteries was reported in 1985 by Norregaard and Moskowitz.[137] It was found that while sensory denervation of these vessels by trigeminal ganglionectomy caused a complete depletion of SP-immunoreactive nerve fibers, there was only a 55% reduction in the total vessel SP content. Immunocytochemical studies have revealed that about one in ten endothelial cells from the coronary (Fig. 2), mesenteric, and femoral arteries in the rat contain SP-immunoreactivity.[117,125] Recently, SP levels have been measured in isolated endothelium from human cerebral arteries and aorta.[115,116] Thus, endothelial cells provide an alternative source for SP. Since 45% of the SP is left in cerebral arteries after denervation, this provides an indication of the highly significant contribution that may be made by endothelial cells to the total supply of SP within the vascular wall.

SP has also been measured in freshly isolated bovine aortic endothelial cells. However, when primary cultures were prepared from the same source and assayed, SP was no longer detectable.[115] This emphasizes the caution that is needed in the extrapolation of data from cell culture studies to in vivo mechanisms, although endothelial cell cultures are undoubtedly an important tool in the investigation of endothelial cell biology. In the case of bovine cerebral microvessel endothelial cells, SP was still detectable in cultured cells, although at levels of only 20% of that of freshly isolated cells.[116] The fact that consecutive passages of these cells revealed similar levels of SP suggested that SP was being synthesized in the cells. Attempts to identify preprotachykinin mRNA, which encodes SP, within endothelial cells were unsuccessful.[115,116] However, the possibility was not excluded that the mRNA was unstable or subject to rapid turnover resulting in low levels of expression below the sensitivity of the technique used to identify it. If this were the case, then SP would be more readily detected than its corresponding mRNA.[116] The loss or reduction of SP in cultured endothelial cells could result from down-regulation of SP synthesis. Alternatively, since less than 10% of endothelial cells exhibit staining for SP,[117,125] it is possible that this subpopulation of endothelial cells may have been selected against by the culturing procedures.[116]

Adenosine Triphosphate (ATP)

There are high levels of ATP in the red blood cells and platelets within the circulation. Extracellular catabolism of circulating nucleotides has been shown to be an extremely rapid and efficient process.[151] Adenosine, produced by the breakdown of adenine nucleotides, is rapidly taken up by endothelial cells by a high-affinity transport process.[29,50,148,151] Breakdown of ATP and uptake of adenosine are two processes that have been recognized as important factors in the maintenance of circulatory homeostasis. If the only contribution by the endothelial cells was in limiting the vasoactive effects of ATP and adenosine, then it might be expected that, once inside the endothelial cells, adenosine would be catabolized further to inosine and hypoxanthine, which are not vasoactive. However, it has been shown that over 90% of the adenosine taken up by porcine aortic endothelial cells in culture is rapidly synthesized into adenine nucleotides, mainly ATP.[148]

In another study that used intact aortic and pulmonary endothelial cells in culture, no evidence could be found for adenosine deaminase activity which converts adenosine to inosine. Adenosine was phosphorylated by the action of adenosine kinase.[50] Adenosine deaminase activity has also been described as very low in coronary endothelial cells.[133,134] In a study of the isolated perfused porcine lung, a changing pattern of pulmonary intracellular adenosine metabolism has been described in which primarily synthesis of ATP occurs at low adenosine concentrations, whereas at high adenosine concentrations, adenosine is broken down via adenosine deaminase.[81,151] Thus, endothelial cells have a marked ability to synthesize their own

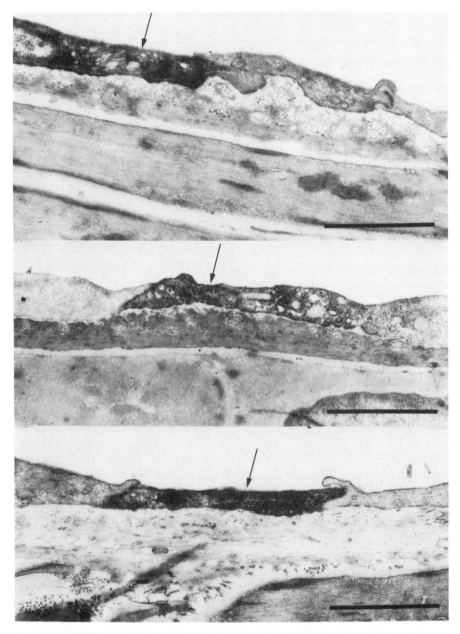

Figure 2: Ultrastructural localization of substance P-like immunoreactivity in endothelial cells of rat coronary arteries (arrows). Note that in all three examples the adjacent cells are completely unlabeled. Calibration bar = 1 μm. Used with permission from: Milner P., Ralevic V., Hopwood A.M., et al.: Experientia 45:121–125, 1989.

stores of ATP. Therefore, the potential for such endothelial stores to be involved in the local regulation of blood flow by causing vasodilatation under certain conditions needs to be considered in addition to the role of the endothelium in restricting vasodilatation by circulating stores of ATP.

Neurosecretory and Locally Produced Hormones

Vassopressin (VP)

The antidiuretic hormone VP is produced by neurosecretory neurons within the hypothalamo-neurohypophysial system. VP also has marked vasoactive properties, although the response depends on the vascular bed and whether the endothelium is intact.[99,100] It has been demonstrated by immunocytochemistry with electron microscopy that VP immunoreactivity can be localized in the cytoplasm of endothelial cells in the rat mesenteric and renal arteries (Fig. 3).[114] In both of these vessels, about 10% of the endothelial cells were immunoreactive for VP. Recently, a higher frequency of staining for VP has been observed in rat pulmonary endothelial cells. Approximately one in two pulmonary endothelial cells revealed VP immunoreactivity (Loesch, unpublished observations). This raises the possibility that variations in the stores of vasoactive substances between different vascular beds could provide differing mechanisms for the local regulation of blood flow within each bed. Little is known about the capacity of endothelial cells to synthesize VP from its amino acid precursors nor is it known if the hormone can be taken up from the circulation. VP in the circulation has been shown to be unaffected by passage through the lung.[92] Monolayer cultures of bovine brain endothelial cells have been used as an in vitro model of the blood-brain barrier. VP fragments can be transported across the endothelial monolayer. However, transport appears to occur by the paracellular route through tight junctional complexes rather than by a carrier-mediated transport mechanism.[190] It is possible that investigations of the endothelial content of VP in conditions which increase (diabetes mellitus) or decrease (diabetes insipidus) circulating levels of VP may shed some light on this question.

Angiotensin II (AgII)

Classically, the synthesis of AgII has been described as a series of biochemical reactions occurring within the circulation. This renin-angiotensin system functions as a systemic endocrine unit. Renin, secreted by the kidney, converts angiotensinogen, secreted by the liver, to angiotensin I (AgI). Angiotensin-converting enzyme (ACE) breaks AgI down to its vasoactive product, AgII.[53,101] This last reaction occurs primarily at the luminal surface of endothelial cells in the lung,[166,167] although ACE has been localized in endothelial cells of capillaries and large arteries and veins throughout the vasculature of the lung, liver, adrenal cortex, pancreas, kidney, and spleen.[23] Recently, however, an additional pathway for the synthesis of AgII has been described which takes place within the vascular wall.[53] Bovine aortic endothelial cells in culture express renin and are able to synthesize AgII intracellularly.[101,113] It has been demonstrated in our own laboratory that AgII-immunoreactivity can be localized within the cytoplasm of endothelial cells in the rat mesenteric artery (Fig. 3).[114]

It has been emphasized that the properties of endothelial cells at one site will not necessarily be shared with cells from another vascular location and that the local environment will influence these properties.[152] In this context, it is worth noting

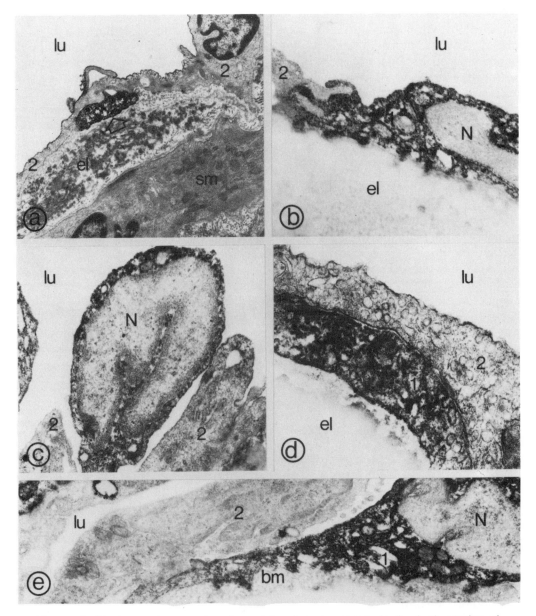

Figure 3: Electron micrographs of renal (a, c) and mesenteric (b, d, e) arteries of control rats labeled for VP, 5-HT, and AgII. (a) Renal artery. A fragment of artery showing the peripheral part of one VP-positive endothelial cell (arrow) and some VP-negative neighboring cells (2). el = elastic lamina; sm = smooth muscle; lu = lumen of the artery. x14,400. (b) Mesenteric artery. A fragment of artery displays the presence of the perinuclear region of one endothelial cell with positive cytoplasmic staining for VP (1). Note unlabeled cell nucleus (N). The neighboring endothelial cell is VP negative (2). x19,000. (c) Renal artery. A 5-HT-positive cell displays immunoprecipitate in perinuclear cytoplasm. The 5-HT-negative neighboring cells are also seen. x21,400. (d) Mesenteric artery. A highly magnified fragment of artery showing one 5-HT-positive endothelial cell (1) which is covered by a 5-HT-negative cell (2) at the luminal aspect of the artery. x78,500. (e) Mesenteric artery. An example of AgII-positive (1) and AgII-negative (2) endothelial cells. bm = basement membrane. x18,000. Used with permission from Lincoln J., Loesch A., Burnstock G.: Cell Tissue Res. 259:341–344, 1990.

that using the same immunocytochemical procedure that visualized AgII in the mesenteric artery, no AgII could be seen in the endothelium of the renal artery.[114] It has previously been suggested that the endothelial cells of the renal glomerulus may be unique among endothelia in that they are not immunoreactive to ACE.[166] In addition, renal proximal tubules were the only parenchymal cells of a variety of organs studied that did demonstrate immunoreactivity to ACE.[23] Efficient uptake of AgII from the circulation has been demonstrated in the systemic circulation, whereas circulating AgII is unaffected by passage through the lung.[9,92] Since both the lung and the kidney play a key role in the production of AgII in the circulation, this may influence the ability of the endothelium within these vascular beds to take up or store AgII.

Biogenic Amines

5-Hydroxytryptamine (Serotonin, 5-HT) and Norepinephrine (NA)

The biogenic amines 5-HT and NA are present both in the circulation and in perivascular nerves. The pulmonary circulation has a marked ability to clear 5-HT from the circulation and it has been shown that uptake rather than degradation to 5-hydroxyindoleacetic acid (5-HIAA) is the rate-limiting step in this process. 5-HT uptake was saturable, temperature-dependent and could be inhibited by cocaine.[93] The endothelial cells of the lung are also able to take up NA. The characteristics of endothelial NA uptake have been shown to be the same as those for uptake into noradrenergic nerves.[14] Isolated endothelial cells from bovine and porcine aorta and from rat adipose capillaries have also been demonstrated to have active, sodium-dependent uptake mechanisms for 5-

HT.[94,150,158] Once again it has been suggested that the ability of the endothelium to take up 5-HT may vary depending on the vascular bed from which the endothelial cells are derived. Further, the mechanism may be lost during culture.[150] The fate of 5-HT once it is taken up has been studied in less detail. In the case of the lung, 5-HT does not appear to be stored, but rather is metabolized rapidly.[93] However, immunocytochemical studies have demonstrated 5-HT within the endothelial cells from the rat mesenteric, renal (Fig. 3), femoral, and coronary arteries.[17,114,117] In the coronary vessels, the number of endothelial cells immunoreactive for 5-HT was greater, being approximately 50% as compared with 10% in the other vessels studied. This provides evidence that some endothelial cells do appear to be able to store 5-HT. Whether or not the endothelium has the capacity to synthesize 5-HT from tryptophan or 5-hydroxytryptophan has not been established.

Histamine

In the case of histamine, systhesis has been demonstrated within endothelial cells. Histidine decarboxylase, the enzyme responsible for the synthesis of histamine, is present in most tissues.[95] Some years ago it was proposed that histamine synthesized in the microcirculation was a primary mechanism in intrinsic microcirculatory regulation.[169,170] A major premise in this proposal was that the endothelium was the principal site of histamine synthesis in the vasculature. Evidence for this was obtained when histidine decarboxylase activity was measured separately in the endothelium and the intima-media of bovine aorta.[83,123] Enzyme activity of the endothelium was found to be about 15 times greater than that of the subjacent intima-media. Intracellular synthesis is not the only source of histamine in endothelial cells; some is derived from plasma.[56] Under normal conditions, the contribution that histidine decarboxylase activity makes to the endogenous levels of histamine within the endothelium appears to be minimal.[140] However, under a variety of different experimental conditions, including in animal models of vascular disease, intracellular histamine synthesis by the endothelial cells increases (see *Changes in Endothelial Neurohumoral Mechanisms in Disease*).

Thus, there is increasing evidence that endothelial cells contain a variety of vasoactive substances that can act via endothelial receptors to modify vascular tone. In certain cases it has been shown that the endothelium is capable of synthesizing its own stores. Many of these substances have already been established as neurohumoral or as neurosecretory hormones. With regard to the endothelial content of such vasoactive agents, there is considerable heterogeneity both within and between different vascular beds.

Release of Neurohumoral Agents from Endothelium

Evidence for the Release of Neurohumoral Agents from Endothelial Cells

In this section, evidence is presented for the release of neurohumoral agents (SP, ATP, 5-HT) from endothelial cells in response to stimulation with increased flow or hypoxia. The effect of an increase in flow rate on the release of substances from the perfused rat hindlimb, isolated perfused rat mesenteric arterial bed, and from columns of cultured human umbilical vein endothelial cells was examined. Hypoxia was used as a stimulus of endothelial cells of the Langendorff heart preparation and of cultured human umbilical vein endothelial

cells. In these studies, fractions of perfusate were collected before and during the induced change in local conditions and were assayed for SP/ATP/5-HT content.

The rat hindlimb was perfused via the aorta with physiological solution (Krebs-Ringer-BSA) with a regulated pulsatile flow ($8-11$ mL/min^{-1}). Fractions of the venous (vena cava) effluent were collected at basal flow and during two consecutive periods of increased flow (threefold increase over basal flow), and were assayed for SP content. This procedure was repeated in (a) rats treated as neonates with capsaicin to cause destruction of primary sensory neurons (the success of this treatment was confirmed by immunohistochemical analysis), and (b) rats in which the endothelium was removed by air treatment[156,157] between the two consecutive periods of increased flow.

Analysis of the fractions for SP content showed that increased flow evoked the release of SP from the preparation. After the recovery period, this release was again elicited by high flow in the control group of rats. Figure 4 shows that the release of SP on each of two consecutive periods of increased flow in capsaicin-treated rats was comparable with that from control rats. Following air treatment to remove endothelial cells, however, there was no significant release of SP. Since SP has been shown by electron microscopic immunocytochemistry to be present within endothelial cells of rat femoral arteries (see *Localization and Synthesis of Neurohumoral Substances in Endothelial Cells*), and since its concentration in plasma is very low, it is likely that the source of the SP released into the perfusate of the rat hindlimb during increased flow is the endothelium. The 5-HT and ATP content of the fractions were also assessed, however, the traces of blood present in the perfusate made it difficult to distinguish between endothelial cell and platelet origin for these substances.

Comparable experiments were performed using an increase in flow to evoke

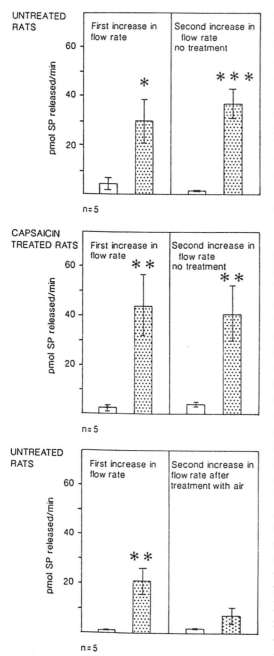

Figure 4: Levels of substance P (SP), expressed as picomoles per minute, released from rat hindlimb vasculature during two periods of low and high flow in untreated (top panel) and capsaicinized rats (middle panel) with no air treatment between the two periods of increased flow. Release from untreated rats with air treatment (to remove endothelium) between the two periods of increased flow (bottom panel). *p<0.05, ** p<0.02, *** p<0.001. Used with permission from Ralevic V., Milner P., Hudlická O., et al.: Circ. Res. 66(5):1178–1183, 1990.

the release of substances into the perfusate of the isolated fat mesenteric arterial bed. In this preparation, the release of SP during high flow was significant, although variable between preparations. In contrast, ATP was consistently released during each of the two consecutive periods of increased flow. To establish the source of the released ATP, sodium deoxycholate[22,155] was used to remove the endothelium between the two periods of high flow; following treatment in this way, there was no significant release of ATP, thus implicating the endothelium as its origin.

Parallel studies have recently been performed in this group to look at the release of substances from columns of human umbilical vein endothelial cells cultured on glass beads. These have the advantage that they represent a population uncontaminated by other cell types. In preliminary experiments, increased flow caused the release of ATP, SP, and ACh from endothelial cells on each of two consecutive occasions. It should be noted that while flow-induced ATP release was consistently observed in cultures prepared from different human umbilical vein specimens, the release of SP and ACh was not consistent. At this stage it is not possible to state whether the expression of SP and ACh in endothelial cells is particularly susceptible to loss during culture, or if the inconsistent release reflects differences in the original umbilical vein specimens from which the endothelial cells were derived. The loss of SP from bovine aortic endothelial cells following culture has been reported[115] and this is discussed in greater detail under the section *Neurohumoral Substances*.

Analysis of the cardiac effluent of the guinea pig Langendorff heart preparation

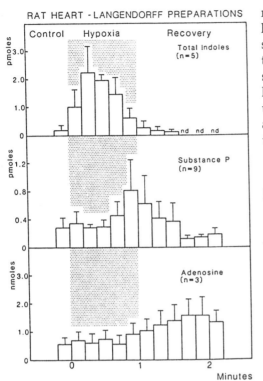

RAT HEART - LANGENDORFF PREPARATIONS

Figure 5: Release of total indoles (5-HT and its breakdown product, 5-hydroxyindole-acetic acid), substance P, and adenosine from Langendorff preparations of the rat heart subjected to a 1-minute period of hypoxia indicated by the shaded area. Both total indole and substance P levels are increased during the hypoxic period when vasodilatation occurs. Adenosine levels are increased after hypoxia, during the recovery period when perfusion pressure returns to basal levels. Results are expressed as pmoles or nmoles per fraction. Each fraction consists of the perfusate collected over a 12-second period. nd = not detectable.

has shown that hypoxic insult causes the release of ATP.[143] In the rat, 5-HT has also been shown to be released during the initial rapid phase of hypoxic vasodilatation (Fig. 5), allowing speculation that 5-HT may have a role, along with ATP, as an initiator of the hypoxic response.[17] Similarly, hypoxia causes the release of SP (Fig. 5) and ACh from the rat heart.[125] 5-HT, SP, and ACh have all been localized in coro-

nary endothelial cells, hence these cells are likely candidates as a source of the substances released in response to local fluctuations in oxygen content. Preliminary studies showing that hypoxia may also release ATP and SP from cultures of human umbilical vein endothelial cells (Milner et al., personal communication) would tend to support this hypothesis.

Physiological Implications

Flow

It is particularly appropriate that endothelial cells have been shown to release neurohumoral substances in response to increases in flow rate, since their position at the luminal surface of blood vessels makes these cells ideally suited to act as sensors and modulators of changes in blood flow. The sensitivity of the endothelium to flow is also illustrated by the morphological and cytoskeletal changes seen to occur in cultured endothelial cells subjected to shear stress.[55,60,102] In some vessels, endothelial cells are subject to pulsatile laminar blood flow, while in other regions, particularly arterial branch sites, blood flow is turbulent,[40,41,109] and it has been suggested that the latter is more important in the predilection of vessels for development of certain lesions such as those that occur in atherosclerosis.

The ability of endothelial cells to sense and regulate changes in blood flow has been demonstrated in large conduit arteries such as the canine femoral, saphenous, and coronary arteries. Removal of the endothelium abolished flow-dependent vasodilatation,[84,88,177] and this was shown to be blocked by methylene blue (via inhibition of cyclic guanosine monophosphate formation and possibly also direct inactivation of EDRF) and eicosatetraynoic acid (ETYA, a nonspecific inhibitor of arachidonate oxygenation), but not by indomethacin,[84,96,163] thus implicating a nonprostaglandin metabolite of arachidonic acid. Flow-dependent vasodilatation has also been demonstrated in resistance vessels[7,71] and is also believed to be mediated by EDRF.

How the endothelium senses and responds to hemodynamic changes is not known. Stretch-activated Ca^{2+} channels[110] and shear activated K^+ channels[139] have separately been implicated in the regulation of vascular tone. The demonstration that shear stress may influence the release of substances endogenous to the endothelium, for example, prostacyclin,[8,60] SP, and ATP, has far-reaching implications with respect to the role of the endothelium in vascular responses to change in flow. Since it has been shown that EDRF participates in this response,[71,163] it is plausible that a neurohumoral substance such as SP may be involved in a primary step of the mechanism. Increased flow may thus trigger an initial release of SP, which would subsequently act on endothelial cell receptors locally or downstream to cause vasodilatation via EDRF. While this mechanism is described in terms of SP, it is likely to be a general one applicable to any of the other neurhumoral substances localized within endothelial cells and capable of inducing EDRF production. For example, flow-induced endothelium-dependent relaxation of isolated canine femoral artery segments can be inhibited by pirenzipine, a muscarinic receptor antagonist, suggesting the involvement of locally produced muscarinic receptor agonists (ACh) in the response (Rubanyi, unpublished observation).

Although these studies have specifically addressed the role of endothelial cells in the regulation of blood vessel tone in response to changes in blood flow, it is important to remember that the situation in vivo is far more complex. The demonstration by Tesfamariam and Cohen of a modulatory effect of shear stress on adrenergic vasoconstriction emphasizes the fact that in practice vessel tone is the result of effects exerted at both the adventitia and the intima.[184]

Hypoxia

Changes in the partial pressure of oxygen (PO_2) of arterial blood are potent stimuli for changes in tone of a number of vascular beds, including the skeletal muscle, brain, coronary, pulmonary, and mesenteric beds.[6,46,104,105,173] While hypoxia generally causes relaxation of most vascular beds and isolated blood vessels, the response of the pulmonary vasculature[105,161] and of isolated canine and porcine coronary arteries[10,108,162,164] is vasoconstriction.

Several studies have indicated that the changes in vascular tone that occur above the "critical" mitochondrial PO_2 are due to the increased production and/or release of vasoactive mediators such as adenosine and prostaglandins[5,162] from smooth muscle cells or endothelial cells. It appears unlikely that vascular smooth muscle cells play a major role in the regulation of vascular tone under physiological fluctuations of PO_2 since an increased formation of adenosine and other purine derivatives in vascular smooth muscle occurs under anoxic conditions[192] and the involvement of prostaglandins in the adjustment of vascular tone during hypoxia or ischemia is controversial.[18] Despite this, since the early 1960s, adenosine has been regarded as the major agent responsible for the vasodilatation seen during hypoxic perfusion, based largely on evidence that it is a potent vasodilator and is released during hypoxia.[5,6,180] Several recent studies have failed to demonstrate a significant role for adenosine in maintaining blood flow or influencing coronary autoregulation during conditions of basal myocardial oxygen requirements or during exercise,[4,67,77,106] which suggests that other agents are likely to be involved in this response.

By virtue of their position at the luminal surface of blood vessels, endothelial cells are ideally situated to function as sensors of fluctuations in oxygen content of the blood. Busse et al. showed that intraluminal hypoxia of rat tail and femoral arteries elicited a dilatation that was abolished after removal of the endothelium, which they concluded was due to the production of endothelial prostaglandins.[19,20] In contrast, Needleman et al. reported that the coronary vasodilatation induced by ischemia or hypoxia is not accompanied by the release of prostaglandins,[132] while Coburn et al. (1986) concluded that hypoxic relaxations of the rabbit thoracic aorta, lamb ductus arteriosus, and canine femoral artery were not dependent on an intact endothelium.[35]

In the guinea pig heart, the EDRF inhibitor hydroquinone[126] significantly reduced the hypoxic response (and also the dilatation to the selective P_{2Y}-purinoceptor agonist 2-methylthioATP, but not the dilatation to adenosine).[85] Pohl and Busse[154] used segments of rabbit aorta and rabbit femoral artery (both virtually insensitive to prostaglandin I_2, thereby excluding this as a mediator of the responses of these vessels to hypoxia) to show that the EDRF inhibitors hemoglobin and dithiothreitol significantly inhibited the hypoxia-induced dilatation of these vessels, as well as those of assay segments perfused with the effluent from hypoxic donors.[154] They also showed that EDRF was released during hypoxia from cultured bovine aortic endothelial cells.

The precise oxygen content appears to be crucial to the production of EDRF since it has been demonstrated that, under anoxic conditions, EDRF is no longer produced[43] and that an endothelium-dependent constricting factor may be released.[164] There also appears to be heterogeneity in the effects of EDRF in different vessel segments since at low oxygen tension or in the presence of sodium cyanide (which inhibits cellular respiration) endothelium-dependent relaxations were markedly inhibited in the rabbit femoral artery, but not in the rabbit jugular vein.[195] Hyperoxia on the other hand, has been re-

ported to contribute to a more rapid inactivation of released EDRF.[21,165]

There is strong evidence that ATP and 5-HT, both of which are released from the guinea pig heart during hypoxia (see *Evidence for the Release of Neurohumoral Agents from Endothelial Cells*), have a role as mediators of the vasodilator response to hypoxia.[17,85] The localization of these substances within endothelial cells makes the endothelium a probable source of the released ATP and 5-HT, and both have been shown to elicit coronary relaxation via specific receptors on the endothelium.[36,85,182] Extracellular ATP has also been measured from endothelial and smooth muscle cells in culture[134,149] and from isolated hypoxic cardiomyocytes.[58] The electron microscopic immunocytochemical localization of SP and ChAT in coronary endothelial cells and the release of SP and ACh from the guinea pig heart during hypoxia suggests that these substances may also participate in the hypoxic response. While the release of adenosine from cardiac endothelial cells has been suggested to account for hypoxic coronary vasodilatation,[46] a separate study showed that adenosine is released after the onset of hypoxic relaxation[91] and a similar finding has been observed in this laboratory (Fig. 5). It has been suggested that ATP and 5-HT may be released in response to hypoxia from endothelial cells to initiate the vascular relaxation, while adenosine produces the longer lasting component of the response.[16,17,85]

pH

There have been relatively few studies on the effects of changes in pH on endothelial cells. There is evidence that Ca^{2+} binding to cell membranes is pH dependent,[72,73,107] thus perturbations affecting the pH near the microenvironment of the cell membrane would be expected to cause the release of bound Ca^{2+}. The exact relevance of this in relation to the Ca^{2+}

dependency of endothelial dilator mechanisms[118] and on the release of vasoactive substances from endothelial cells is difficult to assess.

The effect of hypercapnia (increased CO_2), which causes vasodilatation of some blood vessels, is likely to be dependent on changes in the hydrogen ion concentration, since molecular CO_2 and the bicarbonate ion HCO_3^- do not appear to have inherent vasoactivity.[153] This appears to be quite a specific mechanism, since neither $NaHCO_3$ nor lactic acid (used to change the blood pH) caused changes in cerebral blood flow.[78] While the role of endothelial cells has not been examined in these studies, a suggestion that they contribute to the response comes from the fact that they are prolific producers of prostaglandins[127] and the increase in cerebral blood flow due to hypercapnia has been shown to be attenuated by indomethacin.[153] Hypercapnic acidosis has also been shown to increase coronary blood flow, and the involvement of mediators other than adenosine was suggested by the fact that this was accompanied by only a transient increase in cardiac adenosine production.[46]

The effect of changes in pH on endothelial cells may be particularly relevant for the vascular supply to skeletal muscle, since exercise is often accompanied by a local build-up of lactic acid. In light of the demonstration that various vasoactive substances are contained within endothelial cells, a potential physiological role for these would exist in the regulation of blood flow if they were shown to be released in response to changes in extracellular pH.

Changes in Endothelial Neurohumoral Mechanisms in Disease

Pathological changes in endothelial cells have been implicated in a wide variety of cardiovascular disorders. These include atherosclerosis, diabetic vasculopathy, tumor angiogenesis, thrombosis, hypertension, coronary artery spasm, cerebral vasospasm, and migraine.[152] Many of these disorders will be reviewed in detail in other chapters of this book. As a general rule, endothelium-dependent responses to vasodilator substances are diminished and responses to vasconstrictor substances are increased in clinical and experimental models of hypertension,[193] atherosclerosis,[1,66,80,119,189,196,199] and diabetes.[45,52,59,142] Relative preservation of endothelium-independent vasodilatation has been reported in atherosclerosis[1,196,199] and in diabetes.[45,52,59,142] Alterations to endothelium-independent relaxation responses have been observed in hypertension, although it has been suggested that initially diminished vasodilatation responses are due to alterations in the modulatory function of endothelial cells rather than due to defects in the vascular smooth muscle.[111] The emphasis in this chapter has been on the profound implications that local storage and release of vasoactive substances from endothelial cells may have on the local control of blood flow. Clearly, alterations in such mechanisms could form an integral part of a disease process and it is this particular aspect that will primarily be discussed in relation to disease in the present section.

EDRF(s) and Prostaglandins

The production and release of EDRF and prostacyclin has been studied in vascular disease. The vascular wall produces increased levels of prostacyclin in renovascular hypertension of the rat.[44,128] The release of EDRF and prostacyclin into the vessel lumen induced by exogenous application of ACh is either normal or increased in the aorta from hypertensive rats depending on the model of hypertension studied.[120,191] In atherosclerosis, there are conflicting reports in the literature as to whether EDRF release is normal or decreased.[75,79,196] Overall prostacyclin bio-synthesis in vivo, as assessed by urinary metabolites, is increased in atherosclerosis.[54] In contrast, stimulated prostacyclin production by isolated vessels has been reported to be decreased in clinical and experimental atherosclerosis.[74,176] The discrepancy between these experiments has been reconciled by the suggestion that basal release of prostacyclin may be increased while stimulated release is decreased in atherosclerosis.[119]

Undoubtedly, studies of this type are needed in order to understand the processes involved in altered vascular responses in disease. However, it needs emphasizing that, in the intact organism, EDRF or prostacyclin production is stimulated by vasoactive agents acting on endothelial receptors to produce a response. Whether or not the stimuli for such production are functioning normally in these disorders has received little consideration. Clearly, if there are pathological changes to the endothelial content of vasoactive substances, then altered patterns of their release could provide a mechanism whereby endothelium-dependent responses are disrupted in vivo even when the capacity of the endothelial cells to produce EDRF or prostacyclin is unimpaired. Studies of vascular responses to exogenous application of drugs in vitro are unlikely to detect changes in this part of the overall sequence of events leading to endothelium-dependent vasodilatation. Whether levels of vasoactive agents in endothelial cells are altered in situ in vascular disease requires further examination, although there are already some indications in the literature that this may indeed be the case (see next section).

Endogenous Endothelial Vasoactive Agents

Angiotension II and ACE Inhibitors

The vascular wall renin-angiotensin system, of which endothelial cells are an integral part, has been investigated in two-kidney, one-clip hypertensive rats and in spontaneously hypertensive rats.[131,138] Renin activity was shown to increase in the lung, aorta, and mesenteric bed during the development of hypertension. Further, ACE activity was increased in the vascular wall but not in the plasma of these animals.[138] In addition, renin levels of adrenal and resistance vessels were markedly elevated in spontaneously hypertensive rats.[131] It has been suggested that alterations in the production of AgII by the vascular wall, including the endothelium, may play an important role in the maintenance of high blood pressure in animal models of hypertension. Since the renin-angiotensin system facilitates adrenergic neurotransmission, it has been thought that ACE inhibitors (e.g., captopril), used in the treatment of hypertension, act by interfering with sympathetic activity. However, in a study of spontaneously hypertensive rats, it was found that captopril was able to exert the same effect on cerebral blood flow autoregulation whether or not the hypertensive rats had been sympathetically denervated. Thus it was concluded that reduction in sympathetic nervous activity could not be the only mechanism by which the ACE inhibitor exerted its effects.[197] Inhibition of local synthesis of AgII within the vascular wall with resultant changes in the endothelial control of vascular tone could provide an alternative mechanism for the hypotensive action of captopril. For example, increased synthesis of bradykinin (BK) by ACE inhibitors can contribute to the vasodilator properties of these agents, since BK is a potent endothelium-dependent vasodilator that stimulates the release of PGI_2 and EDRFs from endothelial cells. Both renal and plasma renin activity have been reported to be suppressed in alloxan-diabetic rats,[32] while sensitivity to AgII is increased in diabetic rats[32] and in human diabetics with retinopathy.[33] The contribution of the vascular wall renin-angiotensin system to this process was not investigated in these studies.

Histamine

In the case of histamine, endogenous levels and synthesis have been measured in endothelial cells and vascular smooth muscle in a variety of experimental models of disease, including hypertension, hypercholesterolemia, and diabetes.[82,123,140,141] In all these disease situations, histamine synthesis was increased. In streptozotocin-induced diabetes, increased histamine synthesis together with decreased histamine catabolism resulted in higher intracellular histamine levels in the endothelium of the aorta.[140] Under normal conditions, histidine decarboxylase activity does not appear to be the factor determining endothelial histamine content. However, in diabetes, when the histamine pool expands, this is induced by increased activity of the synthetic enzyme within the vessel wall.[82] Treatment of diabetic rats with insulin reversed the alterations in the histamine pool induced by diabetes.[140]

Vasoconstrictor responses to histamine have been reported to be enhanced in atherosclerosis[97,189] and diseased human coronary arteries contain increased levels of histamine.[97] The number of adventitial mast cells has been observed to increase in a patient with coronary vasospasm.[57] It has therefore been speculated that local release of histamine from mast cells, together with inappropriate vasoconstrictor responses to histamine, could result in coronary vasospasm in atherosclerosis. However, since endothelial cells also contain increased histamine levels in experimental atherosclerosis,[82,123,141] their contribution to coronary artery spasm cannot be ignored. The expanded endothelial and vascular smooth muscle pool of histamine in experimental diabetes and atherosclerosis has been investigated in relation to the increased transmural permea-

bility that is found in these conditions. This was assessed by albumin accumulation in the aorta which increases in streptozotocin-diabetic rats and in hypercholesterolemic rabbits.[82,141] Treatment of diabetic rats with alpha-hydrazinohistidine (a histidine decarboxylase inhibitor) prevented the increased synthesis of histamine. Interestingly, alpha-hydrazinohistidine treatment also prevented the increased aortic albumin accumulation, despite the fact that the diabetic condition persisted.[82] Further, inhibition of histidine decarboxylase activity decreased aortic albumin accumulation and reduced the severity of atherosclerotic plaque formation in hypercholesterolamic rabbits.[141] Thus, manipulation of the endothelial stores of vasoactive substances may prove to be useful in the treatment of vascular disease.

5-HT, ACh, SP, and ATP

Apart from the finding that 5-HT uptake by the pulmonary vascular endothelium is reduced in spontaneously hypertensive rats,[160] little else is known of the changes that may occur in the neurohumoral substances 5-HT, ACh, SP, and ATP that have been shown to be localized and/or synthesized in the endothelium. In the section on *Release of Neurohumoral Agents from Endothelium* evidence has been presented which indicates that acute hypoxia and increased flow can stimulate the release of 5-HT, ACh, ATP, and SP from endothelial cells. Chronic hypobaric hypoxia causes pulmonary hypertension in rats.[89] Both hypoxia and shear stress of the endothelium have been implicated in the pathogenesis of atherosclerosis.[13,40,41,101] The synthesis of histamine has been shown to be increased in rat blood vessels subjected to shear stress.[42] Hypoxic conditions stimulate the synthesis of ACE by pulmonary endothelial cells in culture. However, the form of ACE induced by hypoxia appears to be inactive with regard to the conversion of AgI to AgII.[103] Whether prolonged exposure to hypoxia or shear stress depletes the endothelial supplies of ACh, SP, 5-HT, or ATP or if their turnover is increased is not known. Since EDRF production may be inhibited during hypoxia,[63,147] those agents which, on release from endothelial cells, produce endothelium-dependent vasodilatation via EDRF may no longer be effective under chronic hypoxic conditions. Chronically elevated blood flow has been shown to result in a pattern of increased endothelium-dependent relaxations in femoral arteries and veins.[124]

In a study of porcine coronary arteries with endothelium that had regenerated 4 weeks after its removal, impaired responses to 5-HT and aggregating platelets were reported. At this stage, responses to BK, adenosine diphosphate, and thrombin were unaltered.[174] After longer time intervals of 8 and 16 weeks, responses of previously denuded arteries with regenerated endothelium to all of these agents were depressed.[175] Thus, endothelium-dependent relaxations progressively worsen after regeneration of the endothelium. Evidence has been presented that dysfunction of a pertussin-toxin-sensitive G protein may account in part for dysfunction of chronically regenerated endothelium.[175] As has been discussed previously, the expression of neurohumoral substances within endothelial cells may be altered during culture. Similarly, endothelial cells that regenerate after injury or removal may not recover all their original vasoactive components. This has implications on the long-term control of vascular tone following the treatment of vascular disease by angioplastic techniques.

Trophic Roles of Neurohumoral Factors

Numerous studies have been undertaken to investigate trophic influences between perivascular nerves and vascular smooth muscle, between the endothelium and vascular smooth muscle, and between factors derived from the circulation and the vessel wall. Undoubtedly, many such influences exist and some of the factors involved have been isolated and characterized.[26,28,30,31,38,49,51,68,98,172] A review of these studies is beyond the scope of the present chapter, so discussion in this section will therefore be confined to the concept that neurohumoral substances together with other agents that have been shown to be present in the endothelium may exert trophic effects in addition to their known effects in the modification of vascular tone.

Trophic Interactions between Perivascular Nerves and Endothelial Cells

The discovery in recent years that autonomic nerves contain numerous neurohumoral substances in addition to the classic neurotransmitters, NA and ACh, has led to the consideration of their possible roles. In the case of many peptides, transmitter function has not been established and this has led to the view that one of their roles may be trophic.[15] In arteries and veins, the perivascular nerves are separated from endothelial cells by the vascular smooth muscle. Thus, the possibility of direct neural-endothelial interactions has received little investigation. Indications that such interactions may exist have been provided indirectly by studies of blood vessels following denervation, mechanical injury, and in disease.

Two to eight weeks after sympathetic and sensory denervation of the rabbit ear artery, endothelium-dependent relaxation responses have been shown to be depressed.[121] This was not due to any impairment of the ability of the smooth muscle to relax since the endothelium-independent response to sodium nitroprusside was unaffected by denervation at this stage. Conversely, 3 months after injury to the endothelium in the dog coronary artery, the density of both neuron-specific enolase- and SP-positive perivascular nerve fibers was found to increase.[183] It has been proposed that neuropeptide Y and NA in cerebral vascular nerves, which increase during the development of hypertension in rats, are involved in the protection against cerebral hemorrhage and disruption of the blood-brain barrier caused by hypertension.[48] An increase in the incidence of stroke and increased permeability of the blood-brain barrier occurs if cerebral vessels are sympathetically denervated before the development of hypertension.[129,168] Stress has long been associated with the development of atherosclerosis and its influence appears to be mediated through the sympathetic nervous system. Alterations in endothelial function is widely regarded as the critical initiating factor in atherogenesis.[34,159] The development of atherosclerosis in monkeys fed an atherogenic diet has been shown to be exacerbated by stress.[122] Further evidence of the involvement of the sympathetic nervous system in this process was obtained when it was shown that surgical sympathectomy or long-term adrenoceptor blockade prevented or reduced the induction of atherosclerosis by diet.[112,122]

It is still controversial whether or not capillaries are innervated.[47] Nerve terminal varicosities have been observed in close proximity (approximately 400 nm) to capillary endothelial cells, separated only by basal lamina material.[198] However, morphologlcal proximity alone does not establish that direct neural-endothelial interactions actually take place.

The mounting evidence that endothelial cells contain a wide variety of agents in situ, some of which have previously been thought to be present exclusively in perivascular nerves, has been presented earlier. This means that some neurohu-

moral substances can now be considered in terms of their trophic effects on endothelial cells, even when the spatial separation of nerves and the endothelium in blood vessels appears to make this unlikely.

Trophic Influences of Endothelial Vasoactive Factors

Under normal conditions, in the adult, the endothelial cells of both capillaries and larger blood vessels are a stable population with very low mitotic activity.[86] However, in pathological states such as hyperlipidemia, hypertension, and mechanical stress, the turnover of endothelial cells is increased.[174] Further, capillary growth, of which endothelial cell proliferation is the initiating process, can occur as a result of exercise, hypoxia, and low pH, all of which stimulate vasodilatation and increased blood flow.[86] The factors involved in capillary growth have been divided into two groups; (1) mechanical changes in flow and/or blood pressure, and (2) local chemical factors. It has been suggested that chemical factors may act by the changes they cause in blood flow or permeability rather than by trophic actions on the endothelial cells per se.[86] Damage of endothelial cells by increased shear stress has been implicated in the induction of endothelial cell proliferation in the aorta[27,62] and in culture.[69] It is interesting to note that there is evidence that increased flow, hypoxia, and low pH may all stimulate the release of a variety of substances from the endothelium (see *Release of Neurohumeral Agents from Endothelium*). Thus the two groups of factors considered above may, in fact, be interdependent. Increased blood flow, caused by whatever stimulus, but often mediated by an endothelium-dependent process, may in turn cause the further release of endothelial agents, which, under chronic conditions, could promote endothelial proliferation. Some of the vasoactive substances that have been localized in endothelial cells have been studied in relation to their effects on the growth of capillaries, endothelial cells, and vascular smooth muscle.

Some years ago, it was suggested that histamine was involved in vascular growth during injury,[171,178] although at the time there was little direct evidence for this[86] and it was discussed in the context of mast cells being the source of histamine. In one study, long-term application of histamine resulted in vascularization of the cornea.[200] Histamine has been shown to be mitogenic for bovine aortic endothelial cells.[38,39] Histamine reduces barrier function in endothelial cells in culture.[12] However, endothelial cell migration, which is an integral part of angiogenesis, was found to be inhibited by culturing bovine aortic endothelial cells in the presence of histamine.[11] 5-HT has been shown to induce angiogenesis in the chick chorioallantoic membrane[61] and in the rabbit cornea.[187] Further, 5-HT promotes endothelial cell barrier function and endothelial cell movement in cultures.[11,12] ATP had a small effect on vascular growth in the chick chorioallantoic membrane while ADP, the initial product of ATP degradation, was much more effective in inducing angiogenesis[61] and stimulated endothelial cell growth and migration in culture.[39,185] Long-term administration of adenosine, another breakdown product of ATP, increased capillary growth in skeletal muscle and in the heart.[87] In addition, chronic administration of dipyridamole, which inhibits adenosine uptake, has been shown to cause proliferation of capillary endothelium and increased capillary density in skeletal muscle and heart.[187,188] As has been stated, whether the trophic effects of adenosine and related nucleotides are due to their direct action or as a result of the increased blood flow that they induce is still a matter for debate.[86] ACh stimulates vascular growth in the cornea following long-term application.[200]

Several studies have also investigated the effects of various vasoactive substances on the growth of vascular smooth muscle in culture. Thus, histamine has been shown to increase the migration of bovine aortic smooth muscle cells in vitro.[11] Similarly, 5-HT stimulates the migration of bovine aortic smooth muscle cells in culture[11] and additionally has been reported to stimulate vascular smooth muscle cell mitogenesis.[135] DNA synthesis is stimulated in smooth muscle cells isolated from rat aorta when cultured in the presence of SP, while bombesin has no effect.[136] AgII causes the proliferation of human vascular smooth muscle cells in vitro, while VP either inhibited or stimulated vascular smooth muscle cell growth, depending on the serum used in the culture medium.[24,25]

Synthesis of histamine by endothelial cells and the activity of the vascular wall renin-angiotensin pathway are increased in hypertension (see *Changes in Endothelial Neurohumoral Mechanisms in Disease*), a pathological condition in which there is growth of both the endothelium and vascular smooth muscle. In addition, NA and neuropeptide Y increase in perivascular nerves in spontaneously hypertensive rats.[48] The release of locally synthesized AgII from rat mesenteric arteries has been shown to be mediated by β-adrenoceptors.[130] This raises the possibility of interactions between the release of transmitters and the release of vasoactive substances from endothelial cells. Clearly, the part that endogenous vasoactive substances within endothelial cells play in the growth of the endothelium and vascular smooth muscle requires further investigation, particularly with regard to the pathological changes that occur in vascular disease.

References

1. Aksulu H.E., Cellek S., Türker R.K.: Cholesterol feeding attenuates endothelium-dependent relaxation response to acetylcholine in the main pulmonary artery of chickens. Eur. J. Pharmacol. 129:397–400, 1986.
2. Angus J.A., Cocks T.M.: Endothelium-derived relaxing factor. Pharmacol. Ther. 41:303–351, 1989.
3. Arneric S.P., Honig M.A., Milner T.A., Greco S., Iadecola C., Reis D.J.: Neuronal and endothelial sites of acetylcholine synthesis and release associated with microvessels in rat cerebral cortex: ultrastructural and neurochemical studies. Brain Res. 454:11–30, 1988.
4. Bache R.J., Dai Z.-Z., Schwartz J.S., Homans D.C.: Role of adenosine in coronary vasodilation during exercise. Circ. Res. 62:846–853, 1988.
5. Berne R.M.: Cardiac nucleotides in hypoxia: possible role in regulation of coronary blood flow. Am. J. Physiol. 204:317–322, 1963.
6. Berne R.M., Gidday J.M., Hill H.E., Curnish R.R., Rubio R.: Adenosine in the local regulation of blood flow: some controversies. In: Topics and Perspectives in Adenosine Research, edited by E. Gerlach and B.F. Becker. Berlin: Springer-Verlag, 1987, pp 395–405.
7. Bevan J.A., Joyce E.H.: Flow-dependent dilation in myograph-mounted resistance artery segments. Blood Vessels 25:101–104, 1988.
8. Bhagyalakshmi A., Frangos J.A.: Mechanism of shear-induced prostacyclin production in endothelial cells. Biochem. Biophys. Res. Commun. 158:31–37, 1989.
9. Biron P., Meyer P., Panisset J.-C.: Removal of angiotensins from the systemic circulation. Can. J. Physiol. Pharmacol. 46:175–178, 1968.
10. Borda L.J., Shuchleib R., Henry P.D.: Hypoxic contraction of isolated canine coronary artery. Mediation by potassium-dependent exocytosis of norepinephrine. Circ. Res. 46:870–879, 1980.
11. Bottaro D., Shepro D., Peterson S., Hechtman H.B.: Serotonin, histamine, and norepinephrine mediation of endothelial and vascular smooth muscle cell movement. Am. J. Physiol. 248:C252–C257, 1985.
12. Bottaro D., Shepro D., Peterson S., Hechtman H.B.: Serotonin, norepinephrine, and histamine mediation of endothelial cell barrier function in vitro. J. Cell. Physiol. 128:189–194, 1986.
13. Boxen I.: Mechanisms of atherogenesis: endothelial hypoxia proposed as the major initiator. Med. Hypotheses 18:297–311, 1985.
14. Bryan L.J., O'Donnell S.R., Westwood N.N.: The uptake process for catecholamines in endothelial cells in rat perfused lungs is the same as uptake in noradrenergic neurones. Br. J. Pharmacol. 95:539P, 1988.
15. Burnstock G.: Neuropeptides as trophic factors. In: System Role of Regulatory Peptides, S.R. Bloom, J.M. Polak, E. Lindenlaub (eds.). Schattauer, New York, pp 423–441, 1982.
16. Burnstock G.: Local control of blood pressure by purines. Neurohumoral Control of Blood Vessel Tone. Proc. Int. Symp., Springfield, IL. Blood Vessels 24:156–160, 1986.
17. Burnstock G., Lincoln J., Fehér E., Hopwood A.M., Kirkpatrick K., Milner P., Ralevic V.: Serotonin is localized in endothelial cells of coronary arteries and released during hypoxia: a possible new mechanism for hypoxia-induced vasodilatation of the rat heart, Experientia 44:705–707, 1988.
18. Busse R., Bassenge E.: Endothelium and hypoxic responses. In: Vasodilator Mechanisms, P.M. Vanhoutte, S.F. Vatner (eds). Karger, Basel, pp 21–34, 1984.
19. Busse R., Förstermann U., Matsuda H., Pohl U.: The role of prostaglandins in the endothelium-mediated vasodilatory response to hypoxia. Pflügers Arch. 401:77–83, 1984.
20. Busse R., Pohl U., Kellner C., Klemm U.: Endothelial cells are involved in the vasodilatory response to hypoxia. Pflügers Arch. 397:78–80, 1983.
21. Busse R., Trogisch G., Bassenge E.: The role of endothelium in the control of vascular tone. Basic Res. Cardiol. 80:475–490, 1985.
22. Byfield R.A., Swayne G.T.G., Warner T.J.: A method for the study of endothelial derived relaxing factor (EDRF) in the isolated

perfused rat mesentery. Br. J. Pharmacol. Proc. (Suppl.) 88:438P, 1986.

23. Caldwell P.R.B., Seegal B.C., Hsu K.C., Das M., Soffer R.L.: Angiotensin-converting enzyme: vascular endothelial localization. Science 191:1050–1051, 1976.

24. Campbell-Boswell M., Robertson A.L.: Vasoactive peptides and human smooth muscle cell proliferation. Arteriosclerosis 1:66, 1981.

25. Campbell-Boswell M., Robertson A.L. Jr.: Effects of angiotensin II and vasopressin on human smooth muscle cells in vitro. Exp. Mol. Pathol. 35:265–276, 1981.

26. Campbell J.H., Campbell G.R.: Endothelial cell influences on vascular smooth muscle phenotype. Annu. Rev. Physiol. 48:295–306, 1986.

27. Caplan B.A., Schwartz C.J.; Increased endothelial cell turnover in areas of in vivo Evans blue uptake in the pig aorta. Atherosclerosis 17:401–417, 1973.

28. Castellot J.R. Jr., Rosenberg R.D., Karnovsky M.J.: Endothelium, heparin, and the regulation of vascular smooth muscle cell growth. In: Biology of Endothelial Cells, E.A. Jaffe (ed.). Martinus Nijhoff, Boston, pp 118–128, 1984.

29. Catravas J.D., Bassingthwaighte J.B., Sparks H.V. Jr.: Adenosine transport and uptake by cardiac and pulmonary endothelial cells. In: Endothelial Cells, Vol. I, U.S. Ryan (ed.). CRC Press, Boca Raton, FL, pp 65–82, 1988.

30. Chamley J.H., Campbell G.R.: Tissue culture: interaction between sympathetic nerves and vascular smooth muscle. In: Vascular Neuroeffector Mechanisms, J.A. Bevan, G. Burnstock, B. Johanson, et al. Proc. 2nd Int. Symp., Odense. Karger, Basel, pp 10–18, 1986.

31. Chamley J.H., Campbell G.R., Burnstock G.: Dedifferentiation, redifferentiation and bundle formation of smooth muscle in tissue culture: the influence of cell number and nerve fibers. J. Embryol. Exp. Morphol. 32:297–323, 1974.

32. Christlieb A.R.: Renin, angiotensin, and norepinephrine in alloxan diabetes. Diabetes 23:962–970, 1974.

33. Christlieb A.R., Janka H.-U., Kraus B., Gleason R.E., Icasas-Cabral E.A., Aiello L.M., Cabral B.V., Solan A.: Vascular reactivity to angiotensin II and to norepinephrine in diabetic subjects. Diabetes 25:268–274, 1976.

34. Clarkson T.B., Weingard K.W., Kaplan J.R., and Adams M.R.: Mechanisms in atherogenesis. Circulation 75(Suppl. I):1–20, 1987.

35. Coburn R.F., Eppinger R., Scott D.P.: Oxygen-dependent tension in vascular smooth muscle. Does the endothelilim play a role? Circ. Res. 3:341–347, 1986.

36. Cohen R.A., Shepherd J.T., Vanhoutte P.M.: 5-Hydroxytryptamine can mediate endothelium-dependent relaxations of coronary arteries. Am. J. Physiol. 245:H1077–H1080, 1983.

37. Cohen R.A., Shepherd J.T., Vanhoutte P.M.: Neurogenic cholinergic prejunctional inhibition of sympathetic β-adrenergic relaxation in the canine coronary artery. J. Pharmacol. Exp. Ther. 229:417–421, 1984.

38. D'Amore P.A., Braunhut S.J.: Stimulatory and inhibitory factors in vascular growth control. In: Endothelial Cells, Vol II, U.S. Ryan (ed.). CRC Press, Boca Raton, FL, pp 13–36, 1988.

39. D'Amore P.A., Shepro D.: Stimulation of growth and calcium influx in cultured bovine aortic endothelial cells by platelets and vasoactive substances. J. Cell Physiol. 92:177–184, 1977.

40. Davies P.F.: Endothelial cells, hemodynamic forces, and the localization of atherosclerosis, In: Endothelial Cells, vol. II, U.S. Ryan (ed.). CRC Press, Boca Raton, FL, pp 123–138, 1988.

41. Davies P.F., Remuzzi A., Gordon E.L., Forbes Davey C. Jr., Gimbrone M.A. Jr.: Turbulent fluid shear stress induces vascular endothelial turnover in vitro. Proc. Natl. Acad. Sci. USA 83:2114–2117, 1986.

42. De Forrest J.M., Hollis T.M.: Shear stress and aortic histamine synthesis. Am. J. Physiol. 234:H701–H705, 1978.

43. De Mey J.G., Vanhoutte P.M.: Anoxia and endothelium-dependent reactivity of the canine femoral artery. J. Physiol. Lond. 335:65–74, 1983.

44. Desjardins-Giasson S., Gutkowska J., Garcia R., Genest J.: Release of prostaglandins by the mesenteric artery of the renovascular and spontaneously hypertensive rat. Can. J. Physiol. Pharmacol. 62:89–93, 1984.

45. De Tejada I.S., Goldstein I., Azadzoi K., Krane R.J., Cohen R.A.: Impaired neurogenic and endothelium-mediated relaxation of penile smooth muscle from diabetic men with impotence. N. Engl. J. Med. 320:1025–1030, 1989.

46. Deussen A., Möser G., Schrader J.: Contribution of coronary endothelial cells to

cardiac adenosine production. Pflügers Arch. 406:608–614, 1986.

47. Dhital K.K., Burnstock G.: Adrenergic and non-adrenergic neural control of the arterial wall. In: Diseases of the Arterial Wall, J.P. Camilleri, C.L. Berry, J.N. Fiessinger, et al. (eds.). Springer, London, pp 97–126, 1989.

48. Dhital K.K., Gerli R., Lincoln J., Milner P., Tanganelli P., Weber G., Fruschelli C., Burnstock G.: Increased density of perivascular nerves to the major cerebral vessels of the spontaneously hypertensive rat: differential changes in noradrenaline and neuropeptide Y during development. Brain Res. 444:33–45, 1988.

49. Di Corleto P.E., Fox P.L.: Growth factor production by endothelial cells. In: Endothelial Cells, Vol II, U.S. Ryan (ed.). CRC Press, Boca Raton, FL, pp 51–61, 1988.

50. Dieterle Y., Ody C., Ehrensberger A., Stalder H., Junod A.F.: Metabolism and uptake of adenosine triphosphate and adenosine by porcine aortic and pulmonary endothelial cells and fibroblasts in culture. Circ. Res. 42:869–876, 1978.

51. Dimitriadou V., Aubineau P., Taxi J., Seylaz J.: Ultrastructural changes in the cerebral artery wall induced by long-term sympathetic denervation. Blood Vessels 25:122–143, 1988.

52. Durante W., Sen A.K., Sunahara F.A.: Impairment of endothelium-dependent relaxation in aortae from spontaneously diabetic rats. Br. J. Pharmacol. 94:463–468, 1988.

53. Dzau V.J.: Vascular wall renin angiotensin pathway in control of the circulation. Am. J. Med. 77:31–36, 1984.

54. Fitzgerald G.A., Smith B., Pedersen A.K., Brash A.R.: Increased prostacyclin biosynthesis in patients with severe atherosclerosis and platelet activation. N. Engl. J. Med. 310:1065–1068, 1984.

55. Flaherty J.T., Pierce J.E., Ferrans V.J., Patel D.J., Tucker W.K., Fry D.L.: Endothelial nuclear patterns in the canine arterial tree with particular reference to hemodynamic events. Circ. Res. 30:23–33, 1972.

56. Foldes A., Mead R.J., De La Lande T.S.: Endogenous and exogenous histamine in rabbit thoracic aorta. Aust. J. Exp. Biol. Med. Sci. 55:89–102, 1976.

57. Forman M.B., Oates J.A., Robertson D., Robertson R.M., Roberts L.J., Virmani R.: Increased adventitial mast cells in a patient with coronary spasm. N. Engl. J. Med. 313:1138–1141, 1985.

58. Forrester T., Williams C.A.: Release of adenosine triphosphate from isolated adult heart cells in response to hypoxia. J. Physiol. 268:371–390, 1977.

59. Fortes Z.B., Leme J.G., Scivoletto R.: Vascular reactivity in diabetes mellitus: role of the endothelial cell. Br. J. Pharmacol. 79:771–781, 1983.

60. Frangos J.A., Eskin S.G., McIntire L.V., Ives C.L.: Flow effects on prostacyclin production by cultured human endothelial cells. Science 227:1477–1479, 1985.

61. Frazer R.A., Ellis E.M., Stalker A.L.: Experimental angiogenesis in the chorio al lantoic membrane. Bibl. Anat. 18:25–27, 1979.

62. Fry D.L.: Acute vascular endothelial changes associated with increased blood velocity gradients. Circ. Res. 22:165–197, 1968.

63. Furchgott R.F.: Role of endothelium in responses of vascular smooth muscle. In: Frontiers in Physiological Research, D.G. Garlick, P.I. Korner (eds.). Cambridge University Press, Cambridge, pp 116–133, 1984.

64. Furchgott R.F.: Studies on relaxation of rabbit aorta by sodium nitrite: the basis for the proposal that the acid-activatable inhibitory factor from bovine retractor penis is inorganic nitrite and the endothelium-derived relaxing factor is nitric oxide. In: Vasodilatation: Vascular Smooth Muscle, Peptides, Autonomic Nerves, and Endothelium, P.M. Vanhoutte (ed.). Raven Press, New York, pp 401–414, 1988.

65. Furchgott R.F., Zawadzki J.V.: The obligatory role of endothelial cells in the relaxation of arterial smooth muscle by acetylcholine. Nature 288:373–376, 1980.

66. Ganz P., Ludmer P.L., Leopold J.A., Hollenberg N.K., Shook T.L., Wayne R.R., Mudge G.H., Alexander R.W., Selwyn A.P.: Endothelial dysfunction in vivo: studies in animals and in patients with coronary atherosclerosis. In: Vasodilatation: Vascular Smooth Muscle, Peptides, Autonomic Nerves, and Endothelium, P.M. Vanhoutte (ed.). Raven Press, New York, pp 543–549, 1988.

67. Gewirtz H., Olsson R.A., Brautigan D.L., Brown P.R.: Adenosine's role in regulating coronary arteriolar tone. Am. J. Physiol. 250:H1030–H1036, 1986.

68. Gimbrone M.A. Jr.: Macrophages, neovascularization and the growth of vascular

cells. In: Biology of Endothelial Cells, E.A. Jaffe (ed.). Martinus Nijhoff, Boston, pp 97–107, 1984.

69. Gimbrone M.A. Jr., Cotran R.S., Folkman J.: Human vascular endothelial cells in cultures, growth and DNA synthesis. J. Cell. Biol. 60:673–684, 1974.

70. Gonzalez J.L., Santos-Benito F.F.: Synthesis of acetylcholine by endothelial cells isolated from rat brain cortex capillaries. Brain Res. 412:148–150, 1987.

71. Griffith T.M., Edwards D.H., Davies R.L., Harrison T.J., Evans E.T.: EDRF coordinates the behaviour of vascular resistance vessels. Nature 329:442–445, 1987.

72. Grover A.K., Crankshaw J., Triggle C.R., Daniel E.E.: Nature of norepinephrine-sensitive Ca-pool in rabbit aortic smooth muscle: effect of pH. Life Sci. 32:1553–1558, 1983.

73. Grover A.K., Kwan C.Y., Daniel E.E.: High-affinity pH-dependent passive Ca binding by myometrial plasma membrane vesicles. Am. J. Physiol. 224:C61–C67, 1983.

74. Gryglewski R.J., Dembinska-Kiec A., Zmuda A., Gryglewska T.: Prostacyclin and thromboxane A_2 biosynthesis capacities of heart and platelets at various stages of experimental atherosclerosis in rabbits. Atherosclerosis 31:385–394, 1978.

75. Guerra R., Brotherton A.F.A., Clark C.R., Harrison D.G.: Atherosclerosis decreases production of endothelium derived relaxing factor. Clin. Res. 35:832A, 1987.

76. Hamel E., Assumel-Lurdin C., Edvinsson L., Fage D., MacKenzie E.T.: Neuronal versus endothelial origin of vasoactive acetylcholine in pial vessels. Brain Res. 420:391–396, 1987.

77. Hanley F.L., Grattan M.R., Stevens M.B., Hoffman J.I.E.: Role of adenosine in coronary autoregulation. Am. J. Physiol. 250:H558–H566, 1986.

78. Harper A.M., Bell R.A.: The effect of metabolic acidosis and alkalosis on the blood flow through the cerebral cortex. J. Neurol. Neurosurg. Psychiatr. 26:341–344, 1963.

79. Harrison D.G., Armstrong M.L., Friemann P.C., Heistad D.D.: Restoration of endothelium-dependent relaxation by dietary treatment of atherosclerosis. J. Clin. Invest. 80:1808–1811, 1987.

80. Heistad D.D., Armstrong M.L., Marcus M.L., Piegors D.J., Mark A.L.: Augmented responses to vasoconstrictor stimuli in hypercholesterolemic and athero-

sclerotic monkeys. Circ. Res. 54:711–718, 1984.

81. Hellewell P.G., Pearson J.D.: Metabolism of circulating adenosine by the porcine isolated perfused lung. Circ. Res. 53:1–7, 1983.

82. Hollis T.M., Gallik S.G., Orlidge A., Yost J.C.: Aortic endothelial and smooth muscle histamine metabolism: Relationship to aortic ^{125}I-albumin accumulation in experimental diabetes. Arteriosclerosis 3:599–606, 1983.

83. Hollis T.M., Rosen L.A.: Histidine decarboxylase activities of bovine aortic endothelium and intima-media. Proc. Soc. Exp. Biol. Med. 141:978–981, 1972.

84. Holtz J., Förstermann U., Pohl U., Giesler M., Bassenge E.: Flow-dependent, endothelium-mediated dilation of epicardial coronary arteries in conscious dogs: effects of cyclooxygenase inhibition. J. Cardiovasc. Pharmacol. 6:1161–1169, 1984.

85. Hopwood A.M., Lincoln J., Kirkpatrick K.A., Burnstock G.: Adenosine 5′-triphosphate, adenosine and endothelium-derived relaxing factor in hypoxic vasodilatation of the heart. Eur. J. Pharmacol. 165:323–326, 1986.

86. Hudlicka O.: Development of microcirculation: Capillary growth and adaptation. In: Handbook of Physiology: The Cardiovascular System IV. American Physiological Society, Bethesda, MD, pp 165–216, 1984.

87. Hudlicka O., Tyler K.R., Wright A.J.A., Ziada A.M.: The effect of long-term vasodilatation on capillary growth and performance in rabbit heart and skeletal muscle. J. Physiol. Lond. 334:49P, 1983.

88. Hull S.S., Kaiser L., Jaffe M.D., Sparks H.V.: Endothelium-dependent flow-induced dilation of canine femoral and saphenous arteries. Blood Vessels 23:183–198, 1986.

89. Hung K.-S., McKenzie J.C., Mattioli L., Klein R.M., Menon C.D., Poulose A.K.: Scanning electron microscopy of pulmonary vascular endothelium in rats with hypoxia-induced hypertension. Acta Anat. 126:13–20, 1986.

90. Ignarro L.J., Byrns R.E., Woods K.S.: Pharmacological and biochemical properties of endothelium-derived relaxing factor (EDRF): evidence that it is closely related to nitric oxide (NO) radical. Circulation 74:287, 1986.

91. Ishibashi T., Ichihara K., Abiko Y.: Difference in the time course between in-

creases in coronary flow and in effluent adenosine concentration during anoxia in the perfused rat heart. Jpn. Circ. J. 49:1090–1098, 1985.

92. Johnson A.R.: The metabolism of vasoactive peptides by human endothelial cells. In: Biology of Endothelial Cells, E.A. Jaffe (ed.). Martinus Nijhoff, Boston, pp 302–316, 1984.

93. Junod A.F.: Uptake, metabolism and efflux of ^{14}C-5-hydroxytryptamine in isolated perfused rat lungs. J. Pharmacol. Exp. Ther. 183:341–355, 1972.

94. Junod A.F., Ody C.: Amine uptake and metabolism by endothelium of pig pulmonary artery and aorta. Am. J. Physiol. 232:C88–C94, 1977.

95. Kahlson G., Rosengren E.: New approaches to the physiology of histamine. Physiol. Rev. 48:155–196, 1968.

96. Kaiser L., Hull S.S., Sparks H.V.: Methylene blue and ETYA block flow-dependent dilation in canine femoral artery. Am. J. Physiol. 250:H974–H981, 1986.

97. Kalsner S., Richards R.: Coronary arteries of cardiac patients are hyperreactive and contain stores of amines: A mechanism for coronary spasm. Science 223:1435–1437, 1984.

98. Karnovsky M.J.: Endothelial-vascular smooth muscle cell interactions. Am. J. Pathol. 105:200–206, 1981.

99. Katusic Z.S., Shepherd J.T., Vanhoutte P.M.: Vasopressin causes endothelium-dependent relaxations of the canine basilar artery. Circ. Res. 55:575–579, 1984.

100. Katusic Z., Shepherd J.T., Vanhoutte P.M.: Arginine vasopressin induces endothelium-dependent relaxations of canine basilar and coronary arteries. Fed. Proc. 43:1084, 1984.

101. Kifor I., Dzau V.J.: Endothelial renin-angiotensin pathway: evidence for intracellular synthesis and secretion of angiotensin. Circ. Res. 60:422–428, 1987.

102. Kim D.W., Langille B.L., Wong M.K.K., Gotlieb A.I.: Patterns of endothelial microfilament distribution in the rabbit aorta in situ. Circ. Res. 64:21–31, 1989.

103. King S.J., Booyse F.M., Lin P.-H., Traylor M., Narkates A.J., Oparil S.: Hypoxia stimulates endothelial cell angiotensin-converting enzyme antigen synthesis. Am. J. Physiol. 256:C1231–C1238, 1989.

104. King C.E., Cain S.M.: Peripheral vascular response to hypoxic hypoxia after aortic denervation. Can. J. Physiol. Pharmacol. 63:1197–1201, 1985.

105. Kivity S., Souhrada J.F.: Plasma and platelets potentiate a hypoxic vascular response of the isolated lung. J. Appl. Physiol. 51:875–880, 1981.

106. Kroll K., Feigl E.O.: Adenosine is unimportant in controlling coronary blood flow in unstressed dog hearts. Am. J. Physiol. 249:H1176–H1187, 1985.

107. Kwan C.Y., Grover A.K., Daniel E.E.: Cell membrane and regulation of cytoplasmic levels of Ca^{2+} in vascular muscle. In: Vasodilatation: Vascular Smooth Muscle, Peptides, Autonomic Nerves and Endothelium, P.M. Vanhoutte (ed.). Raven Press, New York, pp 21–27, 1988.

108. Kwan Y.W., Wadsworth R.M., Kane K.A.: Hypoxia- and endothelium-mediated changes in the pharmacological responsiveness of circumflex coronary artery rings from the sheep. Br. J. Pharmacol. 96:857–863, 1989.

109. Langille B.L., Adamson S.L.: Relationship between blood flow direction and endothelial cell orientation at arterial branch sites in rabbits and mice. Circ. Res. 48:481–488, 1981.

110. Lansman J.B., Hallam T.J., Rink T.J.: Single stretch-activated ion channels in vascular endothelial cells as mechanotransducers? Nature 325:811–813, 1987.

111. Lee T.J.-F., Shirasaki Y., Nickols G.A.: Altered endothelial modulation of vascular tone in aging and hypertension. Blood Vessels 24:132–136, 1987.

112. Lichtor T., Davies H.R., Johns L., Vesselinovitch D., Wissler R.W., Mullan S.: The sympathetic nervous system and atherosclerosis. J. Neurosurg. 67:906–914, 1987.

113. Lilly L.S., Pratt R.E., Alexander R.W., Larson D.M., Ellison K.E., Gimbrone M.A. Jr., Dzau V.J.: Renin expression by vascular endothelial cells in culture. Circ. Res. 57:312–318, 1985.

114. Lincoln J., Loesch A., Burnstock G.: Localization of vasopressin, serotonin and angiotensin II in endothelial cells of the renal and mesenteric arteries of the rat. Cell Tissue Res. 259:341–344, 1990.

115. Linnik M.D., Milbury P.E., Moskowitz M.A.: Human cerebrovascular endothelial cells contain the tachykinin substance P. J. Cereb. Blood Flow Metab. 9 (Suppl. 1):S683, 1989.

116. Linnik M.D., Moskowitz M.A.: Identification of immunoreactive substance P in human and other mammalian endothelial cells. Peptides 10(5):957–962, 1989.

117. Loesch A., Burnstock G.: Ultrastructural

localization of serotonin and substance P in vascular endothelial cells of rat femoral and mesenteric arteries. Anat. Embryol. 178:137–142, 1988.

118. Long C.J., Stone T.W.: The release of endothelium-derived relaxant factor is calcium dependent. Blood Vessels 22:205–208, 1985.

119. Lüscher T.F.: Endothelial vasoactive substances and cardiovascular disease. Karger, London, 1988.

120. Lüscher T.F., Romero J.C., Vanhoutte P.M.: Bioassy of endothelium-derived vasoactive substances in the aorta of normotensive and spontaneously hypertensive rats. J. Hypertension 4 (Suppl. 6):81–83, 1986.

121. Mangiarua E.I., Bevan R.D.: Altered endothelium-mediated relaxation after denervation of growing rabbit ear artery. Eur. J. Pharmacol. 122:149–152, 1986.

122. Manuck S.B., Kaplan J.R., Adams M.R., Clarkson T.B.: Effects of stress and the sympathetic nervous system on coronary artery atherosclerosis in the cynomolgus macaque. Am. Heart J. 116:328–333, 1988.

123. Markle R.A., Hollis T.M.: Rabbit aortic endothelial and medial histamine synthesis following short-term cholesterol feeding. Exp. Mol. Pathol. 23:417–425, 1975.

124. Miller V.M., Aarhus L.L.: Vanhoutte P.M.: Modulation of endothelium-dependent responses by chronic alterations of blood flow. Am. J. Physiol. 251:H520–H527, 1986.

125. Milner P., Ralevic V., Hopwood A.M., Feher E., Lincoln J., Kirkpatrick K.A., Burnstock G.: Ultrastructural localisation of substance P and choline acetyltransferase in endothelial cells of rat coronary artery and release of substance P and acetylcholine during hypoxia. Experientia 45:121–125, 1989.

126. Moncada S., Palmer R.M.J., Gryglewski R.J. Mechanism of action of some inhibitors of endothelium-derived relaxing factor. Proc. Natl. Acad. Sci. USA 83:9164–9168, 1986.

127. Moncada S., Palmer R.M.J., Higgs E.A.: Prostacyclin and endothelium-derived relaxing factor: biological interactions and significance. In: Thrombosis and Haemostasis. International Society of Thrombosis and Haemostasis, V. Verstraete, J. Vermylen, H. R. Lijnen, et al. (eds). Leuven University Press, Leuven, pp 597–618, 1987.

128. Morera S., Santoro F.M., Roson M.I., De

129. Mueller S.M., Ertel P.J., Felten D.L., Overhage J.M.: Sympathetic nerves protect against blood-brain barrier disruption in the spontaneously hypertensive rat. Stroke 13:83–88, 1982.

130. Nakamaru M., Jackson E.K., Inagami T.: β-adrenoceptor-mediated release of angiotensin II from mesenteric arteries. Am. J. Physiol. 250:H144–H148, 1986.

131. Naruse M., Inagami T.: Antibody-sensitive renin of adrenal and resistance vessels is markedly elevated in spontaneously hypertensive rats. Clin. Sci. 63:187–189, 1982.

132. Needleman P., Key S.L., Isakson P.C., Kulkarni P.S.: Relationship between oxygen tension, coronary vasodilation and prostaglandin biosynthesis in the isolated rabbit heart. Prostaglandins 9:123–135, 1975.

133. Nees S., Willerhausen-Zönnchen B., Gerbes A.L., Gerlach E.: Studies on cultured coronary endothelial cells. Folia Angiol. 28:64–68, 1980.

134. Nees S., Gerlach E.: Adenine nucleotide and adenosine metabolism in cultured coronary endothelial cells: formation and release of adenine compounds and possible functional implication. In: Regulatory Function of Adenosine, R.M. Berne, T.N. Rall, R. Rubio (eds.). Martinus Nijhoff, Boston, pp 347–355, 1983.

135. Nemecek G.M., Coughlin S.R., Handley D.A., Moskowitz M.A.: Stimulation of aortic smooth muscle cell mitogenesis by serotonin. Proc. Natl. Acad. Sci. USA 83:674–678, 1986.

136. Nilsson J., Von Euler A.M., Dalsgaard C.-J.: Stimulation of connective tissue cell growth by substance P and substance K. Nature 315:61–63, 1985.

137. Norregaard T.V., Moskowitz M.A.: Substance P and the sensory innervation of the intracranial and extracranial feline cephalic arteries. Brain 108:517–533, 1985.

138. Okamura T., Miyazaki M., Inagami T., Toda N.: Vascular renin-angiotensin system in two-kidney, one-clip hypertensive rat. Hypertension 8:560–565, 1986.

139. Olesen S.P., Clapham D.E., Davies P.F.: Haemodynamic shear stress activates a K^+ current in vascular endothelial cells. Nature 331:168–170, 1988.

140. Orlidge A., Hollis T.M.: Aortic endothelial

La Riva I.J.: Prostacyclin (PGI_2) synthesis in the vascular wall of rats with bilateral renal artery stenosis. Hypertension 5 (Suppl. V):38–42, 1983.

and smooth muscle histamine metabolism in experimental diabetes. Arteriosclerosis 2:142–150, 1982.

141. Owens G.K., Hollis T.M.: Relationship between inhibition of aortic histamine formation, aortic albumin permeability and atherosclerosis. Atherosclerosis 34:365–373, 1979.

142. Oyama Y., Kawasaki H., Hattori Y., Kanno M.: Attenuation of endothelium-dependent relaxation in aorta from diabetic rats. Eur. J. Pharmacol. 131:75–78, 1986.

143. Paddle B.M., Burnstock G.: Release of ATP from perfused heart during coronary vasodilation. Blood Vessels 11:110–119, 1974.

144. Palmer R.M.J., Ferrige A.G., Moncada S.: Nitric oxide release accounts for the biological activity of endothelium-derived relaxing factor. Nature 327:524–526, 1987.

145. Parnavelas J.G., Kelly W., Burnstock G.: Ultrastructural localization of choline acetyltransferase in vascular endothelial cells in rat brain. Nature 316:724–725, 1985.

146. Peach M.J., Loeb A.L., Singer H.A., Saye J.: Endothelium-derived vascular relaxing factor. Hypertension (Suppl. I)7:I94–I100, 1985.

147. Peach M.J., Singer H.A., Loeb A.: Mechanisms of endothelium-dependent vascular smooth muscle relaxation. Biochem. Pharmacol. 34:1867–1874, 1985.

148. Pearson J.D., Carleton J.S., Hutchings A., Gordon J.L.: Uptake and metabolism of adenosine by pig aortic endothelial and smooth-muscle cells in culture. Biochem. J. 170:265–271, 1978.

149. Pearson J.D., Gordon J.L.: Vascular endothelial and smooth muscle cells in culture selectively release adenine nucleotides. Nature 281:384–386, 1979.

150. Pearson J.D., Gordon J.L.: Metabolism of serotonin and adenosine. In: Biology of Endothelial Cells, E.A. Jaffe (ed.). Martinus Nijhoff, Boston, pp 330–342, 1984.

151. Pearson J.D., Gordon J.L.: Nucleotide metabolism by endothelium. Annu. Rev. Physiol. 47:617–627, 1985.

152. Petty R.G., Pearson J.D.: Endothelium: the axis of vascular health and disease. J. R. Coll. Physicians London 23:92–102, 1989.

153. Phillis J.W., Delong R.E.: An involvement of adenosine in cerebral blood flow regulation during hypercapnia. Gen. Pharmacol. 18:133–139, 1987.

154. Pohl U., Busse R.: Hypoxia stimulates release of endothelium-derived relaxant factor. Am. J. Physiol. 256:H1595–H1600, 1989.

155. Ralevic V., Burnstock G.: Actions mediated by P_2-purinoceptor subtypes in the isolated perfused mesenteric bed of the rat. Br. J. Pharmacol. 95:637–645, 1988.

156. Ralevic V., Kristek F., Hudlicka O., Burnstock G.: A new protocol for removal of the endothelium from the perfused rat hindlimb preparation. Circ. Res. 64:1190–1196, 1989.

157. Ralevic V., Milner P., Hudlicka O., Kristek F., Burnstock G.: Substance P is released from the endothelium of normal and capsaicin-treated rat hindlimb vasculature, in vivo, by increased flow. Circ. Res. 66(5):1178–1183, 1990.

158. Robinson-White A., Peterson S., Hechtman H.B., Shepro D.: Serotonin uptake by isolated adipose capillary endothelium. J. Pharmacol. Exp. Ther. 216:125–128, 1981.

159. Ross R.: The pathogenesis of atherosclerosis: an update. N. Engl. J. Med. 314:488–500, 1986.

160. Roth R.A., Wallace K.B.: Disposition of biogenic amines and angiotensin I by lungs of spontaneously hypertensive rats. Am. J. Physiol. 239:H736–H761, 1980.

161. Rounds S.S., McMurtry I.F., Reeves J.T.: Glucose metabolism accelerates the decline of hypoxic vasoconstriction in rat lungs. Resp. Physiol. 44:239–249, 1981.

162. Rubanyi G.M., Paul R.J.: Two distinct effects of oxygen on vascular tone in isolated porcine coronary arteries. Circ. Res. 56:1–10, 1985.

163. Rubanyi G.M., Romero J.C., Vanhoutte P.M.: Flow-induced release of endothelium-derived relaxing factor. Am. J. Physiol. 250:H1145–H1149, 1986.

164. Rubanyi G.M., Vanhoutte P.M.: Hypoxia releases a vasoconstrictor substance from the canine vascular endothelium. J. Physiol 364:45–46, 1985.

165. Rubanyi G.M., Vanhoutte P.M.: Superoxide anions and hyperoxia inactivate endothelium-derived relaxing factor. Am. J. Physiol. 250:H822–H827, 1986.

166. Ryan J.W.: The metabolism of angiotensin I and bradykinin by endothelial cells. In: Biology of Endothelial Cells, E.A. Jaffe (ed.). Martinus Nijhoff, Boston, pp 317–329, 1984.

167. Ryan J.W., Ryan U.S., Schultz D.R., Whitaker C., Chung A., Dorer E.E.: Subcellular localization of pulmonary angiotensin-converting enzyme (Kininase II). Biochem. J. 146:497–499, 1975.

168. Sadoshima S., Heistad D.: Sympathetic nerves protect the blood-brain barrier in stroke-prone spontaneously hypertensive rats. Hypertension 4:904–907, 1982.

169. Schayer R.W.: Evidence that induced histamine is an intrinsic regulator of the microcirculatory system. Am. J. Physiol. 202:66–72, 1962.

170. Schayer R.W.: Biogenic amines and microcirculatory homeostasis. In: Biogenic Amines as Physiological Regulators, J.J. Blum (ed.). Prentice Hall, NJ, pp 237–251, 1970.

171. Schoefl G.I.: Studies on inflammation III. Growing capillaries: their structure and permeability. Virchows Arch. Pathol. Anat. Physiol. 337:97–114, 1963.

172. Schumacher B.L., Grant D., Eisenstein R.: Smooth muscle cells produce an inhibitor of endothelial cell growth. Arteriosclerosis. 5:110–115, 1985.

173. Shepherd A.P.: Intestinal O_2 consumption and ^{86}Rb extraction during arterial hypoxia. Am. J. Physiol. 234:E248–E251, 1978.

174. Shimokawa H., Aarhus L.L., Vanhoutte P.M.: Porcine coronary arteries with regenerated endothelium have a reduced endothelium-dependent responsiveness to aggregating platelets and serotonin. Circ. Res. 61:256–270, 1987.

175. Shimokawa H., Flavahan N.A., Vanhoutte P.M.: Natural course of the impairment of endothelium-dependent relaxations after balloon endothelium removal in porcine coronary arteries: possible dysfunction of a pertussis toxin-sensitive G protein. Circ. Res. 65:740–753, 1989.

176. Sinzinger H., Feigl W., Silberbauer K.: Prostacyclin production in atherosclerotic arteries. Lancet ii:469, 1979.

177. Smiésko V., Kozik J., Dolozél S.: Role of the endothelium in the control of arterial diameter by blood flow. Blood Vessels 22:247–251, 1985.

178. Smith R.S.: The development of mast cells in the vascularized cornea. Arch. Ophthalmol. 66:383–390, 1961.

179. Soffer R.L., Reza R., Caldwell P.R.B.: Angiotensin-converting enzyme from rabbit pulmonary particles. Proc. Natl. Acad. Sci. USA 71:1720–1724, 1974.

180. Sparks H.V. Jr., Gorman M.W.: Adenosine in the local regulation of blood flow: current controversies. In: Topics and Perspectives in Adenosine Research, E. Gerlach, B.F. Becker (eds.). Springer-Verlag, Berlin, pp 406–415, 1987.

181. Stephenson J.A., Summers J.R.: Autoradiographic analysis of receptors on vascular endothelium. Eur. J. Pharmacol. 134:35–43, 1987.

182. Stewart D.J., Holtz J., Pohl U., Bassenge E.: Balance between endothelium-mediated dilating and direct constricting actions of serotonin on resistance vessels in the isolated rabbit heart. Eur. J. Pharmacol. 143:131–134, 1987.

183. Taguchi T., Ishii Y., Matsubara F., Tenaka K.: Intimal thickening and the distribution of vasomotor nerves in the mechanically injured dog coronary artery. Exp. Mol. Pathol. 44:138–146, 1986.

184. Tesfamariam B., Cohen R.A.: Inhibition of adrenergic vasoconstriction by endothelial cell shear stress. Circ. Res. 63:720–725, 1988.

185. Teuscher E., Weidlich E.: Adenosine nucleotides, adenosine and adenine as angiogenesis factors. Biomed. Biochim. Acta 44:493–495, 1985.

186. Toda M.: Endothelium-dependent relaxation induced by angiotensin II and histamine in isolated arteries of dog. Br. J. Pharmacol. 81:301–307, 1984.

187. Tornling G.: Capillary neoformation in the heart of dipyridamole treated rats. Acta Pathol. Microbiol. Scand. Sect. A. 90:269–271, 1982.

188. Tornling G., Ungf G., Skoog L., Ljungqvist A., Carlsson S., Adolfsson J.: Proliferative activity of myocardial capillary wall cells in dipyridamole-treated rats. Cardiovasc. Res. 12:692–695, 1978.

189. Tozzi C.A., Dorrel S.G., Merrill G.F.: Evidence of histamine-induced myocardial ischaemia: reversal by chlorpheniramine and potentiation by atherosclerosis. Cardiovasc. Res. 19:744–753, 1985.

190. Van Bree J.B.M.M., De Boer A.G., Verhoef J.C., Danhorf M., Breimer D.D.: Transport of vasopressin fragments across the blood-brain barrier: in vitro studies using monolayer cultures of bovine brain endothelial cells. J. Pharmacol. Exp. Ther. 249:901–905, 1989.

191. Van De Voorde J., Leusen I.: Endothelium-dependent and independent relaxation of aortic rings from hypertensive rats. Am. J. Physiol. 250:H711–H717, 1986.

192. Van Harn G.L., Rubio R., Berne R.M.: Formation of adenosine nucleotide derivatives in isolated hog carotid artery strips. Am. J. Physiol. 233:H299–H304, 1977.

193. Vanhoutte P.M., Lüscher T.F.: Peripheral mechanisms in cardiovascular regulation:

transmitters, receptors and the endothelium. In: Handbook of Hypertension, vol. 8, Physiology and Pathophysiology of Hypertension Regulatory Mechanisms, R.C. Tarazi, A. Zanchetti (eds.). Elsevier, Amsterdam, pp. 96–123, 1987.

194. Vanhoutte P.M., Miller V.M.: Heterogeneity of endothelium-dependent responses in mammalian blood vessels. J. Cardiovasc. Pharmacol. 7 (Suppl. 3):S12–S23, 1985.

195. Vedernikov Y.P., Hellstrand P.: Effects of reduced oxygen tension on endothelium-dependent relaxation induced by acetylcholine differ in rabbit femoral artery and jugular vein. Acta Physiol. Scand. 135:343–348, 1989.

196. Verbeuren T.J., Jordaens F.H., Zonnekeyn L.L., Van Hove C.E., Coene M.-C., Herman A.G.: Effect of hypercholesterolemia on vascular reactivity in the rabbit I. Endothelium-dependent and endothelium-independent contractions and relaxations in isolated arteries of control and hypercholesterolemic rabbits. Circ. Res. 58:552–564, 1986.

197. Waldemar G., Paulson O.B., Barry D.I.: Angiotensin-converting enzyme (ACE) inhibition and CBF autoregulation after acute sympathetic denervation. J. Cereb. Blood Flow Metab. 9(Suppl.1):S36, 1989.

198. Wharton J., Gulbenkian S., Merighi A., Kuhn D.M., Jahn R., Taylor K.M., Polak J.M.: Immunohistochemical and ultrastructural localisation of peptide-containing nerves and myocardial cells in the human atrial appendage. Cell Tissue Res. 254:155–166, 1988.

199. Yamamoto H., Bossaller C., Cartwright J. Jr., Henry P.D.: Videomicroscopic demonstration of defective cholinergic arteriolar vasodilation in atherosclerotic rabbit. J. Clin. Invest. 81:1752–1758, 1988.

200. Zauberman H., Michaelson I.C., Bergmann F., Maurice D.M.: Stimulation of neovascularization of the cornea by biogenic amines. Exp. Eye Res. 8:77–83, 1969.

Part II

Endothelial Control of Special Vascular Beds in Health and Disease

5

Impaired Endothelial Vasodilator Function in Human Coronary Arteries

Peter Ganz, Vladimir I. Vekshtein,
Alan C. Yeung, Charles B. Treasure,
Franz F. Weidinger, Joseph A. Vita,
Thomas J. Ryan, Jr., James M. McLenachan,
Andrew P. Selwyn

The Importance of Coronary Vasoconstriction as a Mechanism of Myocardial Ischemia

The traditional view that coronary stenoses cause myocardial ischemia by limiting increases in blood flow is now thought to be incomplete. Convincing evidence has accumulated that atherosclerotic coronary narrowings play an active role in causing ischemia by intermittently interfering with coronary blood flow not only among the rare patients with Prinzmetal's variant angina but also in nearly all patients with unstable and stable forms of angina pectoris.[3,5,10,17,19,41] Studies of Chierchia and colleagues[5] in patients with unstable angina demonstrated a fall in coronary sinus oxygen saturation that could not be explained by a simultaneous increase in myocardial oxygen demand. Selwyn[41] used radionuclides to monitor myocardial perfusion in patients with stable angina during rapid atrial pacing and found a net fall in myocardial blood flow in regions distal to coronary stenosis. More recently, positron emission tomography was used to assess changes in regional myocardial perfusion in patients with stable angina using rubidium-82. These studies also demonstrated decreases in regional blood flow which accompanied ischemia triggered by exercise, cold pressor stimulation, or mental stress.[10,11] Ganz and colleagues,[20] in patients with unstable angina, measured coronary stenosis resistance directly by simultaneously determining pressure gradients and blood

Rubanyi G.M.: Cardiovascular Significance of Endothelium-Derived Vasoactive Factors, Futura Publishing Co., Inc., Mount Kisco, NY, © 1991.

flow across moderately severe coronary narrowings and demonstrated increases in stenosis resistance preceding and at the onset of episodes of ischemia.

Introduction into the catheterization laboratory of quantitative methods for assessing luminal caliber has permitted a closer examination of vasomotor responses of epicardial arteries in response to external stimuli known to trigger ischemia during daily life, such as exercise, cold, mental stress, and isometric exercise.[3,18,21,22,32] Through the use of quantitative angiography, Gordon,[21] Nabel,[32] and Gage[18] have demonstrated that there are important differences in the reactions of angiographically normal arteries and those containing atherosclerotic narrowings. In patients with clinically stable angina, atherosclerotic arteries generally constrict during the same stimuli (exercise, cold pressor testing) that cause dilation of arteries that are angiographically normal. This paradoxical constriction (vasospasm) of atherosclerotic narrowings likely contributes to the development of myocardial ischemia in this patient population.

Mechanism(s) of Coronary Vasospasm: Focus of Early Studies

The initial focus of investigations into the mechanisms of coronary vasospasm consisted of generally futile attempts to demonstrate that there is an excess of a circulating vasoconstrictor compound in the coronary circulation. For instance, in patients with vasospastic angina, arterial and coronary sinus concentrations of norepinephrine and epinephrine obtained early in ischemia were not elevated above baseline and rose only late in ischemia.[39] In addition, sympathetic nervous system function was investigated in patients with variant angina pectoris by sampling of peripheral venous norepinephrine in supine and upright postures, by measuring urinary excretion of catecholamines, and by assessing they physiological responses to sympathetic stimuli such as the Valsalva maneuver, the isometric hand grip test, and the cold pressor test. No differences were found in these measurements in normal subjects and in patients with variant angina.[38] Thus, these studies suggested that excessive sympathetic nervous system activation is not likely to be an important cause of coronary artery spasm. The weight of the evidence to date suggests that vasospastic angina also cannot be attributed primarily to an excess of the circulating constrictor agonists thromboxane A_2 and serotonin or to a deficiency of the vasodilator prostacyclin.[19]

Mechanism(s) of Coronary Vasospasm: Role of Endothelium and Atherosclerosis

In 1980, two seminal studies were published that helped to shift the emphasis of investigations of vasospasm away from the neurohumoral systems and instead focused the attention on local disturbances in the arterial wall. First, Henry observed that the isolated aortas of rabbits rendered atherosclerotic by a high cholesterol diet were hypersensitive to contraction induced by ergonovine and by serotonin.[27] This study suggested that the augmented vascular responsiveness can be related directly to the biology of the atherosclerotic process. This hypothesis was particularly appealing as it was paralleled by the clinical observations that vasopastic angina almost invariably occurs in the setting of coronary atherosclerosis, although the degree of luminal narrowing varies widely.[37] It was appreciated that even patients thought to have normal coronary arteries at angiography may at autopsy have evidence of atherosclerosis in the same segment of the vessel that was affected by vasospasm.

The second seminal observation was the demonstration by Furchgott that endothelial cells, when appropriately stimulated, release a potent vasodilator substance, called endothelium-derived relaxing factor (EDRF), which causes relaxation of the underlying vascular smooth muscle.[16] Furchgott resolved a long-standing paradox that acetylcholine (ACh) was a vasodilator in vivo yet it frequently induced constriction of arterial strips in vitro. In the presence of endothelium, increasing doses of ACh produced dose-dependent relaxation of isolated strips of rabbit aorta that had been preconstricted with norepinephrine. If the endothelium had been removed, as inadvertently happened during routine handling of isolated vessels, and which Furchgott accomplished by gently rubbing the intimal surface of the arterial strip, then only constriction was induced by ACh. It was therefore suggested that ACh has two distinct and opposite actions on blood vessels: direct constriction of vascular smooth muscle and an indirect vasodilator action that is mediated by endothelium. In most intact arteries, the net effect of these two actions is vasodilation, especially at lower concentrations of ACh (i.e., $\leq 10^{-5}$M).

It was subsequently established that release of EDRF was a mode of action of most other vasodilators including histamine, bradykinin, substance P, ATP, ADP, thrombin, and increasing blood flow. Even substances that act as vasoconstrictors can release EDRF, such as catecholamines, serotonin, and vasopressin.[34] Although the net effect on blood vessels may not be vasodilation, the presence of the endothelium-dependent vasodilating influence will attenuate severe constriction in these vascular beds.

Studies of Endothelium-Dependent Relaxation to Acetylcholine in Humans: Effects of Atherosclerosis and of Coronary Risk Factors

The observations of Henry on the hypercontractility of atherosclerotic arteries and of Furchgott on the importance of endothelium to vasodilation provided new directions in clinical and basic research on the mechanisms of vasospasm. Ludmer et al.[30] addressed the hypothesis that constrictor hyperresponsiveness of atherosclerotic human coronary arteries is caused, wholly or in part, by a loss of endothelial vasodilator function. To test this concept, acetylcholine (endothelium-dependent agent) and nitroglycerin (endothelium-independent agent) were administered directly into the left anterior descending coronary artery of patients undergoing cardiac catheterization and vasomotor responses were assessed by quantitative angiography. ACh induced dose-dependent dilation of human epicardial coronary arteries in the majority of patients free from any evidence of atherosclerosis. As in many animal preparations with intact endothelium, this dilatation was best observed in the ACh range of 10^{-9} to 10^{-6}M. Higher concentrations, which have since been employed by some investigators, are more likely to favor constriction of presumably normal arteries. The ACh-induced dilation of human coronary arteries likely involves an endothelium-dependent mechanism, as the administration of methylene blue, an inhibitor of the actions of EDRF, abolishes this response.[28]

Ludmer also demonstrated that atherosclerotic arteries paradoxically constrict in response to ACh and that this abnormal constriction may be related to disturbed endothelial vasodilator function. Arterial segments from patients with advanced coronary stenoses (greater than 70% luminal narrowing) constricted in a dose-dependent manner to increasing concentrations of ACh in the same dose range in which normal arteries dilated. The ability of these atherosclerotic segments to dilate in response to nitroglycerin, an agent that acts directly on vascular smooth muscle, was preserved, suggesting that the paradoxical response to ACh was indeed related to endothelial dysfunction.

In addition, coronary arterial segments from patients with angiographic evidence of only minor intimal irregularities also constricted to ACh. This indicates that endothelium-dependent vasodilation is impaired early in the atherosclerotic process. Such disturbances in endothelial vasodilator function have been recently shown to exist in angiographically smooth ("normal") arteries of patients with risk factors for the development of atherosclerosis or in arteries with a high likelihood of presence of early atherosclerosis. Thus, angiographically smooth coronary arteries in patients who have a significant narrowing in another coronary artery are likely constrict to ACh.[30,49] Studies of Vita[47] and Yasue[51] have shown that there is an important correlation between the presence of coronary risk factors and the response to ACh in patients with angiographically normal arteries. In Vita's study, a constrictor response to ACh was independently associated with elevated serum cholesterol, male gender, family history of coronary artery disease, and patient age. The overall number of coronary risk factors was the best predictor of the response to ACh. In Yasue's study, the response to ACh matched the expected distribution of occult atherosclerosis; the proximal segments were more likely to constrict to ACh than the distal segments. In addition, impairment of endothelium-dependent dilation has been shown to also be particularly marked at branch points of coronary arteries. These segments are sites of disturbed blood flow patterns at which atherosclerosis is particularly likely to develop.

Thus abnormal vasomotor responses to ACh have served as convenient functional markers of endothelial dysfunction in both early and advanced stages of atherosclerosis. This endothelial vasodilator dysfunction is likely to be an important pathophysiological link between atherosclerosis and associated vasospasm.

Measurements of EDRF in Atherosclerosis

EDRF has been shown to be nitric oxide or a closely related compound, derived from arginine. While insights into endothelium-dependent relaxation in the clinical setting have been obtained using the test agent acetylcholine, more direct assays of EDRF have not been practical in patients. However, EDRF activity can be determined in arteries with experimental atherosclerosis. Several groups of investigators have demonstrated in bioassay studies a depressed release or diminished activity of EDRF from atherosclerotic arteries in response to acetylcholine and serotonin.[23,43,44]

Endothelial Vasodilator Function and Patterns of Responses to Stimuli Known to Trigger Myocardial Ischemia During Daily Life

ACh, an extremely useful test agent of endothelial function, is not likely to be an important physiological regulator of vascular tone. It is interesting, however, that the patterns of vasomotor reactions to ACh are mirrored by the reaction of smooth, irregular, and stenosed coronary arteries to the types of common stimuli that are known to trigger ischemia in daily life such as supine bicycle exercise and the cold pressor test.[18,21,32,52] Thus, during exercise or cold pressor stimulation, angiographically smooth arteries dilate while arteries with evidence of early and advanced atherosclerosis paradoxically constrict. Moreover, an excellent agreement exists in the responses (dilation/constriction) of individual arterial segments to ACh and in the responses of the same segments to exercise[21] or the cold pressor stimulation,[52] suggesting that endothelial function may modulate vasomotion during these activities, in health and in disease. While the responses to dynamic exercise and the cold pressor test are of relevance to the pathophysiology of ischemia during daily life, they are difficult to interpret in light of simultaneous changes in multiple parameters such as activation of the sympathetic nervous system, augmentation of coronary blood flow, and increases in heart rate and blood pressure. With the aim of understanding the responses during these complex daily activities, vasomotion of epicardial coronary arteries has been examined in relation to each parameter individually, i.e., increasing blood flow and changes in catecholamines.

Studies of Flow-Mediated Dilation in Humans: Effects of Atherosclerosis

While the release of EDRF was initially described using pharmacological agents that act through activation of specific membrane receptors on endothelial cells, it was shown subsequently that mechanical stimuli, including blood flow and pulsatility, can also stimulate the release of EDRF.[36,40] Dilatation of the conduit arteries in response to increasing blood flow was first described in 1933, but the mechanism re-

mained unknown until the recent demonstration by Bassenge and colleagues[36] that endothelial cells act as mediators of flow-dependent dilation. Mechanical removal of endothelial cells from the canine femoral artery abolished dilatation in response to increased blood flow. Use of the bioassay techniques demonstrated that increased flow and ACh release a relaxing substance with the same characteristics (EDRF).[40] In humans, coronary arteries free of atherosclerosis (as judged by angiography) have also been shown to dilate in response to increased blood flow.[8,12,33] This flow-mediated response is impaired by atherosclerosis. In these studies, increases in blood flow were induced by the administration of dilators of the resistance vessels such as adenosine and papaverine. Epicardial arteries free of angiographic evidence of atherosclerosis dilated by approximately 16% in response to a threefold increase in blood flow,[8] while arteries with even mild angiographic evidence of atherosclerosis failed to dilate or even constricted.[8,33] This impaired response to increasing blood flow may in part explain the abnormal vasomotor behavior of atherosclerotic epicardial coronary arteries during daily activities such as exercise. During exercise, normal arteries dilate and atherosclerotic arteries fail to dilate appropriately as the demand for blood flow increases with increased metabolic requirements.

The Role of Endothelial Function in Modulating the Effects of Catecholamines on Human Coronary Arteries

Stimuli for myocardial ischemia such as exercise and exposure to cold are associated with sympathetic (adrenergic) activation and increases in the concentration of circulating catecholamines. Catecholamines exert their effects on vascular smooth muscle by α_1-, and α_2-adrenergic mediated constriction and by β-adrenergic mediated dilation. Healthy endothelium is capable of modulating the constrictor effects of catecholamines by several mechanisms. Stimulation of α_2-adrenergic receptors on endothelial cells can lead to a release of EDRF. Cocks[6] demonstrated that stimulation of α_2-receptors on endothelial cells leads to release of EDRF and attenuation of the constrictor effects of norepinephrine. In addition, Martin and Furchgott observed that removal of endothelium from arterial rings markedly increased the sensitivity of arteries to constriction by phenylephrine which lacks significant α_2-agonist properties at the doses administered.[31] They were able to attribute their findings to removal of the tonic dilator influence resulting from the continuous basal release of EDRF.

Vita[48] demonstrated in patients undergoing a cardiac catheterization that coronary segments exhibiting evidence of endothelial dysfunction (assessed by acetylcholine) had a constrictor response to phenylephrine at a 100-fold lower concentration than segments that had normal endothelial function. These results suggest that the endothelial dysfunction that characterizes early and advanced atherosclerosis is associated with a marked increase in sensitivity to the constrictor effects of catecholamines. These results could also in part explain the observation that atherosclerotic coronary arteries constrict during exercise, the cold pressor stimulation, and other stimuli associated with elevated catecholamines.

Treatment of Endothelial Vasodilator Dysfunction in Atherosclerosis

Endothelium overlying atherosclerotic plaques is physically present but exhibits distinct morphological abnormalities. In experimental atherosclerosis, these atypical cells are often cuboidal rather than flat and lack the typical orientation in the direction of blood flow.[50] Similar abnormalities of the endothelial morphology have been found in human coronary arteries.[9] As endothelial cells in atherosclerosis are not absent, it might be feasible to find treatments that restore their function. Such treatments could involve approaches that directly address the biology of atherosclerosis (e.g., cholesterol lowering, fish oil administration) or could more narrowly focus on restoring EDRF (e.g., administration of large amounts of the EDRF precursor arginine, or administration of N-acetylcysteine to increase the potency of residual EDRF).

Effects of Cholesterol Lowering

Harrison,[25] Heistad,[26] and their colleagues have shown in monkeys that endothelium-dependent relaxation to acetylcholine and serotonin is impaired in diet-induced atherosclerosis[25] and that cholesterol lowering will return endothelial vasodilator function to normal in association with histologic evidence of plaque healing (i.e., the inflammatory and cellular components of lesions diminish) and without the need for complete regression of atherosclerotic plaques to occur.

In humans, the efficacy of cholesterol lowering in restoring endothelium-dependent relaxation is not yet known. However, Vita and colleagues[47] have shown in patients with preclinical stages of coronary atherosclerosis that the level of serum cholesterol (and of other coronary risk factors) relates closely to the abnormal constriction elicited by the endothelium-dependent dilator agent acetylcholine.

Effects of Fish Oil Administration

Treatment of atherosclerosis with fish oils has been of considerable interest in view of the findings of reduced rates of cardiovascular disease reported in populations consuming a diet rich in fish oil and in view of the ability of fish oils to reduce atherosclerosis in experimental models. With respect to the ability of fish oils to improve regulation of vascular tone in atherosclerosis, Shimokawa[42] demonstrated in a pig model that a brief course of dietary supplementation with fish oil reverses the impaired endothelium-dependent relaxation in experimental coronary atherosclerosis.

Vekshtein and colleagues[46] have shown in patients that fish oil administration for 6 months can restore dilation of atherosclerotic coronary arteries to acetylcholine. This improved response to acetylcholine occurred without any change in response to the endothelium-independent agent nitroglycerin, suggesting that the beneficial effect of fish oils can be attributed to improved endothelial vasodilator function.

Endothelial Dysfunction and Accelerated Coronary Atherosclerosis in the Transplanted Heart

Accelerated coronary atherosclerosis following cardiac transplantation is a major cause of graft failure. It occurs with similar incidence regardless of whether the original indication for transplantation was coronary artery disease or cardiomyopathy. While there may be several contributing factors in the development of transplant atherosclerosis, the principal cause appears to be an immune-mediated damage to the coronary endothelium[1] and the endothelium appears to actively participate in this process. Thus, while healthy endothelium has on its surface only a limited number of major histocompatibility complex class I antigenic sites and no class II

sites, under pathological conditions relevant to transplantation, it can express an increased number of class I antigenic sites and newly expresses class II antigenic sites and may thus become a target for destruction by the immune system.[35] Endothelial cells can also enhance the immune-mediated rejection process by induced expression of leukocyte-adhesion molecules on their surface, a finding recently demonstrated in the biopsy specimen of human cardiac allografts.[2]

Transplant coronary atherosclerosis is difficult to detect by conventional angiography, since the disease process is diffuse and normal segments against which atherosclerotic stenoses are conventionally judged may be absent. Fish et al.[15] have shown that the majority of coronary arteries of transplanted hearts demonstrate a loss of endothelium-dependent dilatation to acetylcholine and show paradoxical constriction, suggestive of endothelial dysfunction, before angiographic abnormalities are evident. This early emergence of endothelial dysfunction appears to predict the subsequent development of atherosclerotic narrowings. The use of acetylcholine as a test agent of endothelial function may prove to be a useful way of monitoring the activity of the mechanism (endothelial dysfunction) which contributes to the development of accelerated atherosclerosis.

Endothelial Dysfunction in the Microvasculature of Patients with Dilated Cardiomyopathy

The cause(s) of dilated cardiomyopathy in patients remain largely unknown. However, in an experimental model of dilated cardiomyopathy, the hereditary cardiomyopathy in Syrian hamsters, microvascular spasm appears to play an important role.[13,14] Silicone rubber perfusion studies demonstrated microvascular spasm associated with adjacent areas of myocytolytic necrosis in the early stages of this disease. Administration of the calcium channel blocker verapamil, an agent effective in the treatment of vasospasm, halted the progression of myocardial necrosis and prevented the development of cardiomyopathy. In patients with dilated cardiomyopathy, normal epicardial coronary arteries and history of chest pain, Cannon[4] found that ergonovine induced anginal symptoms in nearly all such patients. The apparent increased sensitivity to the vasoconstrictor stimulus ergonovine suggested an intrinsic functional abnormality of the coronary microvasculature.

Treasure and colleagues[45] determined whether endothelium-dependent vasodilator function is abnormal in patients with dilated cardiomyopathy and whether this abnormality could contribute to the disturbed coronary flow regulation found in this disease. Severely impaired relaxation of the microvasculature to the endothelium-dependent vasodilator acetylcholine was demonstrated in all patients with idiopathic or hereditary forms of dilated cardiomyopathy while a milder impairment was present in patients with alcohol-related cardiomyopathy. The loss of relaxation to acetylcholine with a relatively intact relaxation to the endothelium-independent agent adenosine suggests that extravascular factors do not explain the pronounced differences in acetylcholine responses between normal and cardiomyopathic patients and suggests a role for endothelial dysfunction in the microvasculature of hearts with dilated cardiomyopathy. Such endothelial dysfunction could lead not only to abnormal increases in the microvascular tone but also to disturbances in the trophic support that the endothelium provides to the surrounding tissues by producing a variety of growth factors.[7,24,29]

Conclusions

Studies over the last decade have revealed that healthy endothelial cells produce a relaxing substance, EDRF, which is pivotally involved in the local regulation of vascular tone. This substance is similar to the active principle of nitroglycerin, nitric oxide, and can thus be thought of as the "endogenous nitroglycerin." In human and experimental atherosclerosis, the activity of EDRF is diminished, a condition that predisposes to arterial vasospasm and thereby to myocardial ischemia. Impaired endothelium-dependent relaxation may also play a role in patients with dilated cardiomyopathy. Treatments directed at restoring endothelial vasodilator function and thereby improving ischemia should be tested in the clinical setting.

References

1. Bowyer D.E., Reidy M.A.: Scanning electron-microscope studies of the endothelium of aortic allografts in the rabbit: Morphologic observations. J. Pathol. 123:237–243, 1987.

2. Briscoe D.M., Schoen F.J., Rice G.E., Bevilacqua M.P., Ganz P., Pober J.S.: Induced expression of endothelial-leukocyte adhesion molecules in human cardiac allografts: Correlation with CD3+ T cell infiltration. Transplantation (in press).

3. Brown B.G., Lee A.B., Bolsen E., Dodge H.T.: Reflex constriction of significant coronary stenosis as a mechanism contributing to ischemic left ventricular dysfunction during isometric exercise. Circulation 70:18–24, 1984.

4. Cannon R.O., Cunnion R.E., Parrillo J.E.,

Palmeri S.T., Tucker E.E., Schenke W.H., Epstein S.E.: Dynamic limitation of coronary vasodilator reserve in patients with dilated cardiomyopathy and chest pain. J. Am. Coll. Cardiol. 10:1190–1200, 1987.

5. Chierchia S., Lazzari M., Freedman B., Brunellis C., Maseri A.: Impairment of myocardial perfusion and function during painless myocardial ischemia. J. Am. Coll. Cardiol. 16:1359–1373, 1983.

6. Cocks T.M., Angus J.A.: Endothelium-dependent relaxation of coronary arteries by noradrenaline and serotonin. Nature 305:627–630, 1983.

7. Collins T., Pober J.S., Gimbrone J.A. Jr., Hammacher A., Betsholtz C., Westermark B., Heldin C.H.: Cultured human endothelial cells express platelet-derived growth factor A chain. Am. J. Pathol. 126:7–12, 1987.

8. Cox D.A., Vita J.A., Treasure C.B., Fish R.D., Alexander R.W., Ganz P., Selwyn A.P.: Impairment of flow-mediated dilation coronary dilation by atherosclerosis in man. Circulation 80:458–465, 1989.

9. Davies M.J., Woolf N., Rowles A.M., Pepper J.: Morphology of the endothelium over atherosclerotic plaques in human coronary arteries. Br. Heart J. 60:459–464, 1988.

10. Deanfield J., Maseri A., Selwyn A.P., Ribeiro P., Cherchia S., Krikler S., Morgan M.: Myocardial ischemia during daily life in patients with stable angina: Its relation to symptoms and heart rate changes. Lancet 2:753–761, 1983.

11. Deanfield J.E., Kensett M., Wilson R.A., Shea M., Horlock P., deLandsheere C.M., Selwyn A.P.: Silent myocardial ischemia due to mental stress. Lancet 2:1001–1004, 1984.

12. Drexler H., Zeiher A.M., Wollschlager H., Meinertz T., Just H., Bonzel T.: Flow-dependent coronary artery dilatation in humans. Circulation 80:466–474, 1989.

13. Factor S.M., Cho S., Scheuer J., Sonnenblick E.H., Malhotra A.: Prevention of hereditary cardiomyopathy in the Syrian hamster with chronic verapamil therapy. J. Am. Coll. Cardiol. 12:1599–1604, 1988.

14. Figulla H.R., Vetterlein F., Glaubitz M., Kreuzer H.: Inhomogeneous capillary flow and its prevention by verapamil and hydralazine in the cardiomyopathic Syrian hamster. Circulation 76:208–216, 1987.

15. Fish R.D., Nabel E.G., Selwyn A.P., Ludmer P.L., Mudge G.H., Kirshenbaum J.M., Schoen F.J., Alexander R.W., Ganz P.: Responses of coronary arteries of cardiac transplant patients to acetylcholine. J. Clin. Invest. 81:21–31, 1988.

16. Furchgott R.F., Zawadzki J.V.: The obligatory role of endothelial cells in the relaxation of arterial smooth muscle by acetylcholine. Nature 288:373–376, 1980.

17. Fuster V.: Insights into the pathogenesis of acute ischemic syndromes. Circulation 77:1213–1220, 1988.

18. Gage J.E., Hess O.M., Murakami T., Ritter M., Grimm J., Krayenbuehl H.P.: Vasoconstriction of stenotic coronary arteries during dynamic exercise in patients with classic angina pectoris: reversibility by nitroglycerin. Circulation 73:865–867, 1986.

19. Ganz P., Alexander R.W.: New insights into the cellular mechanisms of vasospasm. Am. J. Cardiol. 56:llE-15E, 1985.

20. Ganz P., Abben R.P., Barry W.H.: Dynamic varations in resistance of coronary arterial narrowings in angina pectoris at rest. Am. J. Cardiol. 59:66–70, 1987.

21. Gordon J.B., Ganz P., Nabel E.G., Zebede J., Mudge G.H., Alexander R.W., Selwyn A.P.: Atherosclerosis and endothelial function influence the coronary vasomotor response to exercise. J. Clin. Invest. 83:1946–1952, 1989.

22. Gould K.L.: Quantification of coronary artery stenosis in vivo. Circ. Res. 57:341–353, 1985.

23. Guerra R., Brotherton A.F.A., Goodwin P.J., Clark C.R., Armstrong M.L., Harrison D.G.: Mechanisms of abnormal endothelium-dependent vascular relaxation in atherosclerosis. Blood Vessels 26(5):300–314, 1990.

24. Hannsson H.A., Jennische E., Skottner A.: Regenerating endothelial cells express insulin-like growth factor-I immunoreactivity after arterial injury. Cell Tissue Res. 250:499–505, 1987.

25. Harrison D.G., Armstrong M.L., Freiman P.C., Heistad D.D.: Restoration of endothelium-dependent relaxation by dietary treatment of atherosclerosis. J. Clin. Invest. 80:1808–1811, 1987.

26. Heistad D.D., Mark A.L., Marcus M.L., Piegors D.J., Armstrong M.L.: Dietary treatment of atherosclerosis abolishes hyperresponsiveness to serotonin: Implications for vasospasm. Circ. Res. 61:346–351, 1987.

27. Henry P.D., Yokoyama M.: Supersensitivity of atherosclerotic rabbit aorta to ergonovine. Mediation by a serotonergic mechanism. J. Clin. Invest. 66:306–313, 1980.

28. Hodgson J.M., Marshall J.J.: Direct vaso-

constriction and endothelium-dependent vasodilation; mechanisms of acetylcholine effects on coronary flow and arterial diameter in patients with nonstenotic coronary arteries. Circulation 79:1043–1051, 1989.

29. Lobb R., Sasse J., Sullivan R., Shing Y., D'Amore P., Jacobs J., Klagsburn M.: Purification and characterization of heparin-binding endotheial cell growth factors. J. Biol. Chem. 261:1924–1928, 1986.

30. Ludmer P.L., Selwyn A.P., Shook T.L., Wayne R.R., Mudge G.H., Alexander R.W., Ganz P.: Paradoxical vasoconstriction induced by acetylcholine in atherosclerotic coronary arteries. N. Engl. J. Med. 315:1046–1051, 1986.

31. Martin W., Furchgott R.F., Villani G.M., Jothianandan D.: Depression of contractile responses in rat aorta by spontaneously released endothelium-derived relaxing factor. J. Pharmacol. Exp. Ther. 237:529–538, 1986.

32. Nabel E.G., Ganz P., Gordon J.B., Alexander R.W., Selwyn A.P.: Dilation of normal and constriction of atherosclerotic coronary arteries caused by the cold pressor test. Circulation 77:43–52, 1988.

33. Nabel E.G., Selwyn A.P., Ganz P.: Large coronary arteries in humans are responsive to changing blood flow: An endothelium-dependent mechanism that fails in patients with atherosclerosis. J. Am. Coll. Cardiol. 16(2):349–356, 1990.

34. Peach M.J., Loeb A.L., Singer H.A., Saye J.: Endothelium-derived vascular relaxing factor. Hypertension 7(Suppl. 1):I-94–I-100, 1985.

35. Pober J.S., Collins T., Gimbrone M.A., Libby P., Reiss C.S.: Inducible expression of class II major histocompatibility complex antigens and the immunogenicity of vascular endothelium. Transplantation 41:141–146, 1986.

36. Pohl U., Holtz J., Busse R., Bassenge E.: Crucial role of endothelium in the vasodilator response to increased flow in vivo. Hypertension 8:37–44, 1986.

37. Roberts W.C.: Morphologic cardiac findings in coronary arterial spasm. In: Coronary Artery Spasm: Pathophysiology, Diagnosis and Treatment, Conti C.R. (ed.). Marcel Dekker, New York, pp 23–47, 1986.

38. Robertson D., Robertson R.M., Nies A.S., Oates J.A., Friesinger G.C.: Variant angina pectoris: Investigation of indexes of sympathetic nervous system function. Am. J. Cardiol. 43:1080–1085, 1979.

39. Robertson R.M., Bernard Y., Robertson D.: Arterial and coronary sinus catecholamines in the course of spontaneous coronary artery spasm. Am. Heart J. 105:901–906, 1983.

40. Rubanyi G.M., Romero J.C., Vanhoutte P.M.: Flow-induced release of endothelium-derived relaxing factor. Am. J. Physiol. 250:H1145-H1149, 1986.

41. Selwyn A.P., Forse G., Fox K., Jonathan A., Stiner R.: Patterns of disturbed myocardial perfusion in patients with coronary artery disease. Circulation 64:83–90, 1981.

42. Shimokawa H., Lam J.Y.T., Chesebro J.H., Bowie E.J.W., Vanhoutte A.M.: Effects of dietary supplementation with cod-liver oil on endothelium-dependent responses in porcine coronary arteries. Circulation 76:898–905, 1987.

43. Shimokawa H., Vanhoutte A.M.: Impaired endothelium-dependent relaxation to aggregating platelets and related substances in porcine coronary arteries in hypercholesterolemia and atherosclerosis. Circ. Res. 64:900–914, 1989.

44. Sreeharan N., Jayakody R.L., Senaratne M.P.J., Thomson A.B.R., Kappagoda C.T.: Endothelium-dependent relaxation and experimental atherosclerosis in the rabbit aorta. Can. J. Physiol. Pharmacol. 64:1451–1453, 1986.

45. Treasure C.B., Vita J.A., Cox D.A., Fish R.D., Gordon J.B., Mudge G.H., Colucci W.S., St. John Sutton M.G., Selwyn A.P., Alexander R.W., Ganz P.: Endothelium-dependent dilation of the coronary microvasculature is impaired in dilated cardiomyopathy. Circulation 81:772–779, 1990.

46. Vekshtein V.I., Yeung A.C., Vita J.A., Nabel E.G., Fish R.D., Bittl J.A., Selwyn A.P., Ganz P.: Fish oil improves endothelium-dependent relaxation in patients with coronary artery disease (Abstr.) Circulation 80:II-434A, 1989.

47. Vita J.A., Treasure C.B., Nabel E.G., McLenachan J.M., Fish R.D., Yeung A.C., Vekshtein V.I., Selwyn A.P., Ganz P.: The coronary vasomotor response to acetylcholine relates to risk factors for coronary artery disease. Circulation 81:491–497, 1990.

48. Vita J.A., Treasure C.B., Fish R.D., Yeung A.C., Vekshtein V.I., Ganz P., Selwyn A.P.: Endothelial dysfunction leads to increased coronary constriction to catecholamines in patients with early atherosclerosis (Abstr.) J. Am. Coll. Cardiol. 15:158A, 1990.

49. Werns S.W., Walton J.A., Hsia H.H., Nabel E.G., Sanz M.L., Pitt B.: Evidence of en-

dothelial dysfunction in angiographically normal coronary arteries of patients with coronary artery disease. Circulation 79:287–291, 1989.

50. Weidinger F.F., McLenachan J.M., Cybulski M.I., Gordon J.B., Rennke H.G., Hollenberg N.K., Fallon J.T., Ganz P., Cooke J.P.: Persistent dysfunction of regenerated endothelium after balloon angioplasty of rabbit iliac artery. Circulation 16670–1679, 1990.

51. Yasue H., Matsuyama K., Matsuyama K., Okumara K., Morikami Y., Ogawa H.: Responses of angiographically normal human coronary arteries to intracoronary injection of acetylcholine by age and segment. Possible role of early coronary atherosclerosis. Circulation 81:482–490, 1990.

52. Zeiher A.M., Drexler H., Wollschlaeger H., Saurbier B., Just H.: Coronary vasomotion in response to sympathetic stimulation in humans: Importance of the functional integrity of the endothelium. J. Am. Coll. Cardiol. 14:1181–1190, 1989.

6

Endothelium and Cerebrovascular Diseases

J. Jeffrey Marshall, Hermes A. Kontos

Introduction

Since the discovery of endothelium-dependent relaxing factor by Furchgott in 1980,[15] investigators have demonstrated the presence of endothelium-dependent relaxation in a number of vascular beds including the cerebral circulation.[41,42,45,57,63,67,78,88,94] Endothelium-dependent dilators, such as acetylcholine, stimulate functional endothelium to produce a labile factor which rapidly diffuses into vascular smooth muscle to activate the cytosolic guanylate cyclase enzyme.[11,16,86] This enzyme hydrolyzes guanine triphosphate (GTP) to cyclic guanosine 3′,5′-monophosphate (cGMP) and the resultant increases in cGMP within vascular smooth muscle stimulate a cascade of enzymatic events that results in smooth muscle relaxation. Nitroglycerin (NTG), sodium nitroprusside (NP), and other nitrodilators elicit smooth muscle relaxation by generating the free radical nitric oxide that may directly activate the cytosolic guanylate cyclase enzyme.[7,22,37] It is therefore evident that both endothelium-dependent relaxation and vasorelaxation due to nitrodilators share a common final biochemical pathway involving activation of the soluble guanylate cyclase enzyme (Fig. 1).

The endothelium of various blood vessels has also been shown to generate endothelium-derived constricting factors (EDCF(s)),[39,44,92,99] Endothelin is a recently identified potent vasoconstrictor polypeptide derived from endothelium.[123] The purpose of this chapter is to review the data that support the role of the endothelium in the cerebral vascular circulation in health and in disease.

Endothelium-Dependent Function in Cerebral Arteries

Large Cerebral Arteries

The canine basilar artery is one of the best studied large cerebral arteries; it displays some unusual endothelium-dependent responses. It is one of a handful of

Rubanyi G.M.: Cardiovascular Significance of Endothelium-Derived Vasoactive Factors, Futura Publishing Co., Inc., Mount Kisco, NY, © 1991.

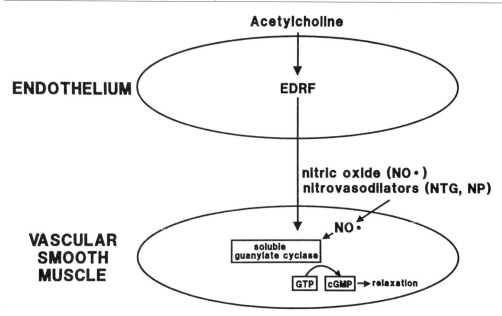

Figure 1: Mechanism of vasodilation from direct acting nitrodilators and the endothelium-dependent dilator acetylcholine. GTP = guanosine triphosphate; cGMP = cyclic 3',5'-guanosine monophosphate.

arteries that does not have muscarinic endothelium-dependent dilation.[115] Indeed, common endothelium-dependent dilators like acetylcholine, the calcium ionophore, A23187, and arachidonic acid, were shown by some to elicit constriction in the canine basilar artery.[44] Others have demonstrated endothelium-dependent dilation from A23187.[78] Despite these uncommon and variable responses, the study of endothelium-dependent dilation in the dog basilar artery has yielded a number of important observations. Most of these studies have been done in vitro, using organ chamber experiments where endothelium-dependent dilation was demonstrated by the absence of vasodilation from an endothelium-dependent agonist after the mechanical removal of the endothelium. Katusic and colleagues[42,116] have clearly shown that the canine basilar artery demonstrates endothelium-dependent dilation to vasopressin,[116] oxytocin,[41,42] and bradykinin.[41] Other large cerebral arteries have also been shown to have endothelium-dependent di-

lation. Lee showed that vasodilation of cat basilar, middle cerebral, anterior cerebral, and internal carotid arteries occurred in response to low concentrations of acetylcholine in vitro.[63] This effect could be blocked by atropine, potentiated by physostigmine, and abolished by the removal of the endothelium. In addition, he showed that high concentrations of acetylcholine caused vasoconstriction via direct action on the vascular smooth muscle. A number of others have confirmed the endothelium-dependent dilation of large cerebral arteries,[30,78] and a recent, preliminary report demonstrated endothelium-dependent dilation from acetylcholine in the rat basilar artery in situ.[13]

Endothelium-dependent constriction of large cerebral arteries has also been demonstrated in vitro. Katusic showed that isolated canine basilar arteries contracted in an endothelium-dependent fashion to acetylcholine, A23187, and arachidonic acid.[44] These contractions could be blocked with the cyclooxygenase inhibitor, indomethacin.[44] Therefore these chemical agonists generate constricting factors by activating the cyclooxygenase enzyme in the endothelium. Furthermore, the thromboxane synthetase inhibitor, dazoxiben, inhibited the endothelium-dependent contractions from the calcium ionophore and arachidonic acid.[44] Thus endothelium-dependent contractions from arachidonic acid are due to, in part, the production of thromboxane A_2. Other experiments clarify that the EDCF from A23187 in the canine basilar artery is the superoxide anion.[39] The EDCF from acetylcholine has not been identified with confidence[44] (and Katusic, personal communication).

In addition to chemical stimulators of endothelium-dependent contraction in large cerebral vessels, physical stimuli have also been shown to cause endothelium-dependent contraction. Two investigators independently showed that stretch or increased intraluminal pressure in cerebral arteries resulted in endothelium-dependent contraction. Harder,[26] studying isolated middle cerebral arteries of the cat, showed that elevation of transmural pressure resulted in electrical depolarization of vascular smooth muscle and vasoconstriction. After treatment of these vessels with collagenase and elastase, which was shown by electron microscopy to remove the endothelium, the vessels no longer contracted in response to increased transmural pressure. Katusic studied canine basilar arteries and showed that vessels with endothelium contracted when stretched, but vessels without endothelium did not.[43] This active contraction could be blocked with indomethacin or diltiazem.[43] However, neither of these two studies could distinguish between contraction from inhibition of EDRF production or contraction due to production of a constricting factor.

To differentiate between these two possibilities, bioassay experiments are necessary. Rubanyi[97] utilized a bioassay apparatus to study endothelium-dependent contraction in isolated canine carotid arteries. He found that endothelium-dependent contraction from increases in transmural pressure were due to depression or inhibition of the synthesis and release of EDRF.[97] On the other hand, Harder and his colleagues,[27] studying cat middle cerebral arteries in a bioassay system, showed that endothelium-dependent contractions from increased intraluminal pressure were due to the secretion of an endothelium-dependent constricting factor, and not a decrease in the secretion of EDRF. These divergent findings may be explained by species, vessel, and model differences. For example, tonic EDRF secretion was present in one model[97] but not in the other.[27] Thus, large cerebral arteries of a number of species have been shown to secrete both endothelium-dependent relaxing factors as well as endothelium-dependent constricting factors. It is noteworthy that there appear to be significant differences in endothelium-dependent responses between species and between specific cerebral vessels within the same species.

Cerebral Microvessels

Unlike the case with large cerebral vessels where the endothelium may be removed easily by simply rubbing the inner surface, this cannot be done easily with cerebral microvessels. In vitro experiments attempting to demonstrate endothelium-dependent dilation of cerebral microvessels have proven difficult. Dacey[8] studied isolated penetrating arteriolar branches of the middle (30–70 μm) cerebral artery in vitro. He was able to show the presence of cholinergic vasodilation after these vessels had been preconstricted. However, when attempts to remove the endothelium were made, significant alterations in muscle function occurred which prevented establishing the endothelium-dependence to this cholinergic dilation.[8] In a similar fashion, Hardebo,[24] studying medium-size cerebral arteries (150–1000 μm), found that uridine triphosphate and uridine diphosphate elicited smooth muscle relaxation of preconstricted arteries from rats and humans. Again, when attempts were made to remove the endothelium, the smooth muscle layer was damaged, as evidenced by loss in maximal constriction to direct-acting vasoconstrictors. Thus, it has been difficult to demonstrate endothelium-dependent dilation of cerebral microvessels in vitro.

Early suggestions that endothelium-dependent function was present in cerebral microvessels came from Wei and colleagues.[121] Before an episode of acute hypertension, acetylcholine caused dose-dependent relaxation of cat pial arterioles. However, after experimental hypertension, acetylcholine caused vasoconstriction.[121] Since it was shown that acute hypertension generated oxygen radicals[49,54,56] and that oxygen radicals destroyed the EDRF from large vessels in vitro,[22a,101] it was hypothesized that the dilation from acetylcholine in these microvessels was due to the release of an endothelium-dependent relaxing factor.[121]

This hypothesis was confirmed by a series of experiments performed by Rosenblum and his colleagues.[84,88,94] Rosenblum's experiments used two light and dye techniques that selectively damaged the vascular endothelium of pial arterioles. These techniques use a light source and a dye administered intravenously that can absorb the radiation of the specific light source. Two techniques were utilized: (1) ultraviolet radiation from a mercury lamp and intravenous fluorescein dye,[84,88] or (2) a helium-neon laser and intravenous Evans blue dye.[89,94] In Rosenblum's experiments, cerebral microvessels were exposed to the light/dye treatment using open cranial window techniques. At baseline, cerebral microvessels demonstrated dilation to acetylcholine, A23187, and arachidonic acid.[84,93–95] However, after dye

administration and light exposure, these microvessels constricted or showed no vasomotor response to these endothelium-dependent agonists.

On the other hand, these vessels dilated in response to topical direct acting dilators such as sodium nitroprusside[94,117] and papaverine[88] to the same extent before and after the light/dye treatment. Thus, this technique appeared to inhibit endothelium-dependent dilation selectively. Examination of vessels treated with the light/dye techniques by electron microscopy revealed selective and minimal damage to the endothelium.[83,84,94,95] The damage consisted of blebs and vacuoles on the endothelium but no endothelial denudation was seen.

Other investigators have successfully utilized this technique in other microvascular beds.[47] As of yet, the exact mechanism by which the light/dye technique prevents the action of EDRF-mediated dilation is not known. The two leading hypotheses are that the light/dye technique generates free radicals that damage the endothelium or that it produces heat that damages the endothelium, thereby preventing the generation of EDRF. Whatever the exact mechanism of the endothelial damage, it is known to be transient. Cerebral microvessels regain their normal dilator response to endothelium-dependent agonists over approximately 4 hours.[91] Another feature of this injury is the graded degree of injury along the length of the vessel. The area on the microvessel where the radiation was focused demonstrates complete loss of endothelium-dependent function, whereas areas more distant to the focal spot, in both directions, have variable responses to endothelium-dependent agonists[94] (Fig. 2). This is one of the features of this technique that has not been explained fully. One explanation might be the local release of agents, like free radicals that destroy EDRF once it is secreted. Rosenblum investigated this possibility by pretreating the pial vessels with SOD and catalase. These scav-

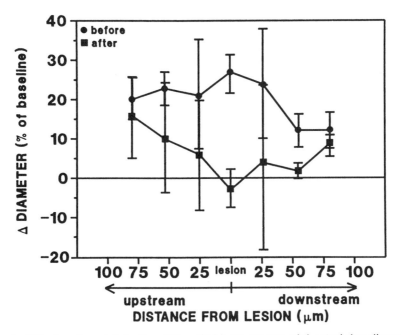

Figure 2: Effects of acetylcholine (80 μg/mL) on mouse pial arteriolar diameter at different sites along the length of a vessel before and after light/dye treatment (Luer/ Evans blue). The figure shows mean ± SD of vessel diameter as a percent of baseline induced by topical application of acetylcholine. "Lesion" is the site on the pial arteriole where the laser was focused. The responses to acetylcholine were also tested up to 80 μm upstream and downstream from the site of endothelial lesion. Each pair of points represents cumulative data from five mice.

engers did not restore the loss of endothelium-dependent function from the vessels treated with the light/dye technique (Rosenblum, personnel communication). Another possibility is the release of EDCF(s). Another concern regarding this technique is that the EDRF from acetylcholine is known to be a very diffusible substance.[57] It is therefore puzzling why EDRF secreted from adjacent segments of the vessel does not diffuse into the area damaged by the light/dye technique to elicit relaxation. This could be easily explained if smooth muscle damage occurred at the site of the injury. However, this has been excluded by the normal response to direct-acting vasodilators and extensive electron microscopy in these vessels.[94] Thus, no satisfying explanation for these features has been found yet.

Another aspect of the light/dye technique that deserves further investigation is the fact that this technique causes sustained dilation of the irradiated microvessels in some species. This varies among the diffrent species in which the technique is utilized. In the cat, illumination of microvessels with the mercury light, after the injection of fluorescein, produces sustained dilation. In the rat, however, the cremaster microvessels dilated initially in response to the light and dye, but this dilation subsided over a period of time.[47] In mice no dilation occurs in most cases. The etiology of this prolonged dilation in some species is unknown. However, knowledge of this prolonged dilation must be considered when making conclusions regarding endothelium-dependent function using this technique.

Finally, most studies that have been done with the light/dye technique utilize single doses of endothelium-dependent agonists instead of dose-response curves. Using single doses of agonists could create the situation where one agonist appears to be blocked when in actuality it is simply on a different part of the dose-response curve when compared to a direct-acting agonist. Results such as these are most likely to occur with the endothelium-dependent agonist that have direct-acting vasoconstrictor effects, as is the case with acetylcholine.[14]

We have recently used a bioassay technique to study endothelium-dependent relaxation from acetylcholine in the cerebral microcirculation of the cat in vivo.[57] We were able to show the generation of a transferable labile EDRF. The technique uses two symmetrically placed cranial windows installed over adjacent parietal cortices of a single animal. One window (the assay window) is subjected to muscarinic blockade by the topical application of atropine. This inhibits any direct effects of acetylcholine. The other window (donor window) is then superfused with cerebrospinal fluid containing acetylcholine. This superfusate is then pulsed to the assay window by either a long route of 2 minutes transit time, or a short route with a transit time of 6 seconds. Using this technique, we have shown that acetylcholine generates a short-lived factor that can be transferred from the donor window to the assay window when the transit time of 6 seconds is selected.[57] However, the factor does not survive the 2-minute transit time when superfusion is performed through the long route. Properties of this short-lived factor from acetylcholine are shown in Table 1. These properties are similar to the properties of the EDRF from acetylcholine in in vitro studies, except that SOD fails to prolong the half-life of EDRF in vivo. This difference can be easily explained by the fact that there is no baseline superoxide generation in the cerebral microcirculation in

Table 1.

Properties of EDRF Generated by Acetylcholine in Cerebral Microvessels of the Cat

Microvessels of the Cat
1. Destroyed by extending transit time to 2 minutes
2. Release prevented by blocking muscarinic receptors with atropine
3. Vasodilator action blocked by methylene blue or by hemoglobin
4. Destroyed by oxygen radical-generating agents or interventions
5. Unaffected by superoxide dismutase

vivo.[56,121] This is not the case in vitro, where a number of investigators have shown that oxygen radicals are produced under baseline in in vitro experimental conditions.[22a,101] Therefore, this difference is an expected one.

Some hypothetical shortcomings of this technique deserve mention. It has recently been shown that EDRF-like material can be secreted from glutaminergic neurons in brain tissue,[19] and thus EDRF produced in the in vivo bioassay could conceivably originate from neuronal sources. This is not the case in this system. We have shown that the EDRF from acetylcholine in the cerebral microcirculation has a vascular origin. First, perturbations that have purely vascular effects, such as acute hypertension,[54,56,121] inhibit the generation of EDRF from acetylcholine. Additionally, in chronically instrumented, conscious rabbit, topical application of acetylcholine on the surface of the brain causes no perceptible change in the behavior or motor function of the animal; thus these neurons are not activated by acetylcholine (unpublished observations).

Oxygen radicals are well known to inhibit endothelium-dependent dilation in vitro[22a,100,101] and in vivo.[67] Therefore, systems that generate oxygen radicals are often utilized as EDRF antagonists and such studies further support the presence of EDRF in the cerebral microcirculation. A variety of techniques have been used including topical arachidonic acid,[55,59] topical methylene blue,[67] and topical hemoglobin.[66] In addition, the pathophysiological interventions of hypertension,[54,70,121] fluid-percussion brain injury,[119] and ischemia and reperfusion[53] have also been utilized. These techniques demonstrate two mechanisms that interfere with endothelium-dependent dilation. The first involves direct injury to the endothelium with inability to generate EDRF. This is the case with high concentrations of topically applied arachidonic acid.[59] Endothelium-dependent dilation from acetylcholine is abolished following pretreatment with arachidonate, and bioassay experiments demonstrate a lack of EDRF generation.[59] Yet these vessels dilate when cross-perfused with fluid containing EDRF from another bioassay source.[59] This indicates that the vascular smooth muscle can respond normally to EDRF. It was shown that high concentrations of arachidonic acid generate superoxide anion within endothelial cells of the cerebral microcirculation.[55] Superoxide so produced can then escape, through the anion channel, into the CSF where hydroxyl radicals are generated via the iron catalyzed Haber-Weiss reaction.[23] Topical application of arachidonic acid was shown to damage endothelium by electron microscopy.[55] Thus, arachidonic acid inhibits endothelium-dependent dilation by damaging the endothelium through an oxygen radical-dependent process and this prevents the generation of EDRF. The second mechanism by which radicals inhibit endothelium-dependent dilation is by destruction of EDRF after its generation and secretion from histologically and functionally normal endothelium. This is the case with hemoglobin[66] and methylene blue[67] in the cerebral microcirculation. Methylene blue[2,67] and hemoglobin[71] are known to generate oxygen radicals by autoxidation. Simultaneous application of either hemo-globin or methylene blue with acetylcholine results in blockade of the vasodilation usually elicited from acetylcholine in cat pial arterioles.[66,67] However, when hemoglobin or methylene blue are flushed from the window, the dilation from topical acetylcholine is restored. Pretreatment or simultaneous treatment with SOD and catalase, or the iron chelator, deferoxamine, restores the dilation to acetylcholine despite the presence of hemoglobin or methylene blue.[66,67] These data indicate that methylene blue and hemoglobin do not damage the endothelium, but instead block the acetylcholine-mediated dilation instantaneously by the generation of free radicals that oxidize EDRF before it can activate the soluble guanylate cyclase enzyme. Additionally, since SOD and catalase are large molecules, thereby unable to gain quick access to intracellular domains, it is safe to assume that methylene blue and hemoglobin are producing the putative oxygen radicals that interact with EDRF extracellularly.

Topical hydrogen peroxide can work by either of these two mechanisms depending on the concentration and the duration of exposure selected.[118] Three micromolar hydrogen peroxide abolishes the response to acetylcholine, and EDRF generation is not detected by bioassay. Treatment of the vessels with SOD and catalase does not restore endothelium-dependent dilation.[118] However, after exposure of the vessels to 1 μM hydrogen peroxide, the vasodilation to acetylcholine is eliminated but can be restored in the presence of SOD and catalase. Thus, with hydrogen peroxide, high dose oxidant damage permanently impairs the ability of the endothelium to generate and secrete EDRF, whereas a lower dose of oxidant destroys the secreted EDRF.[118]

It is important to note that the radical-mediated mechanisms by which some of these agents inhibit endothelium-dependent relaxation depend on the experimental conditions of the preparation used. For instance, methylene blue is known to inhibit activation of the isolated soluble guanylate cyclase enzyme in isolated enzyme systems. In vitro isolated vessel studies demonstrate that methylene blue may partially work through this mechanism. If this were the exclusive mechanism by which methylene blue inhibited vasodilation in vitro, one would expect equivalent blockade of nitrodilator and endothelium-dependent agonist induced-dilation. This, however, is not the case. Martin[68] and Ignarro[32] have documented the superior ability of methylene blue to block acetylcholine-mediated dilation compared to the dilation induced by nitrodilators. In Martin's in vitro experiments, it took a three-to sixfold increase in pretreatment time in order to partially inhibit nitroglycerin induced dilation, whereas, acetylcholine-mediated dilation was completely abolished with the minimal incubation time.[68] Ignarro showed that pretreatment of bovine pulmonary arteries, for 15 minutes with methylene blue, abolished acetylcholine-mediated relaxation, but only partially inhibited the relaxation from nitroglycerin or sodium nitroprusside.[32] Martin proposed that methylene blue could have a direct inhibitory action on EDRF as well an inhibitory action on the guanylate cyclase enzyme.[68] In the cerebral microcirculation of the cat, in vivo, methylene blue selectively blocks acetylcholine-mediated dilation but has no effect on the dilation from nitroglycerin, sodium nitroprusside or nitric oxide.[67] If the permeability of the vascular smooth muscle is increased in the microvessels by pretreatment with a detergent, sodium dodecyl sulfate,[12] then methylene blue can enter the smooth muscle cells and can inhibit the guanylate cyclase enzyme (unpublished observations). Under these conditions, the effect of nitrodilators and acetylcholine are inhibited but the effect of adenosine which causes dilation via adenylate cyclase is unaffected (unpublished observations). Therefore, one important variable that may determine

the mechanism of action of different radical-generating agents is cellular permeability. The differences between the in vivo and in vitro actions of methylene blue can be easily explained by the fact that permeability is increased in some in vitro preparations and allows methylene blue access to the cytosolic guanylate cyclase enzyme, whereas in vivo methylene blue is denied that access.

Chemical Nature of Endothelium-Derived Factors in the Cerebral Circulation

There have been very few studies investigating the chemical nature of EDRFs or EDCFs in the cerebral circulation. In addition, most of these studies have come from a few laboratories and thus the results have not been confirmed by a large number of investigators. Keeping this limitation in mind, we discuss below the possible identities of endothelium-derived factors in large cerebral arteries as well as in the cerebral microcirculation.

Large Cerebral Arteries

Katusic and colleagues,[45] studying the canine basilar artery in vitro, have recently gathered evidence showing that the EDRF from bradykinin has several pharmacological similarities to nitric oxide. The responses to bradykinin were similar to the responses to authentic nitric oxide when the following pharmacological inhibitors were utilized: (1) methylene blue, which is a chemical inactivator of EDRF as well as an inhibitor of the guanylate cyclase enzyme, (2) M&B 22984, an inhibitor of cyclic GMP phosphodiesterase, (3) hemoglobin, a chemical inactivator of nitric oxide, (4) superoxide dismutase and catalase, which act via enzymatic inactivation of superoxide anion and hydrogen peroxide, respectively. These studies show that the EDRF from the canine basilar artery, generated by bradykinin, was not an oxygen radical, a finding divergent from findings in the cerebral microcirculation (see the following section, *Cerebral Microvessels*). The similar responses elicited by the EDRF from bradykinin and authentic nitric oxide in the presence of these pharmacological inhibitors suggest that the EDRF from bradykinin, in the canine basilar artery, may be nitric oxide or a nitric oxide containing compound.[45] Furthermore, preliminary data from Katusic indicates that the endothelium-dependent nitric oxide produced is probably dependent on an arginine-containing pathway since the arginine biosynthesis inhibitor L-N^G-monomethyl arginine inhibits the actions of EDRF in this preparation.[40] Several authors have studied endothelium-dependent contraction in cerebral arteries. They have found that the endothelium-dependent contractions from a number of chemical or physical stimuli are inhibited by indomethacin or other cyclooxygenase inhibitors. Attempts at identifying this EDCF by bioassay have failed to demonstrate a transferable factor (Katusic, unpublished observations). In the canine basilar artery, the calcium ionophore A23817 caused dose-dependent contractions in vessels with endothelium.[39,44] These endothelium-dependent contractions could be inhibited with SOD (150 U/mL) but not by catalase or desferoxamine.[39] The interpretation of these data are complicated by the fact that the calcium ionophore was also shown to increase the production of vasoactive prostanoids including 6-keto PGF$_{1\alpha}$ (stable metabolite of prostacyclin), PGF$_{2\alpha}$, PGE$_2$ and thromboxane B$_2$ (stable metabolite of thromboxane A$_2$). However, SOD and catalase did not reduce the increased production of these prostanoids when stimulated with A23187 and endothelium-dependent contraction was unaffected.[39]

This strongly suggests that one of the endothelium-derived constricting factors is the superoxide anion. The origin of this superoxide is likely to be the hydroperoxidase activity of prostaglandin synthetase since EDCF activity could be blocked with indomethacin.[39,44] It has been shown in vitro that the hydroperoxidase activity of cyclooxygenase is a potent generator of superoxide anions.[61] Others have suggested that endothelium-dependent constriction from arachidonic acid and PGH$_2$ is due to vasoconstrictor prostaglandins.[111] Still others have suggested that endothelium-dependent contraction from acetylcholine and arachidonic acid is mediated by thromboxane A$_2$.[107] Thus, in canine cerebral arteries, there are divergent findings regarding the identity of endothelium-derived constricting factor(s) which could easily be explained by the existence of multiple EDCFs.

Cerebral Microvessels

Endothelium-dependent dilation from acetylcholine and bradykinin in the cerebral microcirculation is mediated by different EDRFs. The separate identities of these two EDRFs are fairly well established. The evidence that supports the distinct chemical nature of these two EDRFs and the identity of the EDRF from bradykinin are presented below. Dilation from acetylcholine is not affected by indomethacin[60] whereas this cyclooxygenase inhibitor abolishes the dilation from bradykinin.[55] Superoxide dismutase plus catalase has no effect on the dilation from acetylcholine[55] whereas the dilation from bradykinin is completely inhibited by these enzymes.[55] This demonstrates that the EDRF from bradykinin in the cerebral microcirculation must be an oxygen radical. The iron chelator deferoxamine has no effect on the dilation from acetylcholine; however, the dilation from bradykinin is partially inhibited in the cat[122] and completely inhibited in mice.[90] This suggests that the EDRF from bradykinin is the hydroxyl radical which is formed from the iron catalyzed Haber-Weiss reaction from precursor superoxide anion and hydrogen. 3-Aminotriazole, which inhibits superoxide production from the cyclooxygenase enzyme by combining with the intermediate radical form of the enzyme, has no effect on the dilation elicited by acetylcholine.[58] 3-Aminotriazole, however, abolishes the dilation from bradykinin.[58] In bioassay experiments, the EDRF from acetylcholine is easily transferable from the donor to the assay window, when the 6-second transit time is used, but the EDRF from bradykinin does not survive transfer via the same 6 second route. This would be expected if the EDRF from bradykinin is an oxygen radical which is too short-lived to survive the 6-second transit time.[60] Finally, co-application of bradykinin and acetylcholine have no effect on the caliber of the cerebral microcirculation whereas individual application of these agonists causes reproducible vasodilation.[60] This would be the expected result if bradykinin produced hydroxyl radical which inactivates the EDRF from acetylcholine. These data strongly suggest that bradykinin induces the production of an oxygen radical via cyclooxygenase-mediated metabolism of arachidonic acid. Specifically, this oxygen radical is most likely the hydroxyl radical. Similar conclusions can be made from Rosenblum's data in the cerebral microcirculation of the mouse.[90]

Strong evidence exists to support the hypothesis that the EDRF generated by acetylcholine in isolated large blood vessels is nitric oxide. This is supported by pharmacological similarities between EDRF and nitric oxide;[18,33,34] by similar effects of inhibition by hemoglobin and methylene blue on nitric oxide and EDRF; by the demonstration of the release of nitric oxide from endothelial cells by a chemiluminescent assay;[79] and by inhibition of the production of EDRF and nitric oxide from precursor arginine by L-N[G]-monomethyl arginine.[87]

Other recent data have suggested that EDRF and nitric oxide may not be identical. These studies have shown that the amount of nitric oxide released from isolated vessels by acetylcholine is not sufficient to account for the observed vasodilation.[72] Others have identified pharmacological differences between nitric oxide from the EDRF from acetylcholine[4,64,106]; still others have been unable to find a release of nitric oxide using electron spin resonance techniques.[103] Thus, there is skepticism concerning the true identity of EDRF from acetylcholine.[114] This has prompted some to suggest that EDRF from acetylcholine may be a nitric oxide-containing compound such as a nitrosothiol.[73,118] We have recently collected data that would suggest that the EDRF in the cerebral microcirculation is a nitrosothiol. The following data support this suggestion. Topical methylene blue and hemoglobin abolish the dilator action of acetylcholine in the cerebral microcirculation. However, these agents have no effect on the vasodilation elicited by nitroglycerin, sodium nitroprusside, or authentic nitric oxide.[67] On the other hand, nitroblue tetrazolium blocks the vasodilation from nitroglycerin, sodium nitroprusside, and nitric oxide, but it has no effect on the vasodilation from acetylcholine.[67] This shows that the EDRF from acetylcholine is not nitric oxide. Since nitroblue tetrazolium interacts with thiol groups,[10] we proposed that nitroblue tetrazolium inhibited the dilation from nitrodilators by oxidizing necessary sulfhydryl groups in the vascular smooth muscle.[67] The sulfydryl requirement for nitrodilator activation has been proposed by Needleman[75,76] and by Ignarro.[31] Their data show that nitrodilators must interact with reduced thiols in order to generate nitrosothiols that are the direct activators of the soluble guanylate cyclase enzyme. Thus by oxidizing a critical sulfhydryl pool, all nitrodilators dependent on sulfhydryl groups for activation can be inhibited by a sulfhydryoxidizing agent. Data utilizing hydrogen peroxide in low concentrations also support the hypothesis that the EDRF from acetylcholine in the cerebral microcirculation of cats is a nitrosothiol.[118.] Hydrogen peroxide is also capable of oxidizing reduced sulfhydryl groups, but because of its molecular size and its lipid solubility, it can penetrate the cell membrane with greater ease and presumably enter both endothelial cells and vascular smooth muscle. Topical application of 1 μM hydrogen peroxide abolishes the response to acetylcholine.[118] Bioassay experiments demonstrate an absence of EDRF production.[118] Similarly, the dilator responses to sodium nitroprusside and nitric oxide were also blocked, as would be expected, if the hydrogen peroxide oxidized the thiols in vascular smooth muscle. The dilation from L-cysteine-S-nitrosothiol applied topically or from EDRF from another source was unaffected by pretreatment of pial arterioles with hydrogen peroxide.[118] These data suggest that the EDRF from acetylcholine in the cerebral microcirculation is a nitrosothiol.

Rosenblum and colleagues have recently demonstrated endothelium-dependent constriction in mouse cerebral arterioles in situ. They showed that constrictor responses from serotonin and arachidonic acid were abolished after the endothelium was damaged with a light and dye technique.[92] The light/dye technique did not alter the expected direct constrictor response from acetylcholine following endothelial damage, thus the smooth muscle was undamaged. Additionally, the cyclooxygenase inhibitors acetylsalicylic acid and indomethacin blocked the endothelium-dependent contractions to serotonin and arachidonic acid when the endothelium was intact.[92] These data show that the endothelium-dependent constriction from serotonin is mediated by arachidonic acid release from endothelial cells with subsequent cyclooxygenase-dependent vasoconstricting prostanoid production.

Rosenblum has also shown that a single vasoactive agonist can produce either vasodilation or vasoconstriction depending on a balance between simultaneous release of an endothelium-derived constricting factor and a direct smooth muscle relaxing action. This is the case with histamine in the cerebral microcirculation of the mouse.[96] High doses of histamine applied topically produced constriction that was converted to dilation when selective endothelial injury was produced from a light/dye technique. The constriction was also abolished by either H_1 blockers or by the cyclooxygenase inhibitor indomethacin.[86] Thus, histamine can stimulate endothelial cells via an H_1 receptor to produce a vasoconstrictor prostanoid. On the other hand, H_2 blockade inhibited the relaxation seen when a low dose of histamine was applied to the pial arterioles. Thus a direct smooth muscle relaxing action of histamine is mediated by an H_2 receptor on the vascular smooth muscle. Therefore, the available data suggest that there are multiple endothelium-dependent vasoactive factors present in the cerebral vascular bed and that the distribution of these factors may be dependent on the anatomic location within the vascular bed.

Physiological Significance of Endothelium-Derived Factors in the Cerebral Circulation

We discuss below possible contributions that endothelium-derived factors may have in the regulation of cerebral vascular tone and hence in the control of blood flow to the brain. Some important mechanisms which mediate physiological adjustment in blood flow are known not to be mediated by endothelium-dependent function. For example, vasodilation in response to hypercapnia is endothelium-independent.[112] Also, changes in blood flow in response to increased metabolic demands of the brain parenchyma appear to be mediated by adenosine,[104] an endothelium-independent dilator.

The resting tone of cerebral vessels depends on a complex balance between a number of vasoconstrictor and vasodilator substances. In many in vitro studies of peripheral arteries, the presence of basal EDRF secretion is a usual occurrence.[20,102] But in vitro studies with cerebral vessels have given divergent results on basal EDRF secretion. Harder and colleagues,[27] studying the middle cerebral arteries of cat, showed that basal EDRF secretion was absent by bioassay. On the other hand, Rubanyi,[97] studying the canine carotid artery, showed the presence of EDRF secretion under baseline conditions. In the cerebral microcirculation of the cat, basal secretion of EDRF is absent by bioassay[57] and known inhibitors of EDRF fail to cause vasoconstriction.[67] Thus, in large cerebral vessels, basal secretion of EDRF may depend on species and specific artery differences; basal EDRF secretion has not been shown in cerebral microvessels in vivo.

Hypoxia is a profound stimulus of cerebral vasodilation. The mechanisms of these vascular responses may be numerous and include alterations in membrane hyperpolarization,[9] adenosine-dependent mechanisms,[5,81,82] changes in sodium/potassium exchange,[9] generation of cyclooxygenase and lipoxygenase products,[35,98] as well as the generation of classic endothelium-derived factors. Katusic showed anoxia-induced vasoconstriction of canine basilar arteries in vitro and augmented constriction to direct-acting agonists.[38] These contractions induced by anoxia could not be blocked with alpha-adrenergic or serotonin antagonists. Apyrase and inhibitors of cyclooxygenase also had no effect on these contractions. The anoxia-induced contractions, however, were abolished with calcium channel blockers.[38] This suggested that these contractions were dependent on the release of an EDCF which is not a product of cyclooxygenase. Pearce and colleagues[80] studied the effects of graded hypoxia on the rabbit common carotid, internal carotid, and basilar arteries in vitro. They showed that arteries denuded of endothelium displayed direct vasoconstrictor responses to hypoxia but that this was modulated by the simultaneous release of both an EDCF and an EDRF.[80] The authors noted varying ratios of EDCF to EDRF release during hypoxia among the different intracranial and cranial vessels. The balance between the release of EDCF and EDRF dictated the resultant response to the vessel during periods of hypoxia.

We have recently investigated the effects of arterial hypoxia on vasodilation in the cerebral microcirculation of the cat. We found that hypoxic vasodilation was unaffected by topical methylene blue, an agent that eliminates the EDRF from acetylcholine (unpublished observations), and thus is not mediated by the release of EDRF from acetylcholine.

Bayliss[1] first described vasoconstriction of arteries in response to increases in transmural pressure. This physiological effect, which now carries his name, is a mechanism that does rely on an intact endothelium. Katusic and colleagues[43] showed that isolated canine basilar arteries responded to stretching with development of active tension but only in rings that had an intact endothelium. Rings of basilar artery that had the endothelium removed by rubbing did not respond to stretching with vasoconstriction.[43] This development of active tension in response to stretching in vessels having an intact endothelium could be blocked with diltiazem or indomethacin. Harder,[25] studying the isolated cat middle cerebral artery in a myograph preparation, demonstrated that increases in intramural pressure resulted in vasoconstriction only if the endothelium was intact. Rubanyi[97] studied the mechanism of pressure-induced constriction in the isolated canine carotid artery with a bioassay apparatus. Elevations in transmural pressure depressed basal, acetylcholine-induced, and flow-induced effects of EDRF. In addition, methylene blue abolished the pressure-mediated constriction.[97] These data are consistent with the notion that pressure-induced vasoconstriction is mediated by a reduction in the generation of EDRF. Harder and colleagues[27] likewise investigated the mechanism of pressure-induced vasoconstriction in the middle cerebral arteries of cats. Using bioassay, they showed that these endothelium-dependent, pressure-induced vasoconstrictor responses were due to the release of a transferable endothelium-derived constricting factor.[27] Oxyhemoglobin did not alter the pressure-induced vasoconstrictor action and therefore a depression of EDRF synthesis as a mediator of this response could not be implicated.[27] From these studies, it is obvious that the endothelium plays an important role in the autoregulation of the cerebral microcirculation; however, there appear to be significant differences in the mechanisms between species and possibly between the different cerebral arteries.

In the cerebral microcirculation, autoregulatory vasodilation induced by arterial hypotension was unaffected by topical methylene blue (unpublished observations).

Pathophysiological Implications of Endothelium-Derived Factors in the Cerebral Circulation

Below we discuss the influence of the pathophysiological mechanisms of hypertension, subarachnoid hemorrhage, ischemia/reperfusion, and brain injury on endothelium-derived factors.

Hypertension

Both chronic[29] and acute[50] hypertension have been shown to cause morphological changes in cerebrovascular endothelial cells. Infusion of vasopressor drugs or fluid percussion brain injury both cause severe acute hypertension, and both have been shown to damage both the endothelium and vascular smooth muscle of cerebral vessels.[54,119,121] Following an episode of severe hypertension, pial arterioles develop pronounced and prolonged vasodilation. This vasodilation can be minimized by the topical application of superoxide dismutase and catalase.[49,54,121] Thus, hypertension causes vasodilation of the cerebral microcirculation through an oxygen radical-mediated process. The generation of superoxide in response to acute hypertension was shown by the demonstration of SOD-inhibitable reduction of nitroblue tetrazolium[121] and by histochemical techniques.[85] In addition to direct damage to cerebral microvessels, the free radicals produced by acute hypertension also have deleterious effects on cerebral vasomotor tone, mediated by the destruction of EDRF.[121] The vasodilator action of acetylcholine on the cerebral microcirculation was converted to vasoconstriction 30 minutes after an episode of severe hypertension induced by the intravenous infusion of norepinephrine. Subsequent treatment with topical SOD and catalase partially restored the acetylcholine-mediated dilation, suggesting that the oxyradicals produced from acute hypertension were destroying EDRF[121] and the direct vasoconstrictor action of acetylcholine on the vascular smooth muscle.[14] Other experiments have confirmed that hydroxyl radicals destroy the EDRF from acetylcholine in the cerebral microcirculation in the cat.[55,67,122]

Chronic hypertension is also known to elicit damage to endothelial cells. Most of the studies investigating the effects on chronic hypertension of endothelium-dependent function have been in noncerebral arteries. Results of the mechanisms of reduced endothelium-dependent function have varied. Some investigators have found that chronic hypertension results in the production of EDCFs that antagonize the effect of endothelium-dependent agonists.[65] Others have shown that the endothelium-dependent responses of vessels from chronically hypertensive animals are attenuated while effects of direct-acting agonists remain intact.[28,48,113]

Mayhan and colleagues[70] have studied endothelium-dependent dilation of pial arterioles in stroke-prone spontaneously hypertensive (SHRSP) rats. They showed that the vasodilator action of acetylcholine and methacholine were absent in SHRSP rats.[70] On the other hand, normotensive (WKY) rat cerebral microvessels dilated to these cholinergic agonists in a dose-dependent fashion.[70] The responses to adenosine and nitroglycerin, two direct-acting vasodilators were no different between WKY and SHRSP rats.[70] This suggests that the pial arterioles from chronically hypertensive rats have impaired production of EDRF. The nature of this impairment is not known with confidence. Yang has reported that the endothelium-dependent responses to bradykinin are also impaired in the chronically hypertensive rat.[124] This is important since the EDRFs from acetylcholine and bradykinin in the cerebral microcirculation are not identical.[60] Thus, chronic hypertension appears to impair the ability of the endothelium to generate EDRFs in a generalized fashion. These mechanisms may be important in the evolution of further vascular pathology that can predispose to cerebral vascular insufficiency.

Subarachnoid Hemorrhage

Subarachnoid hemorrhage following rupture of a cerebral aneurysm may lead to the life-threatening complication of cerebral vasospasm. This complication is associated with high morbidity and mortality rates. The exact mechanisms underlying vasospasm in this condition are not known with certainty. A number of mechanisms, however, have been proposed: (1) decreased production of the vasodilator prostaglandin prostacyclin;[110] (2) inactivation of sodium-potassium ATPase;[109] (3) secretion of endothelin from damaged endothelium;[36] (4) direct free radical-mediated damage of cerebral vessels;[112] (5) and hemoglobin-induced blockade of endothelium-dependent dilation.[66] Our discussion will focus on the effects of hemoglobin in the alterations in cerebral vasomotor tone.

There is evidence that free radical generation occurs in subarachnoid hemorrhage. This is supported by the fact that lipid peroxidation has been demonstrated in vasospasm associated with subarachnoid hemorrhage.[77,105,108] Also, hemoglobin is capable of producing superoxide anion by autoxidation.[71]

It is well established that hemoglobin inhibits endothelium-dependent dilation in large vessels in vitro. Furchgott had suggested that hemoglobin could interfere with endothelium-dependent relaxation and cause or potentiate vasoconstriction thus leading to cerebral vasospasm.[71] Nakogomi and colleagues[74] used a chronic model of experimental subarachnoid hemorrhage in rabbits to demonstrate impairment of endothelium-dependent vasodilation. Experimental subarachnoid hemorrhage was produced by injections of rabbit blood into the cisterna magna. Animals were then sacrificed at different times following these injections and the basilar arteries were dissected and studied in vitro. Subarachnoid hemorrhage impaired endothelium-dependent dilation from acetylcholine and adenosine triphosphate.[74] In addition, pretreatment of some of the more normal vessels with hemoglobin inhibited the vasodilation from acetylcholine in vitro.

Byrne and colleagues[6] studied the effects of subarachnoid hemorrhage on the pig cerebral circulation in vivo. Using angiographic techniques, they showed that intrathecal arteries constricted following experimental subarachnoid hemorrhage whereas extrathecal arteries retained the vasodilator action to acetylcholine.[6] The mechanisms by which hemoglobin interferes with endothelium-dependent dilation is not known with certainty. Some have suggested that the hemoglobin present in the subarachnoid space acts as a "sink" that binds the released EDRF extracellularly and promotes vasospasm.[6] Since hemoglobin is known to autooxidize and thereby generate superoxide,[71] we have recently investigated whether hemoglobin acts through oxygen radical-mediated processes to inhibit endothelium-dependent dilation. Topical applications of low doses of hemoglobin inhibited the vasodilator action of acetylcholine in the pial microcirculation of cats.[66] This low dose of hemoglobin, however, had no effect on the vasodilation from nitroglycerin, nitroprusside, or nitric oxide. Pretreatment with SOD and catalase or deferoxamine restored the vasodilator action of acetylcholine in the presence of hemoglobin.[66] This indicates that hemoglobin blocks endothelium-dependent dilation via an oxygen radical-mediated process. A higher dose of hemoglobin (50 μM) inhibited acetylcholine-mediated dilation, but this could not be reversed with radical scavenging agents. Unlike the lower dose of hemoglobin, 50 μM hemoglobin also blocked the dilation from nitrodilators.[66] This indicates that hemoglobin may have a dual mechanism of inhibiting cerebral vasodilation; an oxygen radical-mediated destruction of EDRF and an unidentified second mechanism. Investigators studying effects of hemoglobin on pig coronary arteries have also noted a dual effect of hemoglobin on vasomotor tone.[3] Thus, the free hemoglobin liberated into the cerebrospinal fluid from subarachnoid hemorrhage could at least partially mediate deleterious vasospasm through the destruction of EDRF in the cerebral circulation.

Ischemia/Reperfusion Injury

Cerebral ischemia followed by re-establishment of blood flow is known to generate oxygen radicals.[46,51,53] These radicals have been shown to cause histologic damage to cerebral endothelium,[56,120,121] to cause vasodilation[53] and hyperemia[21,62] with eventual breakdown of the blood-brain barrier.[62] The initial hyperemic phase is followed by a period of hypoperfusion. The production of free radicals during this pathophysiological process has been confirmed by: (1) the demonstration of SOD-inhibitable reduction of nitroblue tetrazolium;[53] (2) histochemical techniques that show superoxide production within cerebral microvessels;[85] and; (3) by the use of spin traps and electron spin resonance techniques.[46] Wei et al.[50] have shown that the vasodilator action of acetylcholine is abolished after ischemia/reperfusion injury in vivo. Topical SOD plus catalase or deferoxamine preserved the endothelium-dependent dilation to acetylcholine following ischemia/reperfusion injury. Endothelium-independent dilation was not affected by ischemia reperfusion.[50] Similar results have been obtained by Mayhan and colleagues.[69] The exact consequences of the loss of EDRF in ischemia/reperfusion are not known. However, the destruction of EDRF, by free radicals, during reperfusion could certainly potentiate vasoconstrictor stimuli and might serve to worsen ongoing ischemia.

Traumatic Brain Injury

It has long been documented that traumatic brain injury causes the production of oxygen radicals. The immediate mediator of the cellular damage in brain injury is the hydroxyl radical. This radical is produced through the accelerated metabolism of arachidonic acid metabolites via the cyclooxygenase enzyme [56,120] similar to what happens in acute hypertension.[54] Indeed, the pathophysiology of traumatic brain injury is linked closely to severe hypertension. If one prevents the abrupt rise in blood pressure following concussive brain injury in cats, the initial phase of this injury can be prevented.[119] Thus, traumatic brain injury results in release of arachidonic acid from cell membranes probably through the activation of kallikrein, bradykinin, and phospholipases.[52]

The free radicals so produced cause a number of pathological changes in the function of the central nervous system. Additionally, endothelium-dependent dilation to acetylcholine is abolished following fluid-percussion brain injury.[52] The vasodilation toacetylcholine can be partially restored by the topical application of free radical scavengers.[52]

Acknowledgments: Supported by grants HL 21851, HL 07580, NS19316, and NS25630 from the National Institutes of Health and by a grant from the Jeanette and Eric Lipman Foundation.

References

1. Bayliss W.M.: On the local reaction of the arterial wall to changes in internal pressure. J. Physiol. (Lond) 28:220–231, 1902.
2. Beauchamp C., Fridovich I.: Superoxide dismutase: improved usage applicable to acrylamide gels. Anal. Biochem. 44:276–287, 1971.
3. Beny J.L., Brunet P.C., Van der Bent V.: Hemoglobin causes both endothelium-dependent and endothelium-independent contraction of the pig coronary arteries, independently of an inhibition of EDRF effects. Experientia 45:132–134, 1989.
4. Berkowitz B.A., Ohlstein E.H.: Progress on the characterization and identification of endothelium-derived relaxing factor(s). Drug. Dev. Res. 7:291–297, 1986.
5. Berne R.M., Rubio R., Curnish R.R.: Release of adenosine from ischemic brain: effect on cerebral vascular resistance and incorporation into cerebral adenine nucleotides. Circ. Res. 35:262–271, 1974.
6. Byrne J.V., Griffith T.M., Edwards D.H., Harrison T.J., Johnston K.R.: Investigation of the vasconstrictor action of subarachnoid haemoglobin in pig cerebral circulation in vivo. Br. J. Pharmacol. 97:669–674, 1989.
7. Craven P.A., DeRubertis F.R.: Restoration of the responsiveness of purified guanylate cyclase to nitrosoguanidine, nitric oxide, and related activators by heme and hemoproteins. J. Biol. Chem. 253:8433–8443, 1990.
8. Dacey G. Jr., Bassett J.E.: Cholinergic vasodilation of intracerebral arterioles in rats. Am. J. Physiol. 253:H1253–H1260, 1987.
9. Detar R.: Mechanism of physiological hypoxia-induced depression of vascular smooth muscle contraction. Am. J. Physiol. 232:H761–H769, 1980.
10. Deguchi Y.A.: Histochemical method for demonstrating protein-bound sulfhydryl and disulfide groups with nitroblue tetrazolium. J. Histochem. Cytochem. 12:261–265, 1964.
11. Diamond J., Chu E.B.: Possible role for cyclic GMP in endothelium-dependent relaxation of rabbit aorta by acetylcholine. Comparison with nitroglycerine. Res. Commun. Chem. Pathol. Pharmacol. 41:369–381, 1983.
12. Ellison M.D., Povlishock J.T., Merchant R.E.: Blood-brain barrier dysfunction in cats following recombinant interleukin-2 infusion. Cancer Res. 47:5765–5770, 1987.
13. Faraci W.G., Mayhan W.G., Heistad D.D.: Endothelium-dependent responses of the basilar artery in vivo (Abstract). J. Vasc. Med. Biol. 1:85, 1989.
14. Furchgott R.F.: Role of endothelium in responses of vascular smooth muscle. Circ. Res. 53:557–573, 1983.

15. Furchgott R.F., Zawadzki J.V.: The obligatory role of endothelial cells in the relaxation of arterial smooth muscle by acetylcholine. Nature Lond. 288:373–376, 1980.
16. Furchgott R.F., Cherry P.D., Zawadzki J.V., Jothianandan D.: Endothelial cells as mediators of vasodilation of arteries. J. Cardiovasc. Pharmacol. (Suppl.)2:S336–S343, 1984.
17. Furchgott R.F., Martin W., Cherry P.D.: Blockade of endothelium-dependent vasodilation by hemoglobin: a possible factor in vasospasm associated with hemorrhage, Vol. 15. In: Advances in Prostaglandin, Thromboxane and Leukotriene Research, Hayaishi O., Yamamoto S. (eds.). Raven Press, New York, p 499–502, 1985.
18. Furchgott R.F., Khan M.T., Jothianandan D.: Comparison of endothelium dependent relaxation and nitric oxide induced relaxation in rabbit aorta (Abstract). Fed. Proc. 46:385, 1987.
19. Garthwaite J., Charles S.L., Chess-Williams R.: Endothelium-derived relaxing factor release on activation of NMDA receptors suggests role as intercellular messenger in brain. Nature 336:385–388, 1988.
20. Griffith T.M., Edwards D.H., Lewis M.J., Newby A.C., Henderson A.H.: The nature of endothelium-derived vucular relaxant factor. Nature 308:645–647, 1984.
21. Grogaard B., Schurer L., Gerdin B., Arfors K.E.: Involvement of neutrophils in the cortical blood flow impairment after cerebral ischemia in the rat; effects of antineutrophil serum and superoxide dismutase. In: Superoxide and Superoxide Dismutase in Chemistry, Rotilio G. (eds.). Elsevier Science Publishers, New York, p 608, 1986.
22. Gruetter C.A., Barry B.K., McNamara D.B., Gruetter D.Y., Kadowitz P.I., Ignarro L.J.: Relaxation of bovine coronary artery and activation of coronary arterial guanylate cyclase by nitric oxide, nitroprusside and a carcinogenic nitrosamine. J. Cyclic Nucleotide Res. 5:211–224, 1979.
22a. Gryglewski R.J., Palmer R.M.J., Moncada S.: Superoxide anion is involved in breakdown of endothelium-derived vascular relaxing factor. Nature 320:454–456, 1986.
23. Haber F., Weiss J.: The catalytic decomposition of hydrogen peroxide by iron salts. Proc. R. Soc. Lond. A 147:332–351, 1934.
24. Hardebo J.E., Kahrstrom J., Owman C., Salford L.G.: Endothelium-dependent relaxation by uridine tri- and diphosphate in isolated human pial vessels. Blood Vessels 24:150–155, 1987.
25. Harder D.R.: Pressure-dependent membrane depolarization in cat middle cerebral artery. Circ. Res. 55:197–202, 1984.
26. Harder D.R.: Pressure-induced myogenic activation of cat cerebral arteries is dependent on intact endothelium. Circ. Res. 60:120–107, 1987.
27. Harder D.R., Sanchez-Ferrer C., Kauser K., Stekiel W.J., Rubanyi G.M.: Pressure releases a transferable endothelial contractile factor in cat cerebral arteries. Circ. Res. 65:193–198, 1989.
28. Harrison D.G., Freiman P.C., Armstrong M.L., Marcus M.L., Heistad D.D.: Alterations of vascular reactivity in atherosclerosis. Circ. Res. 61(Suppl. II):II-74–II-80, 1987.
29. Hazama F., Amano S., Ozaki T.: Pathological changes of cerebral vessel endothelial cells in spontaneously hypertensive rats, with special reference to the role of these cells in the development of hypertensive cerebrovascular lesions. Adv. Neurol. 20:359–369, 1978.
30. Hongo K., Nakagomi T., Kusell N.F., Sasaki T., Lehamn M., Vollmer D.G., Tsukahara T., Ogawa H., Torner J.: Effects of aging and hypertension on endothelium-dependent vascular relaxation in rat carotid artery. Stroke 19:892–987, 1988.
31. Ignarro L.J., Lippton H.L., Edwards J.C., Baricos W.H., Hyman A.L., Kadowitz P.J., Gruetter C.A.: Mechanisms of vascular smooth muscle relaxation by organic nitrates, nitrites, sodium nitroprusside and nitric oxide evidence for involvement of S-nitrosothiols as active intermediates. J. Pharmacol. Exp. Ther. 21:739–749, 1981.
32. Ignarro L.J., Harbison R., Wood K.S., Kadowitz P.J.: Dissimilarities between methylene blue and cyanide on relaxation and cyclic GMP formation in endothelium-intact intrapulmonary artery caused by nitrogen oxide-containing vaodilators and acetylcholine. J. Pharmacol. Exp. Ther. 236:30–36, 1985.
33. Ignarro L.J., Byrns R., Wood K.S.: Pharmacological and biochemical properties of EDRF: evidence that EDRF is closely related to nitric oxide radical (Abstract). Circ. Res. 74(Suppl. II):II-287, 1986.
34. Ignarro L.J., Byrns R., Buga G.M., Wood K.S., Chaudhuri G.: Pharmacologic evidence that endothelium-derived relaxing

factor is nitric oxide: use of pyrogallol and superoxide dismutase to study endothelium-dependent and nitric oxide-elicited vascular smooth muscle relaxation. J. Pharmacol. Exp. Ther. 244:181–189, 1987.

35. Jackson W.F.: Lipoxygenase inhibitors block O_2 responses of hamster cheek pouch arterioles. Am. J. Physiol. 255:H711–H716, 1988.

36. Katsuhisa I., Yamakawa K., Nakagomi T., Sasaki T., Saito I., Kurihara H., Yosizumi M., Yazaki Y., Takakura K.: The role of endothelin in the pathogenesis of vasospasm following subarachnoid haemorrhage. Neurol. Res. 11:101–104, 1989.

37. Katsuki S., Arnold W.P., Mittal C.K., Murad F.: Stimulation of guanylate cyclase by sodium nitroprusside, nitroglycerin and nitric oxide in various tissue preparations and comparison to the effects of sodium azide and hydroxylamine. J. Cyclic Nucleotide Res. 3:23–35, 1977.

38. Katusic Z.S., Vanhoutte P.M.: Anoxic contractions in isolated canine cerebral arteries: contribution of endothelium-derived factors, metabolites of arachidonic acid, and calcium entry. J. Cardiovasc. Pharmacol. 8 (Suppl. S):S97–S101, 1986.

39. Katusic Z.S., Vanhoutte P.M.: Superoxide anion is an endothelium-derived contracting factor. Am. J. Physiol. 257:H33–H37, 1989.

40. Katusic Z.S., Vanhoutte P.M.: Endothelium-dependent contractions to N^G-monomethyl-L-arginine in the canine basilar artery (Abstract). J. Vasc. Med. Biol. 1:95, 1989.

41. Katusic Z.S., Shepherd J.T., Vanhoutte P.M.: Vasopressin causes endothelium-dependent relaxations of the canine basilar artery. Circ. Res. 55:575–579, 1984.

42. Katusic Z.S., Shepherd J.T., Vanhoutte P.M.: Oxytocin causes endothelium-dependent relaxations of canine basilar arteries by activating V_1-vaspressinergic receptors. J. Pharmacol. Exp. Ther. 236:166–170, 1986.

43. Katusic Z.S., Shepherd J.T., Vanhoutte P.M.: Endothelium-dependent contraction to stretch in canine basilar arteries. Am. J. Physiol. 252:H671–H673, 1987.

44. Katusic Z.S., Shepherd J.T., Vanhoutte P.M.: Endothelium-dependent contractions to calcium inonphore A23187, arachidonic acid, and acetylcholine in canine basilar arteries. Stroke 19:476–479, 1988.

45. Katusic Z.S., Marshall J.J., Kontos H.A., Vanhoutte P.M.: Similar responsiveness

of smooth muscle of the canine basilar artery to EDRF and nitric oxide. Am. J. Physiol. 257:H1235–H1239, 1989.

46. Kirsch J.R., Phelan A.M., Lange D.G., Traystman R.J.: Free radicals detected in brain during reperfusion from global ischemia (Abstract). Fed. Proc. 46:799, 1987.

47. Koller A., Messini E.J., Wolin M.S., Kaley G.: Endothelial impairment inhibits prostaglandin and EDRF-mediated dilation in vivo. Am. J. Physiol. 257(6, Pt. 2):H1966–H1970, 1989.

48. Konishi M., Su C.: Role of endothelium in dilator responses of spontaneously hypertensive rat arteries. Hypertension 5:881–886, 1983.

49. Kontos H.A.: Oxygen radicals in cerebral vucular injury. Circ. Res. 57:508–516, 1985.

50. Kontos H.A.: Oxygen radicals in cerebral ischemia. In: Cerebrovascular Diseases, Ginsberg M.D., Dietric W.D. (eds.). Raven Press, New York, p 365–371, 1989.

51. Kontos H.A.: Oxygen radicals in CNS damage. Chem.-Biol. Interactions 72:229–255, 1989.

52. Kontos H.A.: Oxygen radicals in experimental brain injury. In: Intracranial Pressure, Hoff J.T., Betz A.L. (eds.). Springer-Verlag, Berlin, pp 787–798, 1989.

53. Kontos H.A., Wei E.P.: Oxygen radicals in cerebral ischemia (Abstract). Physiologist 30:122, 1987.

54. Kontos H.A., Wei E.P., Dietrich W.D., Navari R.M., Povlishock J.T., Ghatak N.R., Ellis E.F., Patterson J.L. Jr.: Mechanism of cerebral arteriolar abnormalities after acute hypertension. Am. J. Physiol. 240:H51 1-H527, 1981.

55. Kontos H.A., Wei E.P., Povlishock J.T., Christman C.W.: Oxygen radicals mediate the cerebral arteriolar dilation from arachidonate and bradykinin in cats. Circ. Res. 55:295–303, 1984.

56. Kontos H.A., Wei E.P., Ellis E.F., Jenkins L.W., Povlishock J.T., Rowe G.T., Hess M.L.: Appearance of superoxide anion radical in cerebral extracellular space during increased prostaglandin synthesis in cats. Circ. Res. 57:142–151, 1985.

57. Kontos H.A., Wei E.P., Marshall J.J.: In vivo bioassay of endothelium-derived relaxing factor. Am. J. Physiol. 255:H1259–H1262, 1988.

58. Kontos H.A., Marshall J.J., Wei E.P.: Oxyradicals and endothelium-dependent dilation. In: Oxy-Radicals in Molecular Biology and Pathology, Alan R. Liss, Inc., New York, p 3–10, 1988.

59. Kontos H.A., Wei E.P., Povlishock J.T., Kukreja R.C., Hess M.L.: Inhibition by arachidonate of cerebral arteriolar dilation from acetylcholine. Am. J. Physiol. 256:H665–H671, 1989.

60. Kontos H.A., Wei E.P., Kukreja R.C., Ellis E.F., Hess M.L.: Differences in endothelium-dependent cerebral dilation by bradykinin and acetylcholine. Am. J. Physiol. 1990.

61. Kukreja R.J., Kontos H.A., Hess M.L., Ellis E.F.: PGH synthase and lipoxygenase generate superoxide in the presence of NADH or NADPH. Circ. Res. 59:612–619, 1986.

62. Kuroiwa T., Ting P., Martinez H., Klatzo I.: The biphasic opening of the blood-brain barrier to proteins following temporary middle cerebral artery occlusion. Acta Neuropathol. 68:122–125, 1985.

63. Lee T.J.: Cholinergic mechanism in the large cat cerebral artery. Circ. Res. 50:870–879, 1982.

64. Long C.J., Shikano K., Berkowitz B.A.: Anion exchange resins discriminate between nitric oxide and EDRF. Eur. J. Pharmacol. 142:317–318, 1987.

65. Lüscher T.F., Vanhoutte P.M.: Endothelium-dependent contractions to acetylcholine in the aorta of the spontaneously hypertensive rat. Hypertension 8:344–348, 1986.

66. Marshall J.J., Kontos H.A.: Independent mechanisms of blockade of endothelium-dependent and nitroprusside-induced dilation by hemoglobin (Abstract). FASEB J. 2:A710, 1988.

67. Marshall J.J., Wei E.P., Kontos H.A.: Independent blockade of cerebral vasodilation from acetylcholine and nitric oxide. Am. J. Physiol. 255:H847–H854, 1988.

68. Martin W., Villani G.M., Jothianandan D., Furchgott R.F.: Selective blockade of endothelium-dependent and glycerol trinitrate-induced relaxation by hemoglobin and by methylene blue in the rabbit aorta. J. Pharmacol. Exp. Ther. 232:708–716, 1984.

69. Mayhan W.G., Amundsen S.M., Faraci F.M., Heistad D.D.: Responses of cerebral arteries after ischemia and reperfusion in cats. Am. J. Physiol. 255:H879–H884, 1988.

70. Mayhan W.G., Faraci F.M., Heistad D.D.: Impairment of endothelium-dependent responses of cerebral arterioles in chronic hypertension. Am. J. Physiol. 253:H1435–H1440.

71. Misra H.P., Fridovlch I.: The generation of superoxide radical during the autoxidation of hemoglobin. J. Biol. Chem. 247:6960–6962, 1972.

72. Myers P.R., Guerra R. Jr., Harrison D.G.: Release of NO and EDRF from cultured bovine aortic endothelial cells. Am. J. Physiol. 256:H1030–H1037, 1989.

73. Myers P.R., Guerra R. Jr., Bates J.N., Harrison D.G.: Studies on the properties or endothelium-derived relaxing factor (EDRF), nitric oxide, and nitrosothiols: Similarities between EDRF and S-nitroso-L-cysteine (cys NO) (Abstract). J. Vasc. Med. Biol. 1:106, 1989.

74. Nakagomi T., Kassell N.F., Sasaki T., Fujiwaua S., Lehman R.M., Torner J.C.: Impairment of endothelium-dependent vasodilation induced by acetylcholine and adenosine triphosphate following experimental subarachnoid hemorrhage. Stroke 18:482–489, 1987.

75. Needleman P., Johnson E.M.: Mechanism of tolerance development to organic nitrates. J. Pharmacol. Exp. Ther. 184:709–715, 1973.

76. Needleman P., Jadschik B., Johnson E.M.: Sulfhydryl requirement for relaxation of vascular smooth muscle. J. Pharmacol. Exp. Ther. 187:324–331, 1973.

77. Ohta S., Satoh K., Kuwabara H.: Changes in concentrations in lipid peroxides and activities of their scavengers in the cerebrospinal fluid and in the basilar arteries following experimental subarachnoid hemorrhage. J. Cereb. Blood Flow Metab. 7 (Suppl. 1):S654–S659, 1987.

78. Onoue H., Nakamura H., Toda N.: Endothelium-dependent and -independent responses to vasodilators of isolated dog cerebral arteries. Stroke 19:1388–1394, 1988.

79. Palmer R.M.J., Ferrige A.G., Moncada S.: Nitric oxide release accounts for the biological activity of endothelium-derived relaxing factor. Nature 327:524–526, 1987.

80. Pearce W.J., Ashwal S., Cuevas J.: Direct effects of graded hypoxia on intact and denuded rabbit cranial arteries. Am. J. Physiol. 257:H824–H833, 1989.

81. Phillis J.W., Preston G., DeLong R.E.: Effects of anoxia on cerebral blood flow in the rat brain: evidence for a role of adenosine in autoregulation. J. Cereb. Blood Flow Metab. 4:586–592, 1984.

82. Phillis J.W., DeLong R.E., Towner J.K.: Adenosine deaminase inhibitors enhance cerebral anoxic hyperemia in the rat. J.

Cereb. Blood Flow Metab. 5:295–299, 1985.

83. Povlishock J.T., Rosenblum W.I.: Injury of brain microvessels with a helium-neon laser and Evans blue can elicit local platelet aggregation without endothelial denudation. Arch. Pathol. Lab. Med. 111:415–421, 1987.

84. Povlishock J.T., Rosenblum W.I., Sholley M.M., Wei E.P.: An ultrastructural analysis of endothlial change paralleling platelet aggregation in a light/dye model of microvascular insult. Am. J. Pathol. 110:148–160, 1983.

85. Povlishock J.T., Williams J.I., Wei E.P.: Histochemical demonstration of superoxide in cerebral vessels (Abstract). FASEB J. 2:A835, 1988.

86. Rapoport R.M., Murad F.: Agonist-induced endothelium-dependent relaxation in rat thoracic aorta may be mediated through cGMP. Circ. Res. 52:352–357, 1983.

87. Rees D.D., Palmer R.M.J., Moncada S.: Role of endothelium-derived nitric oxide in the regulation of blood pressure. Proc. Natl. Acad. Sci. USA 86:3375–3378, 1989.

88. Rosenblum W.I.: Endothelial dependent relaxation demonstrated in vivo in cerebral arterioles. Stroke 17:494–497, 1986.

89. Rosenblum W.I.: Laser and Evans blue induced endothelial injury causes focal elimination of EDRF from brain microvessels in vivo (Abstract). Fed. Proc. 45:239, 1986.

90. Rosenblum W.I.: Hydroxyl radical mediates the endothelium-dependent relaxation produced by bradykinin in mouse cerebral arterioles. Circ. Res. 61:601–603, 1987.

91. Rosenblum W.I.: Loss of endothelium-dependent relaxation in mouse cerebral microvessels may be rapidly reversible. Microvasc. Res. 35:132–138, 1988.

92. Rosenblum W.I., Nelson G.H.: Endothelium-dependent constriction demonstrated in vivo in mouse cerebral arterioles. Circ. Res. 63:837–843, 1988.

93. Rosenblum W.I., Nelson G.H.: Endothelium dependence of dilation of pial arterioles in mouse brain by calcium ionophore. Stroke 19:1379–1382, 1988.

94. Rosenblum W.I., Nelson G.H., Povlishock J.T.: Laser-induced endothelial damage inhibits endothelium-dependent relaxation in the cerebral microcirculation of the mouse. Circ. Res. 60:169–176, 1987.

95. Rosenblum W.I., Povlishock J.T., Wei E.P., Kontos H.A., Nelson G.H.: Ultra-structural studies of pial vascular endothelium following damage resulting in loss of endothelium-dependent relaxation. Stroke 18:927–931, 1987.

96. Rosenblum W.I., Nelson G.H., Weinbrecht P.: Histamine elicits competing endothelium-dependent constriction and endothelium-independent dilation in vivo in mouse cerebral arterioles. Stroke 21(2):305–309, 1990.

97. Rubanyi G.M.: Endothelium-dependent pressure-induced contraction of isolated canine carotid arteries. Am. J. Physiol. 255:H783–H788, 1988.

98. Rubanyi G.M., Paul R.J.: Two distinct effects of oxygen on vascular tone in isolated porcine coronary arteries. Circ. Res. 56:1–10, 1985.

99. Rubanyi G.M., Vanhoutte P.M.: Hypoxia releases a vasoconstrictor substance from the canine vascular endothelium. J. Physiol. (Lond) 364:45–56, 1985.

100. Rubanyi G.M., Vanhoutte P.M.: Oxygen-derived free radicals, endothelium and responsiveness of vascular smooth muscle. Am. J. Physiol. 250:H815–H821, 1986.

101. Rubanyi G.M., Vanhoutte P.M.: Superoxide anions and hyperoxia inactivate endothelium-derived relaxing factor. Am. J. Physiol. 250:H822–H827, 1986.

102. Rubanyi G.M., Lorenz R.R., Vanhoutte P.M.: Bioassay of endothelium-derived relaxing factor(s): inactivation by catecholamines. Am. J. Physiol. 249:H95–H101, 1985.

103. Rubanyi G.M., Wilcox D.E., Greenberg S.: Studies on endothelium-derived relaxing factor (EDRF) released from canine femoral arteries by acethylcholine (ACh) and its identity as nitric oxide (NO) (Abstract) J. Vasc. Med. Biol. 1:111, 1989.

104. Rubio R., Berne R.M., Brockman E.L., Curnish R.R.: Relationship between adenosine concentration and oxygen supply in rat brain. Am. J. Physiol. 228:896–902, 1975.

105. Sakaki S., Kuwabara H., Ohta S.: Biological defense mechanism in the pathogenesis of prolonged cerebral vasospasm in the patients with ruptured intracranial aneurysms. Stroke 17:196–199, 1986.

106. Shikano K., Ohlstein E.H., Berkowitz B.A.: Differential selectivity of endothelium-derived relaxing factor and nitric oxide in smooth muscle. Br. J. Pharmacol. 92:483–485, 1987.

107. Shirahase H., Usui H., Kurahashi K., Fujiwara M., Kiyoshi F.: Possible role of en-

dothelial thromboxane A_2 in the resting tone and contractile responses to acetylcholine and arachidonic acid in canine cerebral arteries. J. Cardiovasc. Pharmacol. 10:517–522, 1987.

108. Sano K., Asano T., Tanishima T., Suaki T.: Lipid peroxidation as a cause of cerebral vasospasm. Neurol. Res. 2:253–258, 1980.

109. Sugita T., Endoh S., Iwai I., Kamiyama T., Ohtuji T., Takaku A.: Pathological mechanism of experimental cerebral vasospasm induced by oxyhemoglobin. J. Cereb. Blood Flow Metab. 7 (Suppl. 1):S661–S664, 1987.

110. Toda N.: Hemolysate inhibits cerebral artery relaxation. J. Cereb. Blood Flow Metab. 8:46–53, 1988.

111. Toda N., Inoue T., Okamura T.: Endothelium-dependent and independent responses to prostaglandin H_2 and arachidonic acid in isolated dog cerebral arteries. J. Pharmacol. Exp. Ther. 244:297–302, 1988.

112. Toda N., Hatano Y., Mori K.: Mechanisms underlying response to hypercapnia and bicarbonate of isolated dog cerebral arteries. Am. J. Physiol. 257:H141–H146, 1989.

113. Van de Voorde J., Leusen I.: Endothelium-dependent and independent relaxation of aortic rings from hypertensive rats. Am. J. Physiol. 250:H711–H717, 1986.

114. Vanhoutte P.M.: The end of the quest? Nature 327:459–460, 1987.

115. Vanhoutte P.M.: Endothelium and control of vascular function. Hypertension 13:658–667, 1989.

116. Vanhoutte P.M., Katusic Z.S., Shepherd J.T.: Vasopressin induces endothelium-dependent relaxations of cerebral and coronary, but not of systemic arteries. J. Hypertens 2(Suppl. 3):421–422, 1984.

117. Watanabe M., Rosenblum W.I., Nelson G.H.: In vivo effect of methylene blue on endothelium-dependent and endothelium-independent dilations of brain microvessels in mice. Circ. Res. 62:86–90, 1988.

118. Wei E.P., Kontos H.A.: H_2O_2 and endothelium-dependent cerebral arteriolar dilation: implications for the identity of EDRF generated by acetylcholine. Hypertension 16(2):162–169, 1990.

119. Wei E.P., Dietrich W.D., Navari R.M., Kontos H.A.: Functional, morphologic, and metabolic abnormalities of cerebral microcirculation after concussive brain injury in cats. Circ. Res. 46:37–47, 1980.

120. Wei E.P., Kontos H.A., Kiil F., Povlishock J.T., Inoue T.: Inhibition by free radical scavengers and by cyclooxygenase inhibitors of pial arteriolar abnormalities from concussive brain injury in cats. Circ. Res. 48:95–103, 1981.

121. Wei E.P., Kontos H.A., Christman C.W., DeWitt D.S., Povlishock J.T.: Superoxide generation and reversal of acetylcholine-induced cerebral arteriolar dilation after acute hypertension. Circ. Res. 57:781–787, 1985.

122. Wei E.P., Povlishock J.T., Kontos H.A.: Role of hydroxyl radical in the cerebral arteriolar abnormalities from arachidonate (Abstract). Proc. Int. U. Physiol. Sci. 16:449, 1986.

123. Yanagisawa M., Kurihara H., Kimura S., Tombe Y., Kobayashi M., Mitsui Y., Yazaki Y., Goto K., Masaki T.: A novel potent vasoconstrictor peptide produced by vascular endothelial cells. Nature 332:411–415, 1988.

124. Yang S.T., Mayhan W.G., Heistad D.D.: Responses of pial arterioles to bradykinin, nitric oxide and nitroglycerin during chronic hepertension (Abstract). FASEB J. 3:A846, 1989.

7

Endothelial Control of the Pulmonary Circulation

Philip J. Kadowitz, Sidney Cassin, Dennis B. McNamara, Robert K. Minkes

Introduction

The presence of adrenergic and cholinergic vasomotor nerves and the influence of adrenergic and efferent vagal stimulation on the pulmonary vascular bed have been documented.[25,29,39,43,45,56] The pulmonary vascular beds of the cat and the dog have alpha$_1$ and postjunctional alpha$_2$ adrenoceptors mediating vasoconstriction and beta$_2$ and muscarinic receptors mediating vasodilation.[21,22,24,29] Adrenergic nerve stimulation increases pulmonary vascular resistance (PVR), and when tone is elevated and alpha receptors are blocked, nerve stimulation elicits a vasodilator response, indicating that neuronally released norepinephrine can act on beta$_2$ receptors.[25,29,39] When vascular tone is elevated by an active process, efferent vagal stimulation elicits vasodilator responses that are related to stimulus frequency.[56] The vasodilator responses to vagal stimulation and to acetylcholine injections are blocked by atropine and enhanced by physostigmine, suggesting that they are muscarinic in nature.[56] Pulmo-

nary vasodilator responses to acetylcholine are not modified by cyclooxygenase or lipoxygenase inhibitors, indicating that arachidonic acid metabolites do not play an important role in mediating or modulating vasodilator responses to acetylcholine in the pulmonary vascular bed of the cat or rabbit.[24,26] Although pulmonary vasodilator responses to acetylcholine are blocked by atropine, neither low doses of pirenzipine nor gallamine and pancuronium had an influence on these responses, suggesting that they are mediated by muscarinic receptors that are neither of the M$_1$ nor of the M$_2$ subtype.[24,26]

The mechanism by which acetylcholine relaxes vascular smooth muscle has been the subject of intense investigation in recent years.[10,11,15,68] Relaxation of isolated arterial smooth muscle by muscarinic receptor agonists is dependent on an intact endothelial cell layer.[12] The relaxation in response to acetylcholine and nitrovasodilators is associated with an increase in cGMP levels, and this effect can be blocked by methylene blue, an agent that inhibits soluble guanylate cyclase activator and prevents the rise in smooth muscle cGMP

Rubanyi G.M.: Cardiovascular Significance of Endothelium-Derived Vasoactive Factors, Futura Publishing Co., Inc., Mount Kisco, NY, © 1991.

levels.[8,14,31,32–34,48] Moreover, lipophilic analogues of cGMP have marked relaxant activity on isolated arterial vascular smooth muscle and evidence has been presented for the involvement of nitrosothiols in response to nitrovasodilators.[34,57] The vasodilator responses to acetylcholine in the feline pulmonary vascular bed can be blocked by methylene blue, suggesting that the response may be mediated by a rise in cGMP in resistance vessels, perhaps through an endothelium-dependent mechanism.[27,42] Prostacyclin (PGI$_2$) is a major product of arachidonic acid metabolism in pulmonary endothelium and has marked vasodilator activity in the lung.[19,33,38] PGI$_2$ is an endothelial-derived relaxing factor and may play an important role in maintaining the pulmonary vascular bed in a dilated state.[19,33,38] The prostaglandin precursor, arachidonic acid, is rapidly converted into vasoactive products, including prostacyclin, in the pulmonary vascular bed.[30,33,62] In addition to releasing relaxing factors, the endothelium releases contractile factors.[68] Endothelin is a peptide released from cultured endothelial cells.[73] The activities of this peptide and related peptides and their roles in physiological and pathophysiological processes are being intensively investigated at the present time. The purpose of the studies presented in this chapter is to review the role of the endothelial-derived factors in the control of the pulmonary vascular bed and to compare responses to endothelial-derived factors in the pulmonary and peripheral vascular beds.

Endothelium-Derived Vasoactive Factors in the Pulmonary Circulation

Endothelium-Derived Relaxing Factor(s)

The effects of acetylcholine on isolated ring preparations of bovine intrapulmon-

ary artery as reported by Ignarro et al.[31] are illustrated in Figure 1. When the endothelium was undamaged and the arterial rings were submaximally contracted with phenylephrine, addition of acetylcholine in the range of concentration of 10^{-9} to 10^{-6} M relaxed the artery in a concentration-dependent manner (Fig. 1). The response to acetylcholine was blocked by the addition of atropine to the bath in a concentration of 10^{-7} M, indicating that the response was mediated by muscarinic receptors (Fig. 1). The relaxant response to acetylcholine was also blocked by methylene blue, suggesting that it was mediated by activation of soluble guanylate cyclase and an elevation in smooth muscle cGMP levels.[31] The measurement of cGMP levels and the time-course of the accumulation of the cyclic nucleotide is illustrated in Figure 2. The results of these experiments show that acetylcholine elicited a time-dependent increase in cGMP levels in the bovine intrapulmonary artery ring preparations[31] (Fig. 2). The increase in intracellular cGMP levels correlated closely with the vasorelaxant response to acetylcholine (Fig. 2). The onset of the cGMP level rise preceded the onset of relaxation (Fig. 2). The studies of Ignarro et al. provide evidence in support of the hypothesis that the endothelial-dependent relaxant response to acetylcholine in the bovine intrapulmonary arterial preparation is mediated by an increase in cGMP levels in smooth muscle cells.[31]

The majority of studies on the mechanism of action of endothelium-dependent vasodilator agents has been carried out in isolated vascular smooth muscle preparations and it would be difficult technically, if not impossible, to study the role of the endothelial cell layer and of cGMP level changes in small resistance vessels that regulate tone in the vascular bed of an intact organ system. However, the discovery that methylene blue inhibited vasorelaxant responses to nitrovasodilators and acetylcholine and prevented the rise in smooth muscle cGMP levels provided a chemical

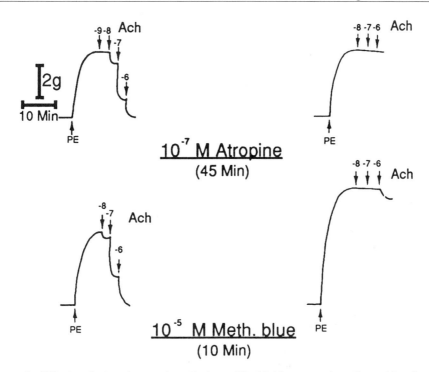

Figure 1: Effects of atropine and methylene (Meth) blue on relaxation of bovine intrapulmonary arterial rings elicited by acetylcholine (Ach). Arterial rings were isolated with an intact endothelium and after the induction of submaximal contractions with 10^{-5} M phenylephrine (PE), Ach was added in cumulatively increasing concentrations. The numbers corresponding to Ach concentrations are shown as exponents to the base power 10. Ring preparations were washed and allowed to equilibrate for 45 to 60 minutes after obtaining the tracings shown on the left-hand side of the figure. Atropine and Meth blue were then added to baths for the periods of time indicated and rings were contracted with PE followed by the addition of Ach. All concentrations are expressed as final bath concentrations. Redrawn from Ignarro et al.[31]

probe by which the mechanism of action of vasodilator agents may be approached in the intact vascular bed.[14,31–34]

In the studies of Hyman and co-workers,[27,42] vasodilator responses to acetylcholine, nitroglycerin, and isoproterenol were compared when tone in the feline pulmonary vascular bed was raised to similarly high values with U46619, a stable prostaglandin endoperoxide analogue that has marked pulmonary vasoconstrictor activity,[40] and with methylene blue.[27,42] When vascular tone was raised to a high steady value with U46619, the three vasodilator drugs caused dose-dependent decreases in lobar arterial pressure (Fig. 3).

However, when lobar arterial pressure was raised to a similarly high level by intralobar infusion of methylene blue, vasodilator responses to acetylcholine and nitroglycerin were reduced markedly (Fig. 3). The baseline levels of lobar arterial pressure attained during intralobar infusions of U46619 and methylene blue were not different, and vasodilator responses to isoproterenol were similar when vascular tone was elevated with U46619 or with methylene blue (Fig. 3). Thirty to 45 minutes after the end of the methylene blue infusion period, when tone was again raised to a high steady level with an infusion of U46619, pulmonary vasodilator

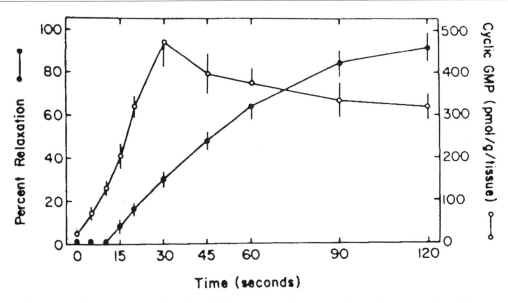

Figure 2: Time-course of cyclic GMP accumulation and relaxation in bovine intra-pulmonary arterial rings elicited by acetylcholine. Arterial rings were isolated with an intact endothelium and were submaximally contracted with 10^{-5} M phenylephrine before exposure to acetylcholine (10^{-6} M). Rings were freeze-clamped at the times indicated. Values represent the mean $\pm$ SE using 6 to 12 arterial rings isolated from three to six separate animals. Relaxation and cyclic GMP levels were determined in the same arterial rings. Relaxation is expressed as the percentage of decrease in phenylephrine-induced tone. Reprinted from Ignarro et al.[31] with permission.

responses to acetylcholine and nitroglycerin were not different from control responses (Fig. 3). In these same experiments, pulmonary vasopressor responses to angiotensin II and BAY K8644, an agent that enhances calcium entry, were compared when tone was raised with U46619 infusion and with methylene blue infusion.[27,42] There was no difference in the pressor response to angiotensin II or the calcium entry promoting agent, BAY K8644, when tone was raised with the prostaglandin endoperoxide analogue or with methylene blue (Fig. 3).

In another series of experiments using a similar experimental design, pulmonary vasodilator responses to acetylcholine, bradykinin, epinephrine, and 8-bromo-cGMP were compared when tone in the feline pulmonary vascular bed was elevated with U46619 and with methylene blue (Fig. 4). During the methylene blue infusion when lobar arterial pressure was raised to a high steady level, pulmonary vasodilator responses to acetylcholine and bradykinin were reduced markedly, whereas vasodilator responses to epinephrine and 8-bromo-cGMP were not altered.[27,42] In these studies, methylene blue infusion had no significant effect on systemic hemodynamic parameters in the cat.[27,42]

The studies of Hyman et al.[27] show that methylene blue inhibits vasodilator responses to acetylcholine, bradykinin, and nitroglycerin in the pulmonary vascular bed of the intact-chest cat. The actions of methylene blue in these studies were selective and responses to the endothelium-dependent vasodilators and nitrovasodilators were reduced by more than 50% at a time pulmonary vasodilator responses to isoproterenol, epinephrine, and the lipophilic cGMP analogue, 8-bromo-cGMP,

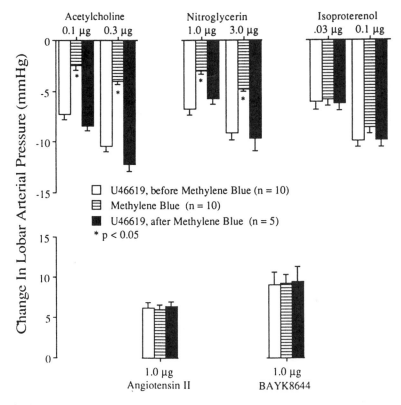

Figure 3: Upper panel: effects of methylene blue infusion on decreases in lobar arterial pressure in response to acetylcholine, nitroglycerin, and isoproterenol. Lower panel: effects of methylene blue infusion on increases in lobar arterial pressure in response to angiotensin II and BAY K8644. Responses to all pressor and depressor agents were obtained during a control period when lobar arterial pressure had been increased to approximately 30 mm Hg by intralobar infusion of U46619. The U46619 infusion was stopped and the methylene blue infusion was started. After an infusion period of 52 minutes in which the infusion rate of methylene blue was 715 μg/min and lobar arterial pressure had attained a steady value of 32 mm Hg, responses to the five agonists were again determined. The methylene blue infusion was terminated and when lobar arterial pressure had fallen to a value near baseline value, the U46619 infusion was again started. When lobar arterial pressure attained a value of 33 mm Hg, responses to the agonist were again obtained. n indicates number of animals and the asterisk indicates that responses are significantly different from control responses. Redrawn from Hyman et al.[27]

were not altered.[27] Furthermore, in these studies methylene blue had no apparent effect on pulmonary vasoconstrictor responses to the peptide hormone, angiotensin II, or the calcium entry promoting agent, BAY K8644.[27] In addition to being selective, the inhibitory effect of methylene blue in these studies was reversible and responses to the endothelium-dependent vasodilators and nitroglycerin returned to control value after the methylene blue infusion.[27] In these experiments, methylene blue increased vascular resistance in the pulmonary vascular bed of the intact-chest cat in a dose-dependent manner.[27] These data provide support for the hypothesis that the basal level of cGMP is important in maintaining the pulmonary vascular bed

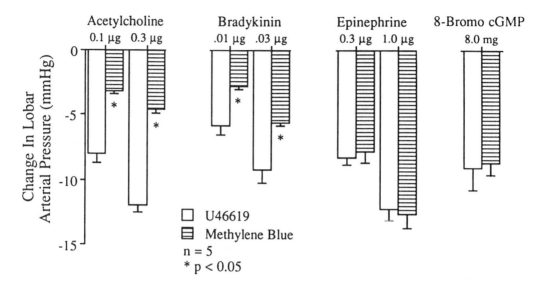

Figure 4: Effects of methylene blue infusion on decreases in lobar arterial pressure in response to acetylcholine, bradykinin, epinephrine, and 8-bromo-cGMP. Responses were compared during infusion of U46619 and during infusion of methylene blue. Responses to the four agents were determined during the control period when lobar arterial pressure had been raised to a mean value of 31 mm Hg by infusion of U46619 and 32 mm Hg 44 minutes after the onset of the methylene blue infusion at which time the final infusion rate was 530 μg/min. n indicates the number of experiments and the asterisk indicates that the responses were significantly different from control responses. Redrawn from Hyman et al.[27]

in a dilated state under resting conditions.[27]

Responses to acetylcholine in the feline pulmonary vascular bed are tone-dependent.[24] Under low resting tone conditions, acetylcholine elicited dose-dependent increases in lobar arterial pressure and lobar vascular resistance (Fig. 5). However, when tone in the pulmonary vascular bed was raised to a high steady level with U46619, injection of acetylcholine in the identical range of doses caused dose-dependent decreases in lobar vascular resistance (Fig. 5). These tone-dependent responses to acetylcholine were blocked by atropine (Fig. 5), indicating that they are mediated by muscarinic receptors.[24] The mechanism by which these novel tone-dependent responses are mediated was investigated in the intact-chest cat.[24] The increase in vascular resistance under low-tone conditions was blocked by low doses

of pirenzepine, indicating that the pressor response was mediated by a muscarinic M_1 type receptor.[24] The vasodilator responses under high-tone conditions were not blocked by low doses of pirenzepine or doses of gallamine or pancuronium up to 10 mg/kg IV.[24] These results suggest that vasodilator responses under high-tone conditions are mediated by muscarinic receptors that are neither M_1 high-affinity nor M_2 low-affinity subtype.[24] The mechanism by which acetylcholine induces vasoconstriction under low resting tone conditions has not yet been determined.[24] It is not known if this response is endothelial-dependent or is mediated by muscarinic receptors on smooth muscle cells of resistance vessels in the lung.[24] This pressor response is not blocked by cyclooxygenase or lipoxygenase inhibitors, suggesting that vasoconstrictor metabolites in the cyclooxygenase or lipoxygenase path-

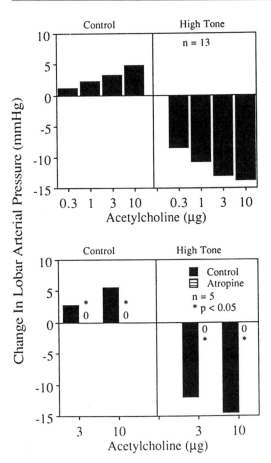

Figure 5: Upper panels: influence of the level of vasoconstrictor tone on responses to acetylcholine in feline pulmonary vascular bed. Under low resting tone (control) conditions acetylcholine in doses of 0.3–10 μg caused a dose-related increase in lobar arterial pressure. However, when the baseline level of tone was raised to a high level with U46619 infusion, acetylcholine caused marked dose-dependent decreases in lobar arterial pressure. n = number of experiments. Lower panels: effect of atropine on increases in lobar arterial pressure in response to acetylcholine under low resting tone (control) conditions and under high-tone conditions. Responses to acetylcholine are compared before and after administration of atropine, 1 mg/kg IV. n indicates number of animals; the asterisk indicates responses that were significantly different from control. Vascular tone was raised with U46619 infusion. Redrawn from Hyman and Kadowitz.[24]

way are not involved.[24] The pressor response could be dependent on the release of an EDCF. However, it is probably not an EDCF-type mediated response modified by cyclooxygenase inhibitors.[68] The question of whether the release of an endothelin-like peptide is important in the mediation of the pressor response to acetylcholine is uncertain, although endothelin (ET-1) has modest vasoconstrictor activity in the feline pulmonary vascular bed.[47,49,68]

It is unlikely that acetylcholine functions as a circulating humoral factor, since cholinesterase activity is high in plasma and tissue. However, the pulmonary vascular bed of the cat is innervated by both the sympathetic and the parasympathetic divisions of the autonomic nervous system.[25,29,39,43,45,56] Moreover, the studies of Nandiwada et al.[56] show that stimulation of the parasympathetic nerves to the lung decreases vascular resistance when vascular tone is high (Fig. 6) When tone is high and the animals are treated with 6-hydroxydopamine to destroy the integrity of the adrenergic neurons which run in the cervical vagus, efferent vagal stimulation at stimulus frequencies of 2–16 cycles/sec caused marked stimulus-related decreases in lobar arterial pressure and lobar vascular resistance (Fig. 6).[56] The dramatic pulmonary vasodilator responses to efferent vagal stimulation are blocked by atropine, indicating that they are mediated by muscarinic receptors.[56] The question of whether these vasodilator responses are endothelial-dependent cannot be answered at the present time. However, the pulmonary vascular bed is functionally innervated by the parasympathetic system, and cholinergic-like nerve terminals are present in the adventitial-medial junction of small arteries in the lung.[45,56] It seems unlikely, however, that acetylcholine could diffuse through the media and interact with muscarinic receptors on endothelial cells, although this possibility cannot be excluded.[45,56]

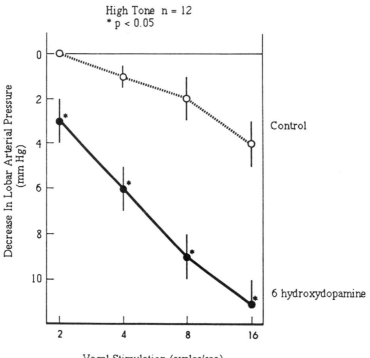

High Tone n = 12
* p < 0.05

Vagal Stimulation (cycles/sec)

Figure 6: Effects of vagal nerve stimulation on the pulmonary vascular bed of the intact-chest cat under high-tone conditions. When tone was raised to a high steady level with U46619 infusion, vagal stimulation at 2–16 cycles/sec caused a stimulus frequency-dependent decrease in lobar arterial pressure (control, open circles and broken line). In animals pretreated with 6-hydroxy-dopamine to destroy the integrity of the adrenergic nerve terminals, vagal stimulus at 2–16 cycles/sec caused significantly greater decreases in lobar arterial pressure (solid circles and line). Redrawn from Nandiwada et al.[56]

The vasodilator response to injected acetylcholine is blocked in a reversible manner by methylene blue, suggesting the involvement of a soluble guanylate cyclase cGMP-related mechanism.[27] However, the site at which exogenous acetylcholine acts to elicit vasodilation and the involvement of the endothelium are uncertain in the intact pulmonary vascular bed.[27]

Products of Arachidonic Acid Metabolism

The lung is a major organ for synthesis, release, and metabolism of products in the cyclooxygenase pathway.[15,30,65,66] The products of the cyclooxygenase pathway have marked effects on the airways and on the pulmonary vascular bed.[20,38,40,41,62,65–67] PGI_2 is a major product of arachidonic acid metabolism in endothelial cells and has marked pulmonary vasodilator and bronchodilator activity.[15,20,36,63] PGI_2, therefore, can be considered to be an endothelial-derived relaxing factor.[15] The effects of PGI_2 on the pulmonary vascular bed of the closed-chest cat have been studied by Hyman and Kadowitz[20] and are illustrated in Figure 7. Under low resting tone (control) conditions, PGI_2 decreased lobar arterial pres-

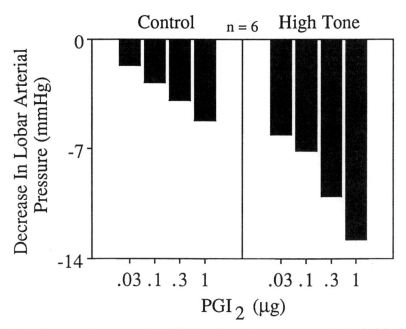

Figure 7: Influence of prostacyclin (PGI₂) on the pulmonary vascular bed of the intact-chest cat. Under low resting tone (control) conditions (left panel), intralobar injections of PGI₂ in doses of 0.03–1.0 μg caused dose-related decreases in lobar arterial pressure. When tone in the pulmonary vascular bed was raised to a high steady level (high tone) vasodilator responses to PGI₂, 0.03–1.0 μg were greatly enhanced (right panels). Redrawn from Hyman and Kadowitz.[20]

sure and lobar vascular resistance in a dose-dependent manner (Fig. 7). However, when tone was raised to a high steady value by infusion of U46619, PGI_2 caused much larger dose-dependent decreases in lobar arterial pressure (Fig. 7). PGI_2 is the only product in the cyclooxygenase pathway known to have marked vasodilator activity in the pulmonary vascular bed of the mature animal.[20,38] The effects of $PGF_{2\alpha}$, PGE_2, and endoperoxide analogue (U46619), whose actions have been shown to mimic those of thromboxane A_2, have vasoconstrictor activity in the pulmonary vascular bed of the intact-chest dog (Fig. 8) and cat.[40,41] The prostaglandin precursor, arachidonic acid, has cyclooxygenase-dependent pressor activity (Fig. 8). The endoperoxide analogue (U46619) is among the most potent pressor agents in the pulmonary vascular bed of the dog and

cat, and PGE_2 has modest pulmonary pressor activity (Fig. 8).

Endothelins

The role of the endothelium in regulating vascular tone and vasomotor responses has been intensively studied in recent years.[10,11,15,68] In addition to releasing relaxing factors, endothelial cells produce contractile factors.[13,16,73] Porcine/human endothelin has been identified as the protease-sensitive contractile substance released from cultured endothelial cells.[73] This 21 amino acid peptide containing two disulfide linkages was initially reported to possess potent contractile activity on isolated vascular smooth muscle and to cause a sustained rise in systemic arterial pres-

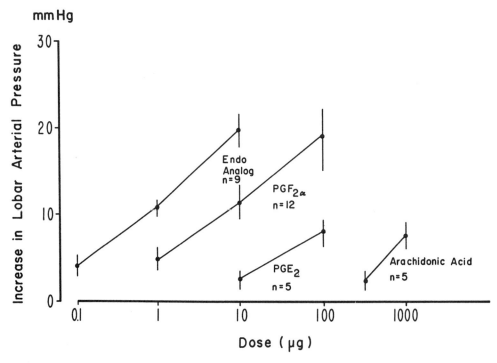

Figure 8: Comparative effects of the endoperoxide analogue (U46619), $PGF_{2\alpha}$, PGE_2, and the prostaglandin precursor, arachidonic acid, on the pulmonary vascular bed of the intact-chest dog under constant flow conditions. Redrawn from Kadowitz and Hyman.[40]

sure in the chemically denervated rat.[73] A second 21 amino acid peptide differing in six amino acid residues and possessing similar blood pressure and smooth muscle contractile activity, although less potent than porcine/human endothelin, has been discovered and was named rat endothelin.[72] It has now been established that there are three human endothelin genes and the products predicted by these genes have been designated ET-1, ET-2, and ET-3.[35]

The effects of ET-1, ET-2, and ET-3 on pulmonary vascular pressures were investigated in the cat, and responses to mid-range doses of the three peptides are illustrated in Figure 9. ET-1, ET-2, and ET-3 injections at a dose of 0.3 nmol/kg IV increased mean pressure in the pulmonary artery in the cat (Fig. 9). There were small

changes in LAP, and CO increased (Fig. 9). The changes in PVR were usually biphasic with an initial decrease in PVR, which was followed by a secondary increase in PVR (Fig. 9). The decrease in PVR was associated with an increase in CO and may be passively mediated. In contrast to the effects of ET-1, ET-2, and ET-3 on the pulmonary vascular bed, an ET-1 analogue, which has only one disulfide bridge and an amidated carboxy terminus, when injected in the cat at a dose of 30 nmol/kg IV had no significant effect on PAP, LAP, or PVR.

The mechanisms by which ET-1 changes systemic vascular resistance (SVR) and pulmonary vascular resistance (PVR) were explored in the cat. In these experiments, the role of arachidonic acid metabolites, autonomic reflexes, and activation

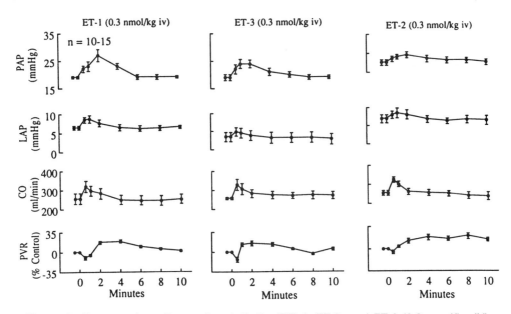

Figure 9. Comparative effects of endothelin (ET)-1, ET-2, and ET-3 (0.3 nmol/kg IV) on pulmonary arterial pressure (PAP), left atrial pressure (LAP), cardiac output (CO), and pulmonary vascular resistance (PVR) in the cat. The peptide was injected at time zero.

of beta-adrenoceptors in cardiovascular and pulmonary responses to ET-1 were investigated in three series of experiments and these data are summarized in Figure 10. In the first group of animals, the changes in SVR and PVR in response to the midrange dose of ET-1 were not modified after administration of meclofenamate, 2.5 mg/kg IV (Fig. 10). However, the fall in AP in response to the prostaglandin precursor, arachidonic acid (300 μg IV), was reduced significantly by the cyclooxygenase inhibitor (control -18 ± 2 mm Hg, meclofenamate -2 ± 1 mm Hg; n=5; p<0.05).

In the second group of animals, the effects of propranolol, 2.5 mg/kg IV, on responses to ET-1 were investigated. Propranolol significantly reduced the fall in SVR and the decrease in AP in response to isoproterenol, 0.3 μg/kg IV (control -27 ± 2 mm Hg, propranolol -2 ± 1 mm Hg; n=6; p<0.05). However, changes in SVR and PVR in response to ET-1 were not

changed after administration of the beta receptor blocking agent (Fig. 10). Although changes in SVR in response to ET-1 were not altered by propranolol, the increases in heart rate (HR) in response to the peptide were reduced significantly. In order to determine if autonomic reflexes are involved in responses to ET-1, the effects of hexamethonium were investigated in a third group of animals. The changes in SVR and PVR in response to ET-1 were not modified after administration of the ganglionic blocking agent in a dose of 5 mg/kg IV (Fig. 10). This dose of hexamethonium significantly reduced the increase in HR in response to ET-1 and blocked the increase in AP in response to bilateral carotid occlusion.

The effects of sarafotoxin 6b (S6b), a toxin in the venom of the snake, *Atractaspis engaddensis,* were also investigated in the anesthetized cat. S6b differs from ET-1 by 7 amino acid residues and is reported to be highly lethal and causes cardiac arrest and

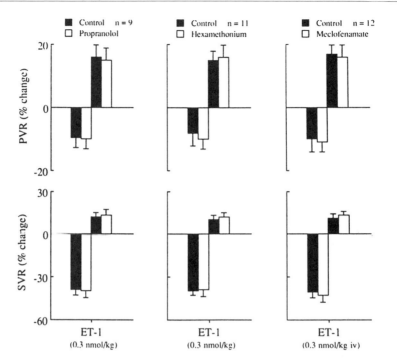

Figure 10: Influence of propranolol, hexamethonium, and meclofenamate on changes in pulmonary vascular resistance (PVR) and systemic vascular resistance (SVR) in response to the midrange dose of endothelin (ET-1) in the cat. Left panel: the response to ET-1, 0.3 nmol/kg IV, was determined before and after administration of propranolol, 2 mg/kg IV. Middle panel: responses to ET-1 were determined before and after administration of hexamethonium, 5 mg/kg. Right panel: responses to ET-1 were determined before and after sodium meclofenamate, 2.5 mg/kg IV. Redrawn from Minkes et al.[49]

death in mice within minutes of IV administration.[44] S6b at a dose of 0.3 nmol/kg IV increased pulmonary arterial pressure and produced a small increase in left atrial pressure (Fig. 11). S6b caused a significant biphasic change in calculated pulmonary vascular resistance, and systemic vascular resistance decreased (Fig. 11).

The effects of ET-1 on blood flow in the regional vascular bed of the cat were also investigated, and the effects of ET-1 on distal aortic blood flow in the cat are summarized in Figure 12. The injection of ET-1 in a dose of 0.03 nmol/kg IV caused a small but significant reduction in systemic arterial pressure and a significant increase in distal aortic blood flow (Fig. 12). Injection of ET-1 at a dose of 0.1 nmol/kg

IV caused a greater reduction in systemic arterial pressure and a larger increase in distal aortic flow than was observed at the small dose of the peptide. The increase in blood flow had a longer duration at the 0.1 nmol dose, and arterial pressure and aortic flow returned toward control value over a 2–4 minute period (Fig. 12). In contrast to responses observed at lower doses of the peptide, injection of ET-1 at a dose of 0.3 nmol/kg IV elicited biphasic changes in arterial pressure and in distal aortic flow. The initial response was characterized by a significant reduction in arterial pressure and an increase in distal aortic flow which peaked at approximately 1 minute (Fig. 12). The initial response was followed by a secondary slowly developing increase in

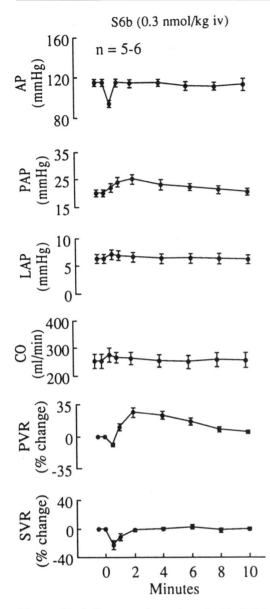

S6b (0.3 nmol/kg iv)

n = 5-6

Figure 11: Influence of sarafotoxin 6b (S6b) on arterial pressure (AP), pulmonary arterial pressure (PAP), left atrial pressure (LAP), cardiac output (CO), pulmonary vascular resistance (PVR), and systemic vascular resistance (SVR) in the cat. The peptide was injected at time zero.

arterial pressure and decrease in distal aortic blood flow. The T 1/2 of secondary changes in pressure and flow were greater than 10 minutes in duration (Fig. 12).

When blood flow to the hindquarters (distal aortic) vascular bed was maintained constant with a pump, injection of ET-1 into the perfusion circuit in a dose of 0.03 nmol caused only a reduction in perfusion pressure (Fig. 13). However, at doses of 0.1, 0.3, and 1 nmol ET-1 elicited biphasic responses that were characterized by an initial decrease in perfusion pressure which was followed by a secondary increase in pressure (Fig. 13). The secondary increase in perfusion pressure was dose-dependent (Fig. 13), and at the two higher doses studied, the T 1/2 on the secondary pressor response was greater than 10 minutes in duration. Since it has been suggested that ET-1 may act to promote calcium entry through voltage-dependent dihydropyridine-sensitive channels, the effects of the calcium entry blocking agent nisoldipine on the pressor component of the response to the 1 nmol dose of ET-1 was investigated. Injections of ET-1 (1 nmol) and BAY K8644 (3 μg), a nifedipine analogue that promotes calcium entry through voltage-dependent channels, both increased hindquarters perfusion pressure, and responses to both agents were reduced significantly during infusion of nisoldipine, 1 μg/min, into the hindquarters vascular bed (Fig. 14). Pressor responses to endothelin and BAY K8644 returned toward control value 60 minutes after the termination of the infusion of the dihydropyridine calcium entry blocking agent (Fig. 14). In other experiments, the pressor component of the response to ET-1 was compared with responses to angiotensin II and neuropeptide Y in order to determine relative pressor activity.[53] When increases in hindquarters perfusion pressure in response to the three peptides were compared on a nanomole basis, angiotensin II was more potent than ET-1 by a factor of about 10, whereas ET-1 was more potent than neu-

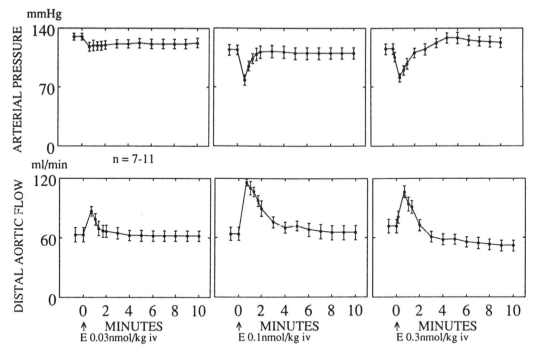

Figure 12: Influence of IV injections of endothelin-1 (E) on arterial pressure and distal aortic blood flow in the cat. The peptide was injected at time zero. The peak changes in arterial pressure and blood flow were statistically significant; n = number of cats. Reprinted from Minkes et al.[53] with permission.

ropeptide Y by a factor of approximately 3 (Fig. 15).

These results show that porcine/human endothelin (ET-1) elicits vasodepressor or biphasic changes in systemic arterial pressure in the anesthetized cat. The characteristics of the response to this novel peptide were dependent on dose, and at doses of 0.03 and 0.1 nmol/kg IV, the decreases in systemic arterial pressure in response to ET-1 were associated with increases in distal aortic blood flow. At the highest dose studied, ET-1 elicited a biphasic response characterized by an initial vasodepressor response that was associated with an increase in blood flow, which was followed by a slowly developing, long duration increase in arterial pressure and a sustained decrease in distal aortic flow. The effects of ET-1 on systemic arterial pressure in the cat differ markedly from

those reported in the rat, where the peptide elicited a marked and sustained rise in arterial pressure when injected in a dose of 1 nmol/kg IV.[73] The reason for the difference in the cat and in the rat were uncertain but may be related to species, dose, or the fact that the rat was pretreated with blocking agents.[53,73] At the two lower doses studied, ET-1 increased distal aortic blood flow by 44% and 82%. The increases in aortic blood flow occurred at a time systemic arterial pressure was decreased and indicate that ET-1 has marked vasodilator activity in resistance vessels of the distal aortic vascular bed of the cat.[53] The mechanism by which ET-1 elicits vasodilation is uncertain, but this response could still be elicited when blood flow was maintained constant and the hindquarters vascular bed was denervated.[53] Moreover, when blood flow was maintained constant, bi-

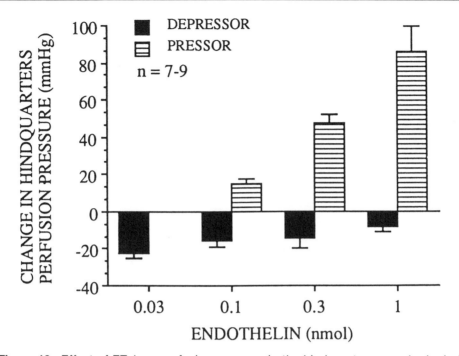

Figure 13: Effect of ET-1 on perfusion pressure in the hindquarters vascular bed of the cat. The peptide was injected into the perfusion circuit in doses of 0.03–1.0 nmol. At the 0.03 nmol dose, only a depressor response was observed, whereas at doses of 0.1–1.0, nmol biphasic responses were observed. The depressor and the biphasic responses were significant. n indicates number of animals. Reprinted from Minkes et al.[53] with permission.

phasic responses with a substantial pressor component could be demonstrated at higher doses of the peptide. The observation that pressor and depressor responses could be elicited in preparations in which the sympathetic pathways were interrupted suggests that these responses were for the most part not dependent on neurogenic mechanisms and were not reflex in origin.[53]

In terms of relative activity in the distal aortic vascular bed, when compared with other peptides, angiotensin II was tenfold more potent than ET-1 whereas ET-1 was approximately threefold more potent than neuropeptide Y.[53] The relative potency of the pressor effects of ET-1 is different in the hindquarters vascular bed and in isolated porcine coronary artery where the EC_{50} for the peptide was found to be at least one order of magnitude lower than

the reported value for angiotensin II, vasopressin, or neuropeptide Y.[73] The reason for the differences in potency in isolated coronary arteries and in the hindquarters vascular bed is uncertain but may reflect differences in species or differences between large arteries and resistance vessel elements which respond to ET-1 in the hindquarters vascular bed in vivo. In the hindquarters vascular bed, the vasoconstrictor component of the response to ET-1 was inhibited by nisoldipine, a dihydropyridine calcium entry blocking agent, and the inhibitory effects of nisoldipine on responses to ET-1 and to BAY K8644 were similar. Since BAY K8644 enhances calcium entry through voltage-dependent calcium channels, the observation that nisoldipine blocks pressor responses to ET-1 and BAY K8644 in a parallel manner may suggest that ET-1 in high doses increases

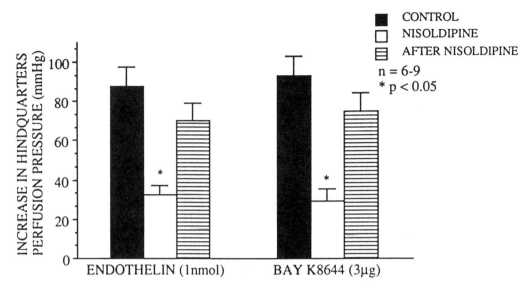

Figure 14: Comparative effects of the calcium entry antagonist, nisoldipine, on the pressor component of the hindquarters response to the 1 nmol dose of ET-1 and to BAY K8644, 3 μg, an agent that promotes calcium entry. Responses to ET-1 and BAY K8644 were determined before and during infusion of nisoldipine and again 60 minutes after the termination of the nisoldipine infusion. n indicates number of animals and the asterisk indicates that responses are significantly different from control responses. Reprinted from Minkes et al.[53] with permission.

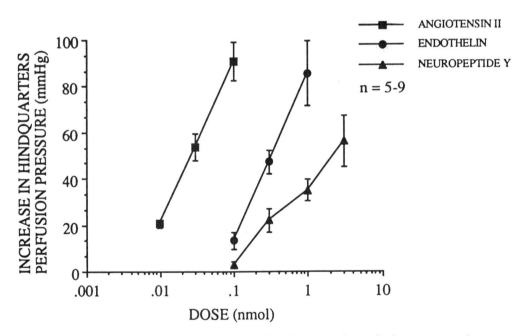

Figure 15: Dose-response curves comparing increases in perfusion pressure in response to human angiotensin II, porcine/human endothelin, and human neuropeptide Y in the hindquarters vascular bed. Only the pressor component of the response to ET-1 was analyzed, and doses of the three peptides were expressed on a nanomole basis. n indicates number of animals. Reprinted from Minkes et al.[53] with permission.

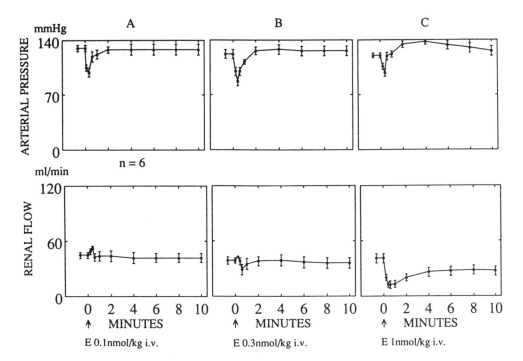

Figure 16: Effects of human/porcine endothelin (E) on arterial pressure and renal blood flow in the cat. ET-1 was injected in doses of 0.1 nmol/kg IV (A), 0.3 nmol/kg IV (B), and 1 nmol/kg IV (C) in the cat. Reprinted from Minkes and Kadowitz[51] with permission.

vascular resistance in the distal aortic bed by a mechanism that involves enhanced calcium entry. The present data with nisoldipine are consistent with previous studies with nicarpidine in isolated arterial smooth muscle and support the concept that ET-1 enhances calcium entry through dihydropyridine-sensitive calcium channels.[53,73]

The effects of ET-1 on renal and superior mesenteric arterial blood flow were also investigated in the anesthetized cat. Injection of the peptide in a dose of 0.1 nmol/kg IV caused a significant decrease in arterial pressure and a small but significant increase in renal blood flow (Fig. 16). The increase in blood flow was transient (T 1/2 <1 min), and systemic arterial pressure returned to control value over a 2- to 3-minute period. When injected at a dose

of 0.3 nmol/kg IV, ET-1 caused a significant fall in arterial pressure and a significant decrease in renal blood flow (Fig. 16). Both parameters returned rapidly to control value, and a small increase in pressure was observed 4 minutes after the injection.[51] Administration of ET-1 at a dose of 1 nmol/ kg IV caused a biphasic change in mean arterial pressure and a marked sustained decrease (T 1/2 >30 min) in renal blood flow (Fig. 16). The change in arterial pressure was characterized by an initial short-lived fall (T 1/2 <1 min) followed by a sustained increase (T 1/2 >10 min) (Fig. 16).[51]

In experiments in which mesenteric blood flow was measured, the peptide, in doses of 0.1–1.0 nmol/kg IV, elicited similar changes in arterial pressure as observed in studies with the renal vascular bed. However, injections of ET-1 at 0.1,

0.3, and 1 nmol/kg IV caused only decreases in blood flow in the superior mesenteric artery (Fig. 17). The decreases in mesenteric blood flow were dose-related and had T 1/2s ranging from 12 to 40 minutes and in some experiments at the 1 nmol/kg IV dose, blood flow did not return to baseline value.

In five other animals, the effects of ET-1 on carotid blood flow were measured, and injection of the peptide in doses of 0.1, 0.3, and 1 nmol/kg IV caused only increases in blood flow. The increases in flow averaged 26 ± 6, 36 ± 7, and 49 ± 9% at the three doses, and blood flow returned to control value over a 45-second to 2-minute period. Baseline flow averaged 40 ± 6 mL/min in the carotid artery.[51]

These experiments in the anesthetized cat demonstrate that ET-1 causes a decrease or a biphasic change in mean arterial pressure.[51,53] At the 0.1 nmol/kg IV dose, the effects of ET-1 on renal and mesenteric blood flow were different, and at this dose, the peptide caused a transient increase in renal blood flow. The increase in flow occurred at a time when arterial pressure was decreased and renal vascular resistance fell by 32%. In contrast, only a reduction in blood flow in the superior mesenteric artery was observed in response to the low dose of the peptide and mesenteric vascular resistance increased by 35%. At the 0.3 nmol/kg IV dose, the peptide decreased both renal and mesenteric blood flow.[51] However, the fall in arterial pressure was greater than the fall in renal flow so that renal vascular resistance was not increased. In contrast, the fall in mesenteric blood flow at the 0.3 nmol/kg dose was greater than the fall in arterial pressure and mesenteric vascular resistance was in-

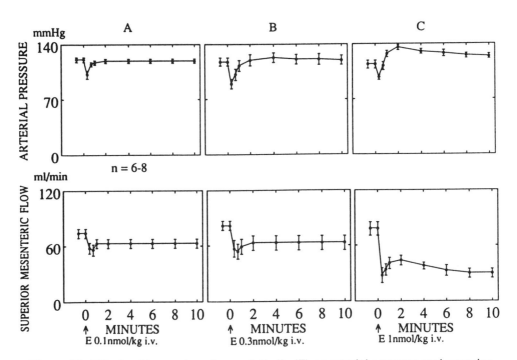

Figure 17: Effects of human/porcine endothelin (E) on arterial pressure and superior mesenteric blood flow in the cat. ET-1 was injected in doses of 0.1 nmol/kg IV (A), 0.3 nmol/kg IV (B), and 1 nmol/kg IV (C) in the cat. Reprinted from Minkes and Kadowitz[51] with permission.

creased. The reduction in blood flow in the superior mesenteric artery in response to the 0.3 nmol/kg dose was sustained. At the 1 nmol/kg IV dose of the peptide, both renal and mesenteric flows were decreased markedly, and these responses were long-lived with T 1/2s greater than 35 minutes.[51] Ten minutes after administration of the peptide at the 1 nmol/kg dose when blood flow was at a steady state, renal vascular resistance was increased by 60% whereas mesenteric vascular resistance was increased by 190%. In the carotid vascular bed, only increases in blood flow and decreases in vascular resistance were observed in response to ET-1.

The present data are consistent with previous studies and support the concept that ET-1 can act as both an endothelial-derived vasodilator hormone and as a vasoconstrictor hormone. This concept differs from the notion that the novel endothelial-derived peptide is one of the most potent vasoconstrictor substances known.[73] The present data, along with results from other studies, suggest that the dose used and the regional vascular bed studied are important determinants of the vascular response to ET-1.[49-53,71]

The effects of ET-3 on regional blood flow in the cat were investigated and these data are summarized in Figure 18. Injection of ET-3 in doses of 0.1, 0.3, and 1 nmol/kg IV caused dose-related decreases in arterial pressure (Fig. 18). The peak decrease occurred within 20–30 seconds and pressure returned to control value over a 2- to 6-minute period. The fall in arterial pres-

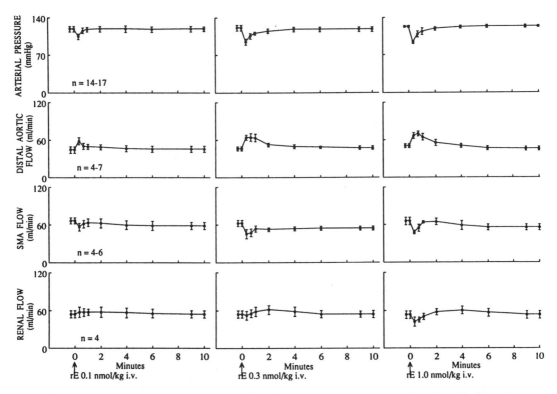

Figure 18. Influence of rat endothelin (rE) on arterial pressure, distal aortic blood flow, superior mesenteric (SMA) blood flow, and renal blood flow in the anesthetized cat. Rat endothelin (ET-3) was injected in doses of 0.1, 0.3, and 1 nmol/kg IV at the arrow (time zero). Reprinted from Minkes and Kadowitz[52] with permission.

sure was associated with a significant increase in distal aortic blood flow and a significant reduction in distal aortic vascular resistance (Fig. 18). Blood flow in the distal aorta returned to control value over a 2- to 4-minute period (Fig. 18). A small but significant secondary reduction in distal aortic flow and an increase in distal aortic vascular resistance were observed 10 minutes after administration of the 1 nmol/kg dose (Fig. 18). Although ET-3 in doses of 0.1 and 0.3 nmol/kg IV increased blood flow in the distal aorta, blood flow in the superior mesenteric artery was decreased in response to the three doses of ET-3 (Fig. 18). Since decreases in pressure were proportionally less than decreases in flow, mesenteric vascular resistance increased significantly at doses of 0.1–1.0 nmol/kg IV of the peptide. In the renal vascular bed, changes in blood flow were biphasic at the 0.3 and 1 nmol/kg IV doses of the rat peptide (Fig. 18). Renal vascular resistance was decreased in response to the 0.1 and 0.3 nmol/kg IV doses and was changed in a biphasic manner at the high dose. At the 1 nmol dose, the fall in renal resistance was followed by a secondary increase in resistance which occurred 4 minutes after injection of ET-3.[52]

These results show that ET-3 in doses of 0.1–1.0 nmol/kg IV decreased arterial pressure in the anesthetized cat. The reductions in arterial pressure were associated with regional changes in blood flow and vascular resistance that were dependent on the vascular bed studied and to a lesser extent on the dose administered. The decreases in arterial pressure were associated with increases in blood flow and decreases in resistance in vascular beds supplied by the distal aorta. A small secondary slowly developing increase in vascular resistance was observed in response to the 1 nmol/kg IV dose of the peptide in the hindquarters vascular bed. These data suggest that vasodilation is a predominant response to ET-3 in vascular beds supplied

by the distal aorta, and responses to ET-3 and ET-1 are quite similar with the exception that ET-1 is about three- to tenfold more potent than ET-3. In the mesenteric vascular bed, only decreases in blood flow and increases in vascular resistance were observed. These data suggest that ET-3 has modest vasoconstrictor activity in the mesenteric vascular bed when injected in doses of 0.1–1.0 nmol/kg IV in the anesthetized cat.

The response to ET-3 was either vasodilator or biphasic in the renal vascular bed.[52] At the low dose, a small increase in blood flow and a significant decrease in vascular resistance was observed, whereas at the 0.3 nmol/kg IV dose, an initial reduction in resistance was followed by a secondary reduction in renal resistance which occurred 2 minutes after the injection. At the high dose, the initial fall in resistance was followed by a small secondary increase in renal resistance. The present data indicate that vascular responses to ET-3 are dependent on the vascular bed studied and to a lesser extent on dose when injected IV in the cat. These results are consistent with studies in the spontaneously hypertensive rat and cat where responses to ET-1 are dependent on the dose and the vascular bed studied.[51,71]

The effects of ET-1 were investigated in the pulmonary circulation of fetal sheep under conditions in which blood flow was maintained constant with a pump.[4] In the fetal (high tone) state, injections of ET-1 in doses of 100, 300, and 1000 ng decreased perfusion pressure and pulmonary vascular resistance when the lungs were ventilated with N_2 (Fig. 19). However, when the lung was ventilated with 93% O_2 and 7% CO_2 and vascular resistance decreased, the vasodilator response to the 300 ng dose of ET-1 was greatly diminished and at doses of 1000 and 3000 ng, significant increases in pulmonary vascular resistance were observed (Fig. 19).

The studies with endothelin isopep-

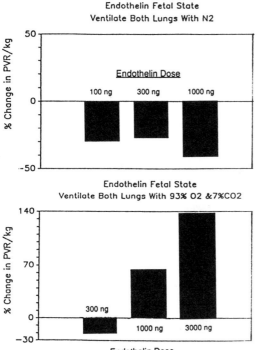

Figure 19: Comparison of effects of ET-1 during ventilation with nitrogen (upper panel) and during ventilation with 93% O_2 and 7% CO_2 (lower panel) in the sheep fetal pulmonary vascular bed. Injection of ET-1, 100, 300, and 1000 ng during ventilation with N_2 caused decreases in pulmonary vascular resistance (upper panel). Injection of ET-1, 300 ng, during ventilation with 93% O_2/7% CO_2, caused a small vasodepressor response and injection of 1000 and 3000 ng caused a marked pressor response (lower panel). Redrawn from Cassin et al.[4]

tides show that these endothelial-derived substances have significant activity in the pulmonary circulation of the adult cat and the fetal sheep and both vasodilator and vasoconstrictor responses have been observed.[47,49] However, the role these peptides play in the regulation of the pulmonary vascular bed under physiological and pathophysiological conditions has not yet been determined, although pathophysiol-

ogical stimuli, such as thrombin infusion, release an ET-like peptide from the lung.[54]

Physiological Significance

Alveolar Hypoxia-Induced Pulmonary Vasoconstriction

Although the rise in pulmonary artery pressure in response to alveolar hypoxia originally documented by von Euler and Liljestrand in 1946 has been extensively studied, the mechanism by which the hypoxic stimulus induces pulmonary hypertension remains unknown.[18,19] Moreover, it is uncertain whether the effects of oxygen deficit are due to a direct action on pulmonary arterial smooth muscle cells or to an effect on other cell types in the lung, including the endothelium, which could result in the release of vasoconstrictor factor(s) EDCFs or decreased release of an EDRF.[1-3,18,19,37,59] A number of putative mediators for the response to alveolar hypoxia have been proposed, including histamine and the leukotrienes; however, none have stood the test of time. Recent work suggests that cGMP may play a role in regulating vascular tone and mediating vascular responses in arterial smooth muscle preparations from the pulmonary and systemic vascular beds.[1,2,8,14,31-34] Most studies on the role of cGMP have been carried out in isolated arterial smooth muscle preparations, and it would be technically difficult to investigate the role of cGMP level changes in small resistance vessels in an intact vascular bed. The observation that methylene blue inhibits soluble guanylate cyclase, prevents the rise in cGMP, and blocks relaxant responses to nitrovasodilators and acetylcholine in arterial smooth muscle preparations provides a means by which the role of cGMP can be assessed in the intact vascular bed.[14,31-34]

Studies in isolated bovine intrapulmonary arteries have shown that hypoxia increases tone in serotonin precontracted vessels and that the response to hypoxia is associated with a reduction in arterial cGMP levels.[1,2] In those studies, the increase in tone in response to hypoxia was reduced by methylene blue.[1,2]

The effects of methylene blue on pulmonary vascular responses to hypoxia and to pressor agents were investigated in a recent study in the pulmonary vascular bed of the intact-chest cat.[23] Responses to ventilatory hypoxia were compared when pulmonary vascular tone was elevated to similar high steady levels with U46619 infusion and with methylene blue infusion.[23] When lobar arterial pressure was increased to a high steady level with infusion of U46619, ventilation with a hypoxic gas mixture caused a significant increase in lobar arterial pressure.[23] After the hypoxic challenge, the cat was again ventilated with an enriched O_2 mixture and pulmonary vascular resistance returned to baseline level.[23] When lobar arterial pressure was raised to a high steady level by methylene blue infusion, the pressor response to hypoxia was reversed and a vasodilator response was observed.[23] The results of these studies show that methylene blue blocks the increase in lobar arterial pressure and pulmonary lobar vascular resistance in response to alveolar hypoxia in the cat and can be interpreted to suggest a relationship between cGMP levels and the pulmonary hypertensive response to hypoxia in the cat.[23]

Published studies in isolated arterial smooth muscle preparations from various organ systems have shown that vasorelaxation in response to nitrogen oxide-containing vasodilators and endothelium-dependent vasodilator agents is associated with a rise in vascular cGMP levels.[8,14,31–34] These findings have led to the hypothesis that cGMP may have an important role in mediating vasodilator responses to endothelium-dependent and nitrogen oxide-containing vasodilator agents.[8,14,31–34] If this hypothesis regarding the role of cGMP is correct, then agents that inhibit guanylate cyclase activation and prevent the increase in vascular cGMP levels should block responses to vasodilator agents that are thought to act by way of this mechanism.[14] In this regard, methylene blue and hemoglobin inhibit the activation of soluble guanylate cyclase by nitrogen oxide-containing and endothelium-dependent vasodilators and block relaxant responses to these agents in isolated arterial smooth muscle preparations.[8,14,31–34,48] Moreover, hemoglobin has been shown to block vasodilator responses to acetylcholine in blood-free lungs of rabbits perfused with Krebs solution, and methylene blue has been shown to reduce vasodilator responses to endothelium-dependent vasodilators and nitroprusside in mouse brain microvessels.[5,70] Moreover, recent studies have shown that methylene blue blocks in a reversible and selective manner vasodilator responses to acetylcholine, bradykinin, and nitroglycerin in the pulmonary vascular bed of the intact-chest cat.[27,42] Methylene blue has been shown to reduce basal vascular cGMP levels, increase tone in isolated intrapulmonary vessels, and increase vascular resistance in a reversible manner in the pulmonary vascular bed of the intact-chest cat.[27,31–34,42]

In isolated bovine intrapulmonary arteries precontracted with serotonin, hypoxia causes a further increase in tone that is associated with a decrease in vascular cGMP levels.[1,2] The increase in isometric force and the decrease in cGMP levels were reduced by methylene blue.[1,2] These data suggest that a reduction in cGMP levels may mediate the force increase in response to hypoxia in isolated intrapulmonary arteries.[1,2] Studies in the cat showing that methylene blue increases vascular tone and blocks the hypoxic pressor response provide support for the hypothesis that changes in cGMP levels may be involved in the response to alveolar hypoxia.[1,2,23,27]

Pathophysiological Significance of Endothelium-Derived Vasoactive Factors in the Control of Pulmonary Circulation

The pulmonary vascular bed was considered to be regulated in a passive manner by changes in blood flow, pulmonary arterial pressure, left atrial pressure, and transpulmonary pressure.[28] However, observations made as early as 1896 suggested that mechanisms are available to permit active regulation of the lesser circulation.[9] It is now known that the pulmonary vascular bed can be regulated by changes in alveolar and mixed venous PO_2, by the autonomic nervous system, and by humoral factors, including the prostaglandins.[18,19,28,30,41] The pulmonary vascular bed is innervated by both the sympathetic and the parasympathetic divisions of the autonomic nervous system.[25,29,39,43,45,56] Resistance vessels, elements that regulate vasomotor tone and responses, possess alpha$_1$ and postjunctional alpha$_2$ receptors mediating vasoconstriction and beta$_2$ and muscarinic receptors mediating vasodilation.[21,22,24,29] Although the autonomic nervous system possesses the ability to regulate vasomotor tone in the pulmonary circulation, the physiological role of the nervous system in regulating this bed is uncertain.[28] Activation of the sympathetic nerves at stimulus frequencies as high as 30 Hz can bring about increases in pulmonary vascular resistance in the range of about 50%.[25,39] Moreover, administration of large doses of norepinephrine brings about similar changes suggesting that the number of alpha receptors on small resistance vessels is limited.[21,46] Although the range of response to sympathetic stimulation is relatively modest, humoral factors can bring about large changes in pulmonary vascular resistance.[40,41]

Arachidonic Acid Metabolites

Of the humoral factors, none are more potent than the prostaglandins and arachidonic acid is rapidly converted into vasoactive products in the lung.[40,41] The prostaglandin endoperoxide analogue, U46619, which is known to mimic the actions of thromboxane A_2, can in low doses cause large increases in pulmonary vascular resistance.[40,41] Thromboxane is released in the lung in a variety of pathophysiological conditions, including adult respiratory distress syndrome and pulmonary embolism.[67] PGI_2 is formed by vascular endothelium and has marked pulmonary vasodilator activity and bronchodilator activity.[20,38,63] It is quite possible that tonic release of PGI_2 from the pulmonary endothelium may also serve to maintain the pulmonary vascular bed in a dilated state, since cyclooxygenase inhibitors increase pulmonary vascular resistance.[20,38]

In regard to the relative importance of regulatory mechanisms in the pulmonary circulation, none is more important than the response of the pulmonary circulation to changes in alveolar and mixed venous PO_2, since without this mechanism, ventilation and perfusion could not be matched and arterial desaturation would result.[15,16] Tone in the pulmonary vascular bed can be altered by changes in alveolar-capillary PO_2 and in mixed venous PO_2.[18,19] The mechanism by which changes in alveolar-capillary and mixed venous PO_2 regulate pulmonary vascular tone is not well understood but may involve changes in cGMP levels.[18,19]

Endothelium-Derived Relaxing Factors and Cyclic GMP

The role of the endothelium in the regulation of vascular tone and vasomotor responses has been extensively investigated, since the discovery of Furchgott and Za- wadzki in 1980 that relaxation of rabbit aor- tic smooth muscle in response to acetyl- choline is endothelium-dependent.[12] It is now clear that the endothelium possesses the ability to modulate the extent of con- traction of underlying vascular smooth muscle.[10,11,15,68] This modulation involves the release of short-lived factors from en- dothelial cells and there are factors that promote relaxation (EDRFs) and factors that promote contraction (EDCFs).[10,11,15,68] While it seems clear that endothelial-de- rived factors have a profound effect on iso- lated arterial and venous smooth muscle preparations, particularly those derived from large conduit vessels, less is known about the regulation of small resistance vessels in the intact vascular bed by en- dothelial-dependent mechanisms.[10,11,15,68] Endothelium-derived relaxing factor (EDRF) stimulates guanylate cyclase of vascular tissue which increases cGMP lev- els and results in relaxation of vascular smooth muscle.[31-34] There is good evi- dence that EDRF is nitric oxide.[68] The rise in cGMP in isolated arterial smooth muscle preparations in response to nitrogen oxide- containing vasodilators (nitroglycerin, ni- troprusside) and endothelial-dependent vasodilators (acetylcholine, bradykinin) can be blocked with methylene blue.[14,31-34] The finding of Gruetter and co-workers in 1980 that methylene blue inhibits coronary arterial relaxation and guanylate cyclase activation by nitrogen oxide-containing va- sodilators has provided a useful probe for the study of cGMP-mediated vasodilator mechanisms.[14] Since it would be techni- cally difficult if not impossible to physically denude the endothelial lining of resistance vessels and still maintain normal barrier function without causing pulmonary edema, the use of methylene blue has ob- vious advantages.[23,27,43] In addition, it would be difficult if not impossible to har- vest small resistance vessels from the intact vascular bed and make meaningful mea-

surements of arterial smooth muscle cGMP levels.[23,27,42] Methylene blue has been used to study the role of cGMP in mediat- ing responses to acetylcholine, bradykinin, and nitroprusside in mouse brain micro- vessels using a cranial window tech- nique.[70] These studies showed that meth- ylene blue inhibited responses to acetyl- choline, bradykinin, and nitroprusside without altering responses to 8-bromo- cGMP.[70]

The effects of methylene blue on va- sodilator responses to endothelial-depen- dent and nonendothelial-dependent va- sodilators were investigated in the pul- monary vascular bed of the intact-chest cat.[23,27,42] These studies showed that methylene blue inhibits pulmonary vaso- dilator responses to acetylcholine, bradyk- inin, and nitroglycerin in the cat.[27,42] The inhibitory effects of methylene blue were selective and responses to the endothe- lium-dependent vasodilators and nitro- glycerin were significantly reduced at a time vasodilator responses to isoproter- enol, epinephrine, and 8-bromo-cGMP were not changed.[27,42] In these experi- ments, methylene blue had no effect on pulmonary vasoconstrictor responses to angiotensin II or the calcium entry pro- moting agent, BAY K8644.[27,42] The inhib- itory effects of methylene blue were re- versible and responses to the endothelium- dependent vasodilators and nitroglycerin returned to control levels 30–45 minutes after the end of the methylene blue infu- sion.[27,42] Studies in isolated pulmonary vessels have shown that relaxation in re- sponse to nitrogen oxide-containing or ni- trovasodilators and endothelium-depen- dent vasodilators is associated with a rise in cGMP levels.[8,31-34] If cGMP mediates re- laxant responses elicited by endothelium- dependent vasodilators and nitroglycerin, then agents that inhibit guanylate cyclase activation should block these vasodilator responses.[8,14,31-34] Methylene blue and hemoglobin inhibit guanylate cyclase activation by endothelial-dependent vaso-dilators and nitroglycerin.[14,48] Further-more, hemoglobin has been shown to in-hibit vasodilator responses to acetylcholine in the lungs of rabbits perfused with Krebs solution, and methylene blue has been shown to reduce vasodilator responses to endothelium-dependent vasodilators and nitroprusside in brain microvessels of the mouse.[5,70]

The finding that responses to endo-thelial-dependent vasodilators and nitro-glycerin are reduced by about 50% may be interpreted to suggest that other mecha-nisms may also be involved in the vaso-dilator response.[27,42] The experiments of Hyman et al.[27,42] provide support for the hypothesis that cGMP may be involved in mediation of vasodilator responses in small resistance vessels that regulate va-somotor tone and responses in the intact pulmonary vascular bed. Although meth-ylene blue infusion increases pulmonary lobar vascular resistance in a dose-depen-dent manner, systemic arterial pressure was not changed in these experiments in the cat.[27,42] These results indicate that basal levels of cGMP may be important in the regulation of vascular tone in the pul-monary vascular bed under baseline (nor-mal resting tone) conditions. Thus the lev-els of vascular tone and cGMP may be in-versely related as they appear to be in isolated intrapulmonary arteries.[27,31–34,42] Moreover, when methylene inhibits guan-ylate cyclase and cGMP levels fall, pul-monary vascular resistance would be ex-pected to rise, and it does in the cat.[27,42] Experiments in isolated intrapulmonary vessels and in the intact-chest cat provide strong evidence in support of this hypoth-esis.[27,31–34,42] The mechanism by which cGMP levels are regulated by changes in O_2 tension in pulmonary vascular smooth muscle have been intensively investigated by Burke-Wolin and Wolin.[1,2] Precon-tracted arterial smooth muscle prepara-tions display a decrease in isometric force with increasing O_2 tension that is antago-nized by way of an inhibition of soluble guanylate cyclase activation with methyl-ene blue.[1,2] The O_2 tension-dependent re-laxation is associated with an increase in intracellular H_2O_2 metabolism through cat-alase.[1,2] This work suggests that an acti-vation of soluble guanylate cyclase involv-ing the metabolism of H_2O_2 by catalase ap-pears to function as an O_2 tension sensor in pulmonary arterial smooth muscle.[1,2] The mechanism by which changes in O_2 tension are sensed in the intact pulmonary vascular bed is uncertain. However, ex-periments in the intact-chest cat show that the increase in pulmonary vascular resis-tance in response to alveolar hypoxia is prevented by methylene blue, suggesting that the response may involve a reduction in cGMP levels in resistance vessels.[23]

The role of the endothelium in the re-sponse to hypoxia is uncertain. In the stud-ies of Burke-Wolin and Wolin[1,2] an in-crease in force in serotonin precontracted bovine intrapulmonary arteries could be elicited by a reduction in O_2 tension in ves-sels without an intact endothelial cell layer. However, the hypoxic contractions of rat and porcine pulmonary arteries are depen-dent on the presence of an intact endothe-lium.[37,59] These observations, along with recently published work in the rabbit pul-monary artery, suggest that an inhibition of basal EDRF production may be part of the mechanism by which hypoxia induces contraction in isolated pulmonary arter-ies.[3,37,39] In most studies in isolated pul-monary vessels and in the intact-chest cat, responses to hypoxia are blocked by meth-ylene blue, suggesting that a guanylate cy-clase mechanism is involved.[1,2,23,37,39] The mechanism by which guanylate cyclase ac-tivity is reduced by hypoxia remains to be elicited and future studies will have to de-termine whether a reduction in EDRF re-lease or another mechanism, perhaps on smooth muscle as postulated by Burke-Wolin and Wolin, is responsible.[1,2]

Endothelium-Derived Contracting Factors and Endothelins

Two types of endothelium-dependent contractions have been postulated.[10,11,15,68] One type of endothelial-dependent contractile response appears to involve the release of superoxide anion and is dependent on the release of an arachidonic acid metabolite, and the other type may involve the release of a vasoconstrictor peptide such as ET-1.[68] ET-1 is released from endothelial cells in culture by hypoxia and has marked contractile activity in isolated vascular smooth muscle preparations.[73] However, responses to ET-1 are complex in the pulmonary and peripheral vascular beds.[47,49,53,71] ET-1 has moderate pressor activity in the pulmonary vascular bed of the cat,[47,49] and it is tempting to speculate that this peptide may be released by alveolar hypoxia and may mediate the increase in pulmonary vascular resistance with hypoxia. The observation that removal of the endothelial cell layer reduces the response to hypoxia in isolated vessels provides evidence in support of a role for the peptide.[37,59] However, the finding that methylene blue blocks responses to hypoxia in isolated vessels and in the intact-chest cat is not consistent with the involvement of ET-1 in hypoxic pulmonary vasoconstriction.[23,35,59] Moreover, the finding that ET-1 has marked vasodilator activity in the pulmonary vascular bed of the fetal lamb argues against its role as a mediator of hypoxic vasoconstriction in that species.[4]

The results of recent studies show that ET-1 and ET-3 produce complex changes in systemic and pulmonary hemodynamics in the anesthetized cat. In addition to causing biphasic changes in SVR, ET-1 and ET-3 elicit biphasic changes in PVR that may be related to changes in CO.[49] Since changes in pulmonary blood flow (CO) and PVR are related in an inverse manner, the direct effects of the peptides on the pulmonary vascular bed were investigated in the intact-chest cat under conditions of controlled pulmonary blood flow. The results of these studies show that ET-1 and ET-3 have vasoconstrictor activity in the pulmonary vascular bed of the cat. The depressor component of the response to ET-1 and the fall in AP in response to ET-3 were associated with an increase in CO and a decrease in the AP-CVP gradient and in SVR. The secondary increase in AP in response to the higher doses of ET-1 occurred at a time when CO was unchanged or decreased significantly and was associated with an increase in SVR. ET-3 only decreased SVR, and a monocyclic ET-1 analogue had no significant effect on pulmonary or systemic hemodynamics. The results with ET-1 are consistent with recent studies in the hindlimb vascular bed of the cat where ET-1 had vasodilator or biphasic activity.[49,53]

The increase in CO in response to ET-1 was associated with an increase in HR but had no consistent effect on RVCF.[49] The increases in HR in response to ET-1 and ET-3 were blocked by hexamethonium and by propranolol, suggesting that they are reflexively mediated.[49] The absence of a consistent effect of ET-1 on RVCF is at variance with studies on isolated guinea pig atria but is more in agreement with studies on human and rat ventricular muscle and rat papillary muscle where the peptide was found to have little if any effect.[17,36,55]

The mechanism by which ET-1 and ET-3 alter systemic and pulmonary vascular resistance in the cat were investigated in experiments in which autonomic reflexes, beta-adrenoceptors, or prostaglandin synthesis was blocked.[49] After administration of hexamethonium in a dose that blocked the pressor response to bilateral carotid occlusion, the biphasic changes in SVR and PVR in response to the midrange dose of ET-1 were not altered.[49] The decrease in SVR and the biphasic change in PVR in response to the midrange dose of ET-3 were not altered. The administration of meclofenamate in a dose that blocked responses to arachidonic acid and the administration of propranolol in a dose that blocked the response to isoproterenol had no significant effect on changes in SVR and PVR in response to ET-1 or ET-3.[49]

It has been reported that ET-1 releases prostaglandins from the lung and that indomethacin modified the pressor response to the peptide in the pithed rat.[6] It has also been reported that ET-1 releases prostaglandins from the isolated perfused rabbit kidney and spleen.[58] However, in the anesthetized cat, sodium meclofenamate had no effect on pulmonary or systemic responses to ET-1 or ET-3. These studies suggest that the release of metabolites in the cyclooxygenase pathway does not mediate or modulate pulmonary or systemic vascular responses to ET-1 or ET-3 in the cat. The reason for the difference in results in the pithed rat and in the anesthetized cat are uncertain but may be related to species.

Results in the literature suggest that enhanced calcium entry may play a role in the vasoconstrictor component of the response to ET-1; however, the mechanism by which ET-1 and ET-3 decrease vascular resistance is uncertain.[50,53,73] In the isolated perfused rat mesentery, ET-1 and ET-3 in low doses elicited vasodilation that was blocked by removal of endothelial cells or by methylene blue and oxyhemoglobin, suggesting that vasodilator responses to these peptides are mediated by release of EDRF and activation of a soluble guanylate cyclase.[69] In studies in the cat, vasodilator responses to ET-1 and ET-3 were not dependent on autonomic reflexes, activation of beta-adrenoceptors, or release of vasodilator prostaglandins.[49] It is possible that release of an EDRF may be involved; however, this mechanism has not yet been addressed in the cat.[49] The data in the cat are, however, consistent with the notion that different receptors may be involved in vasodilator and vasoconstrictor responses to ET-1.[64,69]

The mechanism by which ET-1 and ET-3 increase CO in the cat is uncertain. The peptides had no consistent effect on RVCF, so that myocardial contractility was not increased. The increase in CO was not dependent on an increase in HR, since similar changes were observed when the increase in HR was blocked by propranolol or hexamethonium. The increase in CO was associated with a fall in AP and an increase in CVP, suggesting that an increase in filling pressure and a decrease in afterload may contribute to the response. The mechanism by which ET-1 and ET-3 increase CVP is uncertain but may be related to an effect on venous tone, since ET-1 has been shown to have potent contractile activity on saphenous, jugular, and mesenteric vein rings.[7,60] These results of experiments in the cat suggest that the actions of ET-1 and ET-3 are not modulated by release of products in the cyclooxygenase pathway and are not dependent on autonomic reflexes or activation of beta-adrenoceptors.[49] This work indicates that cardiovascular and pulmonary responses to these novel endothelial-derived peptides are complex in nature. The importance of ET-1 and related peptides in the regulation of the pulmonary and the systemic circulations in physiological and pathophysiological conditions is uncertain at the present time.

Acknowledgments: The authors' wish to thank Ms. Janice Ignarro for editorial assistance. The authors research was supported by NIH grants HL15580 and HL10834.

References

1. Burke T.M., Wolin M.S.: Hydrogen peroxide elicits pulmonary arterial relaxation and guanylate cyclase activation. Am. J. Physiol. 252:H721-H732, 1987.
2. Burke-Wolin T., Wolin M.S.: H_2O_2 and cGMP may function as an O_2 sensor in the pulmonary artery. J. Appl. Physiol. 66:167–170, 1989.
3. Busse R., Pohl U., Kellner C., Klemm U.: Endothelial cells are involved in the vasodilatory response to hypoxia. Pflugers Arch. 397:78–80, 1983.
4. Cassin S., Kristova V., Davis T., Kadowitz P., Gause G.: Tone-dependent responses to endothelin (ET-1) in the fetal pulmonary circulation. J. Appl. Physiol. (submitted), 1990.
5. Cherry P.D., Gillis C.N.: Evidence for the role of endothelium-derived relaxing factor in acetylcholine-induced vasodilation in the intact lung. J. Pharmacol. Exp. Ther. 241:516–520, 1987.
6. De Nucci G., Thomas R., D'Orleans-Juste P., Atures E., Walder C., Warner T.D., Vane J.R.: Pressor effects of circulating endothelin are limited by its removal in the pulmonary circulation by the release of prostacyclin and endothelium-derived relaxing factor. Proc. Natl. Acad. Sci. USA 85:9597–9800, 1988.
7. D'Orleans-Juste P., de Nucci G., Vane J.R.: Endothelin-1 contracts isolated vessels independently of dihydropyridine-sensitive Ca channel activation. Eur. J. Pharmacol. 165:289–295, 1989.
8. Edwards J C., Ignarro L.J., Hyman A.L., Kadowitz P.J.: Relaxation of intrapulmonary artery and vein by nitrogen oxide-containing vasodilators and cyclic GMP. J. Pharmacol Exp. Ther. 228:33–42, 1983.
9. Francois-Franck C.A.: Etude critique et experimentale de la vasoconstriction pulmonaire reflexe. Arch. Physiol. Norm. Pathol. 8:193–198, 1896.
10. Furchgott R.F.: Role of endothelium in response to vascular smooth muscle. Circ. Res. 53:557–573, 1983.
11. Furchgott R.F., Vanhoutte A.M.: Endothelium-derived relaxing and contracting factors. FASEB J. 3:2007–2018, 1989.
12. Furchgott F.R., Zawadzki J.V.: The obligatory role of endothelial cells in the relaxation of arterial smooth muscle by acetylcholine. Nature (Lond.) 288:373–376, 1980.
13. Gilliespie M.N., Owasoyo J.O., McMurtry K.F., O'Brien R.F.: Sustained coronary vasoconstriction provoked by a peptidergic substance released from endothelial cells in culture. J. Pharmacol. Exp. Ther. 236:339–343, 1986.
14. Gruetter C.A., Kadowitz P.J., Ignarro L.J.: Methylene blue inhibits coronary arterial relaxation and guanylate cyclase activation by nitroglycerin, sodium nitrite, and amyl nitrite. Can. J. Physiol. Pharmacol. 59:150–156, 1980.
15. Gryglewski R.J., Botting R.M., Vane R.J.: Mediators produced by the endothelial cell. Hypertension 12:530–548, 1988.
16. Hickey K.A., Rubanyi G., Paul R.J., Highsmith R.F.: Characterization of a coronary vasoconstrictor produced by cultured endothelial cells. Am. J. Physiol. 248:C550-C556, 1985.
17. Hu J.R., Harsdorf R.V., Lang R.E.: Endothelin has potent inotropic effects in rat atria. Eur. J. Pharmacol. 158:275–278, 1988.
18. Hyman A.L., Higashida R.T., Spannhake E.W., Kadowitz P.J.: Pulmonary vasoconstrictor responses to graded decreases in precapillary blood PO_2 in intact-chest cat. J. Appl. Physiol. 51(4):1009–1016, 1981.
19. Hyman A.L., Kadowitz P.J.: Effects of alveolar and perfusion hypoxia and hypercapnia on pulmonary vascular resistance in the lamb. Am. J. Physiol. 228:397–403, 1975.
20. Hyman A.L., Kadowitz P.J.: Pulmonary vasodilator activity of prostacyclin (PGI^2) in the cat. Circ. Res. 45:404–409, 1979.
21. Hyman A.L., Kadowitz P.J.: Evidence for the existence of postjunctional $\alpha1$- and $\alpha2$-adrenoceptors in the cat pulmonary vascular bed. Am. J. Physiol. 249:H891-H898, 1985.
22. Hyman A.L., Kadowitz P.J.: Enhancement of α- and β-adrenoceptor responses by elevations in vascular tone in pulmonary circulation. Am. J. Physiol. 250:H1109-H1116, 1986.
23. Hyman A.L., Kadowitz P.J.: Methylene blue selectively and reversibly inhibits hypoxic pulmonary vasoconstriction. Circulation 78(II):206, 1988.

24. Hyman A.L., Kadowitz P.J.: Tone-dependent responses to acetylcholine in the feline pulmonary vascular bed. J. Appl. Physiol. 64:2002–2009, 1988.

25. Hyman A.L., Kadowitz P.J.: Analysis of responses to sympathetic nerve stimulation in the feline pulmonary vascular bed. J. Appl. Physiol. 67:371–376, 1989.

26. Hyman A.L., Kadowitz P.J.: Influence of tone on responses to acetylcholine in the rabbit pulmonary vascular bed. J. Appl. Physiol. 67:1388–1394, 1989.

27. Hyman A.L., Kadowitz P.J., Lippton H.L.: Methylene blue selectivity inhibits pulmonary vasodilator responses in cats. J. Appl. Physiol. 66:1513 -1517, 1989.

28. Hyman A.L., Lippton H.L., Dempsey C.W., Fontana C.J., Richardson D.E., Rieck P.W., Kadowitz P.J.: Autonomic control of the pulmonary circulation. In: Pulmonary Vascular Physiology and Pathophysiology, Weir E.K., Reeves J.T. (eds.), Marcel Dekker, Inc., New York, 1988, pp 291–324.

29. Hyman A.L., Nandiwada P., Knight D.S., Kadowitz P.J.: Pulmonary vasodilator responses to catecholamines and sympathetic nerve stimulation in the cat: Evidence that vascular α_2-adrenoceptors are innervated. Circ. Res. 48:407–415, 1981.

30. Hyman A.L., Spannhake E.W., Kadowitz P.J.: Divergent responses to arachidonic acid in the feline pulmonary vascular bed. Am. J. Physiol. 239:H49-H46, 1980.

31. Ignarro L.J., Burke T.M., Wood K.S., Wolin M.S., Kadowitz P.J.: Association between cyclic GMP accumulation and acetylcholine-elicited relaxation of bovine intrapulmonary artery. J. Pharmacol. Exp. Ther. 228:682–690, 1984.

32. Ignarro L.J., Harbison R.G., Wood K.S., Kadowitz P.J.: Activation of purified soluble guanylate cyclase by endothelium-derived relaxing factor from intrapulmonary artery and vein: stimulation by acetylcholine, bradykinin and arachidonic acid. J. Pharmacol. Exp. Ther. 237:893–897, 1986.

33. Ignarro L.J., Harbison R.G., Wood K.S., Wolin M.S., McNamara D.B., Hyman A.L., Kadowitz P.J.: Differences in responsiveness of intrapulmonary artery and vein to arachidonic acid: mechanism of arterial relaxation involves cyclic guanosine 3′:5′-monophosphate and cyclic adenosine 3′:5′-monophosphate. J. Pharmacol. Exp. Ther. 233:560–569, 1985.

34. Ignarro L.J., Lippton H.L., Edwards J.C., Baricos W.H., Hyman A.L., Kadowitz P.J., Gruetter C.A.: Mechanisms of vascular smooth muscle relaxation by organic nitrates, nitrites, sodium nitroprusside and nitric oxide; evidence for involvement of S-nitrosothiols as active intermediates. J. Pharmacol. Exp. Ther. 218:739–749, 1981.

35. Inoue, A., Yanagisawa M., Kimura S., Kasuya Y., Miyauchi T., Goto K., Masaki T.: The human endothelin family: three structurally and pharmacologically distinct isopeptides predicted by three separate genes. Proc. Natl. Acad. Sci. USA 86:2863–2867, 1989.

36. Ishikawa, T., Yanagisawa M., Kimura S., Goto K., Masaki T.: Positive inotropic action of novel vasoconstrictor peptide endothelin on guinea pig atria. Am. J. Physiol. 255:H970-H973, 1988.

37. Johns R.A., Linden J.M., Peach M.J.: Endothelium-dependent relaxation and cyclic GMP accumulation in rabbit pulmonary artery are selectively impaired by moderate hypoxia. Circ. Res. 65:1508–1515, 1989.

38. Kadowitz P.J., Chapnick B.M., Feigen L.P., Hyman A.L., Nelson P.K., Spannhake E.W.: Pulmonary and systemic vasodilator effects of the newly-discovered prostaglandin PGI$_2$. Appl. Physiol. 45: 408–413, 1978.

39. Kadowitz P.J., Hyman A.L.: Effect of sympathetic nerve stimulation on pulmonary vascular resistance in the dog. Circ. Res. 32:221–227, 1973.

40. Kadowitz P.J., Hyman A.L.: Influence of prostaglandin endoperoxide analog on the canine pulmonary vascular bed. Circ. Res. 40:282–287, 1977.

41. Kadowitz P.J., Hyman A.L.: Comparative effects of thromboxane B$_2$ on the canine and feline pulmonary vascular bed. J. Pharmacol. Exp. Ther. 213:300–305, 1980.

42. Kadowitz P.J., Hyman A.L.: Methylene blue selectively inhibits pulmonary vasodilator responses to acetylcholine, bradykinin, and nitroglycerin in the cat. Circulation 78(II):320, 1988.

43. Kadowitz P.J., Knight D.S., Hibbs R.G., Ellison J.P., Joiner P.D., Brody M.J., Hyman A.L.: Influence of 5- and 6-hydroxydopamine on adrenergic transmission and nerve terminal morphology in the canine pulmonary vascular bed. Circ. Res. 39:191–199, 1976.

44. Kloog Y., Ambar I., Sokolovsky M., Kochva E., Wollberg Z., Bdolah A.: Sarafotoxin, a novel vasoconstrictor peptide: phosphoinositide hydrolysis in rat heart and brain. Science 242:268–270, 1988.

45. Knight D.S., Ellison J.P., Hibbs R.G., Hyman A.L., Kadowitz P.J.: A light and

electron microscopic study of the innervation of pulmonary arteries in the cat. Anat. Rec. 201:513–521, 1981.

46. Laher I., Bevan J.A.: Alpha adrenoceptor number limits response of some rabbit arteries to norepinephrine. J. Pharmacol. Exp. Ther. 233:290–297, 1985.

47. Lippton H.L., Hauth T.A., Summer W.R., Hyman A.L.: Endothelin produces pulmonary vasoconstriction and systemic vasodilation. J. Appl. Physiol. 66(2):1008–1012, 1989.

48. Martin W., Villani G.M., Jothianandan D., Furchgott R.F.: Selective blockade of endothelium-dependent and glyceryl trinitrate-induced relaxation by hemoglobin and by methylene blue in the rabbit aorta. J. Pharmacol. Exp. Ther. 232:708–716, 1985.

49. Minkes R.K., Bellan J.A., Saroyan R.M., Kerstein M.D., Coy D.H., Murphy W.A., Nossaman B.D., McNamara D.B., Kadowitz P.J.: Analysis of cardiovascular responses to endothelin-1 and endothelin-3 in the cat. J. Pharmacol. Exp. Ther. 253:1118–1125, 1990.

50. Minkes R.K., Coy D.H., Murphy W.A., McNamara D.B., Kadowitz P.J.: Effects of porcine and rat endothelin and an analog on blood pressure in the anesthetized cat. Eur. J. Pharmacol. 164:571–575, 1989.

51. Minkes R.K., Kadowitz P.J.: Influence of endothelin on systemic arterial pressure and regional blood flow in the cat. Eur. J. Pharmacol. 163:163–166, 1989.

52. Minkes R.K., Kadowitz P.J.: Differential effects of rat endothelin on regional blood flow in the cat. Eur. J. Pharmacol. 165:161–164, 1989.

53. Minkes R.K., MacMillan L.A., Bellan J.A., Kerstein M.D., McNamara D.B., Kadowitz P.J.: Analysis of regional responses to endothelin in hindquarters vascular bed of cats. Am. J. Physiol. 256:H598–H602, 1989.

54. Moon D.G., Horgan M.J., Anderson T.T., Krystek S.R., Fenton II J.W., Malik A.B.: Endothelin-like pulmonary vasoconstrictor peptide release by a-thrombin. Proc. Natl. Acad. Sci. USA 86:9529–9533, 1989.

55. Morevac C.S., Reynolds E.E., Stewart R.W., Bond M.: Endothelin is a positive inotropic agent in human and rat heart in vitro. Biochem. Biophys. Res. Commun. 159(1):14–18, 1989.

56. Nandiwada P.A., Hyman A.L., Kadowitz P.J.: Pulmonary vasodilator responses to vagal stimulation and acetylcholine in the cat. Circ. Res. 53:86–95, 1983.

57. Napoli S.A., Gruetter C.A., Ignarro L.J., Kadowitz P.J.: Relaxation of bovine coronary arterial smooth muscle by cGMP, cAMP, and analogs. J. Pharmacol. Exp. Ther. 212:469–473, 1980.

58. Rae G.A., Trybulec M., de Nucci G., Vane J.R.: Endothelin-1 releases eicosanoids from rabbit isolated perfused kidney and spleen. J. Cardiovasc. Pharmacol. 13(5):S89–S92, 1989.

59. Rodman D.M., Yamaguchi T., O'Brien R.F., McMurtry I.F.: Hypoxic contraction of isolated rat pulmonary artery. J. Pharmacol. Exp. Ther. 248:1–8, 1989.

60. Saroyan R.M., Kvamme P., Webb W.R., Fox L., Kerstein M.D., Mills N.L., McNamara D.B., Kadowitz P.J.: Comparative effects of endothelin (ET-1) on human saphenous vein and gastroepiploic artery. Eur. J. Pharmacol. (submitted), 1990.

61. Snedecor C.W., Cochran W.G.: Statistical Methods. 6th Ed., Ames, Iowa State University Press, pp 258–338, 1987.

62. Spannhake E.W., Hyman A.L., Kadowitz P.J.: Dependency of the airway and pulmonary vascular effects of arachidonic acid upon route and rate of administration. J. Pharmacol. Exp. Ther. 212:584–590, 1980.

63. Spannhake E.W., Levin J.L., Mellion B.T., Hyman A.L., Kadowitz P.J.: Reversal of 5-HT induced bronchoconstriction by PGI_2: distribution of central over peripheral actions. J. Appl. Physiol. 49:521–527, 1980.

64. Spokes R.A., Ghatei M.A., Bloom S.R.: Studies with endothelin-3 and endothelin-1 on rat blood pressure and isolated tissues: evidence for multiple endothelin receptor subtypes. J. Cardiovasc. Pharmacol. 13(5):S191–S192, 1989.

65. Tod M.L., Cassin S.: Perinatal responses to arachidonic acid during normoxia and hypoxia. J. Appl. Physiol. 57:977–983, 1984.

66. Tod M.L., Cassin S.: Thromboxane synthetase inhibition and perinatal pulmonary response to arachidonic acid. J. Appl. Physiol. 58(3):710–716, 1985.

67. Underwood D.C., Kriseman T., McNamara D.B., Hyman A.L., Kadowitz P.J.: Blockade of thromboxane responses in the airway of the cat by SQ 29,548. J. Appl. Physiol. 62:2193–2200, 1987.

68. Vanhoutte A.M.: Endothelium and control of vascular function. State-of-the-art lecture. Hypertension 13:658–667, 1989.

69. Warner T.D., Mitchell J.A., de Nucci G., Vane J.R.: Endothelin-1 and endothelin-3 release EDRF from isolated perfused arterial vessels of the rat and rabbit. J. Cardiovasc. Pharmacol. 13(5):S85–S88, 1989.

70. Watanabe M., Rosenblum W.I., Nelson G.H.: In vivo effect of methylene blue on endothelium-dependent and endothelium-

independent dilations of brain microvessels in mice. Circ. Res. 62:86–90, 1988.

71. Wright C.E., Fozard J.R.: Regional vasodilation is a prominent feature of the haemodynamic response to endothelin in anaestheized, spontaneously hypertensive rats. for. J. Pharmacol. 155:201–203, 1988.

72. Yanagisawa M., Inoue A., Ishikawa T., Kasuya Y., Kimura S., Kumagaye S., Nakajima K., Watanabe T.X., et al.: Primary structure, synthesis, and biological activity of rat endothelin, an endothelium-derived vasoconstrictor peptide. Proc. Natl. Acad. Sci. USA 85:6964–6967, 1988.

73. Yanagisawa M., Kurihara H., Kimura A., Tomobe Y., Kobayashi M., Mitsui Y., Yazaki Y., Goto K., Masaki T.: A novel potent vasoconstrictor peptide produced by vascular endothelial cells. Nature 332:411–415, 1988.

8

Role of Endothelium-Derived Vasoactive Factors in the Control of the Microcirculation

Gabor Kaley, Akos Koller, Edward J. Messina, Michael S. Wolin

Introduction

Understanding the role of endothelium-dependent regulation of vascular tone in the microcirculation has progressed at a slower rate than that developed in isolated larger blood vessels[11,21,61,63] due to the inherent difficulties in examining mechanisms in vivo and in isolated microvessels. However, the recent development of pharmacological probes and novel methods of endothelial removal or functional injury have resulted in substantial evidence for a role for the endothelium in microvascular regulation by certain mediators. The endothelial mediators that have thus far been demonstrated to contribute to the regulation of microvascular tone and hence local blood flow to physiological or pharmacological stimuli include the cGMP-associated endothelium-derived relaxing factor (EDRF) thought to be related to nitric oxide, prostaglandins and reactive

O_2 species. In this chapter the current understanding of the regulation of microvascular tone via endothelium-dependent mediators is reviewed.

Effect of Endothelial Mediators on Microvessels

Prostaglandins

The concept that prostaglandins and related metabolites of arachidonic acid participate in the regulation of microvascular function has been investigated extensively. It is based on the findings that in a variety of vascular beds the administration of prostaglandins or inhibitors of prostaglandin synthesis can affect microvascular tone and reactivity to dilator and constrictor agents.[63,67] Few, if any, prostaglandins are detected in circulating blood, primarily

Rubanyi G.M.: Cardiovascular Significance of Endothelium-Derived Vasoactive Factors, Futura Publishing Co., Inc., Mount Kisco, NY, © 1991.

because of their efficient pulmonary metabolism, thus they can be considered local hormones that are released near or at the site of their action. A wealth of evidence has accumulated to suggest that prostaglandins are released by a variety of pharmacological and physiological stimuli and that, in turn, they mediate or modulate vascular responses.

Prostaglandins are synthesized primarily within endothelial cells of blood vessels.[100] The principal prostaglandin made in large arteries of most species is prostacyclin (PGI_2). Small vessels, however, exhibit pathways of arachidonate metabolism that are quite different; thus, under both basal and stimulated conditions, prostaglandin (PG)E_2 release exceeds that of 6-keto-$PGF_{1\alpha}$, the primary metabolite of PGI_2.[22,70] It is then tempting to speculate that the regulation of microvascular blood flow and resistance is controlled by the locally released PGE_2, rather than by PGI_2.[65,67] In line with this idea, the actions of PGI_2 are directed primarily, but not exclusively, toward the modulation of platelet activation whereas those of PGE_2 are directed toward the modulation of vascular tone and reactivity,[67] and of the release of norepinephrine.[29]

Inhibition of prostaglandin synthesis has been shown to increase microvascular reactivity to constrictor agents (e.g., angiotensin, norepinephrine) in a variety of vascular beds[18,19,66] and to enhance vascular tone and vasomotion frequency in skeletal muscle.[18] On the other hand, blockade of cyclooxygenase reduces the arteriolar dilation to bradykinin (but not to acetylcholine), indicating that prostaglandins mediate, at least in part, the responses to this agent.[66] Interestingly, arteriolar dilation to A23187 is also blocked by pretreatment with indomethacin in contrast to large artery preparations in vitro in which the release of EDRF mediates the A23187-evoked vasorelaxation.[41] Impairment of arteriolar endothelium by a light/dye technique[51] essentially abolishes the dilation to exoge-

nous arachidonic acid, while the dilator responses to PGE_2, adenosine, and sodium nitroprusside remain unaltered (Fig. 1). Moreover, light/dye treatment also reduces dilator responses to ATP and significantly enhances constrictor responses to norepinephrine.[45] These and similar studies[15] indicate that the prostaglandin-mediated arteriolar responses to physiological and pharmacological stimuli are dependent upon an intact endothelial cell layer. Moreover, these studies also demonstrate that the vasoactivity of the so-called nonendothelium-dependent agents does not require vascular prostaglandin synthesis.

Recent studies indicate that products of the lipoxygenase pathway of arachidonate metabolism also have an effect on microvascular tone. Leukotriene (LT)C_4 and D_4 constrict rat skeletal muscle arterioles[64] and generally cause, upon intra-arterial administration decreases in blood flow in many vascular beds.[76] In contrast, cytochrome P450-derived epoxygenase metabolites of arachidonic acid evoke arteriolar dilation in a variety of tissues either directly or indirectly by the release of dilator prostaglandins or cyclooxygenase-dependent oxygen radicals.[82] Nevertheless, because of the small amounts of these substances that appear to be synthesized in microvascular endothelial cells, it is unlikely that products of arachidonic acid metabolism, other than those synthesized via cyclooxygenase, have a major role in the regulation of microvascular tone and reactivity to endothelium-dependent stimuli.

EDRF

The actions of several vasoactive agents thought to produce vasodilation through EDRF based on studies in larger isolated blood vessels have been reported in different in vitro and in vivo microvascular preparations. However, definitive

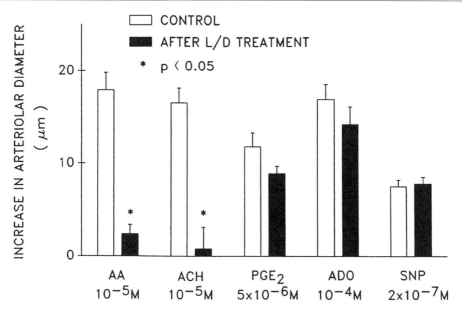

Figure 1: Average vasodilator responses of rat cremasteric arterioles (15–25 μm in diameter) in vivo, before and after local impairment of the vasoactive functions of arteriolar endothelium by light/dye (mercury light/sodium fluorescein; L/D) treatment,[50] to arachidonic acid (AA), acetylcholine (ACH), prostaglandin E_2 (PGE$_2$), adenosine (ADO), and sodium nitroprusside (SNP). All substances were administered onto the Krebs-superfused preparation in 100 μL aliquots. Arteriolar dilation to AA and ACH were essentially abolished, indicating that the vasoactivity of these agents is dependent upon an intact endothelial cell layer. Dilator responses to PGE$_2$, ADO, and SNP were unchanged after endothelial impairment, suggesting that their activity is independent of the endothelium.

evidence for both a role of the endothelium and a mediator with the characteristics of EDRF in the microcirculation has not been reported in every instance. The most extensive investigations of these concepts in in vivo preparations exist in the cat and mouse cerebral circulation and the rat skeletal muscle microcirculation. In these microvascular beds, selective injury to the endothelium employing light/dye techniques has demonstrated that acetylcholine and certain other vasodilators produce endothelium-dependent vasodilation.[45,50–52, 80,86,89–91] (Fig. 1). In these preparations, acetylcholine, nitric oxide, and related nitrovasodilators produce vasodilation; however, only the dilation to acetylcholine is inhibited by methylene blue,[41,62,107] a probe that inhibits the EDRF mechanism.

In the rat skeletal muscle microcirculation, recently identified inhibitors of the biosynthesis of EDRF [N^G-monomethyl-L-arginine (L-NMA) and N^G-nitro-L-arginine (L-NNA)][83,97] antagonize the dilation to acetylcholine (Fig. 2) in an L-arginine reversible fashion.[42] The generation of an endogenously produced transferable factor on exposure to acetylcholine with the characteristics of EDRF has been detected in the cat cerebral microcirculation.[54] Therefore, an endothelium-derived mediator with many of the distinguishing properties of EDRF appears to exist in these microvascular beds which have been most extensively characterized for this mediator.

Study of microvascular preparations in vitro has also resulted in evidence for the importance of EDRF in the control of

ARTERIOLAR
DIAMETER
(μm)

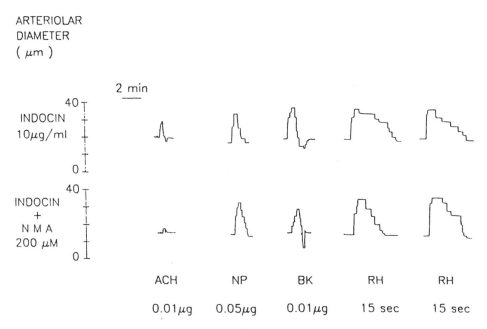

Figure 2: Record of changes in diameter of a rat cremaster muscle arteriole to topical administration of acetylcholine (ACH), bradykinin (BK), sodium nitroprusside (NP), and to 15-second occlusion (RH: reactive hyperemia). Upper panel: following administration of indomethacin (INDOCIN). Lower panel: following additional administration of N^G-mono-methyl-L-arginine (NMA). Response to ACH is eliminated and that to BK is reduced. Dilation to NP and to release of occlusion is unaffected by NMA administration.

arteriolar tone. The microvascular preparations most extensively examined in vitro include the rat mesenteric[21] and skeletal muscle,[41] and coronary resistance vessels[71] from several species. Pharmacological probes that are thought to function via inhibition of the biosynthesis of EDRF,[1,69,83] the generation of superoxide anion, and/or the inhibition of guanylate cyclase activation[5] or the trapping of EDRF (hemoglobin[21,71,102,103]), and methods that appear to selectively impair (e.g., gossypol[5,80] or reactive O_2 species[60,103]) or remove the endothelium,[21,5] inhibit vasodilators thought to act via EDRF in in vitro preparations of resistance arteries from these vascular beds.

Studies of the properties of EDRF in microvascular preparations have contributed to the controversy in determining if EDRF is in fact nitric oxide. In the cat cerebral microcirculation, although acetylcholine releases a transferable mediator with the characteristics of EDRF,[54] pharmacological-type probes clearly distinguish the endogenous mediator released by acetylcholine from the actions of nitric oxide.[62] Vasodilation to acetylcholine is inhibited by methylene blue, but not by nitroblue-tetrazolium. On the other hand, the dilation to topical application of nitric oxide is inhibited by nitrobluetetrazolium, but not by methylene blue.[107] However, in the rat skeletal muscle microcirculation, methylene blue inhibits vasodilation to both acetylcholine and nitric oxide.[41,113] Since inhibitors of the synthesis of EDRF from L-arginine antagonize dilation to acetylcholine in the skeletal muscle microcirculation (and other vascular beds), the mediator involved appears to be the same as the EDRF which was characterized in larger isolated arteries and which possesses many of the properties of nitric oxide.[35,74] Recent studies on isolated coronary microvessels have found a reduction in sensitivity to nitric oxide, but not to acetylcholine, with decreasing arteriolar diameter.[98] These coronary microvessels, however, did not undergo a change in sensitivity to S-nitroso-L-cysteine, a substance that is also under consideration as a mediator of acetylcholine. Recent evidence indicates that the coronary microcirculation releases a hemoglobin-inhibitable mediator that activates guanylate cyclase, since cyclic GMP levels in platelets can be elevated on passage through the rabbit coronary circulation in the presence of acetylcholine.[79] Thus, there is a substantial amount of evidence to indicate that a mediator with the characteristics of the cyclic GMP-associated EDRF contributes to the control of microvascular function; however, the actual identity of this nitric oxide-like mediator remains to be established.

A substantial degree of variability exists in microvascular preparations in the actions of vasodilators that often function via the production of EDRF. Although acetylcholine appears to produce arteriolar vasodilation via EDRF in the microvascular preparations thus far examined, the calcium ionophore A23187, which generally produces EDRF-mediated relaxation of isolated larger arteries, appears to produce endothelium-dependent prostaglandin-elicited microvascular responses in the rat skeletal muscle[41] and mouse cerebral circulation[89] without producing a dilation mediated via EDRF. However, since hemoglobin, but not indomethacin, blocks the dilation to A23187 in the saline-perfused guinea pig coronary circulation,[101] EDRF may mediate its actions in this vascular bed. Bradykinin produces dilator responses that can be attributed to prostaglandins[66] and EDRF[41] in the rat skeletal muscle bed, whereas, reactive O_2 species mediate its action in the cat and mouse cerebral circulation.[53,87] Many other

vasoactive stimuli (e.g., physiological mechanisms, tissue hormones, peptides, etc.) will most likely be found to produce vascular bed and vascular segment-specific EDRF-dependent vascular responses.

O_2 Radicals

Studies on the cerebral microcirculation[90,91] and on isolated endothelial cells[31] have provided evidence that the endothelium may release vasoactive levels of reactive O_2 species. It has been demonstrated in both the cat and the mouse cerebral microcirculation that selective injury to the endothelium employing light/dye techniques attenuates the vasodilation to bradykinin,[90,91] a response that is also inhibited in both preparations by scavengers of reactive O_2 species.[53,87] The metabolism of arachidonic acid via the peroxidase reaction of cyclooxygenase[56] appears to be a source of endothelium-derived superoxide anion in the cat cerebral microcirculation[53] and in cultured human umbilical vein endothelium[31] on exposure to agents such as bradykinin. Stimulation of superoxide anion release from the cat cerebral microcirculation by several stimuli has been detected, and it appears to involve transport via an anion channel.[53] Thus, there is substantial evidence to justify consideration of reactive O_2 species as microvascular, endothelium-derived mediators.

The effects of reactive O_2 species on reactivity of resistance vessels have been examined in several microcirculatory beds. In both the cat and mouse cerebral bed, superoxide anion and hydrogen peroxide appear to produce vasodilation.[85,109] In the rat skeletal muscle microcirculation, hydrogen peroxide produces vasodilation,[115,116] whereas superoxide anion does not appear to affect basal arteriolar tone.[115] Hydrogen peroxide has been shown to produce vasoconstriction in the saline-perfused rat and rabbit lung.[6,105] Lipid or organic peroxides have been shown to produce vasodilation in the rat skeletal muscle bed[114] and to produce vasoconstriction in the mouse cerebral bed[88] and in saline-perfused rabbit lungs.[25] At increased levels of tone, the response to peroxide is converted to vasodilation in the saline-perfused rabbit lungs[9] and in blood-perfused rat lungs.[111] In addition, it has been demonstrated in several vascular beds that reactive O_2 species can alter endothelium-dependent responses to other vasoactive stimuli via injury to the endothelium or by directly interacting with the vasoactive factors released.[41,60,62,103,110,113]

Studies in both in vivo and in vitro preparations have identified several mechanisms through which reactive O_2 species can modulate vascular tone. Superoxide anion can attenuate the actions of the endothelium-derived relaxing factor thought to be nitric oxide[96] and attenuate the actions of catecholamines such as norepinephrine[112] through mechanisms that appear to involve direct chemical reactions with these species in the extracellular environment of the vascular wall. In the rat skeletal muscle microcirculation, the pharmacological probes, hydroquinone and methylene blue, appear to attenuate vasodilation to agents such as acetylcholine through the inactivation of the endothelium-derived relaxing factor thought to be nitric oxide via increased extracellular production of superoxide anion.[41,113]

Hydrogen peroxide and lipid or organic peroxides are excellent stimuli for the production of prostaglandins by tissues, including endothelium.[25] The peroxide-elicited vasoconstrictor responses observed in the mouse cerebral circulation[88] and in the perfused rat[6] and rabbit lung preparations[9,25,105] as well as part of the peroxide-elicited vasodilation in the rat skeletal muscle bed[115,116] are inhibited by antagonists of cyclooxygenase. Thus, peroxides appear to produce the divergent vascular responses described above through a common mechanism involving

the generation of vasoactive prostaglandins (Fig. 3). Although the effects of light/dye injury to the endothelium on prostaglandin-mediated responses to peroxide have not been reported, exposure of the rat skeletal muscle bed to arachidonic acid produces a vasodilation that is mediated completely via prostaglandins and attenuated by light/dye injury.[51] Therefore, the endothelium is the likely source of vasodilator prostaglandins produced on exposure of the rat skeletal muscle bed to peroxides.

Hydrogen peroxide has been suggested to be involved in the stimulation of cGMP-mediated vascular smooth muscle relaxation via two different mechanisms. This O_2 species has been proposed to be involved in the synthesis of the endothelium-derived relaxing factor thought to be nitric oxide[95,96] and in the direct modulation of vascular smooth muscle guanylate cyclase activity through an activation mechanism thought to be mediated through the metabolism of peroxide via catalase.[5,7] In the rat skeletal muscle microcirculation, the prostaglandin-independent portion of the vasodilation to hydrogen peroxide is not altered by L-NMA, suggesting that the cGMP-associated EDRF is not involved in the response.[116] This vasodilation to hydrogen peroxide is inhibited by methylene blue, suggesting that cGMP is involved in the response and that the activation of guanylate cyclase by peroxide metabolism via catalase may play a role in this relaxation mechanism.

There are differences in the stimuli for the production and vasoactive actions of reactive O_2 species between different microvascular beds.[81] For example, bradykinin and arachidonic acid produce vasodilation in the cat cerebral circulation via cyclooxygenase-derived reactive O_2 species.[55] In contrast, in the rat skeletal muscle bed, the extracellular generation of reactive O_2 species is not involved in the observed vascular response to bradykinin or arachidonic acid,[115] and other endothe-

PROSTAGLANDINS AND PEROXIDES IN
SKELETAL MUSCLE REACTIVE HYPEREMIA

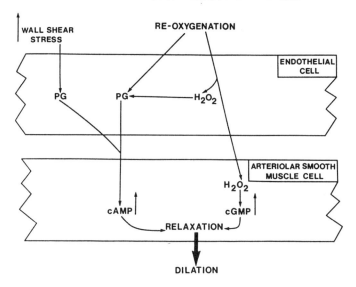

Figure 3: Hypothesized mechanism for the involvement of wall shear stress and hydrogen peroxide produced by restoration of flow and reoxygenation in the generation of reactive hyperemia.

lium-derived mediators (cGMP-associated EDRF and/or prostaglandins) contribute to the observed vasodilation.[41,51] Therefore, there appears to be a considerable variation among vascular beds in (1) the mediators released from endothelium by agonists of specific endothelial receptors and (2) the actions of the mediators released on the vascular smooth muscle segment examined.

Role of Endothelial Factors in the Regulation of Microvascular Tone

Despite mounting evidence suggesting a role for the endothelium in the mediation of vascular responses to various vasoactive agents, little is known about the role of endothelium in the regulation of vascular resistance and blood flow in the microcirculation. The endothelial media-

tors—prostaglandins and EDRF—that were shown to be present in arteriolar endothelium could, however, be involved in the regulation of microvascular function. Studies on large vessels in vitro and cultured endothelial cells indicate the existence of other releasable mediators (e.g., EDCF, EDHF) from these cells (see review by Lüscher[61]) which may also have a physiological role; however, lacking specific inhibitors of these agents, definitive studies have not yet been performed in the microcirculation in vivo. In the following sections we review those physiological responses of arterioles in which endothelial mediators (prostaglandins, EDRF, and oxygen radicals) appear to be involved.

Regulation of Basal Tone

Studies by Rosenblum and his colleagues[86,89–91] on cerebral arterioles, utilizing light/dye treatment to impair the vasoactive functions of endothelium, reveal only a minor role, if any, for the endothelium in the regulation of basal vascular tone. Similar conclusions were drawn by Marshall and Kontos[62] based on the lack of vasoconstriction of cerebral arterioles to topical application of methylene blue, a putative inhibitor of EDRF. The possibility that the endothelium participates in the regulation of basal tone of arterioles in skeletal muscle is indicated by the finding that after impairment of the arteriolar endothelium by light/dye treatment, the tone of the vessels is slightly, but significantly increased.[50-52] Although the decrease in diameter is only about 15%, if such a decrease were to occur in the entire vascular network, it would result in a considerable increase in peripheral vascular resistance.

The role of prostaglandins in the modulation of basal microvascular tone is still controversial. Based on the effects of inhibitors of prostaglandin synthesis, some studies[66,67] suggested the absence for a role, while others[18,26,30,36,51,52] demonstrated significant decreases in arteriolar diameter as well as increase in the frequency of vasomotion.[18] Whether the differences are due to differences in methodology or in the coordinated behavior of microvascular networks has not yet been resolved. Nevertheless, the continuous basal release of prostaglandins may have an important influence on the generation of basal tone by direct vasodilator effects and/or by modulating constrictor stimuli (e.g., myogenic, α-adrenergic).

A role for EDRF (or other endothelial factors) in the basal regulation of arteriolar tone was suspected when, after indomethacin administration, impairment of the arteriolar endothelium by light/dye treatment elicited a further decrease in arteriolar diameter.[51] This idea is strengthened by the findings of recent studies, in which administration of L-NMA, a specific blocker of EDRF synthesis, resulted in an elevation of basal arteriolar tone.[42] In the recent study of Persson et al., L-NMA produced a dose-dependent decrease in microvascular diameter.[75] An interesting, potentially physiological role of EDRF in the regulation of basal vascular tone in microcirculation is offered by a study of Falcone and Bohlen et al.[17] They demonstrated a transfer of EDRF from venules to arterioles in vivo; however, the exact functional role of such a phenomenon[17,106] has not yet been delineated. Since inhibitors of the biosynthesis of EDRF, such as L-NMA, reduced blood flow to several organ systems,[75] EDRF may be quite important in the control of basal microvascular tone.

Despite some conflicting views, it seems likely that the endothelium may continuously modulate the tone of arterioles via the release of endothelium-derived vasoactive factors.

Reactive Hyperemia

In a recent study, impairment of endothelium by light/dye treatment resulted in a decrease in peak reactive dilation of arterioles in skeletal muscle, indicating the possible involvement of endothelium in this autoregulatory response.[46] Also, prior to the discovery of an obligatory role of endothelium in the mediation of vascular reactions to vasoactive agents, a role for prostaglandins in the regulation of microvascular resistance during reactive hyperemia has already been identified. Messina et al. investigated the microvascular effect of prostaglandins[67] and their role in the vascular response following brief occlusions of third-order arterioles in rat cremaster muscle.[68] They found that cyclooxygenase blockade significantly inhibited reactive dilation following arteriole occlusion of 15–60 seconds. The peak dilation was blunted by 50–52% and the duration of responses was reduced by 51–67%. It has been thought for some time that reactive dilation (hyperemia) is the result of multiple mechanisms (i.e., myogenic, metabolic, and passive), elicited in response to changes in intravascular pressure and tissue blood supply; however, a linkage between prostaglandins and these mechanisms has only recently been considered. A plausible explanation for this finding was therefore that reperfusion after exposure to ischemia or hypoxia could elicit or augment prostaglandin release, which then contributes to the mediation of reactive dilation (Fig. 3). Although in previous studies[68] the tissue source of prostaglandins was not yet known, it was suspected that endothelial cells were the primary source of their synthesis.

More recent studies[47,48] indicating the presence of a prostaglandin-dependent "flow sensitivity" of skeletal muscle arterioles, may provide an explanation for the reduced reactive hyperemic response in the presence of inhibitors of prostaglandin synthesis. It seems likely that the release of the arteriolar occlusion results in a sudden increase in blood flow velocity (shear stress) triggering the release of vasoactive prostaglandins which could participate, in concert with other mechanisms, in the final development of reactive dilation of arterioles (Fig. 3). Interestingly, in recent studies, the specific inhibitor of EDRF, L-NMA, while significantly diminishing the dilation to acetylcholine,[42] did not affect reactive dilation of arterioles in cremaster muscle[116] (Fig. 2). These findings indicate that EDRF is not likely to be involved in the generation of reactive hyperemia in the cremaster muscle microcirculation. Interestingly, the nitric oxide-like EDRF was also shown to have no role in functional hyperemia in rabbit skeletal muscle.[75]

Recently, our laboratory has also proposed that the reactive hyperemia that occurs on the release of a brief single arteriolar occlusion of rat skeletal muscle arterioles may involve the intracellular generation of hydrogen peroxide in both the endothelium and smooth muscle[116] (Fig. 3). This hypothesis is based on sim-ilarities observed in the pharmacological modulation of the responses by probes for prostaglandins, the cGMP-associated EDRF, and inhibitors of the activation of guanylate cyclase. An interesting aspect of this proposal is that it may explain the effects of the duration of the occlusion on the magnitude of the hyperemic response because the duration of hypoxia should influence the extent of development of the metabolic state that produces peroxide on reoxygenation (reperfusion).

Oxygen Sensitivity

Much evidence has accumulated indicating that microvessels are sensitive to changes in oxygen tension in their environment.[16,33,37,77,78,108] Besides the well-established indirect effect (via tissue metabolites), there is evidence for a direct effect of oxygen on the vascular wall.[16] In vitro findings of Coburn et al.[12] indicated a minor role for the endothelium in the relaxation of large arteries to hypoxia, and suggested that an endothelial oxygen sensor, affected by low PO_2, may be present in these vessels. It has also been observed that hypoxia stimulates the release of a vasoconstrictor substance from vascular endothelium.[94] Recent in vivo studies of skeletal muscle arterioles examined the question of whether prostaglandins or other arachidonate metabolites may be involved in the response to ischemia or hypoxia. Jackson[36] increased the PO_2 in the superfusion solution from 15 to 150 mm Hg, which resulted in constriction of arterioles. This response, however, was not affected by inhibition of cyclooxygenase with indomethacin. Contrary to these findings, relaxation of coronary vessels to hypoxia is mediated in part via the release of prostaglandins.[10,11,43,84] In more recent studies employing pharmacological probes, Jackson[38] found that leukotrienes (produced via oxidation of arachidonic acid by

5-lipoxygenase) are responsible for the arteriolar constriction to increased PO_2 in hamster cheek pouch. Since 5-lipoxygenase is not known to be expressed in endothelial cells, the question remains as to where the vasoactive leukotrienes are synthesized. However, it should be noted that significant amounts of LTA_4 hydrolase, which produces LTC_4 and LTD_4 from LTA_4, are known to be present in endothelial cells.

The involvement of reactive O_2 species and other endothelial factors in processes related to oxygen-elicited physiological and pathophysiological regulatory mechanisms of microcirculatory blood flow is a potentially important field of study, which remains to be characterized. It is known that the extracellular generation of these species is not involved in the hypoxia-elicited dilation of the hamster cremaster microcirculation.[81] However, it remains to be investigated if the intracellular generation of reactive O_2 species in the endothelium and/or vascular smooth muscle is involved in O_2-dependent microvascular regulation.

Myogenic Response

Since its first description in 1902 (see review by Johnson[39]), it was always assumed that responses of arteries and arterioles to changes in intravascular pressure are inherently dependent on vascular smooth muscle. Indeed, in in vitro experiments, Osol et al.[73] in cat cerebral arteries, Kulik et al.[57] in cat pulmonary arteries, Hwa and Bevan[34] in rabbit ear resistance arteries, and Kuo et al.[58,59] in porcine coronary arterioles found that the myogenic mechanism acts independent of the endothelium. Contrary to the above findings, however, recent in vitro studies of cerebral arteries of various species[27,28,44,92] suggested a role for endothelium, via a transferable contractile factor or depression of EDRF synthesis and/or release, in the pres-

sure-dependent contraction of arteries. These findings could provide an alternate interpretation for myogenic vasoregulation, since during an increase in flow, washout of a constrictor factor could result in vasodilation. It is of note that most of the in vitro studies have been done under "no flow" conditions. In in vivo circumstances, the presence of blood flow may modulate the myogenic response via release of endothelial vasodilator factors (vide infra). Recent in vivo studies by Hill et al.,[30] concerning the role of prostaglandins and EDRF in the myogenic response, showed that blocking prostaglandin synthesis augmented the myogenic response in rat skeletal muscle arterioles. These investigators also observed no changes in the myogenic response when pharmacological probes (methylene blue) were used to block EDRF. Future studies are necessary to clarify the precise role of endothelium in myogenic responses in vivo.

Flow-Dependent Response

In vitro studies on large vessels indicated that an increase in flow itself can elicit relaxation of vascular smooth muscle.[3,4,32,40,93] Our recent in vivo studies in the microcirculation seem to support this finding, since it was found that skeletal muscle arterioles are sensitive to increases in blood flow velocity.[47] Similar results were obtained by Smiesko et al. in arcade vessels of mesentery,[99] indicating the general presence of this phenomenon in the microcirculation. The underlying stimulus for the dilator response is likely to be an increase in wall shear stress upon an increase in blood flow velocity. It was also demonstrated that this phenomenon is mediated by the arteriolar endothelium (Fig. 4) since the dilation to increased flow velocity was inhibited by light/dye treatment of an arteriolar segment.[47] This treatment elicits an impairment of the vasoactive functions of the endothelium while the

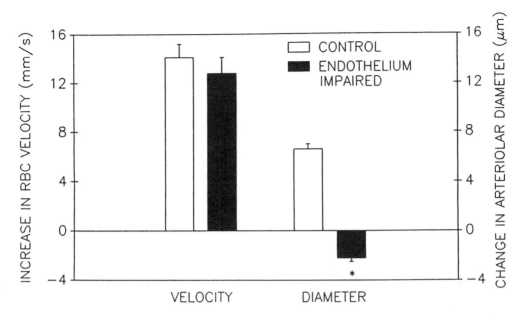

Figure 4: Summary data of peak arteriolar red blood cell velocity (left panel) and diameter (right panel) during parallel occlusion (causing an increase in flow velocity) in control conditions (empty bars) and after endothelial impairment by light/dye technique (black bars) in rat cremaster muscle. N=5–8, *p<0.05. An increase in blood flow velocity evokes an increase in arteriolar diameter in control conditions. Following impairment of the endothelium the increase in blood flow fails to evoke an increase in diameter.

vascular smooth muscle retains its responsiveness to other, nonendothelium-dependent stimuli.[50–52]

The observations of Hill et al.[30] and Kuo et al.[58,59] suggest that myogenic responses of arterioles are still present and even more pronounced after removal of the endothelium or blocking of endothelial mediators. For example, it could be hypothesized that an endothelial factor(s) modulates the myogenic response, but that the actual response is not dependent upon the presence of the endothelium. We recently found that in rat cremaster muscle, the arteriolar dilation to an increase in blood flow velocity was prevented by superfusion of the tissue with indomethacin or meclofenamate. This study[48] indicates that prostaglandins are likely to be responsible for the mediation of the flow velocity-dependent vasodilation in rat skeletal muscle microcirculation. It may be suspected that the presence of constant flow in vivo could elicit a basal release of these (or other) vasoactive factors which could counter myogenic constriction. Microvascular endothelium is a rich source of prostaglandins,[22,100] and studies of endothelial cells in culture already indicated a role for prostaglandins in response to an increase in shear stress.[20,23] Thus, our recent studies[46–48] may also shed light on the physiological role of prostaglandins in skeletal muscle microcirculation. It is known, however, that in vessels of other tissues, or in large conduit vessels, other mechanisms participate in the mediation of "flow-dependent" responses.[13] For example, in the rabbit ear artery studied in vitro, flow-dependent responses were still present after removal of the endothelium,[3,4] and depending on the level of basal tone, an increase in flow could even induce constriction.

Studies by Griffith et al.[24] in the isolated buffer-perfused rabbit ear, employing hemoglobin as a blocker of EDRF, concluded that EDRF may have a role in the flow-sensitive regulation of arterioles by maintaining a fourth-power relationship between flow and diameter. It is of note, however, that hemoglobin itself can cause contraction of vascular smooth muscle.[2] Olesen et al.[72] have suggested that activation of an endothelial K^+ current plays a role in flow velocity-induced vascular changes. It is presently not known whether the size of the vessels or difference in in vitro and in vivo methodology is the underlying reason for these discrepant results. It remains of interest, however, that recent studies indicate the involvement of EDRF and/or a nonprostaglandin product of arachidonic acid metabolism in the flow-sensitive dilation of large arteries.[40,93]

The sensitivity of arterioles to increases in blood flow velocity suggests that increases in diameter might serve to normalize wall shear stress. Since wall shear stress is related to viscosity (η) and wall shear rate (dv/dr), it is likely that if blood flow velocity or blood viscosity changes, a change in wall shear stress[49] will result. In a physiological setting, such as an increase in pressure drop across the microvascular network due to the increase in upstream pressure and/or a decrease in downstream resistance, the participation of flow-dependent mechanisms in the regulation of vessel diameter would be expected to be present. It is possible therefore that one of the primary roles of endothelial prostaglandins in the regulation of the skeletal muscle microcirculation would be to modify vascular resistance in response to a change in wall shear stress. It is likely that such a flow-sensitive mechanism is present at every level of the microcirculation to coordinate changes in vascular resistance. This mechanism, when activated, could

augment the increase in blood flow to tissues in case of increased demand (e.g., during exercise) without the expense of pressure elevation. It could be inferred that the impairment of this mechanism in states characterized by endothelial dysfunction[104] could severely diminish blood flow to parenchymal tissues, contributing further to the pathogenesis of vascular disease.

All of the above findings are consistent with the notion that endothelial mediators, primarily prostaglandins, EDRF, and reactive metabolites of oxygen, have an important role in the regulation of microvascular blood flow and resistance. Of particular interest is the suggestion that the release of PGI_2 and EDRF from endothelial cells is coupled via the mobilization of calcium and activation of phospholipase C.[14] It is also noteworthy that reactive oxygen metabolites are produced in the course of the metabolism of endothelial arachidonic acid, and that they in turn can terminate the activity of EDRF.[96] The interaction among these three classes of mediators at different levels of the circulatory tree may determine the contribution of endothelium to the regulation of vascular tone and blood flow. In addition, marked differences exist among and within species as well as among different vascular beds with regard to the synthesis or release, action, and physiological importance of endothelium-derived mediators. In summary, all the findings suggest that the endothelial cell layer of microvessels, ideally positioned to sense changes within or close to the vessel wall, can affect a variety of vascular reactions, but the precise role of the endothelial mediators in the maintenance of resistance vessel tone remains to be elucidated.

Acknowledgments: We appreciate the excellent secretarial assistance provided by Ms. Annette Ecke. The work described from our laboratories was supported in part by USPHS grants HL37453, HL31069, and PO1-HL-43023. M.S.W. is an Established Investigator of the American Heart Association.

References

1. Amezcua J.L., Palmer R.M.J., de Souza B.M., Moncada S.: Nitric oxide synthesized from L-arginine regulates vascular tone in the coronary circulation of the rabbit. Br. J. Pharmacol. 97:1119–1124, 1989.

2. Bény J.L., Brunet P.C., Van der Bent V.: Hemoglobin causes both endothelium-dependent and endothelium-independent contraction of the pig coronary arteries, independently of an inhibition of EDRF effects. Experientia 45:132–134, 1989.

3. Bevan J.A., Joyce E.H.: Flow-induced resistance artery tone: balance between constrictor and dilator mechanisms. Am. J. Physiol. 258:H663-H668, 1990.

4. Bevan J.A., Joyce E.H., Wellman G.C.: Flow-dependent dilation in a resistance artery still occurs after endothelium removal. Circ. Res. 63:980–985, 1988.

5. Bhardwaj R., Moore P.K.: Endothelium-derived relaxing factor and the effects of acetylcholine and histamine on resistance blood vessels. Br. J. Pharmacol. 95:835–843, 1988.

6. Burghuber O., Mathias M.M., McMurtry I.F., Reeves J.T., Thelkel N.L.: Lung edema to hydrogen peroxide is independent of cyclooxygenase products. J. Appl. Physiol. 56:900–905, 1984.

7. Burke T.M. Wolin M.S.: Hydrogen peroxide elicits pulmonary arterial relaxation and guanylate cyclase activation. Am. J. Physiol. 252:H721-H732, 1987.

8. Burke-Wolin T.M., Wolin M.S.: Inhibition of cGMP-associated pulmonary arterial relaxation to H_2O_2 and O_2 by ethanol. Am. J. Physiol. 258:H1267-H1273, 1990.

9. Burke-Wolin T., Cherry P.D., Gurtner G.H.: Tone-dependent effects of peroxides in rabbit pulmonary artery and isolated perfused lung (abstract). FASEB J. 4:A573, 1990.

10. Busse R., Forstermann U., Matsuda H., Pohl U.: The role of prostaglandins in the endothelium-mediated vasodilatory response to hypoxia. Pflugers Arch. 401:77–83, 1984.

11. Busse R., Trogisch G., Bassenge E.: The role of endothelium in the control of vascular tone. Basic Res. Cardiol. 80:475–490, 1985.

12. Coburn R.F., Eppinger R., Scott D.P.: Oxygen-dependent tension in vascular smooth muscle. Does the endothelium play a role? Circ. Res. 58:341–347, 1986.

13. Davies P.F.: How do vascular cells respond to flow? NIPS 4:22–25, 1989.

14. DeNucci G., Gryglewski R.G., Warner T.D., Vane J.R.: Receptor-mediated release of endothelium-derived relaxing factor and prostacyclin from bovine aortic endothelial cells is coupled. Proc. Natl. Acad. Sci. USA 85:2334–2338, 1988.

15. Doukas J., Hechtman H.B., Shepro D.: Vasoactive amines and eicosanoids interactively regulate both polymorphonuclear leukocyte diapedesis and albumin permeability in vitro. Microvasc. Res. 37:125–137, 1989.

16. Duling B.R.: Microvascular responses to alterations in oxygen tension. Circ. Res. 31:481–489, 1972.

17. Falcone J.C., Bohlen H.G.: EDRF from rat intestine and skeletal muscle venules causes dilation of arterioles. Am. J. Physiol. 258:H1515-H1523, 1990.

18. Faber J.E., Harris P.D., Miller N.: Microvascular sensitivity to PGE_2 and PGI_2 in skeletal muscle of the decerebrate rat. Am. J. Physiol. 243:H844-H851, 1982.

19. Fleming J.T. Harris P.D., Joshua I.G.: Endogenous prostaglandins selectively mask large arteriole constriction to angiotensin II. Am. J. Physiol. 253 (Heart Circ. Physiol. 22):H1573-H1580, 1987.

20. Frangos J.A., Eskin S.G., McIntire L.V., Ives C.L.: Flow effects on prostacyclin production by cultured human endothelial cells. Science 227:1477–1479, 1985.

21. Furchgott R.F., Carvalho M.H., Kahn K.: Evidence for endothelium-dependent vasodilation of resistance vessels by acetylcholine. Blood Vessels 24:145–149, 1987.

22. Gerritsen M.E., Cheli C.D.: Arachidonic acid and prostaglandin endoperoxide metabolism in isolated rabbit coronary microvessels and isolated and cultivated coronary microvessel endothelial cells. J. Clin. Invest. 72:1658–1671, 1983.

23. Grabowski E.F., Jaffee E.A., Weksler B.B.: Prostacyclin production by cultured endothelial cell monolayers exposed to step increases in shear stress. J. Lab. Clin. Med. 105:36–43, 1985.

24. Griffith T.M., Edwards D.H., Davies R.L., Harrison T.J., Evans K.T.: EDRF coordinates the behavior of vascular resistance vessels. Nature 329:442–445, 1987.

25. Gurtner G.H., Knoblauch A., Smith P.L., Sies H., Adkinson N.F.: Oxidant- and lipid-induced pulmonary vasoconstriction mediated by arachidonic acid metabolite. J. Appl. Physiol. 55:949–954, 1983.

26. Guth P.H., Mohler T.L.: The role of endogenous prostanoids in the response of the rat gastric microcirculation to vasoactive agents. Microvasc. Res. 23:336–346, 1982.

27. Harder D.R.: Pressure-induced nyogenic activation of cat cerebral arteries is dependent on intact endothelium. Circ. Res. 60:102–107, 1987.

28. Harder D.R., Sanchez-Ferrer C., Kauser K., Stekiel W.J., Rubanyi G.M..: Pressure releases a transferable endothelial contractile factor in cat cerebral arteries. Circ. Res. 65:193–198, 1989.

29. Hedqvist P.: Basic mechanisms of prostaglandin action on autonomic neurotransmission. Annu. Rev. Pharmacol. Toxicol. 17:259–270, 1977.

30. Hill M.A., Davis M.J., Meininger G.A.: Cyclooxygenase inhibition potentiates myogenic activity of skeletal muscle arterioles. Am. J. Physiol. 258: H127-H133, 1990.

31. Holland J.A., Pappolla M.A., Wolin M.S., Pritchard K.A., Rogers N.J., et al: Bradykinin induces superoxide anion release from human endothelial cells. J. Cell. Physiol. 143:21–25, 1990.

32. Holtz J., Forstermann U., Pohl M., Giesler E.: Flow-dependent, endothelium-mediated dilation of epicardial coronary arteries in conscious dogs: effects of cyclooxygenase inhibition. J. Cardiovasc. Pharmacol. 6:1161–1167, 1987.

33. Hutchins A.M., Bond R.F., Green H.D.: Participation of oxygen in the local control of skeletal muscle microcirculation. Circ. Res. 34:85–93, 1974.

34. Hwa J.J., Bevan J.A.: Stretch-dependent (myogenic) tone in rabbit ear resistance arteries. Am. J. Physiol. 250:H87-H95, 1986.

35. Ignarro L.J.: Biological actions and properties of endothelium-derived nitric oxide formed and released from artery and vein. Circ. Res. 65:1–21, 1989.

36. Jackson W.F.: Prostaglandins do not mediate arteriolar oxygen reactivity. Am. J. Physiol. 250:H1102-H1108, 1986.

37. Jackson W.F., Duling B.R.: The oxygen sensitivity of hamster cheek pouch arterioles. Circ. Res. 53:515–525, 1983.

38. Jackson W.F.: Arteriolar oxygen reactivity is inhibited by leukotriene antagonists. Am. J. Physiol. 257:H1565-H1572, 1989.

39. Johnson P.C.: The myogenic response. In: Handbook of Physiology (2nd Ed.), Bohr D.F., A.F. Somlyo, H.V. Sparks, et al. (eds.). American Physiological Society, Bethesda, p 409–442, 1980.

40. Kaiser L., Hull S. Jr., Sparks V. Jr.: Methylene blue and ETYA block flow-dependent dilation in canine femoral artery. Am. J. Physiol. 250:H974-H981, 1986.

41. Kaley G., Rodenburg J.M., Messina E.J., Wolin M.S.: Endothelium-associated vasodilator mechanisms in the rat skeletal muscle microcirculation. Am. J. Physiol. 256:H720-H725, 1989.

42. Kaley G., Rodenburg J.M., Messina E.J., Wolin M.S.: EDRF in the microcirculation: N^G-monomethyl-L-arginine inhibits acetylcholine and bradykinin-induced arteriolar dilation (abstract). FASEB J. 4:A555, 1990.

43. Kalsner S. Prostaglandins mediate relaxation of coronary artery strips under hypoxia. Prostaglandins Med. 1:231–239, 1978.

44. Katusic Z.S., Shepherd J.T., Vanhoutte A.M.: Endothelium-dependent contraction to stretch in canine basilar arteries. Am. J. Physiol. 252:H671-H673, 1987.

45. Koller A., Wolin M.S., Messina E.J., Kaley G.: Modified arteriolar responses to ATP after impairment of endothelium by light/dye techniques in vivo. Microvasc. Res. In press, 1990.

46. Koller A., Kaley G.: Role of endothelium in reactive dilation of skeletal muscle arterioles. Am. J. Physiol. In press, 1990.

47. Koller A., Kaley G.: Endothelium regulates skeletal muscle microcirculation by a blood flow velocity sensing mechanism. Am. J. Physiol. 258:H916-H920, 1990.

48. Koller A., Kaley G.: Prostaglandins mediate arteriolar dilation induced by increased blood flow velocity in skeletal muscle microcirculation. Circ. Res. 67:529–534, 1990.

49. Koller A., Kaley G.: Endothelial regulation of shear stress and blood flow in skeletal muscle microcirculation. Int. J. Microcirc. Clin. Exp. 9(1):61, 1990.

50. Koller A., Messina E.J., Wolin M.S., Kaley G.: Effects of endothelial impairment on arteriolar dilator responses in vivo. Am. J. Physiol. 257:H1485-H1489, 1989.

51. Koller A., Messina E.J., Wolin M.S., Kaley G.: Endothelial impairment inhibits prostaglandin and EDRF mediated arteriolar dilation in vivo. Am. J. Physiol. 257:H1966-H1970, 1989.

52. Koller A., Holin M.S., Messina E.J., Cherry P.D., Kaley G.: Endothelium-derived vasodilator factors in skeletal muscle microcirculation. In: Endothelium-Derived Relaxing Factors, G.M. Rubanyi, P.M. Vanhoutte (eds.). S. Karger, Basel, pp 309–314, 1990.

53. Kontos H.A., Wei E. P., Ellis E.F., Jenkins L.W., Povlishock J.T., Rowe G.T., Hess M.L.: Appearance of superoxide anion radical in cerebral extracellular space during increased prostaglandin synthesis in cats. Circ. Res. 57:142–151, 1985.

54. Kontos H.A., Wei E.P., Marshall J.J.: In vivo bioassay of endothelium-derived relaxing factor. Am. J. Physiol. 255:H1259–H1262 1988.

55. Kontos H.A., Wei E.P., Povlishock J.T., Christman C.W., Oxygen radicals mediate cerebral arteriolar dilation from arachidonate and bradykinin in cats. Circ. Res. 55:295–303, 1984.

56. Kukreja R.C., Kontos H.A., Hess M.L., Ellis E.F.: PGH synthetase and lipoxygenase generate superoxide in the presence of NADH or NADPH. Circ. Res. 59:612–619, 1986.

57. Kulik T.J., Evans J.N., Gamble W.J.: Stretch-induced contraction in pulmonary arteries. Am. J. Physiol. 255:H1391–H1398, 1988.

58. Kuo L., Chilian W.M., Davis M.J.: The coronary arteriolar myogenic response is independent of the endothelium. Circ. Res. 66:860–866, 1990.

59. Kuo L., Davis M.J., Chilian W.M.: Myogenic activity in isolated subepicardial and subendocardial coronary arterioles. Am. J. Physiol. 255:H1558-H1562, 1988.

60. Lamb F.S., King C.M., Harrell K., Burkel W., Webb R.C.: Free radical-mediated endothelial damage in blood vessels after electrical stinulation. Am. J. Physiol. 252:H1041-H1046, 1987.

61. Lüscher T.F.: Endothelial vasoactive substances and cardiovascular disease. Karger, Basel, 1988.

62. Marshall J.J., Wei E.P., Kontos H.A.: Independent blockade of cerebral vasodilation from acetylcholine and nitric oxide. Am. J. Physiol. 255:H847-H854, 1988.

63. McGiff J.C.: Prostaglandins, prostacyclin and thromboxanes. Annu. Rev. Pharmacol. Toxicol. 21:479–509, 1981.

64. Messina E.J., Rodenburg J., Kaley G.: Microcirculatory effects of leukotrienes, LTC_4 and LTD_4 in rat cremaster muscle. Microcirc. Endoth. Lymph. 5:3S5–375, 1988.

65. Messina E.J., Weiner R., Kaley G.: Microvascular effects of prostaglandins E_1 E_2 and A_1 in the rat mesentery and cremasteric muscle. Microvasc. Res. 8:77–89, 1974.

66. Messina E.J., Weiner R., Kaley G.: Inhibition of bradykinin vasodilation and potentiation of norepinephrine and angiotensin vasoconstriction by inhibitors of prostaglandin synthesis in rat skeletal muscle. Circ. Res. 37:430–437, 1975.

67. Messina E.J., Weiner R., Kaley G.: Prostaglandins and local circulatory control. Fed. Proc. 35:2357–2375, 1976.

68. Messina E.J., Weiner R., Kaley G.: Arteriolar reactive hyperemia: Modification by inhibitors of prostaglandin synthesis. Am. J. Physiol. 232:H571-H575, 1977.

69. Moore P.K., al-Swayeh O.A., Chong N.W.S., Evans R.A., Gibson A.: L-N^G-nitro arginine (L-NOARG), a novel L-arginine reversible inhibitor of endothelium-dependent vasodilation in vitro. Br. J. Pharmacol. 99:408–412, 1990.

70. Myers T.O., Messina E.J., Rodrigues A.M., Gerritsen M.E.: Altered aortic and cremaster muscle prostaglandin synthesis in diabetic rats. Am. J. Physiol. 249:E374-E379, 1985.

71. Myers P.R., Banitt P.F., Guerra R., Harrison D.: Characteristics of canine coronary resistance arteries. Am. J. Physiol. 257:H603-H610, 1989.

72. Olesen S., Clapham D.E., Davies P.F.: Hemodynamic shear stress activates a K+ current in vascular endothelial cells. Nature 331:168–170, 1988.

73. Osol G., Osol R., Halpern W.: Endothelial influence on cerebral artery tone and reactivity to transmural pressure. In: Resistance Arteries, Halpern W., B.L. Pegram, et al. (eds.) Perinatology Press, Ithaca, NY, pp 162–169, 1988.

74. Palmer R.M.J., Ferrige F.A.G., Moncada S.: Nitric oxide accounts for the biological activity of endothelium-derived relaxing factor. Nature 327:524–526, 1987.

75. Persson M.G., Gustafsson L.E., Wiklund N.P., Hedcpist N., Moncada S.: Endogenous nitric oxide as a modulator of rabbit skeletal muscle microcirculation in vivo. Br. J. Pharmacol. 100:463–466, 1990.

76. Piper P.J., Sampson A.P., bin Yaacob H., McLeod J.M.: Leukotrienes in the cardio-

vascular system. In: Advances in Prostaglandin, Thromboxane and Leukotreine Research, B. Samuelsson, et al. (eds.). Raven Press, Ltd., NY, pp 146–152, 1990.

77. Pittman R.N.: Influence of oxygen lack on vascular smooth muscle contraction. In: Vasodilatation, A.M. Vanhoutte, I. Leusen, (eds.). Raven Press, NY, p 181–191, 1989.

78. Pittman R.N.: Interaction between oxygen and the vessel wall. Can. J. Cardiol. 2:124–131, 1986.

79. Pohl U., Busse R.: EDRF increases C&MP in platelets during passage through the coronary vascular bed. Circ. Res. 65:1789–1803, 1989.

80. Pohl U., Dezsi L., Simon B., Busse R.: Selective inhibition of endothelium-dependent dilation in resistance-sized vessels in vivo. Am. J. Physiol. 253:H234-H239, 1987.

81. Proctor K.G.. Duling B.R.: Oxygen-derived free radicals and local control of striated muscle blood flow. Microvasc. Res. 24:77–86, 1982.

82. Proctor K.G., Falck J.R., Capdevila J.H.: Intestinal vasodilation by expoxyeicosatrienoic acids: arachidonic acid metabolites produced by a cytochrome P450 monooxygenase. Circ. Res. 60:50–59, 1987.

83. Rees D.D., Palmer R.M.J., Hodson H.F., Moncada S.: A specific inhibitor of nitric oxide formation from L-arginine attenuates endothelium dependent relaxation. Br. J. Pharmacol. 96:418–424, 1989.

84. Roberts A.M., Messina E.J., Kaley G. Prostacyclin (PGI_2) mediates hypoxic relaxation of bovine coronary arterial strips. Prostaglandins 21:555–569, 1981.

85. Rosenblum W.I.: Effects of free radical generation on mouse pial arterioles: possible role of hydroxyl radical. Am. J. Physiol. 245:H139-H152, 1983.

86. Rosenblum W.I.: Endothelial-dependent relaxation demonstrated in vivo in cerebral arterioles. Stroke 17:494–497, 1986.

87. Rosenblum W.I.: Hydroxyl radical mediates the endothelium-dependent relaxation produced by bradykinin in mouse cerebral arterioles. Circ. Res. 61:601–603, 1987.

88. Rosenblum W.I., Bryan D.: Evidence that in vivo constriction of cerebral arterioles by local application of tert-butyl hydroperoxide is mediated by the release of endogenous thromboxane. Stroke 18:195–199, 1987.

89. Rosenblum W.I. Nelson G.H.: Endothe-

lium-dependent constriction demonstrated in vivo in mouse cerebral arterioles. Circ. Res. 63:837–843, 1988.

90. Rosenblum W.I., Nelson G.H., Povlishock J.T.: Laser-induced endothelial damage inhibits endothelium-dependent relaxation in the cerebral microcirculation of the mouse. Circ. Res. 60:169–176, 1987.

91. Rosenblum W.I., Povlishock J.T., Wei E.P., Kontos H.A., Nelson G.H.: Ultrastructural studies of pial vascular endothelium following damage resulting in loss of endothelium-dependent relaxation. Stroke 18:927–931, 1987.

92. Rubanyi G.M.: Endothelium-dependent pressure induced contraction of isolated canine carotid arteries. Am. J. Physiol. 255:H783-H788, 1988.

93. Rubanyi G.M., Romero J.C., Vanhoutte P.M.: Flow-induced release of endothelium-derived relaxing factor. Am. J. Physiol. 250:H1145-H1149, 1986.

94. Rubanyi G.M., Vanhoutte A.M.: Hypoxia releases a vasoconstrictor substance from the canine vascular endothelium. J. Physiol. (Lond) 364:45–56, 1985.

95. Rubanyi G.M., Vanhoutte P.M.: Oxygen-derived free radicals, endothelium and responsiveness of vascular smooth muscle. Am. J. Physiol. 250:H815-H821, 1986.

96. Rubanyi G.M., Vanhoutte P.M.: Superoxide anions and hyperoxia inactivate endothelium-derived relaxing factor. Am. J. Physiol. 250:H822-H827, 1986.

97. Sakuma I., Stuehr D., Gross S.S., Nathan C., Levi R.: Identification of arginine as a precursor of endothelium derived relaxing factor (EDRF). Proc. Natl. Acad. Sci. USA 85:8664–8667, 1988.

98. Sellke F.W., Myers P.R., Bates J.N., Harrison D.G.: Influence of vessel size on the sensitivity of porcine coronary microvessels to nitroglycerin. Am. J. Physiol. 258:H515-H520, 1990.

99. Smiesko V., Lang D.J., Johnson P.C.: Dilator response of rat mesenteric arcarding arterioles to increased blood flow velocity. Am. J. Physiol. 257:H1958-H1965, 1989.

100. Smith W.L.: Prostaglandin biosynthesis and its compartmentation in vascular smooth muscle and endothelial cells. Annu. Rev. Physiol. 48:251–262, 1986.

101. Stewart A.G., Piper P.J.: Vasodilator actions of acetylcholine, A23187 and bradykinin in the guinea-pig isolated perfused heart are independent of prostacyclin. Br. J. Pharmacol. 95:379–384, 1988.

102. Stewart D.J., Munzel T., Bassenge E.: Re-

versal of acetylcholine-induced coronary resistance vessel dilation by hemoglobin. Eur. J. Pharmacol. 136:239–242, 1987.

103. Stewart D.J., Polh U., Bassange E.: Free radicals inhibit endothelium-dependent dilation in the coronary resistance bed. Am. J. Physiol. 255:H765-H769, 1988.

104. Takahashi M., Yui Y., Yasumoto H., Aoyama T., Morishita H., et al: Liproproteins are inhibitors of endothelium-dependent relaxation of rabbit aorta. Am. J. Physiol. 258:Hl-H8, 1990.

105. Tate R.M., Morris H.G., Schroeder W.R., Repine J.E.: Oxygen metabolites stinulate thromboxane production and vasoconstriction in isolated saline-perfused rabbit lungs. J. Clin. Invest. 74:608–613, 1984.

106. Tingo X.T., Ley K., Proes A.R., Gaehtgens P.: Venulo-arteriolar connunication and propagated response: A possible mechanism for local control of blood flow. Eur. J. Physiol. 414:450–456, 1989.

107. Watanabe M., Rosenblum W.I., Nelson G.H.: In vivo effect of methylene blue on endothelium-dependent and endothelium-independent dilations of brain microvessels in mice. Circ. Res. 62:86–90, 1988.

108. Wei E.P., Ellis E.F., Kontos H.A.: Role of prostaglandins in pial arteriolar response to CO_2 and hypoxia. Am. J. Physiol. 238:H226-H230, 1980.

109. Wei E.P., Christman C.W., Kontos H.A., Povlishock J.T.: Effects of oxygen radicals on cerebral arterioles. Am. J. Physiol. 248:H157-H162 1985.

110. Wei E.P., Kontos H.A., Christman C.W., DeWitt D.S., Povlishock J.T.: Superoxide generation and reversal of acetylcholine-induced cerebral arteriolar dilation after acute hypertension. Circ. Res. 57:781–787, 1985.

111. Weir E.K., Eaton J.W., Chesler E.: Redox status and pulmonary vascular reactivity, Chest 88:249S-252S, 1985.

112. Wolin M.S., Belloni F.L.: Superoxide anion selectively attenuates catecholamine-induced contractile tension in isolated rabbit aorta. Am. J. Physiol. 249:H1127-H1133, 1985.

113. Wolin M.S., Cherry P.D., Rodenburg J.M., Messina E.J., Kaley G.: Methylene blue inhibits vasodilation of skeletal muscle arterioles to acetylcholine and nitric oxide via the extracellular generation of superoxide anion. J. Pharmacol. Exp. Ther. 254:872–876, 1990.

114. Wolin, M.S., Messina E.J., Kaley G.: Involvement of prostaglandins in arteriolar vasodilation to peroxides. Adv. Prostaglandin Thrombox. Leukotr. Res. 19:281–284, 1989.

115. Wolin M.S., Rodenberg J.M., Messina E.J., Kaley G.: Oxygen metabolites and vasodilator mechanisms in rat cremasteric arterioles. Am. J. Physiol. 2S2:H1159-H1163, 1987.

116. Wolin M.S., Rodenburg J.M., Messina E.J., Kaley G.: Similarities in the pharnmcological modulation of reactive hyperemia and vasodilation to H_2O_2 in rat skeletal muscle arterioles: Effects of probes for endothelium-derived mediators. J. Pharmacol. Exp. Ther. 253:508–512 1990.

Part III

Endothelial Dysfunction and Cardiovascular Diseases

9

Endothelial Dysfunction in Hypertension

Thomas F. Lüscher, Paul M. Vanhoutte, Chantal Boulanger, Yasuaki Dohi, Fritz R. Bühler

Introduction

Hypertension is a major cardiovascular risk factor that contributes to the occurrence of coronary artery disease, stroke, and renal failure in a considerable number of patients. The mechanisms of hypertension-induced vascular injury are not well understood. In established hypertension, peripheral vascular resistance is consistently elevated. This vasoconstriction occurring at the resistance artery level could involve an increased activity of sympathetic nerve endings, changes in vascular smooth muscle reactivity to vasoconstrictor and vasodilator substances, and/or alterations in endothelium-dependent control mechanisms of vascular tone.

The endothelium, in particular, is an obvious target organ of hypertension, since—because of its anatomical location—it is that structure of the vascular wall that is most exposed to mechanical forces. Indeed, the endothelium senses the direction of blood flow and can react to changes in shear stress and pressure exerted on it. As the endothelium plays an important protective role in the circulation by the release of substances that inhibit platelet function and evoke vasodilatation, changes in endothelial function occurring in the hypertensive process could contribute importantly to the development of its cardiovascular complications.

This chapter focuses on alterations in endothelium-dependent responses in hypertensive blood vessels and updates previous reviews of that field.[1–5]

Morphological Changes of the Endothelium in Hypertension

Hypertension is associated with distinct morphological changes of the vascular endothelium and the subendothelial

Rubanyi G.M.: Cardiovascular Significance of Endothelium-Derived Vasoactive Factors, Futura Publishing Co., Inc., Mount Kisco, NY, © 1991.

layer.[1] The integrity of the endothelium as a cell layer is well-preserved, but alterations in permeability, shape, replication rate, and density of the cells do occur.[6] Indeed, endothelial cells of hypertensive blood vessels are more voluminous, bulge into the lumen, and exhibit a greater variation in size and shape as compared to those of normal blood vessels. The cell replication rate and number of endothelial cells in the aorta of hypertensive rats is increased. In addition, hypertension is associated with an increased adherence of circulating blood cells to the endothelial cell layer. The adhering cells are mainly granulocytes, monocytes, and lymphocytes and in the cerebral circulation of the rat also platelets.[7,8] Similar morphological changes as in hypertension have been observed in atherosclerosis. In hypertension, however, lipid accumulation in the intima does not occur in the absence of hyperlipoproteinemia.[7] This absence of an increased predisposition to the development of atherosclerotic lesions in most experimental models of hypertension is a major difference to human hypertensive vascular disease.[1]

Endothelium-Derived Substances and Blood Pressure Control

Endothelium-Derived Relaxing Factor

Basal Release of Endothelium-Derived Relaxing Factor

Infusion of hemoglobin, an inhibitor of endothelium-derived relaxing factor (EDRF), increases arterial blood pressure in healthy human subjects.[9] Intravenous infusion of L-N^G-monomethyl arginine (L-NMMA), an inhibitor of the formation of nitric oxide (which most likely is EDRF) from L-arginine,[10,11] augments arterial blood pressure in the rat and in the rabbit.[12,13] Likewise, intra-arterial application of L-NMMA in the forearm of normal subjects increases peripheral vascular resistance and decreases local blood flow (Fig. 1).[14] These observations imply that the continuous release of endothelium-derived nitric oxide contributes to the regulation of peripheral vascular resistance. Thus, alterations in the basal release of endothelium-derived vasoactive factors could contribute to the increase in peripheral vascular resistance characteristic of hypertension.

Stimulated Release of Endothelium-Derived Relaxing Factor

Systemic application of endothelium-dependent vasodilators such as acetylcholine, adenosine diphosphate (ADP), and substance P markedly decreases blood pressure in the rabbit.[15] In the forearm of healthy human subjects, intra-arterial administration of acetylcholine evokes a profound increase in forearm blood flow (Fig. 2).[16] The vasodilator effects of acetylcholine are unaffected by acetylsalicylic acid and phentolamine, indicating that prostacyclin and inhibitory effects of the muscarinic agonist on adrenergic neurotransmission do not contribute significantly.[16] Infusion of L-NMMA blunts the vasodilator effects of acetylcholine in the forearm circulation of normal subjects.[14] This indicates that acetylcholine releases endothelium-derived nitric oxide from the human blood vessel wall in vivo.

Effects on Hormonal Systems of Blood Pressure Control

Endothelium-derived relaxing factor(s) can interfere with the release of sub-

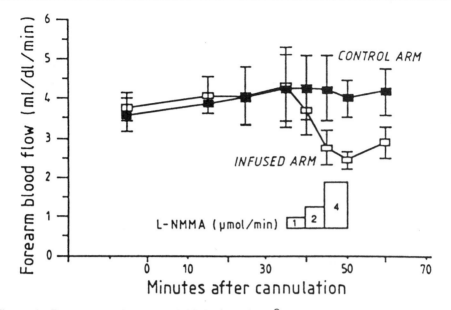

Figure 1: Response to intra-arterial infusion of L-N^G-monomethyl arginine (L-NMMA) into the brachial artery of five human subjects. Changes in forearm blood flow (mL/dL/min) occurring in the control arm (closed symbols) and infused arm (open symbols) during infusion of increasing concentrations of L-NMMA are given. The difference in forearm blood flow between the two arms is statistically significant for each dose of L-NMMA (from ref. 14, by permission).

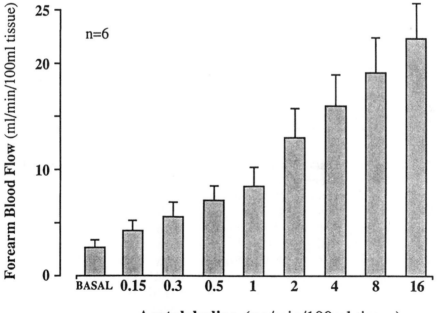

Figure 2: Effects of increasing concentrations of acetylcholine infused intra-arterially into the brachial artery of six human subjects. Note the significant and concentration-dependent increase in forearm blood flow during infusion of acetylcholine (data from ref. 16).

stances involved in blood pressure control such as renin and atrial natriuretic peptide. Endothelium-derived relaxing factor released from perfused canine femoral arteries by acetylcholine or from endothelial cells in culture by bradykinin reduces the production of renin by canine kidney slices.[17,18] Anatomically, endothelial cells and juxtaglomerular cells are closely related to the preglomerular arterioles. Since endothelial cells can respond to physical forces (shear stress, blood flow etc.)[1,5] with an increase in the release of EDRF, modulation of the release of renin by the factor could link changes in perfusion pressure in the afferent arterioles with the release of renin. Thus, the endothelial cells may act as the intrarenal baroreceptor.

Removal of the endocardium in the atrium of the rat with saponin increases the release of atrial natriuretic peptide.[19] Since a similar effect can be obtained with inhibitors of EDRF such as hemoglobin, methylene blue, and hydroquinone, EDRF released from the endocardium or from endothelial cells of the coronary vasculature may modulate the release of natriuretic peptide.

Endothelin

Hemodynamic Effects of Endothelin

In the rat and rabbit, intravenous infusion of endothelin-1 causes a rapid and transient decrease in systemic blood pressure followed by a profound and long-lasting increase in blood pressure.[20] In the human forearm circulation, endothelin increases peripheral vascular resistance and decreases local blood flow.[21,22]

Release of Endothelin from the Vessel Wall

In the porcine aorta, endothelin is continuously released in an endothelium-de-

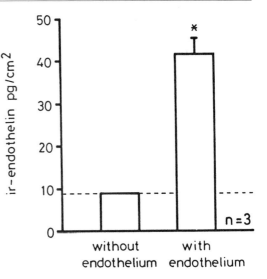

Figure 3: Release of immunoreactive endothelin (ir-endothelin) from intact porcine aortic strips under basal conditions. Note that the peptide is released in preparations with (right column), but not in those without endothelium (left column). The dotted line indicates the limit of detection of the radioimmunoassay (from ref. 23, by permission).

pendent manner as it is in endothelial cells in culture (Fig. 3);[23,24] the fact that endothelin is continuously formed in isolated blood vessels suggests that it may contribute to the long-term regulation of vascular tone. The exact definition of its contribution, however, awaits experiments with specific inhibitors of the peptide.

The release of the peptide can be further stimulated with thrombin (2–4 units/ml) (Fig. 4) and the calcium ionophore A23187.[20,23,24] Since cyclohexamide prevents the formation of the peptide under these conditions, the process must involve de novo protein synthesis.[23] The production of endothelin is regulated further by endothelium-derived nitric oxide which is concomitantly formed during stimulation with thrombin.[5] Hence, the inhibitor of the formation of endothelium-derived nitric oxide L-NMMA augments the thrombin-induced stimulation of endothelin production to a similar degree as

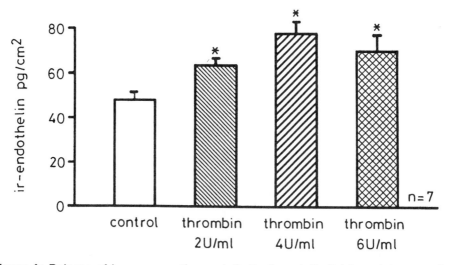

Figure 4: Release of immunoreactive endothelin (ir-endothelin) from intact porcine aortic strips under basal conditions (left column) and during stimulation with increasing concentrations of thrombin. * = indicates statistically significant difference from control. In preparations without endothelium, thrombin did not increase the production of endothelin (data not shown) (from ref. 23, by permission).

the inhibitor of soluble guanylate cyclase methylene blue.[23] On the other hand, superoxide dismutase (which prevents the inactivation of nitric oxide by superoxide radicals) and the stable analogue of cyclic GMP 8-bromo-cyclic GMP inhibits the thrombin-induced formation of the peptide (Fig. 5).[23] This suggests that endothelium-derived nitric oxide inhibits the thrombin-induced formation of endothelin from intact blood vessels via cGMP-dependent mechanisms.

Circulating Endothelin Levels

In humans, the circulating plasma levels of endothelin are very low (1.5 pg/ml).[25–27] The circulating levels of the peptide increase with age.[28]

Effects on Regulation of Blood Pressure

Endothelin increases the release of atrial natriuretic peptide from cultured rat atrial myocytes.[29] In vivo, endothelin increases the release of atrial natriuretic peptide from the rat atrium.[30] Similarly, in bovine adrenal chromaffin cells, endothelin-1 increases the efflux of norepinephrine and epinephrine.[31] In contrast, the peptide reduces the basal and stimulated release of renin from isolated glomeruli of the rat.[32–34] Endothelin also inhibits adrenergic neurotransmission in the guinea pig femoral artery.[35]

Cardiac Effects

In addition, endothelin can interfere with cardiac function. In the atrium of the rat and of the guinea pig, endothelin has potent inotropic and chronotropic effects.[36,37]

Hypertension

Acute Hypertension

In the canine coronary circulation, brief increases in perfusion pressure en-

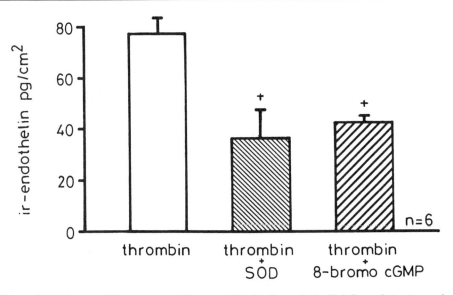

Figure 5: Release of immunoreactive endothelin (ir-endothelin) from intact porcine aortic strips during stimulation with thrombin (4 units/mL) under control conditions (left column) and in the presence of superoxide dismutase (to prevent a breakdown of endothelium-derived nitric oxide) or of 8-bromo-cyclic GMP. Note that both interventions prevent the thrombin-stimulated increase in endothelin release from intact porcine aortic strips (* = $p < 0.05$) (from ref. 23, by permission).

hance the vasoconstrictor response to serotonin, while endothelium-dependent relaxations to acetylcholine remain preserved. These effects of acute hypertension can be prevented by the removal of the endothelium.[38]

In the cerebral circulation of the cat, acute hypertension abolishes endothelium-dependent relaxations to acetylcholine.[39] Since topical application of superoxide dismutase and catalase restores the endothelium-dependent relaxations to acetylcholine in most cases, this indicates that oxygen-derived free radicals are continuously formed after the hypertensive episode has subsided and destroy endothelium-derived relaxing factor.[39]

Chronic Hypertension

Basal Release of Endothelium-Derived Relaxing Factor

In the aorta of the spontaneously hypertensive rat, it is uncertain whether or not the basal release of the endothelium-derived relaxing factor is decreased. A normal basal release of endothelium-derived relaxing factor in the aorta of these hypertensive animals would be in line with the observation that the removal of the endothelium enhances the responsiveness to serotonin and norepinephrine to a similar degree in spontaneously hypertensive and Wistar-Kyoto rats.[1,40,41] However, this is hard to reconcile with the findings that the basal levels of cyclic GMP are decreased in aortas with endothelium from rats with spontaneous renal, DOCA salt hypertension, or coarctation of the aorta.[42,43] In line with these experiments, under bioassay conditions, donor segments of aortas obtained from spontaneously hypertensive rats have a decreased capacity to relax bioassay rings without endothelium as compared to segments obtained from normotensive rats.[44,45]

In perfused and pressurized mesenteric resistance arteries of the spontaneously hypertensive rat, the presence of the endothelium reduces the sensitivity and maximal response to norepinephrine.[46] Since this effect can in large part be prevented by the inhibitor of endothelium-derived nitric oxide L-NMMA, the endogenous nitrate is the most important mediator. In young and even more pronounced in adult spontaneously hypertensive rats, the inhibitory effect of the endothelium is reduced, indicating a diminished basal formation of endothelium-derived nitric oxide in hypertensive mesenteric resistance arteries.[46] A contribution of prostacyclin can be excluded as indomethacin does not affect the response.

Removal of the endothelium enhances the response to sodium nitroprusside in mesenteric resistance arteries, most likely due to an inhibitory effect of basally released endothelium-derived relaxing factor.[47] This augmentation of the response to sodium nitroprusside is reduced in stroke-prone spontaneously hypertensive rats as compared to Wistar-Kyoto rats, again suggesting that the basal release of endothelium-derived relaxing factor is impaired in hypertensive resistance arteries[47] (see also section entitled "Responsiveness of Vascular Smooth Muscle" and Fig. 18).

Endothelium-Dependent Relaxations

Large conduit arteries

The endothelium-dependent relaxations to acetylcholine are attenuated in the aorta of rats with spontaneous hypertension (Fig. 6),[48–50] renal hypertension, salt-induced hypertension, coarctation, and DOCA salt-induced hypertension.[40,51–56] Similar alterations occur in the carotid artery, but not in the renal artery of adult spontaneously hypertensive rats.[41,57] In the aorta of the Dahl rat, the reduction of the endothelium-dependent relaxations to acetylcholine is directly related to the level of arterial blood pressure (Fig. 7).[58] Normalization of blood pressure with

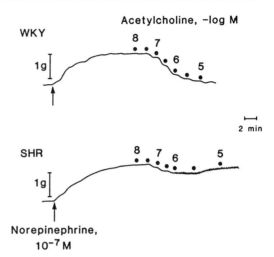

Figure 6: Endothelium-dependent relaxations to acetylcholine in an aortic ring obtained from a normotensive Wistar-Kyoto rat (WKY; top panel) and a spontaneously hypertensive rat (SHR; lower panel). Note the impaired response in the hypertensive rat. NE = norepinephrine (from ref. 2, by permission).

antihypertensive drugs (reserpine, hydrochlorothiazide plus hydralazine) restores endothelium-dependent relaxations in hypertensive Dahl rats (Fig. 8).[59] Similarly, in rats with aortic coarctation, endothelium-dependent relaxations are maintained in the aortic segment distal to the stenosis.[51,52] This suggests that in these forms of hypertension, the impaired endothelium-dependent relaxations are a consequence rather than a cause of the high blood pressure. In contrast to the rat, psychosocial hypertension in the mouse is associated with enhanced endothelium-dependent relaxations to acetylcholine in the aorta.[60] A similar augmentation has been reported in the femoral artery of the spontaneously hypertensive rat.[48] Whether or not these differences between rats and mice are related to differences in the severity, duration, or form of hypertension or reflect true species differences remains to be established.

The endothelium-dependent relaxations to thrombin are reduced in Dahl hypertensive, but not in spontaneously hy-

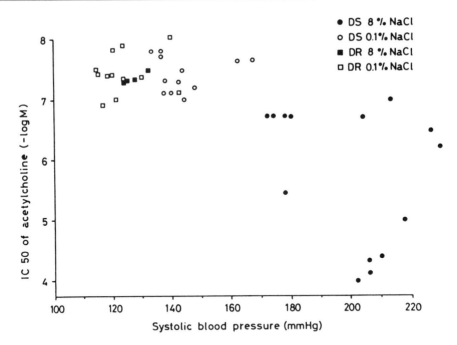

Figure 7: Systolic blood pressure and endothelium-dependent relaxations to ace-tylcholine in Dahl salt-sensitive (DS) and Dahl salt-resistant (DR) rats on different diets. Note that the IC_{50}-value of acetylcholine (negative log M), that is the concentration of the muscarinic agonist required to evoke 50% relaxation of the contraction induced by norepinephrine, is negatively correlated with the level of systolic blood pressure. Closed circle = DS on 8% NaCl; open circle = DS on 0.1% NaCl; closed square = DR on 8% NaCl; open square = DR on 0.1% NaCl (from ref. 58, by permission).

pertensive rats.[1,40,61] In contrast, endothe-lium-dependent relaxations to ADP are impaired in the aorta and in the carotid ar-tery of both hypertensive strains.[40,44,57,61] Serotonin and aggregating platelets do not evoke endothelium-dependent relaxations in the aorta or in the carotid artery of the rat,[41,61] but in the aorta of normotensive rats, the contractions evoked by aggregat-ing platelets are inhibited in the presence of the endothelium.[61] In contrast, in spon-taneously hypertensive rats, the endothe-lium loses its inhibitory capacity against platelet-induced contractions.[61]

The endothelium-dependent relaxa-tion to histamine is reduced in the aorta of renal hypertensive and DOCA salt-hyper-tensive rat, but enhanced in that of spon-taneously hypertensive rats.[55,56] Taken in conjunction with the results obtained with thrombin, these divergent findings illus-trate that endothelium-dependent relaxa-tions can be affected differentially depend-ing on the type of hypertension.

Resistance arteries

In small mesenteric arteries (internal diameter of 100 to 200 μ) of the sponta-neously hypertensive rat studied in a my-ograph system, the endothelium-depen-dent relaxations to acetylcholine and bra-dykinin are reduced (Fig. 9).[47,62–64] As in large arteries, the relaxations are reduced predominantly at higher concentrations of the muscarinic agonist. Similarly, in pres-surized perfused mesenteric resistance, ar-teries contracted with norepinephrine[46,65] and in mesenteric microvessels of the spontaneously hypertensive rat studied in

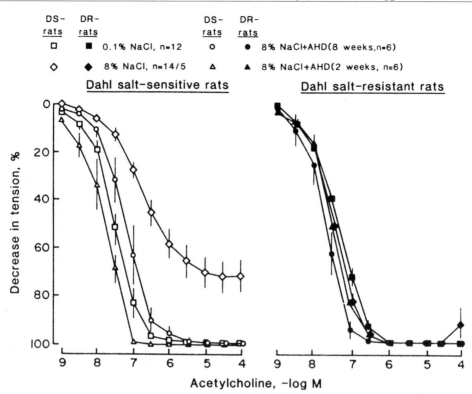

Figure 8: Effect of antihypertensive therapy on systolic blood pressure values in Dahl salt-sensitive (DS; left panel) and Dahl salt-resistant (DR; right panel) rats on a high sodium (8% NaCl) or low sodium diet (0.1% NaCl). Note that the endothelium-dependent relaxations to acetylcholine are reduced in hypertensive rats (i.e., DS rats on a high sodium diet; left panel) and that antihypertensive therapy (with reserpin, hydrochlorothiazide, and hydralazine) for either 8 weeks (to prevent hypertension) or 2 weeks (to reverse hypertension) normalizes the response. In Dahl salt-resistant rats (right panel), the interventions do not significantly affect endothelium-dependent relaxations to acetylcholine (from ref. 59, by permission of the American Heart Association).

vivo,[66] the endothelium-dependent relaxations to acetylcholine are reduced. The defect primarily involves the intraluminal activation of the endothelial cell by acetylcholine, suggesting that the part of the endothelial cell most exposed to high blood pressure and shear stress exerted by the circulating blood becomes dysfunctional in hypertension.[46] Both in perfused mesenteric resistance arteries[46] and in those studied in the myograph system,[62,67] endothelium-dependent relaxations become impaired as blood pressure rises.

In the cerebral microcirculation of the anesthetized, stroke-prone spontaneously hypertensive rat, the vasodilator responses to acetylcholine (but not those to nitroglycerin) and that to ADP and serotonin are attenuated or converted into contraction.[68,69]

In the hindlimb circulation of the rabbit, hypertension does not induce marked changes in vascular reactivity; the maximal relaxation evoked by acetylcholine, however, is reduced.[70] In the perfused hindlimb of rats with psychosocial hypertension, even the endothelium-dependent relaxations to acetylcholine are enhanced.[60]

In the forearm of hypertensive patients, the dilatation evoked by intra-arte-

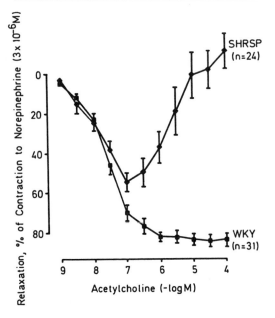

Figure 9: Endothelium-dependent relaxations to acetylcholine in mesenteric resistance arteries obtained from normotensive Wistar-Kyoto rats (WKY) or stroke-prone spontaneously hypertensive rats (SHRSP). Note the reversal of the relaxations induced by acetylcholine at higher concentrations of the muscarinic agonist in the hypertensive animals (from ref. 47, by permission).

rial acetylcholine is attenuated (Fig. 10).[16,71] Since the response to sodium nitroprusside, which as endothelium-derived relaxing factor activates cyclic GMP in vascular smooth muscle, is not significantly reduced, the impaired response to acetylcholine most likely involves an endothelial defect.

Endothelium-Dependent Contractions

Acetylcholine

Acetylcholine causes endothelium-dependent contractions in the aorta of the adult spontaneously hypertensive rat, while the responses are weak or absent in normotensive Wistar-Kyoto rats of the

same age (Fig. 11).[50] In old rats (12 months of age), endothelium-dependent contractions to acetylcholine occur also in normotensive rats and are even more pronounced in spontaneously hypertensive animals.[72] Thus, the occurrence of endothelium-dependent contractions to acetylcholine may reflect the premature aging of the hypertensive arterial wall.

The endothelium-dependent contractions to acetylcholine occur with higher concentrations than those required to trigger the release of endothelium-derived relaxing factor.[50] The endothelial receptor involved is muscarinic in nature, but has not been subtyped. Typically, the endothelium-dependent contractions are associated with rhythmic oscillations in tension, which are prevented by ouabain or potassium-free solution suggesting the involvement of the Na^+, K^+-pump.[1,50] The endothelium-dependent contractions to acetylcholine are abolished by inhibitors of phospholipase A_2 or of cyclooxygenase, demonstrating that the metabolism of endogenous arachidonic acid is involved (Fig. 11).[50]

Most prostaglandins (including prostacyclin) cause contraction of the aorta of the rat and these contractions, particularly those to prostaglandin $F_{2\alpha}$, are enhanced in the spontaneously hypertensive rats.[50,73] Tranylcypromine, an inhibitor of prostacyclin-synthetase, does not reduce the contractions induced by acetylcholine; hence, prostacyclin does not mediate the response.[50] Isolated blood vessels with endothelium of spontaneously hypertensive rats release small amounts of prostaglandin $F_{2\alpha}$, prostaglandin E_2, and—in contrast to normotensive rats—thromboxane B_2.[44] However, infusion of acetylcholine does not significantly stimulate the formation of the prostanoids. Since attempts to bioassay the endothelium-derived contracting factor released by acetylcholine have failed, it is unlikely that stable prostaglandins are involved. Endothelium-dependent contractions could be mediated by

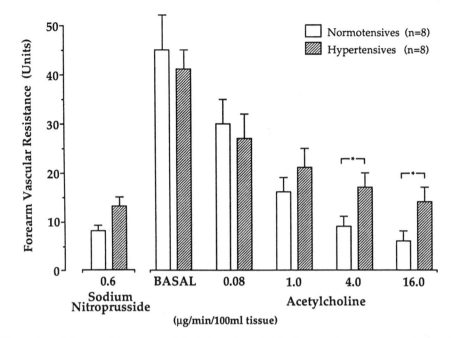

Figure 10: Effects of intra-arterially infused acetylcholine on forearm vascular resistance in normotensive subjects (open bars) and patients with essential hypertension (shaded bars). Note the reduced effects of acetylcholine in the hypertensive patients. * = p < 0.05 (from ref. 16, by permission of the American Heart Association).

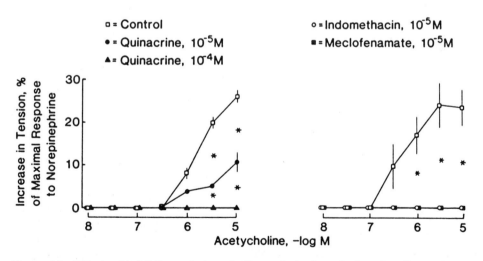

Figure 11: Effects of inhibitors of phospholipase A_2 (quinacrine) and cyclooxygenase (meclofenamate and indomethacin) on endothelium-dependent contractions evoked by acetylcholine in aortas of the spontaneously hypertensive rat. * = significant difference from control (p < 0.05; n = 4) (from ref. 50, by permission of the American Heart Association).

oxygen-derived free radicals formed during the activation of the cyclooxygenase pathway.[74] However, in the aorta of the spontaneously hypertensive rat, scavengers of oxygen-derived free radicals do not prevent endothelium-dependent contractions to acetylcholine.[75] Although inhibitors of thromboxane synthetase are unable to block the endothelium-dependent contractions,[50,76] thromboxane receptor antagonists are effective.[73,76] Similarly, the contractions to exogenous prostaglandin H_2 are prevented by thromboxane receptor antagonists, but unaffected by inhibitors of the synthesis of the prostanoid.[73] Thus, it is likely that prostaglandin H_2 is the endothelium-derived contracting factor released by acetylcholine in the aorta of the rat.

The situation may be somewhat different in mesenteric resistance arteries. Although indomethacin and meclofenamate both normalize the reduced endothelium-dependent relaxations to acetylcholine in mesenteric resistance arteries of the spontaneously hypertensive rat studied in a myograph,[47,62–64] it is difficult to obtain significant endothelium-dependent contractions in quiescent preparations.[47] In pressurized perfused resistance vessels obtained from the same animals, inhibitors of cyclooxygenase do not affect the response to acetylcholine.[46]

Stretch

Isolated aortas obtained from normotensive rats contract when stretched, a response that is larger in arteries from DOCA-hypertensive rats.[77] Removal of the endothelium reduces the stretch-induced increase in tension without affecting contractions to norepinephrine.[77] These observations indicate that hypertension promotes stretch-induced endothelium-dependent contractions.

Platelet-derived products

Release of platelet-derived products: The altered endothelial function, together with the greater aggregability of the platelets from hypertensives[78–84] may favor the occurrence of vasoconstriction and thrombus formation in hypertensive blood vessels. The uptake and content of serotonin of hypertensive platelets, particularly those of older hypertensive men, is reduced.[81] The thrombin-induced release of serotonin from platelets and the aggregation induced by ADP and serotonin are increased in patients with essential hypertension.[83,84]

Vascular reactivity: In the aorta of the spontaneously hypertensive rat contracted with prostaglandin $F_{2\alpha}$, serotonin causes larger contractions in rings with endothelium than in those without endothelium.[61] These differences are particularly apparent in the presence of ketanserin, which blocks $5\text{-}HT_2$-serotonergic receptors on vascular smooth muscle. Under these conditions, a marked inhibitory effect of the endothelium against contractions induced by serotonin is apparent in aortas obtained from normotensive rats, while in hypertensive aortas, the monoamine facilitates contractions induced by serotonin (Fig. 12).[61]

In isolated perfused hearts from normotensive rats, the monoamine induces moderate increases in flow, while marked decreases in flow occur in hearts from spontaneously hypertensive rats (Fig. 13).[85] The constrictor effect of serotonin in the coronary circulation of hypertensive hearts can be blocked by indomethacin. Similarly, in the cerebral microcirculation of hypertensive rats, the dilator effects of adenosine diphosphate and serotonin are lost or converted into contractions, respectively; indomethacin unmasks relaxations in response to the platelet-derived mediators.[68,69] The results of these studies are consistent with the concept that under these conditions, a cyclooxygenase-dependent endothelium-derived contracting fac-

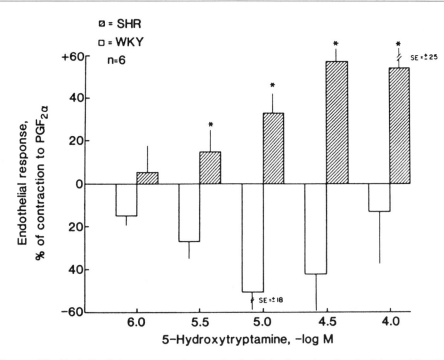

Figure 12: Endothelial response to serotonin (5-hydroxytryptamine) in aortic rings from normotensive Wistar-Kyoto rats (WKY) and spontaneously hypertensive rats (SHR) contracted with prostaglandin $F_{2\alpha}$ ($PGF_{2\alpha}$). In all experiments, the 5-HT_2-serotonergic antagonist ketanserin (10^{-7} M) was present to minimize the direct contractile effects of serotonin on vascular smooth muscle. The endothelial response was calculated as the tension of rings with endothelium minus the tension of rings without endothelium and expressed as percent of the contraction in response to $PGF_{2\alpha}$. * = statistically significant difference between WKY and SHR ($p < 0.05$) (from ref. 61, by permission of the American Heart Association).

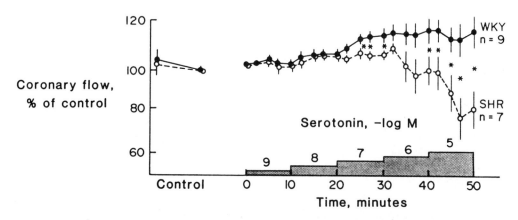

Figure 13: Effects of serotonin on coronary flow in isolated heart perfused by the Langendorff technique from normotensive Wistar-Kyoto rats (WKY; closed circles) and spontaneously hypertensive rat (SHR; open circles). * = statistically significant difference between WKY and SHR (data from ref. 85, figure from ref. 1, by permission).

tor is liberated in response to the platelet products.[1]

Endothelin

Circulating levels: In patients with essential hypertension, the circulating levels of endothelin do not appear to be increased.[28] However, in both normotensive and hypertensive subjects, the levels of the peptide increase with advancing age.[28] On the other hand, plasma levels of endothelin are increased in patients with renal insufficiency, cardiogenic shock, and in the coronary sinus of patients with coronary artery disease.[86-88]

Vascular responsiveness: The first reports on the responsiveness of isolated blood vessels from hypertensive rats to endothelin yielded conflicting results.[89-93] Indeed, while some authors reported a reduced sensitivity to endothelin in the aorta and renal artery and in perfused mesenteric resistance arteries of spontaneously hypertensive rats,[93,94] others reported normal (in mesenteric resistance arteries of stroke-prone spontaneously hypertensive rats studied in the myograph)[90] or augmented responses.[89,92]

Mechanisms of Endothelial Dysfunction in Hypertension

Although endothelium-dependent vascular responses are altered in most types of hypertension, the reasons underlying the dysfunction vary, depending on the cause of the disease and the blood vessel involved (Fig. 14).[2]

Endothelium-derived relaxing factor(s)

As judged from bioassay experiments, in the aorta of spontaneously hyperten-

sive, renal, and DOCA salt-hypertensive rats, the luminal release of endothelium-derived relaxing factor induced by acetylcholine and histamine is normal (Fig. 15).[44,45,56] A reduced abluminal release of the factor, however, cannot be excluded under these experimental conditions. In the Dahl salt-sensitive hypertensive rat, the reduced relaxation to acetylcholine is explained best by the combination of a reduced release of endothelium-derived relaxing factor and a decreased responsiveness of the vascular smooth muscle to the factor (see "Responsiveness of Vascular Smooth Muscle") (see Fig. 18).[40]

In perfused mesenteric resistance arteries of the spontaneously hypertensive rat, less endothelium-derived relaxing factor(s) is released during intraluminal, but not extraluminal stimulation with acetylcholine,[46] suggesting a defective receptor-operated release mechanism of the factor(s). Similarly, in patients with essential hypertension, intra-arterial acetylcholine evokes less vasodilatation, while the response to sodium nitroprusside is not significantly impaired (see Fig. 10).[16,71] Under both conditions, inhibitors of cyclooxygenase (i.e., indomethacin or aspirin intravenously, respectively) do not affect the response evoked by acetylcholine,[16,46] suggesting that under these experimental conditions and in these vascular beds, a contribution of a cyclooxygenase-dependent endothelium-derived contracting factor (EDCF$_2$; see below) is not involved.

As it becomes increasingly obvious that two mediators of endothelium-dependent relaxations are released (endothelium-derived nitric oxide and endothelium-derived hyperpolarizing factor),[1,5] the defect may involve the release of either factor and/or the vascular responsiveness to it. In the aorta of hypertensive rats, the contribution of relative changes in the release of endothelium-derived nitric oxide and/or endothelium-derived hyperpolarizing factor, respectively, has not been delineated. In mesenteric resistance arteries

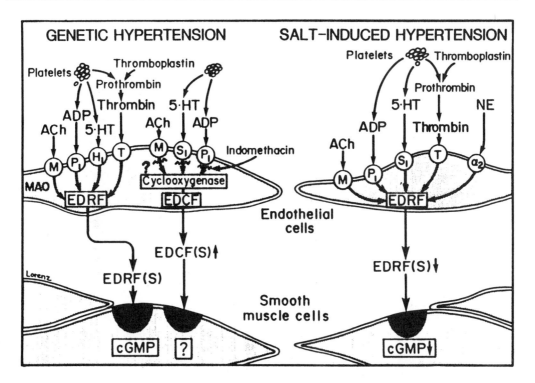

Figure 14: Proposed mechanisms of altered endothelium-dependent relaxations in genetic (spontaneous) and salt-induced hypertension of the rat. In spontaneously hypertensive rats (left), endothelium-dependent relaxations are decreased because of a concomitant release of endothelium-derived relaxing (EDRF) and constricting (EDCF) factors. In salt-induced hypertension (right), a reduced vascular responsiveness to EDRF—and possibly also decreased transit of EDRF—appears to be involved (from ref. 2).

of the rat, endothelium-derived nitric oxide accounts only in part for the endothelium-dependent relaxations to acetylcholine (to judge from the inhibitory effects of L-NMMA), and that part of the response is reduced in adult spontaneously hypertensive rats.[46]

Prostacyclin

The amount of prostacyclin released from the blood vessel wall of hypertensive rats in response to muscarinic activation is similar to that observed in normotensive rats[44,95] (Fig. 15). In most preparations, prostaglandin does not contribute to endothelium-dependent responses.

Endothelium-derived contracting factors

In the aorta of the spontaneously hypertensive rat, the decreased endothelium-dependent relaxations to higher concentrations of acetylcholine are due to the simultaneous release of endothelium-derived relaxing and contracting factors (EDCF$_2$).[12,50] Indeed, inhibitors of cyclooxygenase (i.e., indomethacin or meclofenamate) normalize the impaired endothelium-dependent relaxations (Fig. 16). Similarly, in mesenteric resistance arteries studied in a myograph, inhibitors of cyclooxygenase normalize the response to acetylcholine (Fig. 17).[47,63,64] Thus, in the microvessels, an endothelium-derived

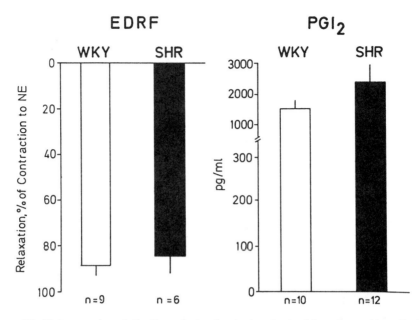

Figure 15: Release of endothelium-derived relaxing factor(s) and prostacyclin from aortic segments obtained from normotensive Wistar-Kyoto rats (WKY) and spontaneously hypertensive rats (SHR) studied under bioassay conditions. Note the similar relaxing effects of perfusate passing through a WKY or SHR aorta during stimulation with acetylcholine (left panel) as well as the comparable amounts of prostacyclin (PGI_2) released by either strain (data from ref. 44).

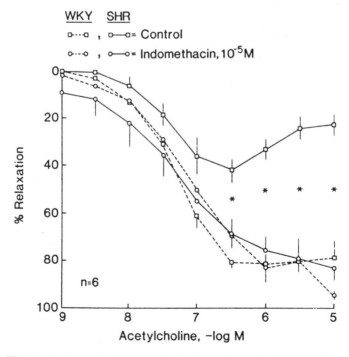

Figure 16: Effect of indomethacin on endothelium-dependent relaxations induced by acetylcholine in rings of aortas from normotensive Wistar-Kyoto rats (WKY) and spontaneously hypertensive rats (SHR) that were contracted with norepinephrine (10^{-8} – 3×10^{-7} M). * = significant difference from control ($p < 0.05$) (from ref. 50, by permission of the American Heart Association).

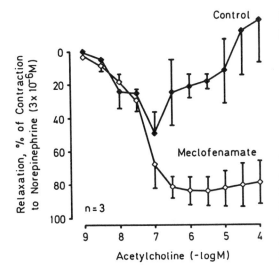

Figure 17: Effect of meclofenamate on endothelium-dependent relaxations induced by acetylcholine in rings of mesenteric resistance arteries (studied in a myograph system) obtained from stroke-prone spontaneously hypertensive rats (SHRSP). Note the normalization of the endothelium-dependent response to acetylcholine in the presence of the inhibitor of cyclooxygenase (from ref. 47, by permission).

product of cyclooxygenase probably interferes either with the release, the half-life, or the action of endothelium-derived relaxing factor.

Subendothelial thickening

A diffusion barrier due to subendothelial thickening in hypertensive blood vessels is unlikely to interfere with the response to acetylcholine (and other endothelium-dependent vasodilators), since endothelium-dependent relaxations to acetylcholine or ADP are impaired at higher rather than low concentrations of the agonists.[1,2] Furthermore, in the carotid artery of normotensive rabbits, extensive intimal thickening occurs after mechanical denudation with a balloon catheter. However, after regeneration of the endothe-

lium, the response to acetylcholine is normal.[96]

Responsiveness of vascular smooth muscle

Sodium nitroprusside is widely used to assess cyclic GMP-dependent relaxation of hypertensive blood vessels; reduced, normal, or even enhanced relaxations have been reported (Figs. 18 and 19).[1,2,40,47, 62,97,98] In any case, depressed endothelium-dependent relaxations are observed in hypertensive arteries despite a normal or even an augmented response to the nitrovasodilators;[47,62,65] even in preparations with a depressed response to sodium nitroprusside, the relaxation to it is impaired less than that to acetylcholine (Fig. 18).[40] Thus, functional alterations of the vascular smooth muscle may contribute to the impaired endothelium-dependent responses in hypertension, but they are not a prerequisite for that phenomenon.

Conclusions

Profound functional alterations of the endothelium occur in hypertensive arteries in vitro. As judged from the vasodilator effects of acetylcholine in forearm circulation of hypertensive subjects, similar changes also occur in vivo. The fact that the degree of functional endothelial alterations and the mechanisms involved differ in various vascular beds and models of hypertension suggests that besides blood pressure, other factors contribute to the impaired endothelium-dependent responses occurring in hypertension.

Alterations in endothelium-dependent control mechanisms of vascular tone and platelet function may contribute to the maintenance of the increased peripheral vascular resistance and/or the pathogen-

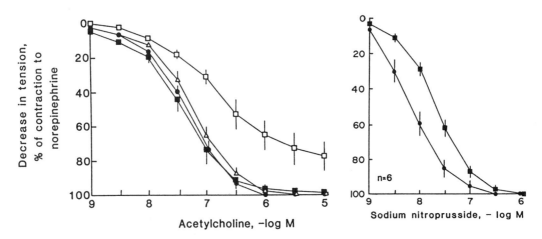

Figure 18: Effects of acetylcholine in rings with endothelium (left panel) and of sodium nitroprusside in rings without endothelium in aortic rings obtained from hypertensive Dahl rats (salt-sensitive on a 8% NaCl diet) and Dahl rats with a normal blood pressure (salt-sensitive on a 0.1% NaCl diet). Note that the response to acetylcholine is much more impaired than that to sodium nitroprusside indicating a predominant endothelial defect (data from ref. 40).

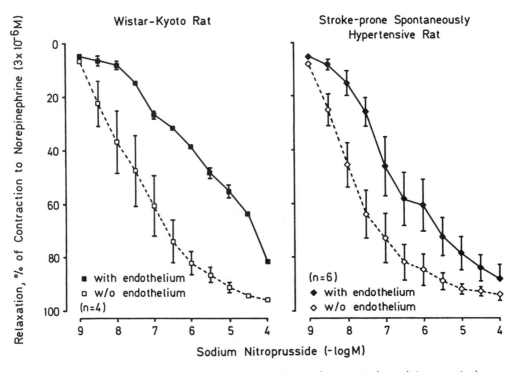

Figure 19: Effects of sodium nitroprusside in rings of mesenteric resistance arteries with (closed symbols) or without endothelium (open symbols) obtained from Wistar-Kyoto rats (left panel) or stroke-prone spontaneously hypertensive rats (right panel). The preparations were studied in a myograph system. Note that removal of the endothelium enhances the response to sodium nitroprusside in both strains, but more so in the normotensive rats. Accordingly, relaxations obtained by sodium nitroprusside are reduced in preparations with endothelium obtained from normotensive rats, while the response in preparations without endothelium was comparable in both strains (from ref. 47, by permission).

esis of the cardiovascular complications of hypertension, such as myocardial infarction, stroke, and peripheral vascular disease.

Acknowledgments: The authors wish to thank Bernadette Libsig and Sabine Bohnert for technical assistance. Original research reported in this manuscript was made possible by grants of the Swiss National Research Foundation (grant no. 32-25468.88), Swiss Cardiology Foundation, the Roche Research Foundation, an educational grant of Janssen Pharmaceutica, Baar, Switzerland, and the National Institutes of Health (grant NIH, #35614). The first author is the recipient of a career development award from the Swiss National Research Foundation (SCORE grant no. 3231-025150).

References

1. Lüscher T.F.: Endothelial vasoactive substances and cardiovascular disease. S. Karger Publisher AG, Basel, pp 1–133, 1988.
2. Lüscher T.F., Vanhoutte P.M.: Mechanisms of altered endothelium-dependent responses in hypertensive blood vessels. In: Relaxing and Contracting Factors, Biological and Clinical Research, P.M. Vanhoutte (ed.). Humana Press, Clifton, NJ, pp 495–509, 1988.
3. Lüscher T.F.: Endothelium-derived relaxing and contracting factors: Potential role in coronary artery disease. Eur. Heart J. 10:847–857, 1989.
4. Lüscher T.F.: Imbalance of endothelium-derived relaxing and contracting factors: A new concept in hypertension? Am. J. Hypertens. 3(4):317–330, 1990.
5. Lüscher T.F., Vanhoutte P.M.: The Endothelium: Modulator of Cardiovascular Function. CRC Press, Florida, 1990.
6. Gabbiani G., Glemes G., Guelpa C., Valloton M.B., Badonnel M.C., Huttner I.: Morphologic and functional changes of the aortic intima during experimental hypertension. Am. J. Pathol. 96:399–422, 1979.
7. Chobanian A.V., Brecher P.I., Haudenschild C.C.: Effects of hypertension and of antihypertensive therapy on atherosclerosis. Hypertension 8(Suppl. I):15–21, 1986.
8. Hazama F., Ozaki T., Amano S.: Scanning electron microscopic study of endothelial cells of cerebral arteries from spontaneously hypertensive rats. Stroke 10:245–252, 1979.
9. Savitsky J.P., Doczi J., Black J., Arnold J.D.: A clinical safety trial of stroma-free hemoglobin. Clin. Pharmacol. Ther. 23:73–80, 1978.
10. Palmer R.M.J., Ashton D.S., Moncada S.: Vascular endothelial cells synthesize nitric oxide from L-arginine. Nature 333:664–666, 1988.
11. Rees D.D., Palmer R.M.J., Hodson H.F., Moncada S.: A specific inhibitor of nitric oxide formation from L-arginine attenuates endothelium-dependent relaxation. Br. J. Pharmacol. 96:418–424, 1989.
12. Rees D.D., Palmer R.M.J., Moncada S.: The role of endothelium-derived nitric oxide in the regulation of blood pressure. Proc. Natl. Acad. Sci. USA 86:3375–3378, 1989.
13. Tolins J.P., Palmer R.M.J., Moncada S., Raij L.: Role of endothelium-derived relaxing factor in the hemodynamic response to acetylcholine in vivo. Am. J. Physiol. 1990, in press.
14. Vallance P., Collier J., Moncada S.: Effects of endothelium-derived nitric oxide on peripheral arteriolar tone in man. Lancet 1:997–1000, 1989.
15. Dudel C., Förstermann U.: Gossypol attenuates selectively the blood pressure lowering effect of endothelium-dependent vasodilators in the rabbit in vivo. Eur. J. Pharmacol. 145:217–221, 1988.
16. Linder L., Kiowski W., Bühler F.R., Lüscher T.F.: Indirect evidence for the release of endothelium-derived relaxing factor in the human forearm circulation in vivo: blunted response in essential hypertension. Circulation 81(6):1762–1767, 1990.
17. Vidal-Ragout M.J., Romero J.C., Vanhoutte P.M.: Endothelium-derived relaxing factor inhibits renin release. Eur. J. Pharmacol. 149:401–402, 1988.
18. Boulanger C., Vidal-Ragout M., Fiksen-Olsen M., Romero J.C., Vanhoutte P.M.: Cultured endothelial cells release a nonprostanoid inhibitor of renin release (abstract). Clin. Res. 36:539, 1988.
19. Lorenz R.R., Sanchez-Ferrer C.F., Burnett J.C., Vanhoutte P.M.: Influence of endocardial-derived factor(s) on the release of atrial natriuretic factor (abstract). FASEB J. 2:1293, 1988.

20. Yanagisawa M., Kurihara H., Kimura S., Mitsui Y., Kobayashi M., Watanabe T.X., Masaki T.: A novel potent vasoconstrictor peptide produced by vascular endothelial cells. Nature 332:411–415, 1988.

21. Brain S.D., Crossman D.C., Buckley T.L., Williams T.J.: Endothelin-1: demonstration of potent effects on the microcirculation of humans and other species. J. Cardiovasc. Pharmacol. 13(Suppl. 5):147–149, 1989.

22. Linder L., Kiowski W., Bühler F.R., Lüscher T.F.: Unpublished observation.

23. Boulanger C.: Lüscher T.F.: Release of endothelin from the porcine aorta: Inhibition by endothelium-derived nitric oxide. J. Clin. Invest. 85:587–590, 1990.

24. Schini V., Hendrickson H., Heublein D., Burnett Jr. J., Vanhoutte P.M.: Thrombin enhances the release of endothelin from cultured porcine aortic endothelial cells. Eur. J. Pharmacol. 165:333–334, 1989.

25. Ando K., Hirata Y., Schichiri M., Emori T., Maruno F.: Presence of immunoreactive endothelin in human plasma. FEBS Lett. 245:164–166, 1989.

26. Hartter E., Woloszczuk W.: Radioimmunoassay of endothelin. Lancet 1:909, 1989.

27. Suzuki N., Matsumoto H., Kitada C., Yanagisawa M., Miyauchi T., Masaki T., Fujino M.: Immunoreactive endothelin-1 in plasma detected by a sandwich-type enzyme immunoassay. J. Cardiovasc. Pharmacol. 13(Suppl. 5):151–152, 1989.

28. Miyauchi T., Yanagisawa M., Suzuki N., Iida K., Sugishita Y., Fujino M., Saito T., et al.: Venous plasma concentrations of endothelin in normal and hypertensive subjects. Circulation 80(Suppl. II):2280, 1989.

29. Fukuda Y., Hirata Y., Yoshimi H., Kojima T., Kobayashi Y., Yanagisawa M., Masaki T.: Endothelin is a potent secretagogue for atrial natriuretic peptide in cultured rat atrial myocytes. Biochem. Biophys. Res. Commun. 155:167–172, 1988.

30. Hu J.R., Berninger U.G., Lang R.E.: Endothelin stimulates atrial natriuretic peptide (ANP) release from rat atria. Eur. J. Pharmacol. 158:177–178, 1988.

31. Boarder M.R., Marriott D.B.: Characterization of endothelin-1 stimulation of catecholamine release from adrenal chromaffin cells. J. Cardiovasc. Pharmacol. 13(Suppl. 5):223–224, 1989.

32. Matsumura Y., Nakase K., Ikegawa R., Hayshi K., Ohyama T., Morimoto S.: The endothelium-derived vasoconstrictor peptide endothelin inhibits renin release in vitro. Life Sci. 44:149–157, 1989.

33. Rakugi H., Nakamaru M., Saito H., Higaki J., Ogihara T.: Endothelin inhibits renin release from isolated rat glomeruli. Biochem. Biophys. Res. Commun. 155:1244–1247, 1988.

34. Takagi M., Matsuoka H., Atarashi K., Yagi S.: Endothelin: a new inhibitor of renin release. Biochem. Biophys. Res. Commun. 157:1164–1168, 1988.

35. Wiklundin N.P., Oehlen A., Cederqvist B.: Inhibition of adrenergic neuroeffector transmission by endothelin in the guinea-pig femoral artery. Acta Physiol. Scand. 134:311–312, 1988.

36. Hu J.R., von Harsdorf R., Lang R.E.: Endothelin has potent inotropic effects in rat atria. Eur. J. Pharmacol. 158:275–278, 1988.

37. Ishikawa T., Yanagisawa M., Kimura S., Goto K., Masaki T.: Positive inotropic action of novel vasoconstrictor peptide endothelin on guinea pig atria. Am. J. Physiol. 255:H970–H973, 1988.

38. Lamping K.G., Dole W.P.: Acute hypertension selectively potentiates constrictor responses of large coronary arteries to serotonin by altering endothelial function in vivo. Circ. Res. 61:904–913, 1987.

39. Kontos H.A.: Endothelium-dependent vasodilatation in the cerebral microcirculation. In: Relaxing and Contracting Factors: Biological and Clinical Research, P.M. Vanhoutte (ed.). Humana Press, Clifton, NJ, pp 417–424, 1988.

40. Lüscher T.F., Raij L., Vanhoutte P.M.: Endothelium-dependent responses in normotensive and hypertensive Dahl rats. Hypertension 9:157–163, 1987.

41. Lüscher T.F., Diederich D., Vanhoutte P.M., Weber E., Bühler F.R.: Endothelium-dependent responses in the common carotid and renal artery of normotensive and spontaneously hypertensive rats. Hypertension 11:573–578, 1988.

42. Otsuko Y., DiPiero A., Hirt E., Brennaman B., Lockette W.: Vascular relaxation and cGMP in hypertension. Am. J. Physiol. 254:H163–H169, 1988.

43. Shirasaki Y., Kolm P., Nickols G.A., Lee T.J.-F.: Endothelial regulation of cyclic GMP and vascular responses in hypertension. J. Pharmacol. Exp. Ther. 245:53–58, 1988.

44. Lüscher T.F., Romero J.C., Vanhoutte P.M.: Bioassay of endothelium-derived vasoactive substances in the aorta of normotensive and spontaneously hypertensive rats. J. Hypertens. 4(Suppl. 6):81–83, 1986.

45. Hoeffner U., Vanhoutte P.M.: Increases in

flow reduce the release of endothelium-derived relaxing factor in the aorta of normotensive and spontaneously hypertensive rats. Am. J. Hypertens. 2(10):762–767, 1989.

46. Dohi Y., Thiel M.A., Bühler F.R., Lüscher T.F.: Activation of the endothelial L-arginine pathway in pressurized mesenteric resistance arteries: Effect of age and hypertension. Hypertension 1990 (submitted).

47. Diederich D., Yang Z., Bühler F.R., Lüscher T.F.: Impaired endothelium-dependent relaxations in hypertensive resistance arteries involve the cyclooxygenase pathway. Am. J. Physiol. 258(Pt 2):H445–H451, 1990.

48. Konishi M., Su C.: Role of endothelium in dilator responses of spontaneously hypertensive rat arteries. Hypertension 5:881–886, 1983.

49. Winquist R.J., Bunting P.B., Baskin E.P., Wallace A.A.: Decreased endothelium-dependent relaxation in New Zealand genetic hypertensive rats. J. Hypertens. 2:536–541, 1984.

50. Lüscher T.F., Vanhoutte P.M.: Endothelium-dependent contractions to acetylcholine in the aorta of the spontaneously hypertensive rat. Hypertension 8:344–348, 1986.

51. Lockette W.E., Otsuha Y., Carretero O.A.: Endothelium-dependent relaxation in hypertension. Hypertension 8(Suppl. II):61–66, 1986.

52. Miller M.J.S., Pinto A., Mullane K.M.: Impaired endothelium-dependent relaxations in rabbits subjected to aortic coarctation hypertension. Hypertension 10:164–170, 1987.

53. Sim M.K., Singh M.: Decreased responsiveness of the aortae of hypertensive rats to acetylcholine, histamine and noradrenaline. Br. J. Pharmacol. 90:147–150, 1987.

54. Van de Voorde J., Cuvelier C., Leusen I.: Endothelium-dependent relaxation effects in aorta from hypertensive rats. Arch. Int. Physiol. Biochem. 92:P10–P11, 1984.

55. Van de Voorde J., Leusen I.: Endothelium-dependent and independent relaxation effects on aorta preparations of renal hypertensive rats. Arch. Int. Physiol. Biochem. 92:P35–P36, 1984.

56. Van de Voorde J., Leusen I.: Endothelium-dependent and independent relaxation of aortic rings from hypertensive rats. Am. J. Physiol. 250:H711–H717, 1986.

57. Hongo K., Nakagomi T., Kassell N.F., Sasaki T., Lehman M., Vollmer D.G., Tsu-kahara T., et al.: Effects of aging and hypertension on endothelium-dependent vascular relaxation in rat carotid artery. Stroke 19:892–897, 1988.

58. Lüscher T.F., Raij L., Vanhoutte P.M.: Effect of hypertension and its reversal on endothelium-dependent relaxations in the rat aorta. J. Hypertension 5(Suppl 5):153–155, 1987.

59. Lüscher T.F., Vanhoutte P.M., Raij L.: Antihypertensive therapy normalizes endothelium-dependent relaxations in salt-induced hypertension of the rat. Hypertension 9(Suppl. III):193–197, 1987.

60. Webb R.C., Vander A.J., Henry J.P.: Increased vasodilator responses to acetylcholine in psychosocial hypertensive mice. Hypertension 9:268–276, 1987.

61. Lüscher T.F., Vanhoutte P.M.: Endothelium-dependent responses to aggregating platelets and serotonin in spontaneously hypertensive rats. Hypertension 8(Suppl. II):55–60, 1986.

62. De Mey J.G., Gray S.D.: Endothelium-dependent reactivity in resistance vessels. Prog. Appl. Microcirc. 88:181–187, 1985.

63. Lüscher T.F., Aarhus L.L., Vanhoutte P.M.: Indomethacin enhances the impaired endothelium-dependent relaxations in small mesenteric arteries of the spontaneously hypertensive rat. Am. J. Hypertens. 3:55–58, 1990.

64. Watt P.A.C., Thurston H.: Endothelium-dependent relaxation in resistance vessels from the spontaneously hypertensive rats. J. Hypertens. 7:661–666, 1989.

65. Tesfamariam B., Halpern W.: Endothelium-dependent and endothelium-independent vasodilation in resistance arteries from hypertensive rats. Hypertension 11:440–444, 1988.

66. Carvalho M.H.C., Scivoletto R., Fortes Z.B., Nigro D., Cordellini S.: Reactivity of aorta and mesenteric microvessels to drugs in spontaneously hypertensive rats: role of the endothelium. J. Hypertens. 5:377–382, 1987.

67. Gray S.D., De Mey J.G.: Vascular reactivity in neonatal spontaneously hypertensive rats. Progr. Appl. Microcirc. 8:173–180, 1985.

68. Mayhan W.G., Faraci F.M., Heistad D.D.: Impairment of endothelium-dependent responses of cerebral arterioles in chronic hypertension. Am. J. Physiol. 253:H1435–H1440, 1987.

69. Mayhan W.G., Faraci F.M., Heistad D.D.: Responses of cerebral arterioles to adeno-

sine diphosphate, serotonin and the thromboxane analogue U-46619 during chronic hypertension. Hypertension 12:556–561, 1988.

70. Wright C.E., Angus J.A.: Effects of hypertension and hypercholesteremia on vasodilatation in the rabbit. Hypertension 8:361–371, 1986.

71. Panza J.A., Quyyumi A.A., Epstein S.E.: Impaired endothelium-dependent vascular relaxation in hypertensive patients (abstract). Circulation 78(Suppl. II):473, 1988.

72. Koga T., Takata Y., Kobayashi K., Takishita S., Yamashita Y., Fujishima M.: Age and hypertension promote endothelium-dependent contractions to acetylcholine in the aorta of the rat. Hypertension 14:542–548, 1989.

73. Kato T., Iwama Y., Okumura K., Hashimoto H., Ito T., Satake T.: Prostaglandin H_2 may be the endothelium-derived contracting factor released by acetylcholine in the aorta of the rat. Hypertension 1990, in press.

74. Katusic Z.S., Vanhoutte P.M.: Superoxide anion is an endothelium-derived contracting factor. Am. J. Physiol. 257:H33–H37, 1989.

75. Auch-Schwelk W., Katusic Z., Vanhoutte P.M.: Contractions to oxygen-derived free radicals are augmented in the aorta of the spontaneously hypertensive rat. Hypertension 13:859–864, 1989.

76. Auch-Schwelk W., Katusic Z.S., Vanhoutte P.M.: Endothelium-dependent contractions in the SHR aorta are inhibited by thromboxane A_2 receptor antagonists (abstract). J. Vasc. Med. Biol. 1:76, 1989.

77. Rinaldi G., Bohr D.: Endothelium-mediated spontaneous response in aortic rings of deoxycorticosterone acetate-hypertensive rats. Hypertension 13:256–261, 1989.

78. Amstein R., Fetkovska N., Lüscher T.F., Kiowski W., Bühler F.R.: Age and the platelet serotonin vasoconstrictor axis in essential hypertension. J. Cardiovasc. Pharmacol. 11(Suppl. 1):35–40, 1988.

79. De Clerck F.: Blood platelets in human essential hypertension. Agents Actions 18:563–580, 1986.

80. Baudouin-Legros M., Dard B., Guicheney P.: Hyperreactivity of platelets from spontaneously hypertensive rats. Hypertension 8:694–699, 1986.

81. Fetkovska N., Amstein R., Ferracin F., Regenass M., Pletscher A., Bühler F.R.: 5-hydroxytryptamine kinetics and activation of blood platelets in patients with essential hypertension. Hypertension 1990, in press.

82. Guicheney P., Legros M., Marcel D., Kamal L., Meyer P.: Platelet serotonin content and uptake in spontaneously hypertensive rats. Life Sci. 36:679–685, 1985.

83. Valtier D., Guicheney P., Baudoin-Legros M., Meyer P.: Platelets in human essential hypertension: in vitro hyperreactivity to thrombin. J. Hypertens. 4:551–555, 1986.

84. Nara Y., Kihara M., Mano M., Horie R., Yamori Y.: Dietary effect on platelet aggregation in men with and without a family history of essential hypertension. Hypertension 6:339–343, 1984.

85. Lüscher T.F., Rubanyi G.M., Aarhus L.L., Vanhoutte P.M.: Serotonin reduces coronary flow in isolated hearts of the spontaneously hypertensive rat. J. Hypertens. 4(Suppl. 5):148–150, 1986.

86. Shichiri M., Hirata Y., Anao K., Emori T., Ohta K., Kimoro S., Inoue A., Marumo F.: Plasma endothelin levels in patients with hypertension and end-stage renal failure. Circulation 80(Suppl. II):0502, 1989.

87. Stewart D.J., Cernacek P.: Plasma endothelin levels are markedly elevated in cardiogenic shock. Circulation 80(Suppl. II):2329, 1989.

88. Emori T., Hirata Y., Aizawa T., Ando K., Shichiri M., Marumo F.: Plasma endothelin levels in patients with coronary artery disease undergoing percutaneous coronary angioplasty. Circulation 80(Suppl. II):2327, 1989.

89. Tomobe Y., Miyauchi T., Saito A., Yanagisawa M., Kimura S., Goto K., Masaki T.: Effects of endothelin on the renal artery from spontaneously hypertensive and Wistar Kyoto rats. Eur. J. Pharmacol. 152:373–374, 1988.

90. Diederich D., Yang Z., Bühler F.R., Lüscher T.F.: Endothelium-derived relaxing factor and endothelin in resistance arteries of hypertensive rats (abstract). J. Vasc. Med. Biol. 1/3:167, 1989.

91. Criscione L., Nellis P., Riniker B., Thomann H., Burdet R.: Reactivity and sensitivity of mesenteric vascular beds and aortic rings of SH and WKY rats to endothelin: Effect of calcium entry blockers. Br. J. Pharmacol. 100:31–36, 1990.

92. Miyauchi T., Ishikawa T., Tomobe Y., Yanagisawa M., Kimura S., Sugishita Y., Ito I., et al.: Characteristics of pressor response to endothelin in spontaneously hypertensive Wistar-Kyoto rats. Hypertension 14:427–434, 1989.

93. Auch-Schwelk W., Vanhoutte P.M.: Contractions to endothelin-1 in the aorta and

renal artery of the spontaneously hypertensive rat. Unpublished observation, 1989.

94. Dohi Y., Lüscher T.F.: Unpublished observations, 1990.

95. Morera S., Santoro F.M., Roson M.I., De la Riva I.J.: Prostacyclin (PGI$_2$) synthesis in the vascular wall of rats with bilateral renal artery stenosis. Hypertension 5(Suppl. V):38–42, 1983.

96. Cocks T.M., Manderson J.A., Mosse P.R.L., Campbell G.R., Angus J.A.: Development of a large fibromuscular intimal thickening does not impair endothelium-dependent relaxations in the rabbit carotid artery. Blood Vessels 24:192–200, 1987.

97. Cohen M.L., Berkowitz B.A.: Decreased vascular relaxation in hypertension. J. Pharmacol. Exp. Ther. 196:396–406, 1976.

98. Shirasaki Y., Su C., Lee T.J.-F., Kolm P., Cline W.H. Jr., Nickols G.A.: Endothelial modulation of vascular relaxation to nitrovasodilators in aging and hypertension. J. Pharmacol. Exp. Ther. 239:861–866, 1986.

10

Endothelial Dysfunction in Diabetes

Galen M. Pieper, Garrett J. Gross

Introduction

Since Furchgott and Zawadski[49] first discovered that the vascular endothelium is a necessary requisite in acetylcholine-induced relaxation of blood vessels, intense interest continues to be generated concerning the exact mechanisms by which the endothelium can mediate vascular relaxation or modulate vascular tone. A number of excellent reviews have been written in this area.[3,10,18,48,56,57,163]

Impairment of endothelium-dependent relaxation has been hypothesized as a mechanism to explain the pathophysiology of certain vascular diseases. For example, recent evidence suggests that endothelium-dependent relaxation is impaired in atherosclerotic vessels derived from human and experimental animals[15,65,72,88] as well as vessels obtained from the genetically hypertensive rat model.[83,92,174] It is well-known that the incidence of both hypertension and atherosclerosis is augmented in diabetic patients.[24,143,175] While there is substantial evidence for impaired endothelium-dependent relaxation in hypertension and atherosclerosis, there remains controversy regarding the role that diabetes per se may play in altered endothelium-mediated functions. Whether diabetes predisposes to injury to endothelium-dependent relaxations in the absence of hypertensive or atherosclerotic disease is an important concern. This chapter reviews the current status of our understanding of the role of the endothelium in the pathophysiology of diabetes-induced vascular disease with special emphasis on alterations in endothelium-dependent vasoactive factors.

Morphology of the Vascular Endothelium in Diabetes

As a prelude to discussions concerning changes in endothelium-dependent relaxations, the morphological alterations of the blood vessel as a consequence of diabetes mellitus will be summarized. Vascular pathology in diabetes has usually

Rubanyi G.M.: Cardiovascular Significance of Endothelium-Derived Vasoactive Factors, Futura Publishing Co., Inc., Mount Kisco, NY, © 1991.

been conveniently categorized into macroangiopathy and microangiopathy since a unified etiology of diabetic angiopathy has not been directly established.

Diabetic macroangiopathy is similar to nondiabetic atherosclerotic lesions except that the lesioning is more diffuse and severe.[71,125] In advanced stages, the pathology consists of fatty streaks, fibrous plaques, calcified lesions, and coronary stenoses. In contrast to atherosclerosis, the morphological lesions in diabetes appear more prominently in peripheral arteries.[31,125,151] For a detailed description of diabetes-induced changes in vascular morphology, the reader is directed to two reviews pertinent to this topic.[9,133]

An early hallmark feature of diabetic microangiopathy is capillary basement membrane thickening.[45,144,172] The subintimal space stains positive for periodic acid Schiff and the endothelial cells proliferate within the arteriolar lumen.[34,55] Furthermore, increased microvascular permeability to large molecules has been demonstrated in diabetic patients and experimental diabetic animals.[14,25,75,78,110,166]

In diabetic retinopathy (for review see ref. 118), endothelial alterations include both acellular and hypercellular capillaries.[79] Endothelial cell proliferation and lumen obstruction has been demonstrated in sural nerve capillaries.[42,159] In contrast, transmission electron microscopic studies have failed to show any specific evidence of cell damage in retinal,[7,12] muscle,[89] skin,[1] or myocardial[138] capillaries. Similarly, light and electron microscopic analysis of rat coronary vessels have failed to show any wall thickening or structural alterations as a result of diabetes.[144]

By scanning electron microscopy of blood vessels from diabetic rabbits, areas of de-endothelialization were observed.[35] Increased numbers of agyrophilic cells and luminal endothelial craters were found in thoracic and abdominal aortas as well as carotid arteries.[35] In cerebral arterioles of the rat, evidence of necrosis of endothelial

cells has been observed.[104] These changes do not appear to be a direct toxic effect of diabetogenic agents such as alloxan[35] or streptozotocin.[6] It appears that advanced stages of vascular disease, including basement membrane thickening and endothelial cell injury, are preceded by a significant reduction in the negative surface charge of the arterial endothelium in diabetic rats.[44,123]

Von Willebrand factor, a marker of endothelial cell function, is elevated in plasma of diabetic patients with[26,27] or without demonstrable vascular disease[29,54] and within 2–4 weeks after induction of diabetes in rats.[173] To date no studies have been performed which correlate defects in endothelium-dependent relaxation with structural modifications, if any, of the diabetic vascular endothelium.

Experimental Models of Diabetes

Several experimental animal models of diabetes mellitus exist (for review see ref. 11). Classically, experimental diabetes has been induced in laboratory animals by either alloxan or streptozotocin.[124]

Streptozotocin is generally preferred as a diabetogenic agent because of its specificity and reduced toxicity. Unfortunately, permanent diabetes is difficult to produce by streptozotocin in certain species such as the rabbit or guinea pig.[85] Thus, alloxan is usually chosen for these species. Studies on dysfunction of the cardiovascular system have been limited primarily to the rat, rabbit, and dog models.

No single animal model mimics all of the clinical manifestations of diabetes mellitus. The diabetic rat has been a standard model used in cardiovascular investigations. It has the advantage of delineating the effects of diabetes without the complications of atherosclerosis and hypertension. The diabetic rabbit model has the advantage in that synergistic actions of atherosclerosis and diabetes can be studied simultaneously. Unfortunately, there is a paradoxical decrease in lesioning in atherosclerotic diabetic rabbits.[16] This is in contrast to the monkey model where diabetes does not limit the progression of atherosclerosis in coconut/peanut oil-fed animals.[61] The diabetic dog model is desirable because of the ability to study functional changes in coronary arteries.

More recently, a genetically prone diabetic rat strain has been developed that is now available for expanded investigations by establishing individual breeding colonies.[107] Three laboratories, including ours, have now studied endothelium-dependent relaxation in this model. Of all the spontaneous diabetic models, only the Chinese hamster and the Bio-Breeding (BB) rat manifest a nonobese, insulin-dependent type of diabetes similar to that which is seen in the human. Another genetically prone rat strain, the NIH-SHR corpulent strain, has recently been developed.[101] This hypertensive-prone strain is a probable candidate as a model of non-insulin-dependent diabetes mellitus. No vascular studies have been performed to date using this strain.

Role of Endothelium in Modulating Vascular Responsiveness to Contracting Agents

In the past, most studies using diabetic blood vessels have focused primarily on vasoconstrictor responses to α-adrenoceptor agonists, serotonin, angiotensin, and potassium ion. For a review, refer to the summary in Table 1. Regarding α-adrenoceptor agonists, most studies show that the pD_2 values of individual agonists are not altered by diabetes regardless of the species or model (i.e., chemical versus genetic models). An exception is one study in female diabetic rat aorta showing increased sensitivity to norepinephrine with no change in maximal response.[94] In contrast, several authors have shown increased maximum contractile tension to norepinephrine and selective α_1- or α_2-adrenoceptor agonists in chemically induced diabetic aorta,[93,95,108,139,167] carotid arteries,[4] mesenteric arteries,[5,93,171] and caudal arteries[122] but not portal veins.[95] Other investigators have shown decreased contractions[68,90,111,122,153] or no change.[109] It has been argued that such discrepancies may be related to the method of calculating tension and the use of vessel ring versus helical strip preparations. While most studies utilize age-matched animals, vessel mass can be smaller in diabetic rat aorta. Thus, contractions should be normalized for either weight or cross-sectional areas as previously suggested.[68,93] Accordingly, some of the reported discrepancies on contractile tension development to constrictor agents in diabetic vessels may be related to the failure to normalize tensions for variations in tissue mass. Our approach has been not only to normalize contractions for cross-sectional area but also to induce diabetes as rats are approaching the plateau phase of growth in order to prevent disproportionate changes in cross-sectional areas of vessels as this might alter the response of diabetic vessels under a given resting tension.

Recent investigations using the spontaneous diabetic rat model indicate that this model may be qualitatively different from the chemically induced model. For example, the contractile responses to norepinephrine or other specific α_1-adrenoceptor agonists were not shown to be altered[5,40,100] despite increased contractions to the α_2-adrenoceptor agonists, BHT-920, and guanabenz.[5] It has not been clearly established whether the endothelium influences this altered α-adrenoceptor response in diabetic vessels. It is known that de-endothelialization augments con-

Table 1.

Effect of Diabetes on Sensitivity (EC_{50}) and Maximum Contractile Responses to Various Agonists in Rat Aorta

Investigator	Phenomenon	NE[1]	PE[2]	ME[3]	Clonidine	BHT920	5HT[4]	K[+]
Owen & Carrier[108]	EC_{50}	→						
	Max tension	→↑						
Turlapathy et al.[160]	EC_{50}	↑						↑
	Max tension	↓						↓
Pfaffman et al.[111]	EC_{50}		↑					↑
	Max tension		↓					↓
Scarborough & Carrier[139]	EC_{50}	→	→	→	→	→		
	Max tension	↓	→	→	↑	↑		
MacLeod[93]	EC_{50}	→						→
	Max tension	↑						→
Ramanadham et al.[122]	EC_{50}	→		→				↓
	Max tension	↓		↓				↓
MacLeod & McNeil[95]	EC_{50}	→					→	→
	Max tension	→					→	→
Head et al.[68]	EC_{50}	→					→	→
	Max tension	↓					↓	↓
Wakabayashi et al.[167]	EC_{50}							
	Max tension				↑			↓

[1] NE (Norepinephrine)
[2] PE (Phenylephrine)
[3] ME (Methoxamine)
[4] 5-HT (5-Hydroxytryptamine)

tractions of normal rat aorta and mesenteric arteries to α-adrenoceptor agonists.[23,40,43,98,105] Morphological[6] and functional[28] damage to the vascular endothelium as a result of diabetes has been reported. Such deterioration could indicate that the increased maximum response of diabetic vessels to α-adrenoceptor agonists arises from a decrease in spontaneous or tonic release of endothelium-derived relaxing factor (EDRF) as a consequence of stimulation of the α_2-adrenoceptor located on vascular endothelium. Therefore, the integrity of the endothelium could not only elicit endothelium-dependent relaxations (see next section) but may also modulate vascular tone in response to α-adrenoceptor stimulation.

Recent studies have addressed the latter suggestion. Removal of endothelium was shown to increase contraction to phenylephrine in diabetic canine femoral arteries[52] and to norepinephrine and other α-adrenoceptor agonists in rat aorta and mesenteric arteries.[64,170] None of these studies showed any impaired relaxation to endothelium-dependent vasodilators. Wakabayashi et al.[167] showed that clonidine-induced contractions were augmented to a greater extent in control than in diabetic rat aorta following removal of the endothelium. Furthermore, no increase in contraction to potassium was seen in either control or diabetic aorta upon removal of the endothelium. Such results suggest that the tonic release of EDRF in diabetic rat aorta is diminished. This hypothesis has not been corroborated by others in which contractions were shown to be enhanced by roughly equivalent degrees in mesenteric arteries from diabetic rats.[170]

The degree of reduction in cGMP levels upon de-endothelialization is regarded as evidence to support tonic release of EDRF. Harris and MacLeod[64] showed that removal of the endothelium decreased cGMP to similar levels in control and diabetic vessels. Therefore, these investigators concluded that a decrease in the release of EDRF is not responsible for increased α-adrenergic responses but rather a change in the reactivity of vascular smooth muscle occurs independent of the endothelium. A similar conclusion was reached, indirectly, by Gebremedhin et al.[53] in diabetic canine coronary arteries in which denudation increased the maximum tension to $PGF_{2\alpha}$, an adrenoceptor-independent agonist, while causing no effect on the sensitivity to this agonist. In contrast, Kamata et al.[76] have recently indicated a significant reduction in basal cGMP levels in diabetic rat aorta.

Endothelium-Independent Vascular Relaxations

Nitrovasodilators produce relaxation of vascular smooth muscle by activation of guanylate cyclase and thus produce an increase in cGMP. Unlike EDRF, the elevation of cGMP in vascular smooth muscle occurs independent of the endothelium. In reports in which endothelium-dependent relaxation was impaired, relaxations to sodium nitroprusside in rat aorta[40,76,109] and canine coronary artery,[53] or nitroglycerin in rat aorta[114] and in rat pial arterioles[99] were not impaired by diabetes. Similarly, no alteration in response to papaverine has been shown in rat mesenteric arteries,[46,155] rat aorta,[117] rat coronary microvasculature,[145] murine cerebral arterioles,[131] or human corpora cavernosa of the penis.[137]

Isoproterenol has also been shown to produce similar vasodilation of control and diabetic rat[70] and canine coronary arteries.[81] In contrast, other investigators have shown reduced vasodilation to isoproterenol in intact diabetic rats[36,74] and in perfused diabetic mesenteric beds.[154,155] Use

of isoproterenol as a test for endothelium-independent relaxation in blood vessels is complicated in diabetes. Takiguchi et al.[155] showed that an attenuated response to isoproterenol could be mimicked by hypothyroidism, which is known to occur in the diabetic rat, and that this response was reversed by thyroxine treatment in vivo.[155] It may be of interest to note that diabetes is not associated with hypothyroidism in the spontaneous BB rat model.[150] Furthermore, in cardiac membranes, several investigators have shown a significant decrease in the number of β-adrenoceptors in diabetic animals.[8,69,87,121,154] This has been attributed to an unspecified uncoupling of adenylate cyclase from the membrane receptor since glucagon-mediated, but not forskolin-mediated, activation of adenylate cyclase was impaired.[8,121]

Adenosine, another vascular smooth muscle vasodilator, increased coronary blood flow to a lesser extent in the intact diabetic lamb[37,39] and in the diabetic monkey.[61] Interestingly, the insulin-induced decrease in coronary vascular resistance was also attenuated in the diabetic lamb model.[38] In contrast, Durante et al.[40] found no altered relaxation to adenosine in isolated aorta taken from the spontaneous diabetic BB rat despite reduced coronary flow responses in isolated perfused diabetic rat hearts.[41] While this may point to a diabetes-induced decrease in the sensitivity of the coronary arteries relative to other vascular beds, this could not be argued to be due to a generalized decrease in the vasodilatory capacity of diabetic coronary artery smooth muscle since challenges to nitroprusside in both instances were not diminished. Caution must be advised in making definitive conclusions about endothelium-independent relaxations when using adenosine as well. While adenosine was originally purported to be an endothelium-independent vasodilator,[32,48] three separate laboratories have since suggested that adenosine can relax rat arterial rings,[83,176] and dog coronary arteries[136] partially, via an endothelium-dependent mechanism. Thus, adenosine, like isoproterenol, must be used cautiously in delineating potential alterations in the vasodilator reactivity of vascular smooth muscle to endothelium-independent agents in diseased vessels.

Endothelium-Dependent Vascular Relaxations

Initial studies on diabetic blood vessels concerning endothelium-dependent relaxation appeared in the literature in a report by Fortes et al.[46] using the alloxan diabetic Wistar rat. These authors showed that relaxations to histamine and bradykinin but not to acetylcholine were impaired in diabetic mesenteric arteries in situ. Since that time, reports have appeared that have either corroborated or refuted the notion of impaired endothelium-dependent relaxation in diabetic blood vessels. Investigations have now been performed in three different species and on six different types of blood vessels. Because of the controversial observations that have arisen, it would appear appropriate that a comprehensive and closer analysis be provided concerning our current understanding of endothelium-dependent relaxation in diabetic blood vessels. Our attempt in this chapter is to summarize these observations as well as to provide some probable insights for current discrepancies.

Most investigations on endothelium-dependent relaxations have been performed using the diabetic rat aorta. A summary of these observations is provided in Table 2. Five independent laboratories including our own (Fig. 1) have shown im-

Table 2.

Endothelium-Dependent Relaxation in Diabetic Rat Aorta

Investigators	Rat Strain	Type of Diabetes	Vasodilator Tested				
			Acetylcholine	Histamine	ADP	A23187	Bradykinin
Fortes et al.[46]	Wistar	ALX[2]	unchanged	unchanged	–	–	unchanged
Oyama et al.[109]	Wistar	STZ[3]	impaired	impaired	–	impaired	–
Head et al.[68]	Sprague[1]	STZ	unchanged	–	–	–	–
Wakabayashi et al.[167]	Wistar	chemical[4]	unchanged	–	–	–	–
Meraji et al.[100]	BB	spontaneous	impaired	impaired	–	–	–
Pieper & Gross[114]	Sprague	STZ	impaired	–	impaired	–	–
Durante et al.[40]	BB	spontaneous	impaired	–	–	impaired	–
Harris & MacLeod[64]	Wistar	STZ	unchanged	–	–	–	–
Kamata et al.[76]	Wistar	STZ	impaired	–	–	–	–
Tanz et al.[157]	Sprague	STZ	–	impaired	–	–	–

[1] Sprague-Dawley

[2] ALX (alloxan)

[3] STZ (streptozotocin)

[4] Diabetogenic agent not delineated

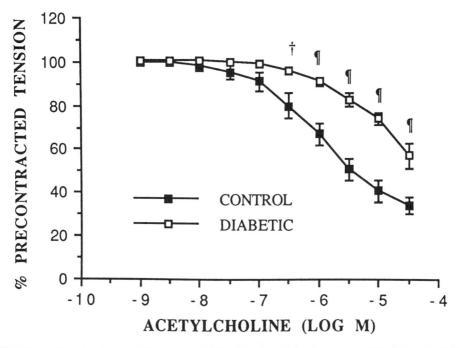

Figure 1: Impaired relaxation to acetylcholine in aortic ring segments from chronic (2 months) streptozotocin-induced diabetic rat. Each point represents the mean ±SE as a percentage of the contraction to 10^{-6}M norepinephrine. Control (n = 28), diabetic (n = 19). †p<0.025; ¶p<0.001.

paired relaxation to acetylcholine in aorta of diabetic rats,[40,76,100,109,114] whereas four other laboratories have reported no change.[46,64,68,167] The reports in which endothelium-dependent relaxations to acetylcholine were shown to be impaired have also presented evidence that relaxations to other endothelium-dependent vasodilators such as histamine,[100,109] ADP,[114] and the calcium ionophore, A23187[40,109] are also impaired.

The observations of reduced endothelium-dependent relaxation to acetylcholine could potentially be related to reduced numbers of muscarinic receptors. This hypothesis is based upon previous reports of reduced myocardial sensitivity to muscarinic agonists[161] which could be attributed to reduced muscarinic receptor density but not affinity in myocardial atrial and ventricular tissue obtained from diabetic animals.[21,22,87] Thus, while it cannot be ex-

cluded that a decrease in muscarinic receptors occurs in diabetic vasculature, the impaired responses to ADP and to histamine suggest that a sole defect in the muscarinic receptor is unlikely. Our initial experience suggests that the impairment may be restricted to receptor-mediated endothelium-dependent vasodilators (Figs. 1 and 2) since we found no impairment to the calcium ionophore, A23187, a receptor-independent endothelium-dependent vasodilator.[58] Oyama et al.[109] alluded to impairment to A23187 in streptozotocin-induced diabetic rat aorta but provided no supporting data. In the spontaneous diabetic BB rat aorta, Durante et al.[40] showed that relaxations to a single concentration of A23187 were impaired; however, studies were performed on a limited sample size (n = 3).

Many other stimulators of EDRF have not yet been tested in diabetic blood ves-

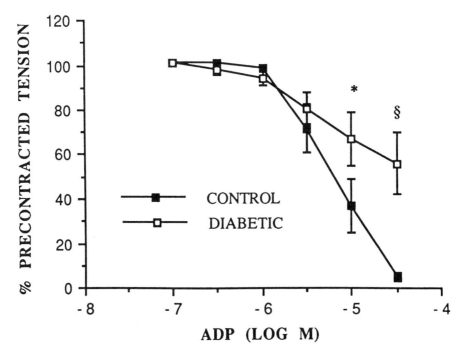

Figure 2: Impaired relaxation to adenosine diphosphate (ADP) in aortic ring segments from chronic diabetic rat. Each point represents the mean ±SE as a percentage of the contraction to norepinephrine. Control (n=10), diabetic (n=9). *p<0.05, ‡p<0.005.

sels. Future studies with other vasodilators may reveal the nature of impaired endothelium-dependent responses in diabetes. For example, the relaxations produced by EDRF-stimulants such as thrombin are not inhibited by the same agents that inhibit acetylcholine responses,[33,84] suggesting that there may be more than one EDRF. Our studies indicate that thrombin-mediated relaxations of diabetic rat aorta are not impaired (Fig. 3). Thus, diabetes-induced defects may be selective to certain pathways of release of EDRF and/or to certain types of EDRFs.

It is not known what influence the choice of the constrictor agent has on the presence or absence of impaired endothelium-dependent relaxations in diabetic blood vessels (Table 3). In most previous reports, the impaired endothelium-dependent responses in diabetic vessels were limited to vessels contracted with mixed α_1- and α_2-adrenergic agonists. Thus it is theoretically possible that diabetic vessels release less basal EDRF when α_2 adrenoceptors on the endothelium are stimulated. In contrast, preliminary studies in our laboratories have been unable to demonstrate impaired relaxations to acetylcholine in diabetic rat aorta when $PGF_{2\alpha}$ was used as the contracting agent. The importance of this latter observation is not fully understood since no other laboratory (except ref. 53 in the canine coronary artery) has performed endothelium-dependent relaxation in diabetic blood vessels using a prostanoid as the agonist. The studies using phenylephrine would tend to suggest that impaired endothelium-dependent relaxation is not limited to studies using α_2-adrenoceptor agonists to produce contraction.

It still remains uncertain why some

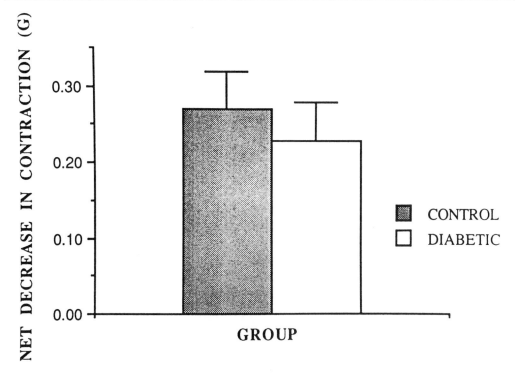

Figure 3: Normal relaxations to thrombin (1 U/mL) by aortic ring segments from strep-tozotocin-induced diabetic rats. Each point represents the mean $\pm$ SE as a percentage of contraction to 3×10^{-7}M norepinephrine. Control (n = 12), diabetic (n = 8).

Table 3.

Relationship of Type of Contracting Agonist on Endothelium-Dependent Relaxation in Diabetic Rat Aorta

Investigators	Contracting Agent	Concentration (M)	Response
Fortes et al.[46]	NE[1]	10^{-7}	unchanged
Oyama et al.[109]	NE	10^{-6}	impaired
Head et al.[68]	NE	3×10^{-7}	unchanged
Wakabayashi et al.[167]	PE[2]	10^{-7}	unchanged
Meraji et al.[100]	NE	10^{-6}	impaired
Pieper & Gross[114]	NE	10^{-6}	impaired
Durante et al.[40]	PE	2.5×10^{-6}	impaired
Harris & MacLeod[64]	NE	5×10^{-7}	unchanged
Kamata et al.[76]	NE	$3 \times 10^{-8} \rightarrow 10^{-7}$	impaired
Tanz et al.[157]	PE	10^{-6}	impaired

[1] NE = norepinephrine

[2] PE = phenylephrine

laboratories have shown impaired relaxations to acetylcholine in diabetic rat aorta while others have not. Those reports showing impairment have been observed in at least two different rat strains as well as in both chemically induced and genetically induced models. Therefore, it is unlikely that the rat strain can explain these apparent discrepancies. Reports using the spontaneous diabetic rat model,[40,100] which has been confirmed in our laboratory (unpublished observations), all showed impaired relaxations to endothelium-dependent vasodilators. In the chemically induced model, it could be argued that the diabetogenic dose and the intensity and progression of the disease might explain the discrepancies in the results. Closer analysis reveals that the blood glucose concentrations of diabetic animals varied widely from 377 ± 3 mg/dL[64] to 738 ± 109 and 668 ± 21 mg/dL, respectively[68,167] in those reports not showing impaired responses to acetylcholine. The possibility exists that single measures of blood glucose at the time of the functional vascular studies may not be a true index of the extent and/or duration of the disease. Perhaps multiple sampling over a period of time as well as measures of glucosylated hemoglobin may be more pertinent criteria to document and compare the extent of the underlying pathology between various studies.

A crucial problem that has yet to be adequately addressed in such comparisons is the optimal diabetogenic dose per se and the relationship of that dose relative to the age at which the animal is given the diabetogenic agent. For example, older rats require less diabetogenic agent to produce the same amount of disease than younger rats.[97] Careful analysis of all studies shows that the dose of streptozotocin given varies from 50 to 80 mg/kg in rats and the time of induction varies from 6 to 12 weeks of age. Thus, it is likely that the combination of dose and age of the animal at the time of induction acting in concert with the du-

ration of the disease are more important interdependent factors to keep in mind when making any rational comparative evaluation between different studies. Furthermore, the failure to show impaired relaxations in diabetic rat aorta in one study[68] could potentially be related to the intraperitoneal administration of streptozotocin rather than the usual intravenous mode since streptozotocin is known to degrade rapidly via the former route.

Most investigations using rats have been performed in males. It is not entirely clear from the reports using spontaneous BB rats whether both genders were used. Accordingly, it is known that the endothelium has a greater capacity to modulate vascular tone in the female rat.[96] Furthermore, estrogen treatment increases the response to acetylcholine.[102] Thus, differences due to gender must be considered. Our preliminary observations suggest that impaired relaxations to acetylcholine can be found in spontaneous diabetic BB rat aorta obtained from female animals (unpublished observations).

From a methodological standpoint, only two laboratories, Harris and Mac-Leod,[64] and ourselves[114] have used neurotransmitter blockers such as β-adrenoceptor antagonists and neuronal and extraneuronal uptake inhibitors routinely in their preparations. It is conceivable that a differential release or uptake of catecholamines by diabetic blood vessels might contribute to the observation of impaired endothelium-dependent relaxation in some preparations. It is unlikely that these are significant factors since we saw impaired relaxations with the use of such blockers while Harris and MacLeod[64] did not. Furthermore, other investigators using rat aorta came to similar conclusions as we did without using these neurotransmitter blockers. For the rat aorta at least, use of such agents is probably not an absolute necessity because of the sparse sympathetic innervation, but it may be a legitimate consideration for species such as rabbit where the innervation is more prominent.[67]

All studies, except one,[76] in which impaired endothelium-dependent relaxation was shown, used vessel rings rather than helical strips. Therefore, it is unlikely that inadvertent damage to endothelium in the helical preparations versus the ring preparations could be argued. Of the various studies cited above, only two studies[100,114] have provided any simultaneous electron microscopic analysis of endothelial structures. These studies showed areas of endothelial cell swelling, some loss of cell margins, and luminal crater formation. Thus, structural integrity of the endothelium is always an important consideration.

An interesting observation (Table 3) is that in those studies in which there was no impairment in responses to acetylcholine, the concentration of the contracting agent, norepinephrine, was somewhat lower (i.e., 10^{-7} to 5×10^{-7}M) compared to most other studies (i.e., 10^{-6}M). Perhaps the diabetic aorta is more sensitive to impaired relaxations to acetylcholine at higher levels of contractile tension. It is known in normal tissue that acetylcholine-mediated relaxations are progressively diminished as one approaches the maximum contraction of an agonist.[48] A more recent study by Kamata et al.,[76] using even lower agonist concentrations of 3×10^{-8} to 10^{-7}M would tend to argue against the hypothesis that impairment in acetylcholine-mediated relaxations is manifested only at higher concentrations of norepinephrine.

A potentially crucial methodological consideration is the influence of the initial resting tension on control versus diabetic vessels which may have disproportionate weights and cross-sectional areas. In our studies, diabetes was induced as rats were approaching the slower plateau phase of growth. Aortic ring weights (control = 3.2 ± 0.2 mg; diabetic = 2.6 ± 0.1 mg; cross-sectional areas of 1.18 ± 0.05 and 1.02 ± 0.03 g/mm², respectively) were not as markedly different as in many other stud-

ies where diabetic vessel cross-sectional areas and weights varied as much as 30%. In this regard, stretching is known to increase Ca^{2+} channel opening in isolated endothelial cells.[86] This stretching could increase intracellular calcium and provide increased basal EDRF release. Thus, the application of the same resting tension (or stretch) to disproportionate diameters of control versus diabetic blood vessels could augment basal EDRF in diabetic blood vessels relative to control and may obscure any detection of impaired endothelium-dependent relaxation.

Three reports have investigated endothelium-dependent relaxations in the diabetic rabbit aorta. Both Head et al.[68] and Jayakody et al.[72] reported no impaired response to acetylcholine in norepinephrine-contracted thoracic aorta taken from alloxan-diabetic rabbits. In contrast, impaired relaxations were observed in diabetic rabbit abdominal aorta that were contracted with phenylephrine.[158] The discrepancies between these reports on diabetic rabbits could be related to differential susceptibility of abdominal versus thoracic aorta. The observed impairment to acetylcholine in the rabbit aorta was reversed by either indomethacin or a thromboxane receptor antagonist, SQ 29548, suggesting that the impaired response might be mediated by the release of vasoconstrictor eicosanoids. Interestingly, we have noted that acetylcholine-induced responses were not impaired in $PGF_{2\alpha}$-contracted aorta from diabetic rats (unpublished observations). In experiments with $PGF_{2\alpha}$, indomethacin was always used in contrast to our earlier studies[114] using norepinephrine as the contracting agent where acetylcholine-induced responses were attenuated. Indomethacin has not been routinely used in most studies on endothelium-dependent relaxations in diabetic vessels. Oyama et al.[109] claimed that indomethacin did not alter impaired responses in the rat aorta but no data was provided. Our studies using pretreatment with indomethacin confirm the observation that indomethacin does not alter the impaired response to acetylcholine in norepinephrine-contracted diabetic rat aorta (Fig. 4).

Tesfamarian et al.[158] observed endothelium-dependent contractions to acetylcholine in quiescent diabetic rabbit aorta. It is not known whether such contractions to acetylcholine are peculiar to the rabbit abdominal aorta since no one has provided corroborating evidence for this observation in any large vessels among the three different species tested to date. In contrast, contractions to acetylcholine have been shown in diabetic renal microvasculature (see below).

Implications of impaired endothelium-dependent relaxations in other blood vessels is of obvious importance for generalized conclusions to be made. A few studies have been conducted in the mesenteric bed in situ,[46] in perfused segments in vitro,[155,156] and in suspended rings in vitro,[64,171] all in the rat model (Table 4). Impaired relaxations have been shown in mesenteric arteries to acetylcholine,[155,156] histamine,[46,155] and bradykinin.[46] In contrast, no impairment to acetylcholine was shown[46,64] and another report cited an augmented relaxation to histamine.[171]

Thirty days of streptozotocin treatment in the rat resulted in impaired relaxations to both acetylcholine and bradykinin in the perfused kidney.[60] It is assumed that these agents produced relaxations in renal microvasculature via endothelium-dependent processes.[30] Interestingly, the same group also showed endothelium-dependent contractions to acetylcholine in perfused diabetic kidneys.

In cerebral arterioles from diabetic

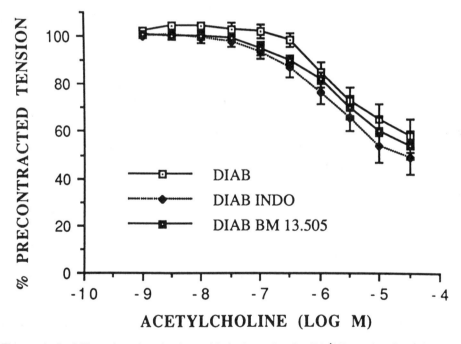

Figure 4: Inability of preincubation with indomethacin (10^{-4}M) or the thromboxane A_2 receptor antagonist, BM 13.505 (3×10^{-5}M) for 15 minutes to reverse the impairment of endothelium-dependent relaxation to acetylcholine in streptozotocin-diabetic rat aorta. Diabetic (n = 13), diabetic plus indomethacin (n = 14), diabetic plus BM 13.505 (n = 11).

Table 4.

Endothelium-Dependent Relaxation in Diabetic Rat Mesenteric Arteries

Investigators	Rat Strain	Type of Diabetes	Endothelium-Dependent Vasodilator				
			Acetylcholine	Histamine	ADP	A23187	Bradykinin
Fortes et al.[46]	Wistar	ALX[1]	unchanged	impaired	–	–	impaired
White & Carrier[171]	Sprague-Dawley	STZ[2]	–	augmented	–	–	–
Takiguchi et al.[155]	Wistar	STZ	impaired	impaired	–	–	–
Harris & MacLeod[64]	Wistar	STZ	unchanged	–	–	–	–

[1] ALX (alloxan)
[2] STZ (streptozotocin)

rats,[99] it was reported that relaxations to ADP were impaired, which is in agreement with the altered responses to ADP in diabetic rat aorta.[114] Furthermore, 5-HT relaxed normal rat cerebral arterioles but contracted diabetic arterioles, suggesting that cerebral endothelium might be damaged in diabetic animals as previously suggested.[104]

One group has studied endothelium-dependent relaxations in three separate vascular beds (i.e., coronary, femoral, and renal arteries) in alloxan diabetic dogs of mixed gender.[51,52,53] In femoral arteries, Gebremedhin et al.[52] showed no impaired relaxations to acetylcholine in vessels that were contracted with phenylephrine. Furthermore, diabetes increased the sensitivity to acetylcholine in phenylephrine-contracted renal arteries.[51] These responses were not altered by cyclooxygenase inhibitors. The same group showed in $PGF_{2\alpha}$-contracted canine coronary arteries that diabetes produced impaired relaxations to both acetylcholine and to the calcium ionophore A23187 but only when indomethacin or ibuprofen was present.[53] These data are in contrast with the results cited by Tesfamarian et al.[158] in which indomethacin reversed the impaired response

to acetylcholine in alloxan-diabetic rabbit aorta. It is possible that these differences result from species differences, differences in the response of the divergent vessel types, or differences in the contractile agents which were chosen in the individual studies. Rosen et al.,[128] using the perfused rat heart, were the first to show that diabetes also attenuates the dilatation to bradykinin in the coronary resistance vessels. Thus, coronary microvessels as well as larger coronary conductance vessels are apparently susceptible to diabetes and develop impaired endothelium-dependent relaxation.

A single in vitro study has recently been reported on human tissue. Acetylcholine-induced relaxation, but not nitroprusside or papaverine-induced responses, were impaired in the corpora cavernosa of the penis.[137]

In summary, despite some controversial findings, impaired endothelium-dependent relaxations to more than one vasodilator have been now demonstrated in at least three different animal species (i.e. rat, rabbit, dog) and five separate vessel types (i.e. aorta, mesenteric artery, renal microvasculature, cerebral arterioles, coronary arteries).

Possible Explanations for Impaired Endothelium-Dependent Relaxation in Diabetes

Diabetes-induced abnormalities in relaxations to endothelium-dependent vasodilators could be explained by changes in either the tonic or agonist-stimulated EDRF production and release. Thus, it is possible that diabetic vessels may produce less EDRF than normal tissue. Since quantitive measures of EDRF per se have not been made in diabetic vessels, it cannot be ascertained whether diabetic vessels actually release less EDRF. Alternatively, alterations in either the transport of EDRF or destruction of EDRF may occur in diabetes. Vascular smooth muscle responsiveness to released EDRF may be decreased by diabetes as well. EDRF is believed to produce relaxation by increasing the content of cGMP in vascular smooth muscle. To date, only two laboratories have published analyses of cGMP in diabetic blood vessels.[64,76] Harris and MacLeod[64] showed no difference in either basal or acetylcholine-stimulated levels of cGMP in diabetic rat aorta, which was consistent with their observations of similar relaxation of control and diabetic aorta to acetylcholine. In contrast, Kamata et al.[76] showed both impaired relaxation to acetylcholine along with decreases in cGMP under basal conditions and after stimulation with acetylcholine.

Impaired relaxation to acetylcholine could also be explained by an augmented sensitivity to the direct contractile effects of acetylcholine on vascular smooth muscle (e.g., via endothelium-derived constricting factor, EDCF) in diabetic rabbit aorta.[158] The role of EDCF has been refuted in two studies[40,109] in which acetylcholine-mediated relaxations were otherwise impaired. We also have not observed constrictor responses to acetylcholine in quiescent rat thoracic aorta (unpublished observations).

A defect in muscarinic receptor signal transduction by the endothelium cannot be excluded; however, a selective defect for muscarinic receptors is unlikely since impaired relaxations to histamine, bradykinin, and ADP have also been shown by others in different vessels. Our data tend to suggest, in lieu of more definite experiments, that the response may be a generalized defect in receptor-mediated transduction of intracellular signals since responses to A23187, a receptor-independent endothelium-dependent vasodilator, are not altered. Further studies will be required to verify this possibility.

Role of Eicosanoids in Impaired Endothelium-Dependent Vascular Relaxation in Diabetes

It is not presently clear how eicosanoids might interact to modulate endothelium-dependent relaxations in diabetic vasculature. It is possible that impaired responses are related to either an augmented release of vasoconstrictor prostanoids or decreased release of vasodilatory prostanoids. The report by Tesfamarian et al.[158] suggests that thromboxane A_2 might mediate the impaired relaxations to acetylcholine in abdominal aorta of diabetic rabbits, while Gebremedhin et al.[53] showed that cyclooxygenase inhibition with indomethacin unmasked an impaired relaxation to acetylcholine in diabetic canine coronary arteries. In paired experiments, we found that neither indomethacin nor the thromboxane A_2 receptor antagonist, BM-13.505, was able to reverse the impaired relaxation to acetylcholine in diabetic rat thoracic aorta (Fig. 4). Thus, it is premature to say whether simultaneous release of vasoactive eicosanoids are uniformly responsible for altering endothelium-mediated relaxations in all diabetic blood vessels. It is possible, but untested, that the augmented relaxations to histamine (a potent stimulator of prostacyclin release) which were shown by White and Carrier[171] could have been mediated by increased release of prostacyclin by diabetic mesenteric arteries. This is potentially important since Fugii et al.[47] showed augmented prostacyclin production in diabetic rat mesenteric arteries unlike that observed by other investigators in other vascular beds (see below). Shimokawa et al.[140] have suggested a synergistic interaction of endothelium-derived relaxations with prostacyclin in normal vessels. Therefore, production rates of prostacyclin might play an important role in endothelium-dependent relaxation in certain diabetic vascular beds but not others.

Data are available concerning prostacyclin production by diabetic blood vessels. Original studies by Silberbauer et al.[142] and Harrison et al.[66] using veins from diabetic patients and age-matched control subjects indicated that diabetic venous tissue synthesizes less prostacyclin. Since these original studies, several authors have reported decreased levels of production of prostacyclin by aorta and arteries from several experimental animal models[20,66,73,106,119,126,132,141,162] and spontaneous diabetic rat models.[152]

Analysis of coronary effluents from isolated perfused hearts has revealed reduced prostacyclin content in diabetic versus control rats.[129,130] However, perfusion with arachidonic acid significantly elevated prostacyclin production even above that seen in normal hearts.[127,130,132] Decreases in basal rates of prostacyclin release may have been influenced by disproportionate rates of coronary flow between the two groups. In contrast, when coronary perfusion flow rates were held constant between control and diabetic hearts, we observed no differences in basal rates of prostacyclin release between control and diabetic groups.[112,115] The difference in prostacyclin production by coronary microvasculature versus larger arteries such as the aorta may indicate that generalizations about a putative decrease in capacity to synthesize prostacyclin cannot be made for all vascular beds (refer to review by Pieper, ref. 113). For example, there are reports of increased prostacyclin production in diabetic canine coronary arteries[147] and the perfused diabetic rat mesenteric microvascular bed.[47] Furthermore, another study showed decreased prostacyclin production in rat aortic segments despite normal production in cerebral microvessels taken from the same animals.[169] Why such differences occur is not fully understood, but it is known that diabetes enhances the endothelial surface area in small arterioles while it diminishes the surface area in larger conductance vessels.[13] In contrast, Koltai et al.[82] have shown no significant differences in prostacyclin production in diabetic canine coronary, femoral, or basilar arteries but they demonstrated augmented production of thromboxane A_2.

Not only is there evidence for altered synthesis of prostacyclin by diabetic blood vessels but there is also evidence for alterations in vascular reactivity to prostanoids. Prostacyclin and PGE_1 have been shown to produce paradoxical constriction in diabetic rabbit carotid arteries[4] in contrast to no response in control vessels. The observation that phentolamine completely blocked the constriction to prostacyclin and partially blocked the response to PGE_1 suggested either a direct effect on postsynaptic α-adrenoceptors or an indirect release of norepinephrine from presynaptic nerve terminals. Prostacyclin, which renlaxes canine coronary and mesenteric arteries, produced constriction in diabetic but not control arteries.[147,148] These constrictions were reversed by either indomethacin, acetylsalicylic acid, or cortisone as well as inhibitors of thromboxane A_2 synthesis, imidazole or L-8027,[148,149] which suggests that such constrictions were mediated by the release of vasoconstrictive eicosanoids such as thromboxanes. These observations would be similar to the report in which the impaired endothelium-dependent relaxation to acetylcholine in the diabetic rabbit abdominal aorta was reversed by indomethacin or a thromboxane receptor antagonist.[158] In diabetic canine basilar, coronary, and femoral arteries,[82] thromboxane A_2 production, but not prostacyclin production, was elevated in phenylephrine-contracted vessels. Treatment with phentolamine doubled prostacyclin production in diabetic coronary arteries while normalizing the elevated thromboxane production rates. These studies suggest a complex interaction between α-adrenoceptors and eicosanoid synthesis which appears altered in certain diabetic blood vessels.

Role of Oxygen-Derived Free Radicals in Impaired Endothelium-Dependent Vascular Relaxation in Diabetes

Initial studies by Rubanyi and Vanhoutte[135] showed that oxygen-derived free radicals could reduce endothelium-dependent relaxations to acetylcholine in canine coronary arteries. This diminished response is probably due to the ability of free radicals to interfere with or destroy released EDRF.[59,168] The nature of free radical interactions with vascular responses is provided in an excellent minireview by Rubanyi.[134]

Additions of superoxide dismutase to norepinephrine-contracted vessels caused concentration-dependent relaxations that were greater in diabetic versus control rat aorta (Fig. 5). This increased relaxation response in diabetic aorta was not prevented by indomethacin. Since superoxide dismutase produced no relaxations in denuded diabetic vessels, the response to superoxide dismutase was obligatory for some factors related to the endothelium. Thus, the possibility exists that superoxide anion may play a significant role in the impaired endothelium-dependent relaxation in diabetes.

We analyzed whether diabetic blood vessels would be more at risk to free radical-mediated injury to the vascular endothelium. In control rat aorta, oxygen-derived free radicals have latent effects on endothelial function;[114,116] if vessels are exposed for a finite period of time to free radicals and the source of free radicals removed by serial washings, a subsequent challenge by acetylcholine produces a diminished response in contracted vessels. Relaxations to the purinergic agonist, ADP, were also impaired but not relaxations that were elicited by the receptor-independent endothelium-dependent vasodilator, A23187, or by the endothelium-independent vasodilators, nitroglycerin or papaverine. Thus, not only may free radicals destroy released EDRF but they may also produce latent damage in the coupling of receptor-dependent endothelium-mediated relaxations of vascular smooth muscle.

While prior free radical exposure impaired endothelium-dependent relaxations to acetylcholine in control rat aorta, the same regimen abolished relaxations to both ADP and acetylcholine in diabetic vessels.[117] Free radical exposure of diabetic vessels only marginally reduced relaxations to the calcium ionophore A23187 and did not alter responses to either papaverine or nitroglycerin, suggesting selectivity

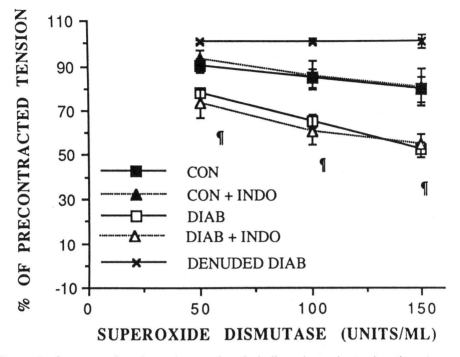

Figure 5: Concentration-dependent and endothelium-dependent relaxations to superoxide dismutase in norepinephrine-contracted aortic ring segments from diabetic rat. Control (n = 6), diabetic (n = 14) in the presence of 10^{-6}M indomethacin (n = 6), denuded diabetic (n = 6). ¶$p < 0.001$.

primarily for receptor-mediated endothelium-dependent processes. The abolition of response to acetylcholine in diabetic rings was attenuated by catalase (a promoter of H_2O_2 catabolism), mannitol (a hydroxyl radical scavenger), dimethylthiourea (a hydroxyl radical scavenger), or desferrioxamine (an iron chelator). This suggested that hydroxyl radicals or iron-mediated hydroxyl radical formation may be the prime initiator of the injury to diabetic endothelium by the free radical-generating system.

Free radicals can also interact in complex ways to limit prostacyclin production by the endothelium. In related studies using the isolated, isovolumically perfused rat heart, brief periods of global ischemia followed by reperfusion stimulated the release of prostacyclin in normal hearts that tended to be slower in onset in acute (48 hr) diabetic hearts.[112] Prostacyclin release could be enhanced in these acute diabetic hearts but not control hearts by co-perfusion with superoxide dismutase plus catalase, suggesting that prostacyclin synthesis in postischemic hearts from acute diabetic animals, unlike nondiabetic hearts, is regulated by concomitant free radical production. Such observations would be consistent with those of Kawamura et al.,[77] who showed that incubations of unsuspended, quiescent rat aorta with *t*-butyl hydroperoxide produced greater inhibition of prostaglandin synthase in diabetic blood vessels. Thus, it appears that generation of endothelium-dependent vasoactive factors (e.g., EDRF and prostacyclin) in diabetic blood vessels are particularly susceptible to free radical-induced modulations.

Implications of Endothelial Cell Alterations in Diabetes-Induced Vascular Complications

An increasing number of studies tend to implicate perturbations in endothelium-dependent modulation of vascular smooth muscle tone in the pathogenesis of cardiovascular disease.[164] There is evidence that diabetes can decrease the release of at least two endothelium-derived vasoactive substances, namely EDRF and prostacyclin. A pictoral diagram of the modulation of vascular tone is summarized for normal (Fig. 6) and diabetic (Fig. 7) blood vessels. Present information suggests that diabetes does not alter all relaxation responses to different stimulants of EDRF release. The defect appears to be specific for receptor-mediated processes. It is important to note that this dysfunction occurs in the rat, which is an atherosclerosis-resistant model. Thus, diabetes per se may be an independent risk factor to impaired endothelium-dependent relaxation. It is possible that this may contribute to the accelerated atherosclerosis[146] and increased risk of hypertension[24,143] in this subpopulation.

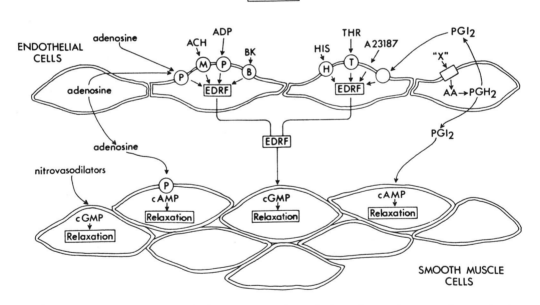

Figure 6. An illustration depicting the normal regulation of vascular smooth muscle tone by endothelium-derived vasoactive factors. Endothelium-derived relaxant factors (EDRF) are released by receptor-independent stimuli (calcium ionophore A23187) or various receptor-dependent vasodilators such as acetylcholine (ACH), adenosine diphosphate (ADP), bradykinin (BK), histamine (HIS), and thrombin (THR). Various stimulants (X), including those that release EDRF, can also release prostacyclin (PGI$_2$) arising from arachidonic acid (AA) within endothelial cells as well. PGI$_2$ can relax vascular smooth muscle directly or indirectly via action on endothelial cells.

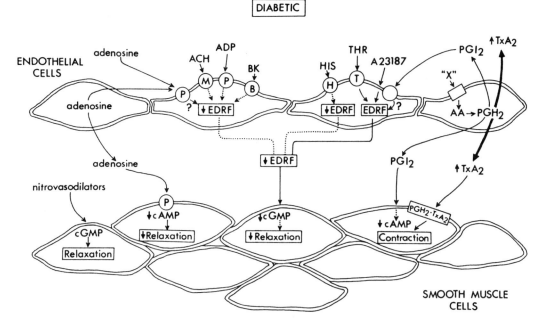

Figure 7: An illustration summarizing the hypothetical modulation of vascular tone by endothelium-derived vasoactive factors in diabetic blood vessels. Dashed lines denote reduced release or diminished response. In general, diabetic vascular tone is altered by diminished production of EDRF with augmented thromboxane A_2 (TxA_2) production favoring a more constricted state. Endothelium-dependent relaxation is impaired to several receptor-dependent stimuli. In contrast, thrombin- and A23187-mediated responses appear unimpaired, indicating potential differentiation in susceptibility of different EDRFs on pathways of EDRF stimulation. Diabetic vascular smooth muscle appears to be subsensitive to relaxation induced by PGI_2 and supersensitive to TxA_2.

In addition to these chronic manifestations, impaired endothelium-dependent relaxation in the diabetic patient may also increase the risk of platelet aggregation in acute myocardial infarction and in coronary vasospasm.[165] Both EDRF and prostacyclin act synergistically to inhibit platelet aggregation.[17,50,103,120] Decreased production of both of these vasoactive substances (Fig. 8) should tend to promote platelet aggregation, which is known to be enhanced in diabetic patients.[28]

The vascular response to platelet aggregation is further complicated in diabetes because of elevated basal thromboxane A_2 levels[19,62,177] and increased sensitivity to thromboxane analogues.[132,149] Further-more, U-46619-mediated stimulation of endogenous prostacyclin release by the myocardium consequent to ischemia plus reperfusion was recently shown to be decreased in diabetes.[113] Thus, the diabetic patient would be at increased risk to vasospasm (Fig. 8) because of enhanced sensitivity of coronary arteries to vasoconstrictors and decreased ability of coronary endothelium to generate compensatory vasodilators, such as EDRF and prostacyclin.

Acknowledgments: This work was supported by funds provided by Coronary Heart Disease Research, a program of the American Health Assistance Foundation, Rockville, Maryland, by grants-in-aid from the American Heart Association and the American Diabetes Association, Inc./Wisconsin Affiliate, and by NIH grant HL08311.

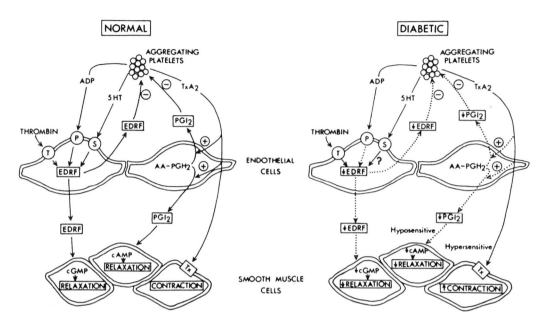

Figure 8: A proposed model depicting the theoretical consequences of products released by aggregating platelets as modified by diabetic endothelial cells. Release of EDRF is diminished in response to ADP-derived from platelet degranulation. This results in diminished relaxation of vascular smooth muscle and a diminished anti-aggregatory response of platelets to EDRF. Prostacyclin release may be reduced along with a subsensitive relaxation response of vascular smooth muscle to prostacyclin. Thromboxane A_2 (TxA_2) released by aggregating platelets produces a hyperreactive constrictor response in diabetic vascular smooth muscle. Furthermore, the compensatory release of PGI_2 as an anti-aggregatory and anti-spasmotic agent in response to TxA_2 is also diminished.

References

1. Aagenaes O., Moe H.: Light and electron microscope study of skin capillaries of diabetic. Diabetes 10:253–259, 1961.
2. Altura B.M., Halevy S., Turlapaty P.D.M.V.: Vascular smooth muscle in diabetes and its influence on the reactivity of blood vessels. Adv. Microcirc. 8:118–150, 1979.
3. Angus J.A., Cocks T.M.: Endothelium-derived relaxing factor. Pharmacol. Ther. 41:303–351, 1989.
4. Agrawal D.K., Bhimji S., McNeill J.H.: Effect of chronic experimental diabetes on vascular smooth muscle function in rabbit carotid artery. J. Cardiovasc. Pharmacol. 9:584–593, 1987.

5. Agrawal D.K., McNeill J.H.: Vascular responses to agonists in rat mesenteric artery from diabetic rats. Can. J. Physiol. Pharmacol. 65:1484–1490, 1987.
6. Arbogast B.W., Berry D.L., Newell C.L.: Injury of arterial endothelial cells in diabetic, sucrose-fed and aged rats. Atherosclerosis 51:31–45, 1984.
7. Ashton N.: Vascular basement membrane changes in diabetic retinopathy. Br. J. Ophthalmol. 58:344–346, 1974.
8. Atkins F.L., Dowell R.T., Love S.: β-adrenergic receptors, adenylate cyclase activity, and cardiac dysfunction in diabetic rat. J. Cardiovasc. Pharmacol. 7:66–70, 1985.

9. Banga J.D., Sixma J.J.: Diabetes mellitus, vascular disease and thrombosis. Clin. Hematol. 15:465–492, 1986.
10. Bassenge E., Busse R.: Endothelial modulation of coronary tone. Prog. Cardiovasc. Dis. 30:349–380, 1988.
11. Bell R.H. Jr., Hye R.J.: Animal models of diabetes mellitus: physiology and pathology. J. Surg. Res. 35:433–460, 1983.
12. Bloodworth J.M.B.: Diabetic microangiopathy. Diabetes 12:99–114, 1963.
13. Bohlen H.G., Niggl B.A.: Arteriolar anatomical and functional abnormalities in juvenile mice with genetic or streptozotocin-induced diabetes mellitus. Circ. Res. 45:390–396, 1979.
14. Bollinger A., Frey J., Jager K.: Capillaries in patients with long-term diabetes. N. Engl. J. Med. 307:1305–1310, 1982.
15. Bossaller C., Habib G.B., Yamamoto H., Williams C., Wells S., Henry P.D.: Impaired muscarinic endothelium-dependent relaxation and cyclic guanosine 5'-monophosphate formation in atherosclerotic human coronary artery and rabbit aorta. J. Clin. Invest. 79:170–174, 1987.
16. Brecker P., Chobanian A.V., Small D.M., VanSickle W., Tercyak A., Baler J.: Relationship of an abnormal plasma lipoprotein to protection from atherosclerosis in the cholesterol-fed diabetic rabbit. J. Clin. Invest. 72:1553–1562, 1983.
17. Busse R., Luckhoff, A., Bassenge E.: Endothelium-derived relaxant factor inhibits platelet activation. Naunyn-Schmiedeberg's Arch. Pharmacol. 336:566–571, 1987.
18. Busse R., Trogisch G., Bassenge E.: The role of endothelium in the control of vascular tone. Bas. Res. Cardiol. 80:475–490, 1985.
19. Butkus A., Skrinska V.A., Schumacher O.P.: Thromboxane production and platelet aggregation in diabetic subjects with clinical complications. Thromb. Res. 19:211–213, 1980.
20. Carreras L.O., Chamone, D.A.F., Klerckx P., Vermylen J.: Decreased vascular prostacyclin (PGI_2) in diabetic rats. Stimulation of PGI_2 release in normal and diabetic rats by the antithrombotic compound BAY g6575. Thromb. Res. 19:663–670, 1980.
21. Carrier G.O., Aronstam R.S.: Altered muscarinic receptor properties and function in the heart in diabetes. J. Pharmacol. Exp. Ther. 242:531–535, 1987.
22. Carrier G.O., Edwards A.D., Aronstam R.S.: Cholinergic supersensitivity and decreased number of muscarinic receptors in atria from short-term diabetic rats. J. Mol. Cell. Cardiol. 16:963–965, 1984.
23. Carrier G.O., White R.E.: Enhancement of alpha-1 and alpha-2 adrenergic agonist-induced vasoconstriction by removal of endothelium in rat aorta. J. Pharmacol. Exp. Ther. 232:682–687, 1985.
24. Christlieb A.R., Warram J.H., Krolewski A.S., Busick E.J., Ganda O.P., Asmal A.C., Soeldner, Bradley R.F.: Hypertension: the major risk factor in juvenile-onset insulin-dependent diabetes. Diabetes 30(Suppl. 2):90–96, 1981.
25. Colantuoni A., Bertuglia S., Donato L: Effects of metformin on microvascular permeability in diabetic Syrian hamsters. Diab. Metab. (Paris) 14:549–553, 1988.
26. Colwell J.A., Lopes-Virella M.L., Halushka P.V.: Pathogenesis of atherosclerosis in diabetes mellitus. Diabetes Care 4:121–133, 1981.
27. Colwell J.A., Winocour P.D., Lopes-Virella M., Halushka P.V.: New concepts about the pathogenesis of atherosclerosis in diabetes mellitus. Am. J. Med. 75:67–80, 1983.
28. Colwell J.A., Halushka P.V., Sarji K.E., Lopes-Virella M.F., Sagel J.: Vascular disease in diabetes. Pathophysiological mechanisms and therapy. Arch. Intern. Med. 139:225–230, 1979.
29. Colwell J.A., Nair R.M.G., Halushka P.V., Rogers C., Whetsell A., Sagel J.: Platelet adhesion and aggregation in diabetes mellitus. Metabolism 28:394–400, 1979.
30. Conger J.D., Robinette J.B., Schrier R.W.: Smooth muscle calcium and endothelium-derived relaxing factor in the abnormal vascular responses of acute renal failure. J. Clin. Invest. 82:532–537, 1988.
31. Crall F.A., Roberts W.C.: The extramural and intramural coronary arteries in juvenile diabetes mellitus: Analysis of nine necropsy patients aged 14–38 years with onset of diabetes before age 15 years. Am. J. Med. 64:221–230, 1978.
32. De Mey J.G., Vanhoutte P.M.: Role of the intima in cholinergic and purinergic relaxation of isolated canine femoral arteries. J. Physiol. 316:347–355, 1981.
33. De Mey J.G., Claeys M., Vanhoutte P.M.: Endothelium-dependent inhibitory effects of acetylcholine, adenosine triphosphate, thrombin and arachidonic acid in the canine femoral artery. J. Pharmacol. Exp. Ther. 222:166–173, 1982.

34. Ditzel J., Bearen D.W., Renold A.E.: Early vascular changes in diabetes mellitus. Metabolism 9:400–407, 1960.

35. Dolgov V.V., Zaikina O.E., Bondarenko M.F., Repin V.S.: Aortic endothelium of alloxan diabetic rabbits: a quantitative study using scanning electron microscopy. Diabetologia 22:338–343, 1982.

36. Dowell R.T., Atkins F.L., Love S.: Integrative nature and time course of cardiovascular alterations in the diabetic rat. J. Cardiovasc. Pharmacol. 8:406–413, 1986.

37. Downing S.E.: Restoration of coronary dilator action of adenosine in experimental diabetes. Am. J. Physiol. 249:H102–H107, 1985.

38. Downing S.E., Lee J.C.: Myocardial and coronary vascular responses to insulin in the diabetic lamb. Am. J. Physiol. 237:H514–H519, 1979.

39. Downing S.E., Lee J.C., Weinstein E.M.: Coronary dilator actions of adenosine and CO_2 in experimental diabetes. Am. J. Physiol. 243:H252–H258, 1982.

40. Durante W., Sen A.K., Sunahara F.A.: Impairment of endothelium-dependent relaxation in aortae from spontaneously diabetic rats. Br. J. Pharmacol. 94:463–468, 1988.

41. Durante W., Sunahara F.A., Sen A.K.: Effect of diabetes on metabolic coronary dilatation in the rat. Cardiovasc. Res. 23:40–45, 1989.

42. Dyck P.J., Hansen S., Karnes J., O'Brien P., Yasuda H., Windebank A., Zimmermann B.: Capillary number and percentage closed in human diabetic sural nerve. Proc. Natl. Acad. Sci. USA 82:2513–2517, 1985.

43. Egleme C.T., Godfraind, T., Miller R.C.: Enhanced responsiveness of rat .isolated aorta to clonidine after removal of the endothelial cells. Br. J. Pharmacol. 81:16–18, 1984.

44. Fischer V.W.: Modification of anionic sites in myocardial capillary basal laminae of diabetic rats. Microvasc. Res. 37:42–52, 1989.

45. Fischer V.W., Barner H.B., Leskiw M.L.: Capillary basal laminar thickness in diabetic human myocardium. Diabetes 28:713–719, 1979.

46. Fortes Z.B., Leme J.G., Scivoletto R.: Vascular reactivity in diabetes mellitus: role of the endothelial cell. Br. J. Pharmacol. 79:771–781, 1983.

47. Fujii K., Soma M., Huang Y.-S., Manku M.S., Horrobin D.F.: Increased release of prostaglandins from the mesenteric vascular bed of diabetic animals: the effects of glucose and insulin. Prost. Leuk. Med. 24:151–161, 1986.

48. Furchgott R.F.: Role of endothelium in responses of vascular smooth muscle. Circ. Res. 53:557–573, 1983.

49. Furchgott R.F., Zawadski J.V.: The obligatory role of endothelial cells in the relaxation of arterial smooth muscle by acetylcholine. Nature 288:373–376, 1980.

50. Furlong B., Henderson A.H., Lewis M.J., Smith J.A.: Endothelium-derived relaxing factor inhibits in vitro platelet aggregation. Br. J. Pharmacol. 90:687–692, 1987.

51. Gebremedhin D., Koltai M.Z., Pogátsa G., Magyar K., Hadházy P.: Altered responsiveness of diabetic dog renal arteries to acetylcholine and phenylephrine: role of endothelium. Pharmacology 38:177–184, 1989.

52. Gebremedhin D., Koltai M.Z., Pogátsa G., Magyar K., Hadházy P.: Differential contractile responsiveness of femoral arteries from healthy and diabetic dogs: role of endothelium. Arch. Int. Pharmacodyn. 288:100–108, 1987.

53. Gebremedhin D., Koltai M.Z., Pogátsa G., Magyar K., Hadházy P.: Influence of experimental diabetes on the mechanical responses of canine coronary arteries: role of endothelium. Cardiovasc. Res. 22:537–544, 1988.

54. Giustolisi R., Lombardo T., Musso R., Cacciola E.: Factor VIII antigen plasma levels in diabetes mellitus. Enhanced endothelial release and storage. Thromb. Haemost. 44:46, 1980.

55. Goldenberg S., Alex M., Joshi R.A., Blumenthal H.T.: Non-atheromatous peripheral vascular disease of the lower extremities in diabetes mellitus. Diabetes 8:261–273, 1959.

56. Greenberg S., Diecke F.P.J.: Endothelium-derived relaxing and contracting factors: new concepts and new findings. Drug Dev. Res. 12:131–149, 1988.

57. Griffith T.M., Lewis M.J., Newby A.C., Henderson A.H.: Endothelium-derived relaxing factor. J. Am. Coll. Cardiol. 12:797–806, 1988.

58. Gross G.J., Pieper G.M.: Impairment of receptor-mediated, endothelium-dependent relaxation in diabetes and enhanced susceptibility to oxygen-derived free radicals. Pharmacologist 30:A209, 1988.

59. Gryglewski R.J., Palmer, R.M.J., Moncada S.: Superoxide anion is involved in the

breakdown of endothelium-derived vascular relaxing factor. Nature 320:454–456, 1986.

60. Ha H., Dunham E.W.: Limited capacity for renal vasodilatation in anesthetized diabetic rats. Am. J. Physiol. 253:H845–H855, 1987.

61. Haider B., Lyons M., Torres R., Oldewurtel H., Regan T.: Effects of diabetes on myocardial perfusion in the atherosclerotic monkey. J. Lab. Clin. Med. 113:123–132, 1989.

62. Halushka P.V., Mayfield R., Colwell J.A.: Insulin and arachidonic acid metabolism in diabetes mellitus. Metabolism 34(Suppl. I):32–36, 1985.

63. Haluska P.V., Rogers R.C., Loadholt C.B., Colwell J.A.: Increased platelet thromboxane synthesis in diabetes mellitus. J. Lab. Clin. Med. 97:87–96, 1981.

64. Harris K.H., MacLeod K.M.: Influence of the endothelium on contractile responses of arteries from diabetic rats. Eur. J. Pharmacol. 153:55–64, 1988.

65. Harrison D.G., Freiman P.C., Armstrong M.L., Marcus M.L., Heistad D.D.: Alterations of vascular reactivity in atherosclerosis. Circ. Res. 61(Suppl. II):II-74–II-80, 1987.

66. Harrison H.E., Reece A.H., Johnson M.: Decreased vascular prostacyclin in experimental diabetes. Life Sci. 23:351–356, 1978.

67. Head R.J., Hempstead J., Berkowitz B.A.: Catecholamines in the vasculature of the rat and rabbit: Dopamine, norepinephrine, epinephrine. Blood Vessels 19:135–147, 1982.

68. Head R.J., Longhurst P.A., Panek R.L., Stitzel R.E.: A contrasting effect of the diabetic state upon the contractile responses of aortic preparations from the rat and rabbit. Br. J. Pharmacol. 91:275–286, 1987.

69. Ingebretsen C.G., Hawelu-Johnson C., Ingebretsen W.R. Jr.: Alloxan-induced diabetes reduces β-adrenergic receptor number without affecting adenylate cyclase in rat ventricular membranes. J. Cardiovasc. Pharmacol. 5:454–461, 1983.

70. Ingebretsen W.R. Jr., Peralta C., Monsher M., Wagner L.K., Ingebretsen C.G.: Diabetes alters the myocardial cAMP-protein kinase cascade system. Am. J. Physiol. 240:H375–H382, 1981.

71. Jarrett R.J., Keen H., Chakrabarti R.: Diabetes, hyperglycemia and arterial disease. In: H. Keen, R.J. Jarrett (eds.). Complications of Diabetes, London, Arnold, 1982, pp 179–204.

72. Jayakody L., Senaratne M., Thomson A., Kappagoda T.: Endothelium-dependent relaxation in experimental atherosclerosis in the rabbit. Circ. Res. 60:251–264, 1987.

73. Jeremy J.Y., Thompson C.S., Mikhailidis D.P., Owen R.H., Dandona P.: Fasting and diabetes mellitus elicit opposite effects on agonist-stimulated prostacyclin synthesis by the rat aorta. Metabolism 36:616–620, 1987.

74. Jobidon C., Nadeau A., Tancréde G., Rousseau-Migneron S.: Diminished hypotensive response to isoproterenol in streptozotocin-diabetic rats. Gen. Pharmacol. 20:39–45, 1989.

75. Joyner W.L., Mayhan W.G., Johnson R.L., Phares C.K.: Microvascular alterations develop in Syrian hamsters after the induction of diabetes mellitus by streptozotocin. Diabetes 30:93–100, 1981.

76. Kamata K., Miyata N., Kasuya Y.: Impairment of endothelium-dependent relaxation and changes in levels of cyclic GMP in aorta from streptozotocin-induced diabetic rats. Br. J. Pharmacol. 97:614–618, 1989.

77. Kawamura K., Dohi T., Ogama T., Shirakawa M., Okamoto H., Tsujimoto A.: Susceptibility of diabetic rat aorta to self-deactivation during prostacyclin synthesis. Prost. Leuk. Med. 28:1–13, 1987.

78. Kilzer P., Chang K., Marvel J., Rowold E., Jaudes P., Ullensvang S., Kilo C., Williamson J.P.: Albumin permeation of new vessels is increased in diabetic rats. Diabetes 34:333–336, 1985.

79. Kohner E.M., Henkind P.: Correlation of fluorescein angiogram and retinal digest in diabetic retinopathy. Am. J. Ophthalmol. 69:403–414, 1970.

80. Koltai M.Z., Jermendy G., Kiss V., Wagner M., Pogátsa G.: The effects of sympathetic stimulation and adenosine on coronary circulation and heart function in diabetes mellitus. Acta Physiol. Hung. 63:119–125, 1984.

81. Koltai M.Z.: Role of adrenergic mechanism in the altered coronary reactivity in diabetes. J. Mol. Cell. Cardiol. 15(Suppl. 1):86, 1983.

82. Koltai M.Z., Rösen P., Hadházy P., Ballagi-Pordány G.Y., Köszeghy A., Pogátsa G.: Relationship between vascular adrenergic receptors and prostaglandin biosyntheses in canine diabetic coronary arteries. Diabetologia 21:681–686, 1988.

83. Konishi M., Su C.: role of endothelium in dilator responses of spontaneously hyper-

tensive rat arteries. Hypertension 5:881–886, 1983.

84. Ku D.: Mechanism of thrombin-induced endothelium-dependent coronary vasodilation in dogs: role of its proteolytic enzymatic activity. J. Cardiovasc. Pharmacol. 8:29–36, 1986.

85. Kusher B., Lazar M., Furman M., Lieberman T.W., Leopold I.H.: Resistance of rabbits and guinea pigs to the diabetogenic effect of streptozotocin. Diabetes 18:542–544, 1969.

86. Lansman J.B., Hallam T.J., Rink T.J.: Single stretch-activated ion channels in vascular endothelial cells as mechanotransducers? Nature (London) 325:811–813, 1987.

87. Latifpour J., McNeill J.H.: Cardiac autonomic receptors: effect of long-term experimental diabetes. J. Pharmacol. Exp. Ther. 230:242–249, 1984.

88. Lefer A.M., Osborne J.A., Yunagisawa A., Sun J.-Z.: Influence of atherosclerosis on vascular responsiveness in isolated rabbit vascular smooth muscle. Cardiovasc. Drugs. Ther. 1:385–391, 1987.

89. Leinonen H., Matikainen E., Juntunen J.: Permeability and morphology of skeletal muscle capillaries in type I (insulin-dependent) diabetes mellitus. Diabetologia 22:158–162, 1982.

90. Longhurst P.A., Head R.J.: Responses of the isolated perfused mesenteric vasculature from diabetic rats: the significance of appropriate control tissues. J. Pharmacol. Exp. Ther. 235:45–49, 1985.

91. Lues I., Schümann H.J.: Effect of removing the endothelial cells on the reactivity of rat aortic segments to different α-adrenoceptor agonists. Naunyn-Schmiedeberg's Arch. Pharmacol. 328:160–163, 1984.

92. Lüscher T.F., Vanhoutte P.M.: Endothelium-dependent contractions to acetylcholine in the aorta of the spontaneously hypertensive rat. Hypertension 8:344–348, 1986.

93. MacLeod K.M.: The effect of insulin treatment on changes in vascular reactivity in chronic, experimental diabetes. Diabetes 34:1160–1167, 1985.

94. MacLeod K.M., McNeill J.H.: Alpha adrenoceptor-mediated responses in aorta from 3-month streptozotocin diabetic rats. Proc. West. Pharmacol. Soc. 25:245–247, 1982.

95. MacLeod K.M., McNeill J.H.: The influence of chronic experimental diabetes on

96. Maddox Y.T., Falcon J.G., Ridinger M., Cunard C.M., Ramwell P.W.: Endothelium-dependent gender differences in the response of the rat aorta. J. Pharmacol. Exp. Ther. 240:392–395, 1987.

97. Marsiella P., DePaoli A., Bergamini E.: Influence of age on the sensitivity of the rat to streptozotocin. Horm. Metab. Res. 11:262–274, 1979.

98. Martin W., Furchgott R.F., Villani G.M., Jothianadan D.: Depression of contractile response in rat aorta by spontaneously released endothelium-derived relaxing factor. J. Pharmacol. Exp. Ther. 237:529–538, 1986.

99. Mayhan W.G.: Impairment of endothelium-dependent dilatation of cerebral arterioles during diabetes mellitus. Am. J. Physiol. 256:H621–H625, 1989.

100. Meraji S., Jayakody L., Senaratne M.P.J., Thomson A.B.R., Kappagoda T.: Endothelium-dependent relaxation in aorta of BB rat. Diabetes 36:978–981, 1987.

101. Michaelis O.E. IV, Carswell N., Hansen C.T., Canary J.J., Kimmel P.L.: A new genetic model of noninsulin-dependent diabetes and hypertension: the spontaneously hypertensive/NIH corpulent rat. In: Frontiers in Diabetic Research: Lessons from Animal Diabetes. E. Shafrin, A.E. Renold (eds.). John Libbey and Co., Ltd, London, pp 257–264, 1988.

102. Miller V.M., Gisclard V., Vanhoutte P.M.: Modulation of endothelium-dependent and vascular smooth muscle responses by oestrogens. Phlebology 3(Suppl. I):63–69, 1988.

103. Moncada S., Higgs E.A., Vane J.R.: Human arterial and venous tissue generate prostacyclin (prostaglandin X) a potent inhibitor of platelet aggregation. Lancet 1:18–20, 1977.

104. Moore S.A., Bohlen H.G., Miller B.G., Evan A.P.: Cellular and vessel wall morphology of cerebral cortical arterioles after short-term diabetes in adult rats. Blood Vessels 22:265–277, 1985.

105. Murakami K., Karaki H., Urakawa N.: Role of endothelium in the contraction induced by norepinephrine and clonidine in rat aorta. Jap. J. Pharmacol. 39:357–364, 1985.

106. Myers T.O., Messina E.J., Rodrigues A.M., Gerritsen M.E.: Altered aortic and cremaster muscle prostaglandin synthesis

in diabetic rats. Am. J. Physiol. 249:E374–E379, 1985.

107. Nakhooda A.F., Like A.A., Chappel C.I., Murray F.T., Marliss E.B.: The spontaneously diabetic Wistar rat. Metabolic and morphologic studies. Diabetes 26:100–112, 1976.

108. Owen M.P., Carrier G.O.: Calcium dependence of norepinephrine-induced vascular contraction in experimental diabetes. J. Pharmacol. Exp. Ther. 212:253–258, 1980.

109. Oyama Y., Kawasaki H., Hattori Y., Kanno M.: Attenuation of endothelium-dependent relaxation in aorta from diabetic rats. Eur. J. Pharmacol. 131:75–78, 1986.

110. Parving H.-H., Noer I., Deckert T., Evrin P.E., Nielsen S.L., Lyngsøe J., Morgensen C.E., Rørth M., Svendsen P.A., Trap-Jensen J., Lassen N.A.: The effect of metabolic regulation on microvascular permeability to small and large molecules in short-term juvenile diabetes. Diabetologia 12:161–166, 1976.

111. Pfaffman M.A., Ball C.R., Darby A., Hilman R.: Insulin reversal of diabetes-induced inhibition of vascular contractility in the rat. Am. J. Physiol 242:H490–H495, 1982.

112. Pieper G.M.: Superoxide dismutase plus catalase improves postischaemic recovery in the diabetic heart. Cardiovasc. Res. 22:916–926, 1988.

113. Pieper G.M.: Alterations in reperfusion-stimulated prostacyclin release by the diabetic heart. In: Diabetic Heart, M. Nagano, N.S. Dhalla (eds.). Raven Press, New York, 1991.

114. Pieper G.M., Gross G.J.: Oxygen free radicals abolish endothelium-dependent relaxation in diabetic rat aorta. Am. J. Physiol. 255:H825–H832, 1988.

115. Pieper G.M., Gross G.J.: Diabetes alters the postischemic response to a prostacyclin-mimetic. Am. J. Physiol. 256:H1353–H1360, 1989.

116. Pieper G.M., Gross G.J.: Selective impairment of endothelium-dependent relaxation by oxygen-derived free radicals. Blood Vessels 26:44–47, 1989.

117. Pieper G.M., Langenstroer P., Gross G.J.: Role of iron and hydroxyl radicals in impaired endothelium-dependent relaxation of diabetic vessels following free radical-induced injury. J. Vasc. Med. Biol. 1:109, 1989.

118. Porta M., La Selva M., Molinatti P., Mol-

inatti G.M.: Endothelial cell function in diabetic microangiopathy. Diabetologia 30:601–609, 1987.

119. Quilley T., McGiff J.C.: Arachidonic acid metabolism and urinary excretion of prostaglandins and thromboxane in rats with experimental diabetes mellitus. J. Pharmacol. Exp. Ther. 234:211–216, 1985.

120. Radomski M.W., Palmer R.M.J., Moncada S.: Comparative pharmacology of endothelium-derived relaxing factor, nitric oxide and prostacyclin in platelets. Br. J. Pharmacol. 92:181–187, 1987.

121. Ramanadham S., Tenner T.E. Jr.: Alterations in the myocardial β-adrenoceptor system of streptozotocin-diabetic rats. Eur. J. Pharmacol. 136:377–378, 1987.

122. Ramanadham S., Lyness W.H., Tenner T.E. Jr.: Alterations in aortic and tail artery reactivity to agonists after streptozotocin treatment. Can. J. Physiol. Pharmacol. 62:418–423, 1984.

123. Raz I., Havivi Y., Yarom R.: Reduced negative surface charge on arterial endothelium of diabetic rats. Diabetologia 31:618–620, 1988.

124. Rerup C.C.: Drugs producing diabetes through damage of the insulin secreting cells. Pharmacol. Rev. 22:485–518, 1970.

125. Robertson W.B., Strong J.P.: Atherosclerosis in persons with hypertension and diabetes mellitus. Lab. Invest. 18:538–551, 1968.

126. Rogers S.P., Larkins R.G.: Production of 6-oxo-prostaglandin $F_{1\alpha}$ by rat aorta. Influence of diabetes, insulin treatment, and caloric deprivation. Diabetes 30:935–939, 1981.

127. Rösen P., Schrör K.: Increased prostacyclin release from perfused hearts of acutely diabetic rats. Diabetologia 18:391–394, 1980.

128. Rösen R., Beck E., Rösen P.: Early vascular alterations in the diabetic rat heart. Acta Physiol. Hungarica 72:3–11, 1988.

129. Rösen P., Rösen R., Hohl C., Reinauer H., Klaus W.: Reduced transcoronary exchange and prostaglandin synthesis in diabetic rat heart. Am. J. Physiol. 247:H563–H569, 1984.

130. Rösen P., Senger W., Feuerstein J., Grote H., Reinauer H., Schrör K.: Influence of streptozotocin diabetes on myocardial lipids and prostaglandin release by the rat heart. Biochem. Med. 30:19–33, 1983.

131. Rosenblum W.I., Levasseur J.E.: Microvascular responses of intermediate-sized arterioles on the cerebral surface of dia-

betic mice. Microvasc. Res. 28:368–372, 1984.

132. Roth D.M., Reibel D.K., Lefer A.M.: Vascular responsiveness and eicosanoid production in diabetic rats. Diabetologia 24:372–376, 1983.

133. Ruderman N.B., Haudenschild C.: Diabetes as an atherogenic factor. Prog. Cardiovasc. Dis. 26:373–412, 1984.

134. Rubanyi G.M.: Vascular effects of oxygen-derived free radicals. Free Radical Biol. Med. 4:107–120, 1988.

135. Rubanyi G.M., Vanhoutte P.M.: Oxygen-derived free radicals, endothelium, and responsiveness of vascular smooth muscle. Am. J. Physiol. 250:H815–H821, 1986.

136. Rubanyi G.M., Vanhoutte P.M.: Endothelium-removal decreases relaxations of canine coronary arteries caused by beta-adrenergic agonists and adenosine. J. Cardiovasc. Pharmacol 7:139–144, 1985.

137. Saenz de Tejada I., Goldstein I., Azadzoi K., Krane R.J., Cohen R.A.: Impaired neurogenic and endothelium-mediated relaxation of penile smooth muscle from diabetic men with impotence. N. Engl. J. Med. 320:1025–1030, 1989.

138. Seager M.J., Singal P.K., Orchard R., Pierce G.N., Dhalla N.S.: Cardiac cell damage: a primary myocardial disease in streptozotocin-induced chronic diabetes. Br. J. Exp. Pathol. 65:613–623, 1984.

139. Scarborough N.L., Carrier G.O.: Nifedipine and alpha adrenoceptors in rat aorta. II. Role of extracellular calcium in enhanced alpha-2 adrenoceptor-mediated contraction in diabetes. J. Pharmacol. Exp. Ther. 231:603–609, 1984.

140. Shimokawa H., Flavahan N.A., Lorenz R.R., Vanhoutte P.M.: Prostacyclin releases endothelium-derived relaxing factor and potentiates its action in coronary arteries of the pig. Br. J. Pharmacol. 95:1197–1203, 1988.

141. Silberbauer K., Clopath P., Sinzinger H., Schernthaner G.: Effect of experimentally induced diabetes on swine vascular prostacyclin (PGI$_2$) synthesis. Artery 8:30–36, 1980.

142. Silberbauer K., Schernthaner G., Sinzinger H., Piza-Katzer H., Winter M.: Decreased vascular prostacyclin in juvenile-onset diabetes. N. Engl. J. Med. 300:366–367, 1979.

143. Simonson D.C.: Etiology and prevalence of hypertension in diabetic patients. Diabetes Care 11:821–827, 1988.

144. Siperstein M.D., Unger R.H., Madison L.L.: Studies of muscle capillary basement membranes in normal subjects, diabetic, and pre-diabetic patients. J. Clin. Invest. 47:1973–1999, 1968.

145. Sjorgren A., Edvinsson L.: Vasomotor changes in isolated coronary arteries from diabetic rats. Acta Physiol. Scand. 134:429–436, 1988.

146. Steiner G.: Diabetes and atherosclerosis. An overview. Diabetes 30(Suppl. 2):1–7, 1981.

147. Sterin-Borda L., Borda E.S., Gimeno M.F., Lazzari M.A., del Castillo E., Gimeno A.L.: Contractile activity and prostacyclin generation in isolated coronary arteries from diabetic dogs. Diabetologia 22:56–59, 1982.

148. Sterin-Borda L.J., Franchi A.M., Borda E.S., del Castillo E., Gimeno M.F., Gimeno A.L.: Prostacyclin, its fatty acid precursor and its metabolites on the inotropic function of and on the prostanoid generation by diabetic arteries. Biomed. Biochim. Acta 43:S257–S264, 1984.

149. Sterin-Borda L., Gimeno M., Borda E., del Castillo E., Gimeno A.L.: Prostacyclin (PGI$_2$) and U-46619 stimulate coronary arteries from diabetic dogs and their action is influenced by inhibitors of prostaglandin biosynthesis. Prostaglandins 22:267–278, 1981.

150. Sternthal E., Like A.A., Sarantis K., Braverman L.E.: Lymphocytic thyroiditis and diabetes in the BB/W rat: a new model of autoimmune endocrinopathy. Diabetes 30:1058–1061, 1981.

151. Strandness J.W., Priest R.W., Gibbens G.E.: Combined clinical and pathological study of peripheral arterial disease. Diabetes 13:336–372, 1964.

152. Subbiah M.T.R., Deitemeyer D.: Altered synthesis of prostaglandins in platelet and aorta from spontaneously diabetic Wistar rats. Biochem. Med. 23:231–235, 1980.

153. Sullivan S., Sparks H.V.: Diminished contractile response of aortas from diabetic rabbits. Am. J. Physiol. 236:H301–H306, 1979.

154. Sundaresar P.R., Sharma V.K., Gingold S.I., Banerjee S.P.: Decreased β-adrenergic receptors in rat heart in streptozotocin-induced diabetes: role of thyroid hormones. Endocrinology 114:1358–1363, 1984.

155. Takiguchi Y., Satoh N., Hashimoto H., Nakashima M.: Changes in vascular reactivity in experimental diabetic rats: comparison with hypothyroid rats. Blood Vessels 25:250–260, 1988.

156. Takiguchi Y., Satoh N., Hashimoto H., Nakashima M.: Reversal effect of thyroxine on altered vascular reactivity in diabetic rats. J. Cardiovasc. Pharmacol. 13:520–524, 1989.

157. Tanz R.D., Chang K.S.K., Weller T.S.: Histamine relaxation of aortic rings for diabetic rats. Agents and Actions 28:1–8, 1989.

158. Tesfamarian B., Jakubowski J.A., Cohen R.A.: Contraction of diabetic rabbit aorta caused by endothelium-derived PGH_2-TxA_2. Am. J. Physiol. 257:H1326–H1333, 1989.

159. Timperley W.R., Boulton A.J.M., Davies-Johnson G.A.B., Jarratt J.A., Ward J.D.: Small vessel disease in progressive diabetic neuropathy associated with good metabolic control. J. Clin. Pathol. 38:1030–1038, 1985.

160. Turlapathy P.D.M.V., Lum G., Altura B.M.: Vascular responsiveness and serum biochemical parameters in alloxan diabetic mellitus. Am. J. Physiol. 239:E412–E421, 1980.

161. Vadlamudi R.V.S.V., McNeill J.H.: Effect of alloxan- and streptozotocin-induced diabetes on isolated rat heart responsiveness to carbachol. J. Pharmacol. Exp. Ther. 225:410–415, 1983.

162. Valentovic M.A., Lubawy W.C.: Impact of insulin or tolbutamide treatment on ^{14}C-arachidonic acid conversion to prostacyclin and/or thromboxane in lungs, aortas, and platelets of streptozotocin-induced diabetic rats. Diabetes 32:846–851, 1983.

163. Vanhoutte P.M., Rubanyi G.M., Miller V.M., Houston D.S.: Modulation of vascular smooth muscle contraction by the endothelium. Ann. Rev. Physiol. 48:307–320, 1986.

164. Vanhoutte P.M. (ed.): Relaxing and Contracting Factors. The Humana Press, Inc., New Jersey, 1988.

165. Vanhoutte P.M., Shimokawa H.: Endothelium-derived relaxing factor and coronary vasospasm. Circulation 80:1–9, 1989.

166. Viberti G.C.: Increased capillary permeability in diabetes mellitus and its relationship to microvascular angiopathy. Am. J. Med. 75:81–84, 1983.

167. Wakabayashi I., Hatake K., Kimura N., Kakishita E., Nagai K.: Modulation of vascular tonus by the endothelium in experimental diabetes. Life Sci. 40:643–648, 1987.

168. Wei E.P., Kontos H.A., Christman C.W., Dewitt D.S., Povlishock J.T.: Superoxide generation and reversal of acetylcholine-induced cerebral arteriolar dilation after acute hypertension. Circ. Res. 57:781–787, 1985.

169. Wey H.E., Jakubowski J.A., Deykin D.: Effect of streptozotocin-induced diabetes on prostaglandin production by rat cerebral microvessels. Thromb. Res. 42:527–538, 1986.

170. White R.E., Carrier G.O.: Enhanced vascular α-adrenergic neuroeffector system in diabetes: importance of calcium. Am. J. Physiol. 255:H1036–H1042, 1988.

171. White R.E., Carrier G.O.: Supersensitivity and endothelium dependency of histamine-induced relaxation in mesenteric arteries isolated from diabetic rats. Pharmacology 33:34–38, 1986.

172. Williamson J.R., Kilo C.: Basement-membrane thickening and diabetic microangiopathy. Diabetes 25(Suppl. 2):925–927, 1976.

173. Winocour P.D., Lopes-Virella M., Laimins M., Colwell J.A.: Effects of insulin treatment in diabetic rats on in vitro platelet function and plasma von Willebrand factor (VIII R:WF) and factor VII-related antigen (VII R:AG). J. Lab. Clin. Med. 106:319–325, 1985.

174. Winquist R.J., Bunting P.B., Baskin E.P., Wallace A.A.: Decreased endothelium-dependent relaxation in New Zealand genetic hypertensive rats. J. Hypertension 2:541–545, 1984.

175. World Health Organization: Vascular Disease in Diabetics. Report of WHO Multinational Study of Vascular Disease in Diabetics. World Health Organization, Geneva, Switzerland, 1982, pp 1–93.

176. Yen M.-H., Wu C.-C., Chiou W.-F.: Partially endothelium-dependent vasodilator effect of adenosine in rat aorta. Hypertension 11:514–518, 1988.

177. Ylikorkala O., Kaila J., Viinikka L.: Prostacyclin and thromboxane in diabetes. Br. Med. J. 283:1148–1150, 1981.

11

Lipoproteins and Endothelial Dysfunction

Mark A. Creager, John P. Cooke, Julie I. Tucker, Victor J. Dzau

Introduction

Abnormalities of the endothelium may promote abnormal platelet-vascular wall interactions, uptake, and activation of circulating macrophages and expression of endogenous mitogens, and thereby contribute to the development of atherosclerosis.[33,40] There is evidence that hyperlipoproteinemia impairs endothelial function even prior to the development of atherosclerosis. The purpose of this chapter is to review, in some detail, those studies that examined the effect of hyperlipoproteinemia on vascular function and to propose mechanisms responsible for the observed abnormalities.

Diet-Induced Atherosclerosis Impairs Endothelial Function

A cholesterol-enriched diet is often used to produce experimental atheroscle-

rosis in certain species. As discussed in greater detail elsewhere in this book, diet-induced experimental atherosclerosis is associated with impaired endothelium-dependent relaxation in vitro and in vivo.[4,15,21,44] Typically, aortae isolated from cholesterol-fed rabbits with atherosclerosis dilate less to the endothelium-dependent vasodilator, acetylcholine, than aortae from control rabbits.[14,44] In contrast, endothelium-independent vasodilation (i.e., direct smooth muscle relaxation) is generally preserved. These alterations are best documented in a recent study of iliac arteries excised from cynomolgus monkeys with diet-induced atherosclerosis.[16] The results showed that the in vitro endothelium-dependent vasodilator responses to acetycholine and thrombin are significantly attenuated in iliac arteries that manifest moderate to severe atherosclerosis. Furthermore, regression of atherosclerosis with dietary treatment restored the endothelium-dependent relaxation response.[16]

The impairment of endothelium-mediated vasodilation has been demonstrated

Rubanyi G.M.: Cardiovascular Significance of Endothelium-Derived Vasoactive Factors, Futura Publishing Co., Inc., Mount Kisco, NY, © 1991.

in vivo also. In cholesterol-fed atherosclerotic rabbits, the vasodilator response to intra-arterial injections of acetylcholine, but not nitroprusside, is significantly depressed.[16] Likewise, atherosclerotic human coronary arteries respond abnormally to intracoronary infusions of acetylcholine, but not nitroglycerin.[13,23] Multivariate analysis suggests that hypercholesterolemia is one of the most important factors that predict abnormal endothelial function in these vessels[45] (Fig. 1).

Effect of Hyperlipoproteinemia on Vascular Function in Vitro

Although one may infer from these studies that hypercholesterolemia impairs endothelial function, interpretation is confounded by the presence of morphological changes of early atherosclerosis. Several groups of investigators have examined the direct effect of lipoproteins on endothelium-dependent vasorelaxation in vitro, thereby circumventing the confounding structural effects of atherosclerosis in animals exposed to prolonged elevation of serum cholesterol. Andrews and others assessed the effect of low density lipoprotein (LDL) on endothelium-dependent relaxation of normal rabbit thoracic aortae.[2,41,42] Levels of LDL, corresponding to those existing in the plasma of hypercholesterolemic patients, inhibited the relaxation of precontracted aortae to the endothelium-dependent vasodilators acetylcholine, calcium ionophore A23187, and adenosine triphosphate (ATP). Inhibition of acetylcholine-induced vasorelaxation was dependent on the time of exposure to LDL, but was virtually complete if the vessel had been incubated with LDL for 30 minutes. In addition, the attenuated response persisted for over 2 hours, despite extensive washing of the vessel. Incubation with

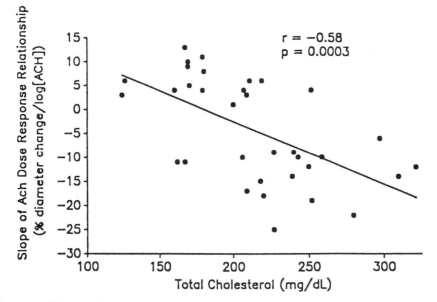

Figure 1: The relation between serum cholesterol level and the vasomotor response to intracoronary infusion of acetylcholine in human subjects. Reproduced with permission.[45]

LDL did not affect relaxation to sodium nitroprusside which is independent of the endothelium.

Similarly, Tomita et al. studied the effect of LDL on endothelium-dependent vasodilation of porcine coronary arteries.[42] Incubation of the vascular strips with LDL essentially abolished the endothelium-dependent vasorelaxant response to thrombin, ADP, calcium ionophore A23187, and platelet activating factor. Both heat and acid denaturation of LDL eliminated its inhibitory effects. High density lipoprotein (HDL) did not inhibit endothelium-dependent vasorelaxation. The response to sodium nitroprusside was not affected by LDL exposure.

The recent study of Takahashi and colleagues examined these effects in further detail.[41] These investigators studied the effect of lipoproteins on endothelium-dependent relaxation of rabbit aortae in vitro. However, rather than incubating the vascular strips with lipoproteins, they added solutions of lipoproteins, as well as phospholipids, to the organ chamber bath *after* endothelium-dependent relaxation was induced by acetylcholine or A23187. Reversibility of endothelium-dependent relaxation occurred when LDL was added to the bath. In addition, very low density lipoprotein (VLDL), HDL, as well as the phospholipids, phosphatidylcholine, phosphatidylinositol, and sphingomyelin reversed endothelium-dependent relaxation. The authors concluded that all lipoproteins are capable of inhibiting endothelium-dependent vasodilation.

Chronic in vivo exposure to high levels of cholesterol also has been shown to inhibit endothelium-dependent vasodilation, even when there is no morphological evidence of atherosclerosis. Cohen and colleagues fed pigs a cholesterol-rich diet for 9 weeks.[6] Light microscopic examination confirmed that arteries from hypercholesterolemic pigs were free of foam cells and intimal thickening. In addition, scanning electron microscopy demonstrated

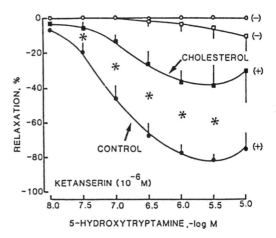

Figure 2: Relaxations of coronary arteries from normal and hypercholesterolemic pigs caused by 5 hydroxytryptamine. Arteries were pretreated with ketanserin and contracted with $PGF_{2\alpha}$. The presence or absence of endothelium is indicated by $(+)$ and $(-)$. Reproduced with permission.[6]

only minor changes in the surface of the endothelial cells, including rare gaps and some microvillus alterations in coronary arteries. These histologic characteristics were present in pigs given a cholesterol-poor diet as well as in those receiving a cholesterol-rich diet. The vasodilator response to serotonin (in the presence of the $5\text{-}HT_2$ receptor antagonist, ketanserin) in vitro was substantially attenuated in the coronary artery rings obtained from the hypercholesterolemic pigs (Fig. 2). Similarly, endothelium-dependent relaxation to substance P was blunted in coronary arteries from the hypercholesterolemic pigs. In contrast, however, both norepinephrine and the calcium ionophore A23187 caused comparable endothelium-dependent vasodilation in rings from both the control and hypercholesterolemic pigs. Relaxation to papavarine and nitroprusside was not affected by hypercholesterolemia. The data from this study suggest that hypercholesterolemia, in the absence of atherosclerosis, impairs endothelium-dependent vasodilation. The exact mechanism of hypercholesterolemia-induced endothelial dysfunction is not completely understood.

Similar results were reported in two studies by Shimokawa and Vanhoutte.[38,39] They too observed that hypercholesterolemia impairs endothelium-dependent relaxation of porcine coronary arteries to serotonin as well as to ADP, but not to bradykinin.[39] In addition, hypercholesterolemia impaired endothelium-dependent relaxation of porcine basilar arteries in response to ADP and aggregating platelets.[38]

Osborne and colleagues reported that endothelium-dependent vasodilation was severely impaired in subepicardial coronary resistance arteries of cholesterol-fed rabbits.[26] Rabbits were fed normal chow or chow enriched with 0.5% or 2.0% cholesterol for 10–12 weeks. The first- and second-order branches of the left anterior descending coronary artery were removed and studied in vitro. Histologic examination of these vessels revealed no atheroma in the hypercholesterolemic rabbits. Both acetylcholine and ADP caused vasodilation in control rabbits, but not in hypercholesterolemic rabbits. In contrast, sodium nitrite relaxed vessels comparably in all rabbit groups.

Effect of Hypercholesterolemia on Vascular Function in Vivo

Several studies have examined endothelium-dependent vasodilation of resistance vessels in vivo.[4,26,48] Using this approach, one can examine the effect of a hypercholesterolemic environment in the absence of atherosclerosis because, unlike the larger arteries, the walls of resistance vessels do not develop atheroma. Wright and Angus examined the effect of acetylcholine and adenosine on rabbit hindlimb resistance vessels following 4 weeks of feeding with a 1% cholesterol diet.[49] They observed that the maximal dilatation caused by acetylcholine was less in cholesterol-fed rabbits than in the control group of rabbits; in contrast, the maximal vasodilatory response to the endothelium-independent vasodilator, adenosine, was comparable in each group. Bossaler and colleagues studied the effects of acetylcholine and nitroprusside, administered via the femoral artery, on hindlimb vascular resistance in rabbits fed a 1% cholesterol diet for 10 weeks.[4] The decrease in hindlimb vascular resistance caused by acetylcholine was significantly less in the hypercholesterolemic rabbits than in the control rabbits. The response of the hindlimb resistance vessels to nitroprusside was similar in hypercholesterolemic and control rabbits.

These findings were corroborated further by our recent in vivo study.[6] The effect of acetylcholine chloride and sodium nitroprusside on hindlimb vascular resistance was examined in rabbits that received a 2% cholesterol diet for 8 weeks and compared to rabbits ingesting normal chow. Each drug was infused intra-arterially, hindlimb blood flow was determined by means of an electromagnetic flow probe, and hindlimb vascular resistance was calculated as a ratio of mean blood pressure to mean hindlimb blood flow. The increase in hindlimb blood flow and decrease in hindlimb vascular resistance caused by acetylcholine was attenuated in the cholesterol-fed rabbits compared to the control rabbits (Fig. 3). In contrast, the effect of nitroprusside on hindlimb vascular resistance did not differ between control and cholesterol-fed rabbits. Thus, in this experimental model, our data indicate that hypercholesterolemia impairs endothelium-dependent vasodilation of the resistance vessels.

Yamamoto and colleagues used a more direct technique to examine the effect of cholesterol on endothelium-dependent vasorelaxation of resistance vessels.[46] Utilizing videomicroscopy, they examined the vascular reactivity of resistance vessels in

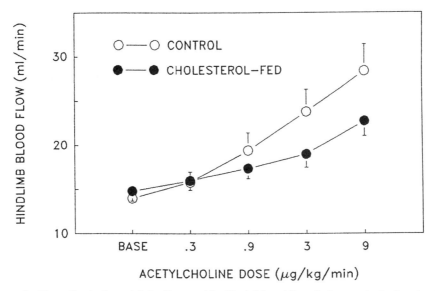

Figure 3: The effect of acetylcholine on hindlimb blood flow in hypercholesterolemic rabbits. The vasodilator response is blunted in the hypercholesterolemic animals when compared to normal rabbits (adapted from ref. 6).

the cremaster muscle of rabbits receiving standard chow or chow containing 1% cholesterol for 12 weeks. Both intra-arterial and topical acetylcholine caused less arteriolar dilation in cholesterol-fed than in control rabbits; the increase in arterial diameter caused by sodium nitroprusside, however, was similar in both groups. Histologic examination of the arterioles was also performed in this study. The authors noted that the endothelial cell lining appeared intact and there was no appreciable thickening of the arteriolar walls in either group, thereby documenting that the altered endothelial-dependent vasorelaxation was not due to the presence of overt atherosclerosis.

Effect of Hypercholesterolemia on Vascular Function in Humans

We have studied vascular reactivity in the forearm resistance vessels of young normal human volunteers and age-matched subjects with hypercholesterolemia.[10] Serum LDL cholesterol was 111 ± 7 mg/dL in the normal subjects and 211 ± 19 mg/dL in the hypercholesterolemic individuals. Each subject received intrabrachial artery infusions of methacholine chloride to assess endothelium-dependent vasodilation, and sodium nitroprusside to evaluate endothelium-independent vasodilation. In addition, maximal vasodilation was determined during reactive hyperemia following 5 minutes of an ischemic stimulus. Forearm blood flow was determined by venous occlusion strain gauge plethysmography and forearm vascular resistance was calculated as the ratio of mean blood pressure to forearm blood flow. Basal forearm vascular resistance was comparable in normal and in hypercholesterolemic subjects. Similarly, minimal forearm vascular resistance during reactive hyperemia did not differ between the two groups. In contrast, the vasodilator response to methacholine in hypercholesterolemic subjects was less than that observed in normal subjects (Fig. 4). In addition, the

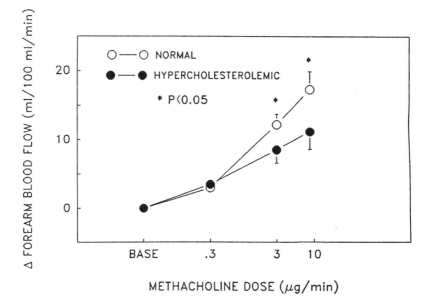

Figure 4: The vasodilator response to methacholine chloride in the forearms of normal subjects and patients with hypercholesterolemia. The increase in forearm blood flow induced by this endothelium-dependent vasodilator was attenuated in hypercholesterolemic individuals (adapted from ref. 10).

vasodilator response to sodium nitroprusside was less in hypercholesterolemic subjects. Thus, in humans with hypercholesterolemia, defects in both endothelium-dependent relaxation as well as direct relaxation of vascular smooth muscle of resistance vessels to nitrovasodilators can be demonstrated.

Mechanisms of Impaired Endothelium-Dependent Relaxation by Lipoproteins

As discerned from the aforementioned studies, hyperlipoproteinemia impairs endothelium-dependent vasorelaxation. The mechanism(s) that underlies this abnormality has not been identified precisely. Possibilities include reduced synthesis of endothelium-derived relaxant factor(s),

modification of membrane receptor-operated pathways affecting release of EDRF, impaired diffusion or transport of relaxing factors through the intima, and/or reduced responsiveness of soluble guanylate cyclase to EDRF in vascular smooth muscle.

Several studies have implicated abnormalities of endothelial membrane receptor function as the cause of reduced endothelium-dependent relaxation. Coronary artery rings excised from hypercholesterolemic pigs display impaired relaxation to serotonin, ADP, and substance P, but not to bradykinin or the calcium ionophore A23187.[6,39] Whereas serotonin, substance P, and ADP release EDRF by activating endothelial receptors, the calcium ionophore acts by a receptor-independent pathway. Kugiyama et al. proposed that oxidized LDL reduced receptor-mediated release of EDRF.[22] They compared the effects of native LDL to LDL modified by incubation with endothelial cells in culture, the latter being oxidized. The vasodilator effect of acetylcholine on isolated normal rabbit aortae was attenuated by oxidized, but not native, LDL (Fig. 5). Furthermore, the investigators reported that lysolecithin, a component of oxidized LDL, also reduced endothelium-dependent vasodilation. The authors suggested that lysolecithin interferes with receptor-mediated release of EDRF, possibly by perturbing G protein-dependent transmembrane signaling.

How may one explain the impaired responsiveness to both methacholine chloride and sodium nitroprusside in hyperlipoproteinemic humans? Both endothelium-derived relaxing factor and sodium nitroprusside induce vasodilation by stimulating the activity of soluble guanylate cyclase within the vascular smooth muscle, thereby elevating tissue levels of cyclic GMP.[18,19,24] A nitrosyl-porphyrin complex, formed during the metabolism of nitrovasodilators, triggers the activation of soluble guanylate cyclase. In addition, sulfhydryl groups associated with guanylate cyclase may modulate its activity.[25,48]

Oxidation of either the heme iron or the associated thiol groups by lipoprotein may inactivate the enzyme resulting in an attenuated response to nitrovasodilation.[5,8,9,48]

Effect of Hyperlipoproteinemia on Vasoconstriction

In addition to impairing vasodilation, hypercholesterolemia may augment the contractile responsiveness of vascular smooth muscle. Yokogama and Henry examined the effect of cholesterol on vasoconstriction in isolated canine coronary arteries.[47] In this in vitro study, cholesterol induced small contractions of canine coronary arteries and enhanced the constrictor effects of extracellular calcium and potassium.[47] Heistad et al. performed an in vivo study that examined the effect of hypercholesterolemia on vasoconstrictive re-

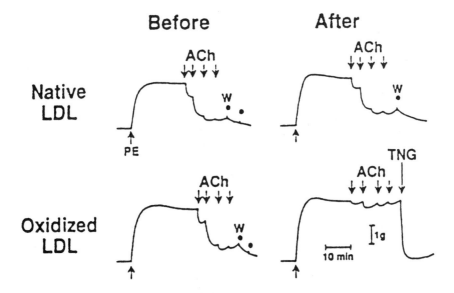

Figure 5: Rabbit aortic strips mounted for recording of isometric tension were contracted with phenylephrine (PE). Relaxation in response to acetylcholine (ACh) was determined before and after incubation with native or oxidized LDL. Oxidized LDL suppressed the response to acetylcholine but not to nitroglycerin (TNG). Reproduced with permission.[22]

sponses in the hindlimb vessels of cynomolgus monkeys.[17] Monkeys were treated with a high cholesterol diet for 4–5 months. Vasoconstrictor responsiveness was determined by measuring hindlimb perfusion pressure during intra-arterial infusion of norepinephrine and serotonin. The vasoconstrictor responses to norepinephrine, but not serotonin, were augmented in the resistance vessels of the hypercholesterolemic monkeys compared to control monkeys. This study corroborated a previous study by Rosendorff et al., who reported that the coronary vasoconstrictor responses to norepinephrine were augmented in dogs fed a high cholesterol diet for 1 month compared to control dogs.[32] These findings have not been confirmed in humans. In this context, we examined the forearm vascular response to intra-arterial phenylephrine in patients with hypercholesterolemia and observed that the vasoconstrictive responsiveness to intra-arterial phenylephrine was not different between normals and hypercholesterolemic subjects.[10]

Is the Impaired Endothelium-Dependent Vasodilation Caused by Hypercholesterolemia Reversible?

The strategies employed to reverse abnormal endothelium-dependent vasodilation caused by hypercholesterolemia have focused either on increasing the synthesis of endothelium-derived relaxant factor, altering the lipid milieu, or reducing the level of serum cholesterol.

Endothelium-derived relaxing factor is nitric oxide or a labile nitroso compound that liberates nitric oxide.[11,20,14,28] L-arginine is the substrate required for formation of nitric oxide and increases synthesis of endothelium-derived relaxing fac-

tor.[29,30,34] It has been demonstrated that release of nitric oxide by acetylcholine may be increased by the administration of L-arginine, and blocked by L-monomethyl arginine (L-NMMA), a specific inhibitor of nitric oxide formation.[1,30] Recently we assessed the effects of L-arginine on the impaired endothelium-dependent vasodilation in hypercholesterolemic rabbits.[7,31] Our results demonstrated that L-arginine restored endothelium-dependent vasodilation in hindlimb resistance vessels of cholesterol-fed rabbits in vivo.[7] This effect was specific since endothelium-independent vasodilation was not affected by L-arginine infusion. Furthermore, endothelium-dependent relaxation was greater in the thoracic aorta excised from hypercholesterolemic rabbits treated with arginine than those from rabbits treated with vehicle.[7] In addition, we have found that L-arginine improves endothelium-dependent relaxation of perfused isolated basilar arteries harvested from hypercholesterolemic rabbits.[31]

Altering the lipid milieu may improve endothelium-dependent vasodilation also. Shimokawa et al. reported that cod liver oil enhanced endothelium-dependent responses in normal porcine coronary arteries.[36] Endothelium-dependent relaxations in response to serotonin, bradykinin, thrombin, and adenosine diphosphate were greater in arteries from pigs treated with fish oil for 4 weeks than in a control group. Endothelium-independent relaxations were not affected by dietary supplementation with fish oil. Thereafter, Shimokawa et al. examined the effect of dietary cod liver oil on endothelium-dependent responses in coronary arteries of Yorkshire pigs fed a 2% high-cholesterol diet for 10 weeks.[37] Addition of cod liver oil increased the plasma levels of eicosapentanoic acid, decreased the level of arachidonic acid, and had no effect on total cholesterol, LDL, VLDL, or HDL. In the hypercholesterolemic pigs whose diet was supplemented with cod liver oil, endothelium-dependent relaxation to bradykinin, serotonin, and ADP were greater than in the cholesterol-fed pigs that did not receive dietary supplementation with fish oil. It is possible that the change in the plasma-free fatty acids affected the composition of membrane phospholipids. In this study, however, some morphological changes of atherosclerosis were evident in the porcine coronary arteries. Thus, it is possible that dietary treatment with cod liver oil also reduced some of the intimal lesions, thereby influencing synthesis, release, or transport of endothelium-derived relaxant factor.

Several studies examined the effect of reduction of serum cholesterol on endothelium-dependent vasodilation.[16] Harrison and co-authors examined three groups of cynomolgus monkeys.[16] One group was fed standard monkey chow, one group was fed an atherogenic diet that contained 0.7% cholesterol and 40% fat for 18 months, and a third group was fed the same atherogenic diet for 18 months followed by standard monkey chow for 18–20 months. The atherogenic diet resulted in atherosclerotic lesions characterized by foam cells and inflammatory cells in the iliac vessels. Reduction in dietary cholesterol and saturated fats resulted in significant regression of the atherosclerotic lesions, although fibrotic plaque was still present. Endothelium-dependent vasorelaxation was studied in ring segments of iliac arteries from each group. Endothelium-dependent relaxation caused by acetylcholine and thrombin was reduced in the atherosclerotic vessels. The responses to these endothelium-dependent vasodilators were normalized in the regression group in which the serum cholesterol levels were significantly decreased. However, this study does not specifically address abnormalities caused by hypercholesterolemia alone since morphological changes of atherosclerosis were clearly present. Osborne and colleagues studied the effect of lovastatin, an inhibitor of hydroxymethylglutaryl-coenzyme A reductase (HMG-

CoA reductase), the rate-limiting enzyme in cholesterol biosynthesis, on endothelium-dependent vasodilation in rabbit fed a 0.5% cholesterol diet for only 2 weeks.[27] Serum cholesterol level in vehicle-treated rabbits approximated 320 mg/dL, whereas in lovastatin-treated animals, it approximated 140 mg/dL. Histologic examination of aortae from both groups revealed no evidence of intimal thickening, fat deposition, or atherosclerosis. The vasodilator response of excised aortic rings to acetylcholine was greater in lovastatin than vehicle-treated rabbits. Moreover, these investigators also examined the coronary resistance vasculature by using an isolated Langendorff-perfused heart. Acetylcholine induced coronary vasoconstricion in the vehicle-treated rabbits and vasodilation in the lovastatin-treated groups. Thus, in the absence of atherosclerosis, lowering of serum cholesterol improves endothelium-dependent relaxation.

Summary and Conclusions

Multiple lines of evidence support the hypothesis that hyperlipoproteinemia impairs endothelium-dependent vasodilation, even in the absence of atherosclerosis. The effect of hyperlipoproteinemia may be seen acutely since exposure of normal arteries to lipoproteins in vitro reduces endothelium-dependent relaxation. In addition, hyperlipoproteinemia may also exert chronic effects on vascular function and structure. Indeed, arteries excised from animals that had been exposed chronically to diets rich in cholesterol also demonstrate impaired relaxation to endothelium-dependent vasodilators. Vasodilator responsiveness of resistance vessels is reduced in vivo in hypercholesterolemic rabbits and humans. The mechanism(s) of impaired vasodilation in hyperlipoproteinemia may involve alterations of membrane receptor-coupled release of EDRF. In humans, lipoproteins also may inhibit the activity of soluble guanylate cyclase in vascular smooth muscle, but this possibility still must be tested.

It appears that abnormalities caused by hyperlipoproteinemia are reversible. Increasing synthesis of EDRF by administration of L-arginine, altering the lipid milieu by enriching the diet with unsaturated fatty acids or reduction of lipoprotein concentration in vitro or in vivo are interventions capable of restoring endothelium-dependent vasodilation. Further exploration of the causes underlying functional disturbances caused by hyperlipoproteinemia may provide further insight into the mechanisms contributing to endothelial injury and atherogenesis in patients with this disorder.

Acknowledgments: This work is supported by NIH grants HL36348, HL35610, HL35792, HL19259, HL35252, HL43131, HL42663, and a grant-in-aid from the American Heart Association, 900871. Dr. Creager is a recipient of an NIH Research Career Development Award, HL01768.

References

1. Amezcua J.L., Palmer R.M.J., De Souza B.M., Moncada S.: Nitric oxide synthetized from L-arginine regulates vascular tone in the coronary circulation of the rabbit. Br. J. Pharmacol. 97:1119–1124, 1989.
2. Andrews H.E., Bruckdorfer K.R., Dunn R.C., Jacobs M.: Low-density lipoproteins inhibit endothelium-dependent relaxation rabbit aorta. Nature 327:237–239, 1987.
3. Bossaller C., Habib G.B., Yamamoto H., Williams C., Wells S., Henry P.D.: Impaired muscarinic endothelium-dependent relaxation and cyclic guanosine 5'-monophosphate formation in atherosclerotic human coronary artery and rabbit aorta. J. Clin. Invest. 79:170–174, 1987.
4. Bossaller C., Yamamoto H., Lichtlen P.R., Henry P.D.: Impaired cholineroic vasodilation in the cholesterol-fed rabbit in vivo. Basic Res. Cardiol. 82:396–404, 1987.
5. Brandwein H.J., Lewicki J.A., Murad F.: Reversible inactivation of guanylate cyclase by mixed disulfide formation. J. Biol. Chem. 256:2958–2962, 1981.
6. Cohen R.A., Zitnay K.M., Haudenschild C.C., Cunningham L.D.: Loss of selective endothelial cell vasoactive functions in pig coronary arteries caused by hypercholesterolemia. Circ. Res. 63:903–910, 1988.
7. Cooke J.P., Andon N.A., Girerd X.J., Hirsch A.T., Creager M.A.: L-arginine normalizes endothelium-dependent responses in hypercholesterolemic rabbits (abstract). Clin. Res. 38:291A, 1990.
8. Craven P.A., DeRubertis F.R.: Effects of thiol inhibitors on hepatic guanylate cyclase activity: evidence for the involvement of vicinal dithiols in the expression of basal and agonist-stimulated activity. Biochim. Biophys. Acta 524:2231–2244, 1978.
9. Craven P.A., DeRubertis F.R.: Restoration of the responsiveness of purified granylate cyclase to nitrosoguanidine, nitric oxide, and related activators by heme and hemeproteins. J. Biol. Chem. 253:8433–8443, 1978.
10. Creager M.A., Cooke J.P., Mendelsohn M.E., Gallagher S.J., Coleman S.M., Loscalzo J., Dzau V.J.: Impaired vasodilation of forearm resistance vessels in hypercholesterolemic humans. J. Clin. Invest. 86:228–234, 1986.
11. Furchgott R.F.: Studies on relaxation of rabbit aorta by sodium nitrite: the basis for the proposal that the acid-activable inhibitory factor from bovine retractor penis is inorganic nitrite and the endothelium-derived relaxing factor is nitric oxide. In: Vasodilation: Vascular Smooth Muscle, Peptides, Autonomic Nerves, and Endothelium, Vanhoute A.M. (ed.). Raven Press, NY, pp 427–435, 1988.
12. Girerd X.J., Hirsch A.T., Cooke J.P., Creager M.A.: L-arginine augments endothelium-dependent vasodilation in cholesterol fed rabbits. Circulation 80:II-280, 1989 (abst).
13. Ginsburg R., Bristow M.R., Davies K., Didiasc A., Billingham M.E.: Quantitative pharmacologic responses of normal and atherosclerotic isolated human epicardial

coronary arteries. Circulation 69:430–440, 1984.

14. Gryglewski R.J., Botting R.D., Vane J.R.: Mediators produced by the endothelial cell. Hypertension 12:530–548, 1988.

15. Habib J.B., Bossaller C., Wells S., Williams C., Morrisett J.D., Henry P.D.: Preservation of endothelium-dependent vascular relaxation in cholesterol-fed rabbit by treatment with the calcium blocker PN 200110. Circ. Res. 58:305–309, 1986.

16. Harrison D.G., Armstrong M.L., Freiman P.C., Heistad D.D.: Restoration of endothelium-dependent relaxation by dietary treatment of atherosclerosis. J. Clin. Invest. 80:1808–1811, 1987.

17. Heistad D.D., Armstrong M.L.I., Marcus M.L., Piegors D.J., Mark A.L.: Augmented responses to vasoconstrictor stimuli in hypercholesterolemic and atherosclerotic monkeys. Circ. Res. 54:711–718, 1984.

18. Ignarro L.J., Kadowitz P.J.: Pharmacological and physiolgoicalrole of cyclic AMP in vascular smooth muscle relaxation. Annu. Rev. Pharmacol. 25:171–191, 1985.

19. Ignarro L.J., Harbison R.G., Wood K.S., Kadowitz P.J.: Activation of purified soluble guanylate cyclase by endothelium-derived relaxing factor from intrapulmonary artery and vein: stimulation by acetylcholine, bradykinin and arachnidonic acid. J. Pharmacol. Exp. Ther. 237:893–900, 1986.

20. Ignarro L.J., Biological actions and properties of endothelium-derived nitric oxide formed and released from artery and vein. Circ. Res. 65:1–21, 1989.

21. Jayakody L., Senaratne M., Thomson A., Kappagoda T.: Endothelium-dependent relaxation in experimental atherosclerosis in the rabbit. Circ. Res. 60:251–264, 1987.

22. Kugiyama K., Kerns S.A., Morrisett J.D., Roberts R., Henry P.D.: Impairment of endothelium-dependent arterial relaxation by lysolecithin in modified low-density lipoproteins. Nature 344:160–162, 1990.

23. Ludmer P.L., Selwyn A.P., Shook T.L., Wayne R.R., Mudge G.H., Alexander R.W., Ganz P.: Paradoxical vasoconstriction induced by acetylcholine in atherosclerotic coronary arteries. N. Engl. J. Med. 315:1046–1051, 1986.

24. Martin W., Villani G.M., Jothianandan D., Furchgott R.F.: Selective blockade of endothelium-dependent and glyceryl trinitrate-induced relaxation by hemoglobin and by methylene blue in the rabbit aorta. J. Pharmacol. Exp. Ther. 232:708–716, 1985.

25. Murad F.: Cyclic guanosine monophosphate as a mediator of vasodilation. J. Clin. Invest. 73:1–5, 1986.

26. Osborne J.A., Siegman M.J., Sedar A.W., Mooers S.U., Lefer A.M.: Lack of endothelium-dependent relaxation in coronary resistance arteries of cholesterol-fed rabbits. Am. J. Physiol. 256(Ce11):C591-C597, 1989.

27. Osborne J.A., Lento P.H., Siegfried M.R., Stahl G.L., Fusman B., Lefer A.M.: Cardiovascular effects of acute hypercholesterolemia in rabbits. Reversal with lovastatin treatment. J. Clin. Invest. 83:465–473, 1989.

28. Palmer R.M.J., Ferridge A.G., Moncada S.: Nitric oxide release accounts for the biological activity of endothelium-derived relaxing factor. Nature 327:524–526, 1987.

29. Palmer R.M.J., Asthon D.S., Moncada S.: Vascular endothelial cells synthesize nitric oxide from L-arginine. Nature 333:664–666, 1988.

30. Rees D.D., Palmer R.M.J., Moncada S.: Role of endothelium-derived nitric oxide in the reguation of blood pressure. Proc. Natl. Acad. Sci. USA 86:3375–3378, 1989.

31. Rossitch E. Jr., Black P. McL., Alexander E. III, Cooke J.P.: L-arginine normalizes endothelial function in hypercholesterolemic basilar arteries (abstract). FASEB J 4:A416, 1990.

32. Rosendorff C., Hoffman J.I.E., Verrier E.D., Rouleau J., Boerboom L.E.: Cholesterol potentiates the coronary artery response to norepinephrine in anesthetized and conscious dogs. Circ. Res. 48:320–329, 1981.

33. Ross R.: The pathogenesis of atherosclerosis: an update. N. Engl. J. Med. 314:488–500, 1986.

34. Sakuma I., Stuehr D., Gross S.S., Nathan C., Levi R.: Identification of arginine as a precursor of endothelium-derived relaxing factor. Proc. Natl. Acad. Sci. USA 85:8664–8667, 1988.

35. Schmidt H.H.H.W., Nau H., Wittfoht W., Gerlach J., Prescher K.-E., Klein M.M., Niroomand F., Bohme E.: Arginine is a physiological precursor of endothelium-derived nitric oxide. Eur. J. Pharmacol. 154:213–216, 1988.

36. Shimokawa H., Vanhoutte A.M.: Dietary cod-liver oil improves endothelium-dependent responses in hypercholesterolemic and atherosclerotic porcine coronary arteries. Circulation 78:1421–1430, 1988.

37. Shimokawa H., Lam J.Y.T., Chesebro J.H., Bowie E.J.W., Vanhoutte A.M.: Effects of dietary supplementation with cod-liver oil on endothelium-dependent responses in

porcine coronary arteries. Circulation 76:898–905, 1987.

38. Shimokawa H., Kim P., Vanhoutte A.M.: Endothelium-dependent relaxation to aggregating platelets in isolated vasilar arteries of control and hypercholesterolemic pigs. Circ. Res. 63:604–612, 1988.

39. Shimokawa H., Vanhoutte A.M.: Impaired endothelium-dependent relaxation to aggregating platelets and related vasoactive substances in porcine coronary arteries in hypercholesterolemia and atherosclerosis. Circ. Res. 64:900–914, 1989.

40. Steinberg D., Parthasarathy S., Carew T.E., Khoo J.C., Witztum J.L.: Beyond cholesterol. Modifications of low-density lipoprotein that increase its atherogenicity. N. Engl. J. Med. 320:915–924, 1989.

41. Takahashi M., Yui Y., Yasumoto H., Aoyama T., Morishita H., Hattori R., Kawai C.: Lipoproteins are inhibitors of endothelium-dependent relaxation of rabbit aorta. Am. J. Physiol. 258(Heart Circ. Physiol. 27):Hl-H8, 1990.

42. Tomita T., Ezaki M., Miwa M., Nakamura K., Inoue Y.: Rapid and reversible inhibition by low density lipoprotein of the endothelium-dependent relaxation to hemostatic substances in porcine coronary arteries. Circ. Res. 66:18–27, 1990.

43. Vallance P., Collier J., Moncada S.: Effects of endothelium-derived nitric oxide on peripheral arteriolar tone in man. Lancet 2:999–1000, 1989.

44. Verbeuren T.J., Jordaens F.H., Zonnekeyn L.L., Van Hove C.E., Coene M.C., Herman A.G.: Effect of hypercholesterolemia on vascular reactivity in the rabbit. I. Endothelium-dependent and endothelium-independent contractions and relaxations in isolated arteries of control and hypercholesterolemic rabbits. Circ. Res. 58:552–564, 1986.

45. Vita J.A., Treasure C.B., Nabel E.G., McLenachan J.M., Fish R.D., Yeung A.C., Vekshtein V.I., et al.: Coronary vasomotor response to acetylcholine relates to risk factors for coronary artery disease. Circulation 81:491–497, 1990.

46. Yamamoto H., Bossaller C., Cartwright J. Jr, Henry P.D.: Videomicroscopic demonstration of defective cholinergic arteriolar vasodilation in atherosclerotic rabbit. J. Clin. Invest. 81:1752–1758, 1988.

47. Yokogama M., Henry P.D.: Sensitization of isolated canine coronary arteries to calcium ions after exposure to cholesterol. Circ. Res. 45:479–486, 1979.

48. Waldman S.C., Murad F.: Biochemical mechanisms underlying vascular smooth muscle relaxation: the guanylate cyclase-cyclic GMP system. J. Cardiovasc. Pharmacol. 12(Suppl. 5):S115-S118.

49. Wright C.E., Angus J.A.: Effects of hypertension and hypercholesterolemia on vasodilation in the rabbit. Hypertension 8:361–371, 1986.

12

Endothelial Dysfunction in Atherosclerosis

David G. Harrison, Robert L. Minor, Ricardo Guerra, James E. Quillen, Frank W. Sellke

Introduction

In 1980, Robert Furchgott and co-workers first showed that the endothelium must be intact for acetylcholine to produce vascular relaxation.[21] Subsequently this was shown to be true for a variety of important neurohumoral and pharmacological agents.[10,12,13,20] As a result of work from several laboratories, it is now recognized that the endothelium releases a potent labile nonprostanoid vasodilating agent in response to numerous vasoactive stimuli that either causes vasodilatation or modulates vasoconstriction.[23,24] This factor, subsequently termed the endothelium-derived relaxing factor, recently has been shown to be either nitric oxide[51] or a compound with a nitric oxide moiety within its structure.[47] There is evidence that there may be multiple EDRFs,[15,44,58] and that the endothelium may also release a substance that causes vascular smooth muscle hyperpolarization.[17]

Shortly after Dr. Furchgott's original observation, several groups became interested in the possibility that this important function of the endothelium is impaired by atherosclerosis. The rationale underlying this hypothesis was that many of the compounds that stimulate the release of EDRF also have a direct constrictor effect on vascular smooth muscle. These include (in some but not all vascular beds) acetylcholine,[12,13,21] serotonin,[9,10] vasopressin,[34] bradykinin,[7] norepinephrine,[6,10] histamine,[67] endothelin,[73] and several other substances. If the endothelium were dysfunctional in atherosclerosis, these compounds might have a predominant, unopposed vasoconstrictor effect. Thus, endothelial dysfunction might play an important role in the several syndromes of vasospasm encountered in patients with atherosclerosis.

In this chapter, abnormalities of endothelial regulation of vasomotor tone in atherosclerosis will be reviewed. Recent observations regarding the production of nitrogen oxides from normal and atherosclerotic vessels will be presented and stud-

Rubanyi G.M.: Cardiovascular Significance of Endothelium-Derived Vasoactive Factors, Futura Publishing Co., Inc., Mount Kisco, NY, © 1991.

ies of endothelial function in the coronary microcirculation will be discussed. Finally, we will speculate as to the mechanisms underlying abnormal endothelium dependent vascular relaxation in atherosclerosis.

Morphological Alterations of the Endothelium in Atherosclerosis

To accurately examine the endothelium of atherosclerotic and normal vessels, it is necessary to perfusion fix the tissue with gluteraldehyde or other suitable fixatives. Because this cannot be performed in humans, there is no accurate description of the effect of atherosclerosis on human endothelial cell morphology. In contrast, several groups have examined the effect of dietary-induced hypercholesterolemia on endothelial cell morphology in experimental animals. Several earlier studies, which suggested that endothelial cell denudation or desquamation was an integral and early result of hypercholesterolemia, suffered from inattention to proper fixation techniques. More recent studies have shown that endothelial cell desquamation does not occur in either unaffected areas or over raised lesions. Faggiotto and co-workers have observed endothelial cell retraction over lesions of cholesterol-fed stump-tail monkeys.[16] This, however, is not a universal finding. Taylor et al. recently examined the effect of cholesterol feeding on the morphology of endothelial cell in Cynomolgus monkeys after 3–6 months on an atherogenic diet.[65] Endothelial cell desquamation was not apparent, even over sites of multilayered plaque. There were, however, marked changes in endothelial cell morphology. Over raised lesions, the usual distinct polarization of endothelial cells in the direction of flow tended to be lost, due mainly to an increase in cell width, while cell length was preserved. Cholesterol feeding decreased the extent of

overlap between adjacent endothelial cells but did not alter endothelial cell number or the number of surrounding endothelial cells in contact with each individual endothelial cell. The presence of raised lesions increased the lumen surface profile of the vessels by approximately 15% and the endothelial cells conformed to the contours of the immediately underlying foam cells. Endothelial cells demonstrated marked thinning and attenuation of their cell bodies over the bulging foam cell profiles. In contrast, endothelial cell thickness was normal or even increased in cells that overlay crevices between adjacent foam cells. On the abluminal surface of the endothelial cells, an abundance of 45–65 Å cytoplasmic filaments were noted to insinuate between foam cells to maintain contact with the underlying internal elastic lamina.

Impaired Endothelium-Dependent Relaxations in Atherosclerosis

Animal Studies

Large Conduit Arteries

Chronic exposure to high cholesterol

In 1986 and 1987, several publications appeared that clearly showed that endothelium-dependent vascular relaxations are impaired in animals with experimentally induced atherosclerosis. Habib and co-workers studied aortic rings from cholesterol-fed rabbits and found that relaxations to acetylcholine were markedly abnormal.[29] Verbuerren and co-workers studied rabbits fed cholesterol for 8 and 16 weeks.[71] These investigators found that relaxations to acetylcholine were dramatically impaired in both groups while relaxations to nitroglycerin were slightly impaired only in the longer term group. These investigators also found that contractions to serotonin were selectively enhanced in cholesterol-fed animals. Jayakody et al. also showed that cholesterol feeding of rabbits caused a decrease in aortic relaxations to acetylcholine.[33] Studies by Freiman et al.,[20] and Harrison et al.,[28] showed that endothelium-dependent vascular relaxations to acetylcholine, thrombin, and the calcium ionophore A23187 were impaired in iliac arteries from monkeys with diet-induced atherosclerosis (Fig. 1), while relaxations to nitroglycerin were normal.

In most of these studies, histologic examination of the endothelium in the experimental groups revealed either no abnormality or only subtle changes in endothelial cell morphology (similar to those mentioned earlier in this chapter). Specifically, endothelial cell denudation was

minimal or absent. Thus, it was generally concluded from these studies that cholesterol feeding and diet-induced atherosclerosis could cause a functional rather than anatomic impairment of the vascular endothelium.

Time course of the effect of hyperlipidemia on endothelial cell function: effect of short-term exposure to high cholesterol/LDL

This defect in endothelial cell function seems to occur very soon after the onset of cholesterol feeding. In the earliest studies by Jayakody and co-workers, endothelium-dependent vascular relaxation to acetylcholine was found to be abnormal after only 4 weeks of cholesterol feeding.[33] More recently, Wines and co-workers have shown that constriction to serotonin is en-

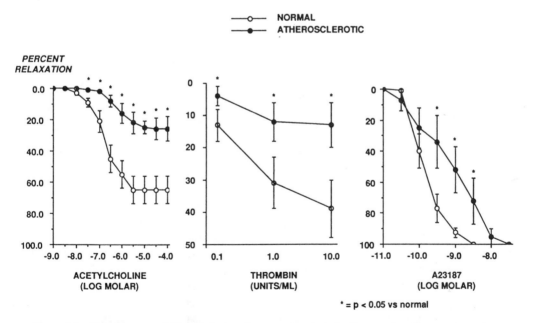

Figure 1: Responses of iliac arteries from normal and atherosclerotic monkeys to acetylcholine, thrombin, and the calcium ionophore A23187. Monkeys were made atherosclerotic by feeding a 0.7% cholesterol diet for 18 months. Iliac vessels were studied in vitro following constriction with prostaglandin $F_{2\alpha}$. Data are redrawn from references 20 and 28, with permission of the American Heart Association.

hanced and relaxation to methylcholine reduced in the aorta of Watanabe heritable hyperlipidemic rabbits at 1 month of age.[76] At this time, only minor microscopic abnormalities of the vascular intima are present, and no gross evidence of atherosclerosis exists.

In 1987, Andrews and co-workers reported that *acute* exposure (in excess of 10 minutes) to relatively high concentrations of purified low density lipoprotein could selectively inhibit relaxations of rabbit aorta to acetylcholine and the calcium ionophore A23187 while not altering relaxations to sodium nitroprusside.[2] Subsequently, Cohen and co-workers have shown in preliminary studies that acute incubations with LDL can inhibit bradykinin-induced endothelium-dependent vascular relaxation in isolated segments of pig coronary arteries.[8] This was corrected by exposure to indomethacin, suggesting a prostanoid-dependent mechanism. These investigators further showed that this perturbation of endothelial cell function could be prevented by the concomitant incubation with specific antibodies for the LDL receptor, suggesting that this effect occurred via unmodified (nonoxidized) LDL. More recent preliminary work by Kugiyama et al. have suggested that oxidized LDL, rather than native LDL impaired endothelium-dependent relaxations of rabbit aorta to acetylcholine.[39] (For further details on this subject, see Chapter 11.)

The Effect of Atherosclerosis/Ischemic Heart Disease on the Coronary Microcirculation

All of the early work relevant to endothelial vascular function involved large conduit vessels (aorta, iliac arteries, proximal coronary arteries) which are not generally involved in the direct regulation of tissue perfusion. The resistance vasculature does not develop overt atherosclerosis. Thus it seemed possible that endothelium-dependent vascular relaxation may be normal in this segment of the circulation despite abnormalities in larger vessels in the setting of chronic hyperlipidemia and atherosclerosis.

Recently, at least three mechanisms have been identified by which atherosclerosis may affect the endothelium of the resistance circulation. These will be reviewed briefly.

Effect of hypercholesterolemia

Two studies have examined the effect of hypercholesterolemia on true resistance vessels. Yamamoto showed that the relaxations to acetylcholine were strikingly abnormal in 25 μm diameter arterioles of the cremaster muscle of cholesterol-fed rabbits.[77] More recently, Sellke et al. have studied resistance arteries (100–200 μm in diameter) of cholesterol-fed primates using a unique in vitro microvessel imaging apparatus.[60] Prior in vivo studies had shown that these vessels were true coronary resistance arteries. Relaxations to the endothelium-independent vasodilators nitroprusside and adenosine were not altered in these vessels. In contrast, endothelium-dependent vascular relaxations to bradykinin, acetylcholine, and the calcium ionophore A23187 were strikingly abnormal in resistance vessels from cholesterol-fed animals (Fig. 2). These studies of the microcirculation clearly show that hypercholesterolemia may affect endothelium-dependent vascular relaxation in vessels that do not develop overt atherosclerosis. Further, these findings likely have important implications regarding neurohumoral regulation of tissue perfusion in atherosclerosis.

Effect of ischemia and reperfusion

Another mechanism by which atherosclerosis may alter endothelial function

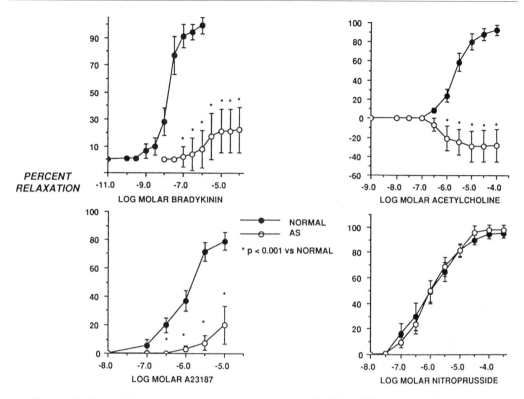

Figure 2: Relaxations of coronary resistance vessels (100–200 microns in diameter) from hearts of normal monkeys and monkeys with diet-induced atherosclerosis. The vessels were studied in vitro using a microvessel imaging apparatus. Drugs were applied after preconstriction with the thromboxane analog U46619. Data are from Sellke et al.[60] Used with permission of the American Heart Association.

within the coronary resistance circulation relates to vascular occlusion and reperfusion which may occur as the result of advanced coronary atherosclerotic narrowing. Ku et al. first suggested that acute, brief occlusions would impair endothelium-dependent relaxations to thrombin in canine left anterior descending coronary arteries while not altering relaxations to nitroglycerin.[38] Subsequently, Van Benthysen and co-workers showed that coronary occlusion followed by reperfusion selectively impaired endothelium-dependent relaxations of the left anterior descending coronary artery to acetylcholine[68] while not altering relaxation to nonendothelium-dependent agents. More recently, Quillen

et al. have examined endothelium-dependent relaxations to acetylcholine, ADP, and the calcium ionophore A23187 in both large coronary arteries (obtuse marginal branches of the circumflex) and coronary microvessels (100–200 microns in diameter) branching from the circumflex after coronary occlusion and reperfusion.[53] Unlike prior studies,[38,68] Quillen et al. found that these epicardial coronary arteries were unaffected by up to 3 hours of ischemia and 1 hour of reperfusion. In contrast, 1 hour of ischemia and 1 hour of reperfusion selectively and markedly impaired endothelium-dependent relaxations of coronary microvessels. This effect was importantly influenced by reperfusion as ischemia alone did not dramatically alter endothelium-dependent vascular relaxations.

Effect of chronic perfusion through collaterals

Finally, the most advanced stages of atherosclerosis lead to total coronary occlusion. In many species, including man, if coronary occlusion occurs gradually, coronary collaterals develop. These prevent the development of myocardial infarction and eventually can restore myocardial perfusion to normal both under resting conditions and in some instances during peak exercise. In our laboratory,[61] we have found that the arterioles perfused by well-developed collaterals have impaired receptor-mediated relaxations to acetylcholine

and ADP while relaxations to the calcium ionophore A23187 are not altered (Fig. 3). In addition, constrictions to vasopressin are markedly enhanced (Fig. 3). Morphologically, the endothelium of these vessels appeared entirely normal. It is conceivable that alterations of perfusion pressure or characteristics of perfusion pressure (such as the pulsatile nature or vascular shear) distal to collaterals may alter endothelial function. While the precise mechanism underlying this phenomenon remain obscure, the findings strongly suggest that neurohumoral regulation of perfusion to collateral-dependent myocardium may be strikingly different than that to normal myocardium.

Thus, there are at least three ways that hypercholesterolemia and atherosclerosis can alter endothelial function within the coronary microcirculation. These include

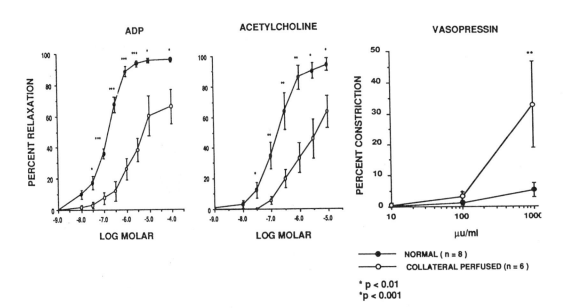

Figure 3: Responses of coronary microvessels obtained from normal and collateral-dependent myocardium. Collaterals were stimulated to develop by gradual occlusion of the circumflex coronary artery of dogs using the ameroid technique. Four to 6 months later coronary microvessels less than 200 microns in diameter were studied in vitro. Vessels from the collateral-dependent myocardium relaxed less to the endothelium-dependent substances ADP and acetylcholine. Constriction to vasopressin was markedly enhanced in collateral perfused coronary microvessels. Data are from Sellke et al.[61] Used with permission of the American Heart Association.

the effects of chronic hypercholesterolemia, ischemia followed by reperfusion, and altered endothelial function related to chronic perfusion through mature collaterals. Given these considerations, it may clearly be concluded that atherosclerosis, in particular coronary atherosclerosis, is not simply a "large vessel disease" but has important direct and indirect effects on the microvasculature that may alter neurohumoral regulation of tissue perfusion.

Studies in Humans

In Vitro Studies

Shortly after the initial observations of impaired endothelium-dependent relaxations in cholesterol-fed animals came evidence that this function of the endothelium is also impaired in humans with atherosclerosis. Two studies examined endothelium-dependent vascular relaxations of human coronary arteries in vitro. Bossaller et al. studied nonatherosclerotic and atherosclerotic ring segments of coronary arteries from patients undergoing cardiac transplantation.[69] Relaxations of atherosclerotic segments to acetylcholine, substance P, and histamine were impaired while relaxations to the calcium ionophore A23187 were preserved. They further found that cyclic GMP accumulation in atherosclerotic segments was impaired to acetylcholine but unaltered in response to calcium ionophore. These investigators proposed that atherosclerosis altered endothelial cell receptor function and that the responses to the calcium ionophore were intact because this agonist bypasses receptor-mediated mechanisms.

More recently Forstermann, and co-workers have examined endothelium-dependent vascular relaxation in strips of coronary arteries removed from patients undergoing heart transplant.[18] These investigators found that responses to all endothelium-dependent vasodilators including substance P, bradykinin, *and* the calcium ionophore A23187 were abnormal in atherosclerotic segments compared to nonatherosclerotic segments (Fig. 4). The reason for the discrepancy between these two studies regarding the effect of the calcium ionophore A23187 remains unclear.

Studies in the Catheterization Laboratory

Several groups have examined the effect of acetylcholine on human coronary arteries at the time of cardiac catheterization. Ludmer et al. showed that acetylcholine, when infused into the left anterior descending coronary artery produced either no response or minimal dilatation of normal coronary vessels, while causing constriction (often severe, near total occlusions) of atherosclerotic coronary arteries.[41] There has been substantial controversy regarding this finding. Okamura and co-workers have reported that somewhat larger concentrations of acetylcholine uniformly caused vasoconstriction.[49] This apparent paradox may be explained by the possibility that the group studied by Okamura et al. may have had minimal, nonobstructive atherosclerosis which caused endothelial cell dysfunction. Indeed, acetylcholine was more likely to produce vasoconstriction of an angiographically normal left anterior descending artery if there was angiographically apparent disease of either of the other two major coronary arteries, suggesting that the left anterior descending likely had undetected atherosclerosis.[41] More recently, Vita et al. have shown that the propensity for vasodilatation versus vasoconstriction produced by intracoronary acetylcholine bears a strong relationship to the individual's number of risk factors for atherosclerosis.[39]

In addition to the large number of neu-

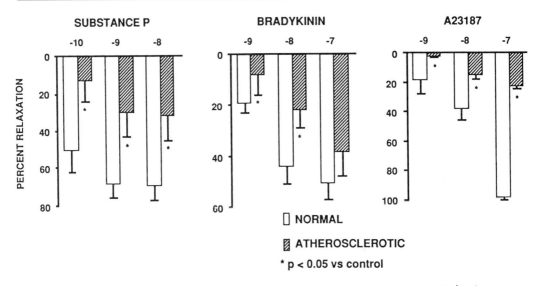

Figure 4: Relaxations of normal and atherosclerotic human coronary arteries to en-dothelium-dependent vasodilator compounds, substance P, bradykinin, and the cal-cium ionophore A23187. Vessels were obtained from patients undergoing cardiac transplantation and studied in vitro. Relaxations to all three substances were signif-icantly impaired in the atherosclerotic vessels. Responses to sodium nitroprusside were not altered by atherosclerosis. Redrawn from data originally presented by For-stermann et al.[18] With permission from the American Heart Association and the au-thors.

rohumoral stimuli that elicit the release of the endothelium-derived relaxing factor, mechanical shear stress also regulates its release.[30–33,57] This may have an important role in maintaining shear stress at rela-tively constant levels during large changes in blood flow. Recently, two groups have shown that this regulatory function of the endothelium is also abnormal in athero-sclerosis.[11,14] In both of these experiments, adenosine was infused into the left ante-rior descending coronary artery of patients at the time of cardiac catheterization. The diameter of the left anterior descending ar-tery proximal to the site of adenosine in-fusion was measured using quantitative techniques. Among the patients with en-tirely normal (smooth) coronary arteries, the proximal left anterior descending ar-tery dilated. Since this portion of the vessel was not exposed to adenosine, the ob-served vasodilatation was assumed to be due to flow-mediated release of EDRF. In contrast, among patients with minimal atherosclerosis, essentially no flow-me-diated vasodilatation was observed. This finding of impaired flow-mediated vascu-lar relaxation in atherosclerosis has re-cently been confirmed in monkeys with diet-induced atherosclerosis.[43]

Based on these in vitro and in vivo studies of human coronary arteries, it is now apparent that atherosclerosis not only alters endothelium-dependent vas-cular relaxation in experimental animals with diet-induced atherosclerosis but also results in a similar defect of endothelial function in the coronary circulation of humans with atherosclerosis. These observations may have important impli-cations regarding the pathogenesis of vas-cular spasm and alterations of neuro-humoral regulation of the circulation in atherosclerosis.

Mechanism of Impaired Endothelium-Dependent Relaxation in Atherosclerotic Blood Vessels

Release and Action of EDRFs

Studies such as those described in the preceding sections, in which intact vessels, intact animals, or the coronary circulation of humans is studied during cardiac catheterization, are not capable of determining if abnormal endothelium-dependent vascular relaxation is due to endothelial dysfunction or if the vascular smooth muscle of atherosclerotic vessels is less responsive to EDRF. To address this question, Guerra et al.[26] have employed a bioassay preparation to examine the amount and effect of EDRF released from normal and atherosclerotic rabbit aorta (6 months of cholesterol feeding). EDRF released from athero-

sclerotic rabbit aorta in response to both acetylcholine and the calcium ionophore A23187 produced only about one-half as much relaxation of denuded normal detector vessel ring segments as in response to EDRF from normal rabbit aorta (Fig. 5). In addition, the autocrine/paracrine function of EDRF in stimulating the production of cyclic GMP within endothelial cells was also impaired by atherosclerosis. Guerra et al. performed additional studies to examine the sensitivity of normal and atherosclerotic vessels to EDRF released from normal rabbit aorta.[26] In these studies, atherosclerotic vessels were found to be supersensitive to EDRF and equally sensitive to nitric oxide compared to normal vessels (Fig. 6). Thus, these bioassay studies clearly showed that the predominant mechanism underlying abnormal endothelium-dependent vascular relaxation is related to either decreased release of EDRF or release of a defective EDRF rather than insensitivity of atherosclerotic smooth muscle to EDRF.

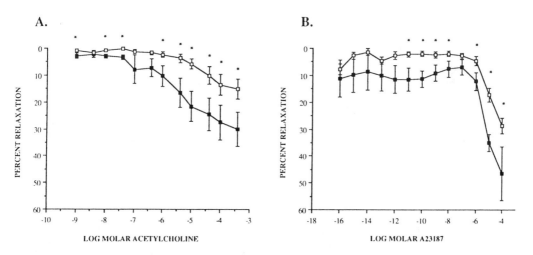

Figure 5: Bioassay of EDRF activity from normal (closed squares) and cholesterol-fed (open squares) rabbit aorta released in response to acetylcholine (A) and the calcium ionophore A23187 (B). Segments of thoracic aorta from normal and cholesterol-fed rabbits were studied in parallel. Studies were performed in the presence of indomethacin. Vessels were perfused with physiological buffer and the effluent allowed to superfuse a segment of normal rabbit aorta denuded of endothelium. Responses were obtained after preconstriction of the detector vessel with $PGF_{2\alpha}$. From Guerra et al.[26] Used with permission from Karger Publishing.

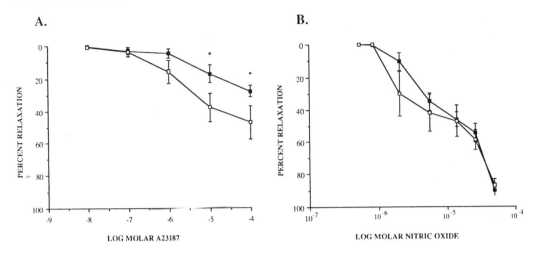

Figure 6: Responses of normal (open squares) and hypercholesterolemic segments (closed squares) of rabbit aorta to EDRF released from normal rabbit aorta (a) and to nitric oxide (b). Segments of either normal or cholesterol-fed rabbit aorta were mounted in a tissue bath so that they could be perfused with the effluent from a segment of normal rabbit aorta. Tension was measured near the midportion of the recipient vessel. Vessels from hypercholesterolemic rabbits were supersensitive to EDRF from normal rabbit aorta and were equally sensitive to nitric oxide. From Guerra et al.[26] Used with permission from Karger Publishers.

Miscellaneous Mechanisms

It is conceivable that other mechanisms may contribute to abnormal endothelium-dependent relaxation in atherosclerosis. The above bioassay studies examined the luminal release of EDRF only. Since the luminal and abluminal release of EDRF may be quantitatively[3] and qualitatively different,[58] it is conceivable that the abluminal diffusion of EDRF may be impaired by the often marked intimal thickening that occurs in the advanced stages of atherosclerosis. It is also possible that EDRF may be degraded by oxygen radicals released from subintimal macrophages and other inflammatory cells present in the atherosclerotic lesion.[25,52,59] Shimokowa and co-workers have shown that intimal thickening developing as a result of vascular trauma may in fact impair endothelium-dependent relaxations to serotonin but not to bradykinin or the calcium ionophore A23187.[62]

It is now apparent that the endothelium releases a variety of constrictor factors including several cyclooxygenase prostanoids,[45,64,65] the superoxide anion,[78] angiotensin II,[15] and the polypeptide endothelin.[26] If these compounds were released in excess in the setting of atherosclerosis, it is conceivable that they may counteract the concomitant release of EDRF. Recent studies of rabbit aorta studied both as intact rings and in bioassay have failed to show any evidence for this phenomenon.[26]

Potential Role of Intimal Inflammatory Cells

The atherosclerotic plaque contains a number of abnormal cellular elements, including leukocytes, macrophages, and adherent platelets, which may release potent vasoactive agents. These include thromboxane A$_2$ from platelets and leukocytes, leukotrienes from leukocytes, oxygen-derived radicals from leukocytes and macrophages, and vasoconstrictor prostanoids from leukocytes.[55,69] Recently, Lopez and co-workers have examined the vascular responses to the peptide fmet-leu-phe (fMLP) infused into the hindlimb of normal and atherosclerotic Cynomolgus monkeys.[40] fMLP did not change large artery resistance in normal monkeys, however, it produced pronounced constriction of large arteries in atherosclerotic monkeys. Furthermore, Lopez et al. found that prostaglandin E_2, which may be released from leukocytes, produced marked constriction of large arteries in atherosclerotic but not in normal monkeys. Thus, not only do atherosclerotic vessels contain a variety of cell types that may release vasoactive agents, but these vessels have increased responsiveness to at least one vasoactive substance released from leukocytes.

The Relationship of Nitric Oxide Production: Biological Activity of EDRF in Normal and Atherosclerotic Vessels

In an effort to further understand abnormalities of endothelium-dependent relaxation of atherosclerosis, we began studies of the release of nitric oxide and related compounds from the vascular endothelium. In an initial study, we compared the release of nitric oxide (detected by chemiluminescence) and the biological activity of EDRF (determined via bioassay) from bovine aortic endothelial cells.[49] To summarize these data, the amount of nitric oxide present in the effluent of superfused aortic endothelial cells was only about 1/5 to 1/8 that necessary to account for the biological activity of the endothelium-derived relaxing factor. Based on these observations, we concluded that either there are multiple EDRFs and that nitric oxide only accounted for a portion of the endothelium-dependent relaxation mediated by the endothelium, or alternatively that the endothelium-derived relaxing factor is not free nitric oxide but nitric oxide incorporated into a parent compound that was substantially more potent than free nitric oxide. In support of this latter hypothesis, we found that the potency of one such nitrosylated compound, S-nitrosocysteine more closely resembled the endothelium-derived relaxing factor than did nitric oxide on a mole-to-mole basis.[47] Subsequently, Rubanyi et al. have shown that the endothelium-derived relaxing factor and S-nitrosocysteine in concentrations sufficient to produce vascular relaxation do not alter the electron paramagnetic resonance shift of hemoglobin while nitric oxide does.[56] Finally, Wei et al. have shown that pial vessels exposed to hydrogen peroxide do not relax to nitric oxide but do relax to either EDRF or S-nitrosocysteine.[74] One effect of hydrogen peroxide is to cross-bridge available sulfhydryl groups. Wei et al. have therefore suggested that nitric oxide requires sulfhydryl groups, whereas the endothelium-derived relaxing factor and S-nitrosocysteine, being nitrosothiols, do not.[74] (See also Chapter 6 in this book.) These studies further support the concept that EDRF is not authentic nitric oxide but is more likely a nitrosylated compound such as a nitrosothiol.

More recently, Minor et al. examined the release of nitric oxide and related compounds from the thoracic aorta of normal and cholesterol-fed rabbits.[46] In addition, these investigators quantified the vasorelaxant activity of EDRF released from these vessels using bioassay. As previously found, the vasorelaxant activity of EDRF from hypercholesterolemic animals was markedly reduced compared to controls. Very surprisingly, however, the quantity of nitric oxide recovered (after reduction preprocessing) from cholesterol-fed rabbit aorta markedly exceeded that from normal rabbit aorta. Further, acetylcholine stimulated additional release of nitric oxide although the biologic activity of EDRF release by acetylcholine from cholesterol-fed animals was minimal. The increment in the increase of nitric oxide release stimulated by acetylcholine was actually greater in cholesterol-fed animals than in normals. This very interesting finding may potentially have very important implications regarding endothelium-dependent vascular relaxation in atherosclerosis. These findings clearly show that there is not a defect in the enzymatic process leading to the production of nitric oxide within atherosclerotic endothelium. Further, these studies do not support the concept that there is a defect in endothelial cell membrane receptors caused by cholesterol feeding as the release of nitric oxide clearly increased (more so than in normals) upon administration of acetylcholine.

Hypothesis

Based on our work and that of others, we have suggested that the endothelium-derived relaxing factor is not simply authentic nitric oxide but is a nitrosylated compound that yields nitric oxide, likely upon one electron reduction (and thus is measured as nitric oxide using chemiluminescence combined with sodium iodide reflux preprocessing). A potential pathway for the formation of such a compound is summarized in Figure 7. The incorporation of nitric oxide into such a compound markedly increases its potency and may provide a "salvage pathway" by which higher oxidation products of nitric oxide can be converted from compounds with essentially no vasodilator activity to potent vasodilators. One such example would be the reaction with cysteine to yield S-nitrosocysteine which is markedly more stable (and thus more potent on a molar basis) than nitric oxide. Several diseases including atherosclerosis, diabetes,[42] acute hypertension,[76] and ischemia with reperfusion[38,53,68] are associated with abnormal endothelium-dependent vascular

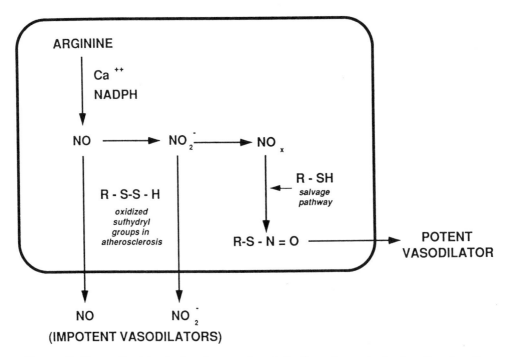

Figure 7: Theoretical basis for abnormal endothelium-dependent relaxation in atherosclerosis. See text for details.

relaxations. One feature potentially common to all these processes is the excessive generation of oxygen-free radicals. These may react with free sulfhydryl groups (or other EDRF substrates) making them unavailable to incorporate the nitrosyl moiety. This would allow the endothelial cell to produce large quantities of nitric oxide while not producing an effective EDRF. This mechanism may underlie abnormal endothelium-dependent responses in many disease states.

Can Alterations of Endothelium-Dependent Relaxation be Prevented or Corrected in Atherosclerotic Vessels?

If alterations of endothelium-dependent responses are important in modulating vasomotor tone in atherosclerosis, correction of this abnormality may have important clinical implications. Several studies have addressed this issue. Habib and co-workers examined endothelium-dependent responses to acetylcholine in three groups of rabbits: a control group, a cholesterol-fed group, and a cholesterol-fed group treated with the calcium antagonist PN200110.[22] Cholesterol feeding markedly elevated both plasma cholesterol levels and the level of cholesterol in the rabbit aorta and impaired endothelium-dependent relaxation to acetylcholine. The plasma cholesterol level of the animals treated with a calcium antagonist were elevated to the same degree as the cholesterol-fed group; however, there was a substantial reduction in the amount of cholesterol within the aortic wall. Endothelium-dependent relaxation to acetylcholine was reduced in this group but not nearly as severely as in the group fed cholesterol alone. Thus it would appear that treatment with calcium antagonist may slow the development of atherosclerosis and partially preserve endothelium-dependent responses.

We have examined the effect of dietary treatment on endothelium-dependent responses to atherosclerosis.[27] Three groups of animals were examined in our study. One was a group of Cynomolgus monkeys fed an atherogenic diet for 18 months. A second group of monkeys received an atherogenic diet for 18 months followed by a normal diet for the ensuing 18 months. A third group of monkeys served as control. Within the cholesterol-fed group, there was marked intimal thickening with lipid-laden foam cells and inflammatory cells present in the intima. After regression of atherosclerosis, the intimal area decreased by about 50% but remained markedly thickened compared to control vessels. In contrast to this modest improvement in intimal thickening, endothelium-dependent responses to both acetylcholine and thrombin were restored entirely to normal. Responses to nitroglycerin were similar among all groups.

Interestingly, in this study, the regression of intimal thickening was far from complete and yet the abnormality of endothelium-dependent relaxation was eliminated by atherosclerosis regression. Morphological evidence of atherosclerosis regression occurs predominantly when lesions contain large quantities of foam cells and intracellular lipids. When atherosclerotic vessels contain predominantly fibrotic plaque without a large amount of intracellular lipid and foam cells, decreases in lesion size are less likely to occur despite improvement or even correction of the serum lipids. In contrast to the concept that anatomic regression may be limited by the presence of fibrosis in the intima of atherosclerotic vessels, the results from our study of regression suggests that dietary treatment may produce an improvement in functional abnormalities of the vessel in atherosclerosis. This "functional regression" may occur despite only modest decreases in intimal thickness or minimal changes in the gross appearance of the lesion. It is interesting to speculate whether the dietary changes or alterations in medical therapy might promote absorption of lipid from the vessel wall, restore endothelial modulation of vascular smooth muscle reactivity toward normal, and result in resolution of abnormal vasomotor phenomenon in the clinical setting.

Shimokawa and Vanhoutte have shown that dietary cod liver oil improves endothelium-dependent responses in a pig model of focal coronary atherosclerosis produced by a combination of balloon denudation and cholesterol feeding.[62] Vekshtein and co-workers have recently presented preliminary data showing that 6 months of therapy with omega-3 fatty acids can reverse the abnormal coronary constriction to acetylcholine in patients with early atherosclerosis.[68]

Summary and Implications

While it has been possible in both experimental animals and humans to show impaired endothelium-dependent modulation of vascular smooth muscle in the setting of atherosclerosis, the significance of this phenomenon in terms of human disease has yet to be clearly defined. Recently it has been shown that the production of endothelium-derived constricting factors increases with age.[37] Since EDRF may play an important role in the maintenance of normal blood pressure,[54] it is conceivable that the loss of EDRF with atherosclerosis, together with the increased production of constrictor factors with age, may predispose to "essential" hypertension, which so commonly develops in the elderly.

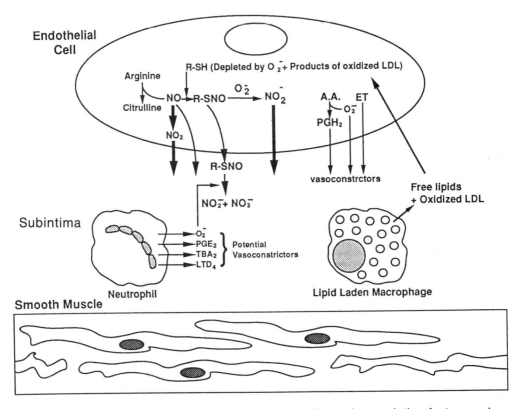

Figure 8: Interactions of endothelium-derived relaxing and constricting factors and factors released from infiltrating cell types in atherosclerosis.

Loss of EDRF may unmask or enhance constrictor effects of both humoral and locally produced substances (some released by subintimal inflammatory cells). This may contribute to several syndromes of altered vasomotion including unstable angina, myocardial infarction, variant angina encountered in the setting of atherosclerosis. The endothelium-derived relaxing factor also inhibits platelet aggregation.[1,5] It is interesting to speculate that the loss of this effect may enhance the propensity for local platelet deposition leading to vascular occlusion and the release of both vasoconstrictor factors and factors that may accelerate the development of atherosclerosis. These considerations are schematically illustrated in Figure 8.

Finally, it is now apparent that the effect of atherosclerosis on the endothelium is not limited to the large vessels but also occurs in the coronary microcirculation. This phenomenon is due to the direct effect of chronic hypercholesterolemia, altered endothelial function due to ischemia and reperfusion which occurs in advanced stages of atherosclerosis, and the effect of perfusion through mature collaterals which are present in the most advanced stages of atherosclerosis when vascular occlusion has occurred. Thus, in addition to predisposing to altered vasomotion of large vessels, endothelial dysfunction in atherosclerosis may dramatically impair neurohumoral regulation of tissue perfusion at the microvascular level.

References

1. Alheid U., Reichwehr I., Förstermann U.: Human endothelial cells inhibit platelet aggregation by separately stimulating platelet cyclic AMP and cyclic GMP. Eur. J. Pharmacol. 164:103–110, 1989.

2. Andrews H.E., Bruckdorfer X.R., Dunn R.C., Jacobs M.: Low-density lipoproteins inhibit endothelium-dependent relaxation in rabbit aorta. Nature 327:237–239, 1987.

3. Bassenge E., Busse R., Pohl U.: Abluminal release and asymmetrical response of the rabbit arterial wall to endothelium-derived relaxing factor. Circ. Res. 61:II-68–II-73, 1987.

4. Bossaller C., Habib G.B., Yamamoto H., Williams C., Wells S., Henry P.D.: Impaired muscarinic endothelium-dependent relaxation and cyclic guanosine 5'-monophosphate formation in atherosclerotic human coronary artery and rabbit aorta. J. Clin. Invest. 79:170–174, 1987.

5. Busse R., Luckhoff A., Bassenge E.: Endothelium-derived relaxant factor inhibits platelets activation. Arch. Pharmacol. 336:566–577, 1987.

6. Carrier G.O., White R.E.: Enhancement of alpha-1 and alpha-2 adrenergic agonist-induced vasoconstriction by removal of endothelium in rat aorta. J. Pharmacol. Exp. Ther. 1985:682–687, 1985.

7. Cherry P.D., Furchgott R.F., Zawadski J.V., Jothianandan D.: Role of endothelial cells in relaxation of isolated arteries by bradykinin. Proc. Natl. Acad. Sci. U.S.A. 79:2106–2110, 1982.

8. Cohen R.A., Cunningham L.D.: Low density lipoproteins inhibit endothelium-dependent relaxations caused by bradykinin in the pig coronary artery. Circulation 78:II-183, 1988.

9. Cohen R.A., Shepherd J.T., Vanhoutte P.M.: Inhibitory role of the endothelium in the response of isolated coronary arteries to platelets. Science 221:273–274, 1983.

10. Cocks T.M., Angus A.R.: Endothelium-dependent relaxation of coronary arteries by noradrenaline and serotonin. Nature 305:627–630, 1983.

11. Cox D.A., Vita J.A., Treasure C.B., Fish R.B., Alexander R.W., Ganz P., Selwyn A.P.: Atherosclerosis impairs flow-mediated dilation of coronary arteries in man. Circulation 80:458–465, 1989.

12. De Mey J.G., Claeys M., Vanhoutte P.M.: Endothelium-dependent inhibitory effects of acetylcholine, adenosine triphosphate, thrombin and arachidonic acid in the canine

femoral artery. J. Pharmacol. Exp. Ther. 222:166–173, 1982.

13. De Mey J.G., Vanhoutte P.M.: Role of the intima in cholinergic and purinergic relaxation of isolated canine femoral arteries. J. Physiol. (Lond.) 316:347–355, 1981.

14. Drexler H., Zeiher A.M., Wollschlager H., Meinertz T., Hanjorg J., Bonzel T.: Demonstration of flow-dependent coronary dilatation in man. Circulation 80:466–474, 1989.

15. Dzau V.J.: Significance of the vascular renin-angiotensin pathway. Hypertension 8:553–559, 1986.

16. Faggiotto A., Ross R., Harker L.: Studies of hypercholesterolemia in the nonhuman primate. II. Fatty streak conversion in fibrous plaque. Arteriosclerosis 4:341–356, 1984.

17. Feletou M., Vanhoutte P.M.: Endothelium-dependent hyperpolarization of canine coronary smooth muscle. Br. J. Pharmacol. 93:515–524.

18. Förstermann U., Mügge A., Alheid U., Haverich A., Frölich J.C.: Selective attenuation of endothelium-mediated vasodilation in atherosclerotic human coronary arteries. Circ. Res. 62:185–190, 1988.

19. Förstermann U., Trogisch G., Busse R.: Species-dependent differences in the nature of endothelium-derived vascular relaxing factor. Eur. J. Pharmacol. 106:639–643, 1984.

20. Freiman P.C., Mitchell G.C., Heistad D.D., Armstrong M.L., Harrison D.G.: Atherosclerosis impairs endothelium-dependent vascular relaxation to acetylcholine and thrombin in primates. Circ. Res. 58:783–789, 1986.

21. Furchgott R.F., Zawadski J.V.: The obligatory role of endothelial cells in the relaxation of arterial smooth muscle by acetylcholine. Nature 228:373–376, 1980.

22. Furchgott R.F.: The role of endothelium in the responses of vascular smooth muscle to drugs. Annu. Rev. Pharmacol. Toxicol. 24:175–197, 1984.

23. Griffith T.M., Edwards D.H., Lewis M.J., Newby A.C., Henderson H.A.: The nature of endothelium derived vascular relaxant factor. Nature 308:645–647, 1984.

24. Gryglewski R.J., Moncada S., Palmer R.M.J.: Bioassay of prostacyclin and endothelium-derived relaxing factor (EDRF) from porcine aortic endothelial cells. Br. J. Pharmacol. 87:685–694, 1986.

25. Gryglewski R.J., Palmer R.M.J., Moncada S.: Superoxide anion is involved in the breakdown of endothelium-derived vascular relaxing factor. Nature 320:454–456, 1986.

26. Guerra R. Jr., Brotherton A.F.A., Goodwin P.J., Clark C.R., Armstrong M.L., Harrison D.G.: Mechanisms of abnormal endothelium-dependent vascular relaxation in atherosclerosis. Blood Vessels (accepted), 1990.

27. Harrison D.G., Armstrong M.L., Freiman P.C., Heistad D.D.: Restoration of endothelium-dependent relaxation by dietary treatment of atherosclerosis. J. Clin. Invest. 80:1808–1811, 1987.

28. Harrison D.G., Freiman P.C., Mitchell G.G., Armstrong M.L., Heistad D.D.: Alterations of vascular reactivity in atherosclerosis. Circ. Res. 61:II-74–II-80, 1987.

29. Habib J.B., Bossaler C., Wells S., Williams C., Morrisett J.D., Henry P.D.: Preservation of endothelium-dependent vascular relaxation in cholesterol-fed rabbit by treatment with the calcium blocker PN 200110. Circ. Res. 58:305–309, 1986.

30. Holtz J., Förstermann U., Pohl U., Giesler M., Bassenge E.: Flow-dependent, endothelium-mediated dilation of epicardial coronary arteries in conscious dogs: Effects of cyclo-oxygenase inhibition. J. Cardiovasc. Pharmacol. 6:1161–1169, 1984.

31. Holtz J., Giesler M., Bassenge E.: Two dilatory mechanisms of anti-anginal drugs on epicardial coronary arteries in-vivo: Indirect, flow-dependent, endothelium-mediated dilation and direct smooth muscle relaxation. Z. Cardiol. 72:98–106, 1983.

32. Inou T., Tomoike H., Hisano K., Nakamura M.: Endothelium determines flow-dependent dilation of the epicardial coronary in dogs. J. Am. Coll. Cardiol. 11:187–191, 1988.

33. Jayakody L., Senaratne M., Thomson A., Kappagoda T.: Endothelium-dependent relaxation in experimental atherosclerosis in the rabbit. Circ. Res. 60:251–264, 1987.

34. Katusic Z.S., Shepherd J.T., Vanhoutte P.M.: Vasopressin causes endothelium-dependent relaxations of the canine basilar artery. Circ. Res. 55:575–579, 1984.

35. Katusic Z.S., Vanhoutte P.M.: Superoxide anion is an endothelium-derived contracting factor. Am. J. Physiol. 257:H33–H37, 1989.

36. Koga T., Takata Y., Kobayashi K., Takishita S., Yamashita Y., Fujishima M.: Age and hypertension promote endothelium-dependent contractions to acetylcholine in the aorta of the rat. Hypertension 14:542–548, 1989.

37. Koga T., Takata Y., Kobayashi K., Takishita S., Yamashita Y., Fujishima M.: Age and hypertension promote endothelium-dependent contractions to acetylcholine in the aorta of the rat. Hypertension 1989 (in press).

38. Ku D.: Coronary vascular reactivity after acute myocardial ischemia. Science 218:576–578, 1982.

39. Kugiyama K., Bucay M., Morrisett J.D., Roberts R., Henry P.D.: Oxidized LDL impairs endothelium-dependent arterial relaxation. Circulation 80:II-278, 1989.

40. Lopez J.A.G., Armstrong M.L., Harrison D.G., Piegors D.J., Heistad D.D.: Vascular responses to leukocyte products in atherosclerotic primates. Circ. Res. 65:1078–1086, 1989.

41. Ludmer P.L., Selwyn A.P., Shook T.L., Wayne R.R., Mudge G.H., Alexander R.W., Ganz P.: Paradoxial vasoconstriction induced by acetylcholine in atherosclerotic coronary arteries. N. Engl. J. Med. 315:1046–1051, 1986.

42. Mayhan W.G.: Impairment of endothelium-dependent dilatation of cerebral arterioles during diabetes mellitus. Am. J. Physiol. 256:H621–H625, 1989.

43. McLenachan J.M., Williams J.K., Ganz P., Selwyn A.P.: Loss of flow-mediated endothelium-dependent dilation in atherosclerosis. Circulation 80:II-279, 1989.

44. Miller V.M., Vanhoutte P.M.: Is nitric oxide the only endothelium-derived relaxing factor in canine femoral veins? Am. J. Physiol. 26:H1910–H1916, 1989.

45. Miller V.M., Vanhoutte P.M.: Endothelium-dependent contractions to arachidonic acid are mediated by products of cyclooxygenase in canine veins. Am. J. Physiol. 248:H432–H437, 1985.

46. Minor R.L. Jr., Myers P.R., Bates J.N., Harrison D.G.: Atherosclerosis impairs release of EDRF, but not nitric oxide from the vascular endothelium. Circulation 80:II-2220, 1989.

47. Myers P.R., Guerra R., Bates J.N., Harrison D.G.: Comparative studies on nitrosothiols: Similarities between EDRF and S-nitroso-1-cysteine (cysNO). FASEB J. (Abst.)3:5336, 1989.

48. Myers P.R., Guerra R., Jr., Bates J.N., Harrison D.G.: Comparative studies on endothelium-derived relaxing factor (EDRF), nitric oxide (NO) and nitrosothiols: Similarities between EDRF and S-nitroso-L-cysteine (cysNO). FASEB J. 3:A1145, 1989.

49. Myers P.R., Guerra R. Jr., Harrison D.G.: Release of NO and EDRF from cultured bovine aortic endothelial cells. Am. J. Physiol. 256:H1030–H1037, 1989.

50. Okumura K., Yasue H., Matsuyama K., Goto K., Miyagi H., Ogawa H., Matsuyama K.: Sensitivity and specificity of intracoronary injection of acetylcholine for the induction of coronary artery spasm. J. Am. Coll. Cardiol. 12:883–888, 1988.

51. Palmer R.M.J., Ferrige A.G., Moncada S.: Nitric oxide release accounts for the biological activity of endothelium-derived relaxation factor. Nature (Lond.) 327:524–526, 1987.

52. Pieper G.M., Gross G.J.: Selective impairment of endothelium-dependent relaxation by oxygen-derived free radicals: Distinction between receptor versus nonreceptor mediators. Blood Vessels 26:44–47, 1989.

53. Quillen J.E., Sellke F.W., Brooks L.A., Harrison D.G.: Ischemia-reperfusion impairs endothelium-dependent relaxation of coronary microvessels while not affecting large coronary arteries. Circulation 80:II-396, 1989.

54. Rees D.D., Palmer R.M.J., Moncada S.: Role of endothelium-derived nitric oxide in the regulation of blood pressure. Proc. Natl. Acad. Sci. U.S.A. 86:3375–3378, 1989.

55. Reiko T., Werb Z.: Secretory products of macrophages and their physiological functions. Am. J. Physiol. 246:C1–C9, 1984.

56. Rubanyi G.M., Johns A., Harrison D.G., Wilcox D.: Evidence that EDRF may be identical with an S-nitrosothiol and not with free nitric oxide. Circulation 80(Suppl. II):II-281, 1989.

57. Rubanyi G.M., Romero J.C., Vanhoutte P.M.: Flow-induced release of endothelium-derived relaxing factor. Am. J. Physiol. 250:H145–H149, 1986.

58. Rubanyi G.M., Vanhoutte P.M.: Nature of endothelium-derived relaxing factor: Are there two relaxing mediators? Circ. Res. 61:II-61–II-67, 1987.

59. Rubanyi G.M., Vanhoutte P.M.: Oxygen-derived free radicals, endothelium and responsiveness of vascular smooth muscle. Am. J. Physiol. 250:H815–H821, 1986.

60. Sellke F.W., Armstrong M.L., Harrison D.G.: Endothelium-dependent vascular relaxation is abnormal in the coronary microcirculation of atherosclerotic primates. Circulation (In Press).

61. Sellke F.W., Quillen J.E., Brooks L.A., Harrison D.G.: Endothelial modulation of the coronary vasculature in vessels perfused via mature collaterals. Circulation (in press), 1990.

62. Shimokawa H., Aarhus L.L., Vanhoutte P.M.: Porcine coronary arteries with regenerated endothelium have a reduced endothelium-dependent responsiveness to aggregating platelets and serotonin. Circ. Res. 61:256–270, 1987.

63. Shimokawa H., Vanhoutte P.M.: Dietary cod-liver oil improves endothelium-dependent responses in hypercholesterolemic and atherosclerotic porcine coronary arteries. Circulation 78:1421–1430, 1988.

64. Shirahase H., Usui H., Kurahashi K., Fujiwara M., Fukui K.: Endothelium-dependent contraction induced by nicotine in isolated canine basilar artery: possible involvement of a thromboxane A_2 (TXA_2) like substance. Life Sci. 42:437–445, 1988.

65. Traylor K.E., Glgov S., Zarins C.K.: Preservation and structural adaptation of endothelium over experimental foam cell lesions. Quantitative ultrastructural study. Arteriosclerosis 9:881–894, 1989.

66. Tesfamarian B., Jakubowski J.A., Cohen R.A.: Contraction of diabetic rabbit aorta caused by endothelium-derived PGH_2-TxA_2. Am. J. Physiol. 257:H1327–H1333, 1989.

67. Toda N.: Mechanisms of histamine-induced relaxation in isolated monkey and dog coronary arteries. J. Pharmacol. Exp. Ther. 239:529–535, 1986.

68. Vanbenthuysen K.M., McMurty I.F., Horowitz L.D.: Reperfusion after acute coronary occlusion in dogs impairs endothelium dependent relaxation to acetylcholine and augments contractile reactivity in vitro. J. Clin. Invest. 79:265–274, 1987.

69. Vanhoutte P.M., Houston D.S.: Platelets, endothelium and vasospasm. Circulation 72:728–734, 1985.

70. Vekshtein V.I., Yeung A.C., Vita J.A., Nabel E.G., Fish R.D., Bittl J.A., et al.: Fish oil improves endothelium-dependent relaxation in patients with coronary artery disease. Circulation 80:II-434, 1989.

71. Verbeuren T.J., Jordaens F.H., Zonnekeyn L.L., Van Hove C.E., Coene M.C., Herman A.G.: Effect of hypercholesterolemia on vascular reactivity in the rabbit. Circ. Res. 58:552–564, 1986.

72. Vita J.A., Treasure C.B., Nabel E.G., Fish R.D., McLenachan J.M., Yeung A.C., Vekshtein V.I., et al.: The coronary response to acetylcholine relates to coronary risk factors. Circulation 80:II-435, 1989.

73. Warner T.D., Mitchell J.A., de Nucci G., Vane J.R.: Endothelin-1 and endothelin-3 release EDRF from isolated perfused arterial vessels of the rat and rabbit. J. Cardiovasc. Pharmacol. 13:S85–S88, 1989.

74. Wei E.P., Kontos H.A.: H_2O_2 and endothelium-dependent cerebral arteriolar dilation: implications for the identity of EDRF from acetylcholine. Hypertension (in press).

75. Wei E.P., Kontos H.A., Christman C.W., DeWitt D.S., Povlishock J.T.: Superoxide generation and reversal of acetylcholine-induced cerebral arteriolar dilation after acute hypertension. Circ. Res. 57:781–787, 1985.

76. Wines P.A., Schmitz J.M., Pfister S.L., Clubb Jr. F.J., Buja L.M., Willerson J.T., Campbell W.B.: Augmented vasoconstrictor responses to serotonin precede development of atherosclerosis in aorta of WHHL rabbit. Arteriosclerosis 9:195–202, 1989.

77. Yamamoto H., Bossaller C., Cartwright J.Jr., Henry P.D.: Videomicroscopic demonstration of defective cholinergic arteriolar vasodilation in atherosclerotic rabbit. J. Clin. Invest. 81:1752–1758.

78. Yanagisawa M., Kurihara H., Kimura S., Tomobe Y., Kobayashi M., Mitsui Y., Yazaki Y., Goto K., Masaki T.: A novel potent vasoconstrictor peptide produced by vascular endothelial cells. Nature 332:411–415, 1988.

13

The Role of the Endothelium in Vascular Remodeling

Victor J. Dzau, Gary H.Gibbons

Introduction

A growing body of evidence supports the concept that the vasculature is an organ capable of sensing changes within its milieu, integrating and modulating these signals by intercellular communication, and responding and adapting by the local production of various mediators that influence function as well as structure. The vasculature as an integrated organ is not only capable of short-term responses to acute stimuli, such as the autoregulatory change in tone in response to changes in perfusion pressure, but it is also capable of responding to chronic stimuli by long-term structural changes that modify function.

Because of its unique localization, the endothelium is ideally situated to sense changes within the circulation. It is capable of transducing the signals to the smooth muscle cells. In addition, the endothelium can release effector substances that mediate structural modification of the vessel wall in response to the changes in the circulation. These effector substances include growth factors, matrix proteins, and vas-

oactive substances. This chapter will examine the role of the endothelium as a signal sensor, transducer, and mediator of vascular modeling.

Endothelium as a Signal Sensor-Transducer and a Producer of Mediators in Vascular Remodeling

Alterations in hemodynamic forces, such as blood flow and pressure, should first affect the endothelium. Similarly, as the major interface with the bloodstream, the endothelium senses changes in humoral factors (e.g., hormones, vasoactive substances, serum electrolytes), which may influence vessel tone or structure. This role as sensor and transducer also extends to the inflammatory response via its interaction with endotoxins, cytokines, and inflammatory cells. Endothelial cells contain receptors, ion channels, and other membrane-bound structures that may function as sensors detecting specific

Rubanyi G.M.: Cardiovascular Significance of Endothelium-Derived Vasoactive Factors, Futura Publishing Co., Inc., Mount Kisco, NY, © 1991.

changes in the milieu and thereby triggering adaptive responses.

The endothelium responds to a variety of ligands by specific receptor-coupled events. Bradykinin, histamine, acetylcholine, ATP, platelet-activating factor, and thrombin all trigger an increase in intracellular calcium within the endothelial cell.[6,12,15,74] Indeed, many of the endothelial cell responses evoked by these ligands can also be elicited by calcium ionophores. The receptor-mediated calcium signal appears to be mediated by an activation of phospholipase C-induced hydrolysis of inositol phospholipids resulting in the generation of inositol 1,4,5-trisphosphate (IP3) and 1,2-diacylglycerol (DAG). IP3 binds to intracellular sites and causes a release of calcium into the cytoplasm whereas DAG activates protein kinase C. Thus, the calcium ion appears to play an important role in the signal transduction function of the endothelium.

There is also evidence to suggest that endothelial cells respond to humoral stimuli via activation of ion channels. Both bradykinin and acetylcholine have been reported to activate potassium channels in endothelial cells.[12,64] Similarly, platelet activating factor, histamine, and thrombin appear to activate endothelial cell ion channels.[15,41] Although there are some conflicting data, voltage-sensitive calcium channels do not appear to play a significant signal transduction role. The precise role of these signals in stimulus-secretion coupling or other functional responses is still not well defined.

Endothelial cells also respond to hemodynamic stimuli. Studies in vivo and in vitro suggest that endothelial cells increase synthesis of prostacyclin, endothelial-derived relaxing factor (EDRF), histamine, and endothelin in response to alterations in flow.[16,22,42,68,73,88] Harder and co-workers have also reported that the autoregulatory increase in vascular tone induced by increased perfusion pressure is an endothelium-dependent response in the cerebral vasculature.[31] In canine carotid arteries, pressure-induced vasoconstriction (Bayliss effect) is also mediated by the endothelium.[72] These data suggest that the endothelial cell can sense changes in flow or pressure and thereby modulate the vascular response by releasing vasoactive substances.

The precise signal-transduction pathway mediating these responses remains to be clarified. The capacity to sense pressure could be transduced by the recently described stretch-activated ion channel on endothelial cells.[48] Flowing blood exerts a tractive force on endothelial cells defined as shear stress. Endothelial cells may sense shear stress via an inwardly rectifying potassium channel recently described by Olesen et al.[65] Moreover, shear stress can also induce an increase in intracellular calcium.[1] The stimulus-secretion coupling events linking shear stress, potassium channels, intracellular calcium, and mediator release (e.g., EDRF, endothelin, etc.) have not been fully characterized. However, such a linkage can be inferred from recent studies in our laboratory in which flow-mediated release of EDRF was inhibited by pharmacological blockade of calcium-activated potassium channels.[13] These data support the postulate that hemodynamic stimuli may activate endothelial cells by signal transduction pathways similar to those employed by vasoactive agents and other agonists. Indeed, it is noteworthy that the calcium ion appears to play a central role in mediating endothelial cell activation in a variety of biological settings such as hemostasis, inflammation, or blood flow control. It is therefore less surprising that rather diverse types of stimuli result in similar secretory responses such as eicosanoid or EDRF release.[6,28,40]

In addition to sensing and transducing the signals, the endothelium can mediate or trigger the blood vessel to undergo structural and geometric changes by the transfer of these signals to underlying vascular smooth muscle by the release of effector molecules. The effector substances may be growth-promoting, growth-inhibitory, vasoactive, or extracellular matrix modulators.

Endothelium-Derived Growth Factors

The endothelium produces several growth regulatory substances that can be divided into growth-promoting or growth-inhibitory factors.

Growth-Promoting Factors

Endothelial-derived growth promoting factors include platelet-derived growth factor (PDGF), basic fibroblast growth factor (FGF), insulin-like growth factor 1 (IGF-1), and interleukin-1 (IL-1).[14,21,29,30,84] Both the A and B chains of PDGF are synthesized by the endothelium such that theoretically all three isoforms of PDGF may be produced. This may be of significance since there are two PDGF receptors, alpha and beta, which have different binding affinities for each isoform.[32] Differences in receptor isoform activation could influence the VSMC response.[5,26] Indeed, studies in our laboratory suggest that the PDGF AA homodimer is a weaker VSMC mitogen compared to the BB homodimer.[26] Production of either the AB or BB isoforms promotes VSMC migration and proliferation and may play a role in some forms of vascular remodeling.

Both the PDGF A and B chain messenger RNA levels are increased in microvascular endothelium in response to phorbol esters, thrombin, and transforming growth factor beta.[14] This response appears to be primarily due to an effect on transcription rate.[80] Increased cyclic AMP appears to block the increased transcription of PDGF B chain induced by these agents.[14] Tissue necrosis factor, interleukin-1 and endotoxin (possibly mediated by IL-1) also promote secretion of PDGF by endothelial cells.[21,29]

The regulation of IL-1, IGF-1, and FGF expression, and the role of these agents in vascular remodeling is poorly defined. IL-1 expression is increased by substances such as endotoxin. Administration of the peptide induces VSMC proliferation only during prostaglandin synthesis blockade.[52] The IL-1 proliferative response appears to be mediated by inducing autocrine production of PDGF-AA.[70] The role of IGF-1 in endothelial cells is poorly defined, but data suggest that it plays a growth-promoting role in microvascular endothelial cells.[45] Regenerating endothelium appears to express IGF-1 after balloon injury[30] and may play a role in endothelial cell migration. In the presence of growth factors such as PDGF or FGF, IGF-1 potentiates VSMC hyperplasia,[10] whereas in the absence of these competence factors it promotes hypertrophy.[51]

FGF is a potent autocrine growth factor for endothelial cells as well as a potent VSMC mitogen.[25,76] In vitro studies with neutralizing antibodies suggest that FGF plays a critical role in endothelial cell proliferation, cell migration, cell invasion, matrix alterations, and angiogenesis.[59,76] FGF-induced production of endothelial plasminogen activators appears to be important in vascular cell invasion into tissues.[59] Thrombin, phorbol esters, and FGF itself appear to increase mRNA levels of FGF in capillary endothelial cells.[86]

Growth-Inhibitory Factors

The endothelium also modulates vascular structure via the production of growth-inhibitory substances. These include heparan sulfate, TGF-β, EDRF, and prostacyclin. Campbell and others have observed that confluent endothelial cells secrete growth-inhibitory substances that appear to maintain VSMC in the most quiescent, differentiated-appearing phenotype.[7] Studies by Karnovsky and colleagues have suggested that heparan sulfate produced by endothelial cells have a growth-inhibitory effect on VSMC.[9,35] The endothelium also produces transforming growth factor beta (TGF).[2] This multifunctional growth factor has the autocrine effects of inhibiting endothelial cell proliferation and migration in some conditions but promoting angiogenesis in other circumstances.[34,71,77] TGF-beta has a bifunctional effect on VSMC in that it either inhibits mitogen-induced proliferation of VSMC or promotes hypertrophy and matrix production of quiescent VSMC.[56,66] Based on the available data, we would speculate that TGF-beta and heparan sulfate produced by the endothelium may also contribute to vascular remodeling. Factors such as TGF-beta may be particularly important in structural changes in which lumen size decreases or vessels undergo rarefaction or regression, i.e., settings in which cell involution and matrix production are important. Recent data suggest that the vasodilatory substances, EDRF and prostacyclin, are both growth inhibitors. Garg and Hassid demonstrated that nitrovasodilators and substances that mimic EDRF effect by releasing nitric oxide intracellularly are capable of inhibiting VSMC proliferation.[23] Since EDRF exerts its intracellular effect via cGMP production, we examined the effect of 8-bromo cGMP on VSMC growth. Indeed, our data showed that cGMP inhibits VSMC growth.[38] The other endothelial-derived vasodilator, prostacyclin, is also a growth inhibitor[55] that exerts its action via cAMP production. This inhibitory effect may be mediated by suppression of autocrine PDGF expression in VSMC.

Vasoactive Substances in Vascular Remodeling

Peptide growth factors such as platelet-derived growth factor (PDGF) and epidermal growth factor (EGF) have been shown to possess vasoconstrictor properties.[3,5] These data suggest that growth factors and vasoactive agents may share similar signal transduction pathways. Indeed, both vasoactive agents and several VSMC mitogens activate phospholipase C and generate IP3 and DAG in association with increased intracellular calcium and cellular alkalinization.[4] Based on these findings, it is not surprising that there is a substantial body of in vitro evidence that vasoactive substances influence VSMC growth.

Studies in our laboratory and others have shown that the vessel wall (including the endothelium) not only contains angiotensin converting enzyme activity but also renin and angiotensinogen as well.[44,53] Hence, there is a paracrine renin-angiotensin system in addition to the circulating hormonal system that may influence vascular structure. This paracrine system may modify vascular reactivity as well as modulate vascular remodeling.

In confluent quiescent vascular smooth muscle cells in culture, angiotensin II induces cellular hypertrophy.[24,61] We have shown that this hypertrophic response is in association with increased mRNA levels of protooncogenes c-fos, c-myc, and the autocrine growth factors PDGF-A chain and transforming growth factor-beta.[27,61] These autocrine growth factors may mediate angiotensin-induced hypertrophy. Angiotensin may also potentiate serum or fibroblast growth factor-induced DNA synthesis.[8,25]

These data suggest that angiotensin may modulate the proliferative response to autocrine/paracrine growth factors. Similarly, other endothelium-derived vasoactive substances also possess growth regulatory properties. We have shown that endothelin induces increased expression of c-myc in association with VSMC proliferation.[19] Growth-promoting effects of vasoconstrictors on VSMC have also been described for thromboxane, leukotrienes, substance P, and serotonin.[37,62,63,67] In contrast, vasodilators such as prostaglandins and nitrovasodilators appear to inhibit VSMC proliferation.[23,38,55] These data suggest that circulating or locally produced vasoactive substances may influence VSMC growth and thereby modulate vascular remodeling. Given that endothelial cells produce prostacyclin and nitrovasodilators, and generate angiotensin and endothelin locally, it is tempting to speculate that the endothelium may contribute to vascular remodeling by the synthesis of these potentially growth-modulating substances.

Extracellular Matrix in Vascular Remodeling

Alterations of vascular structure not only involve cellular hypertrophy, hyperplasia, or regression but must also involve the structural elements and binding elements present within the extracellular compartment of the vessel wall. The endothelium may participate in vascular remodeling by the production of extracellular matrix and proteolytic enzymes. It has become increasingly clear that these matrix proteins play an important role in modulating cell phenotype and function as well as provide structural support.[58,87] For example, the amount of fibronectin or laminin within the extracellular matrix can influence whether VSMCs in culture express a more proliferative "synthetic" phenotype versus the more quiescent "differentiated" phenotype.[7,33] Conversely, the extracellular matrix synthesized by cells in culture is modulated by the cell phenotype.[33,81] Matrix proteins such as thrombospondin are not growth factors per se but they appear to be necessary agents for mitogen-induced proliferation of VSMCs.[57] This growth-promoting role of the matrix protein thrombospondin is in contrast to the growth-inhibiting role of heparan sulfate described above.[9,35] The finding that PDGF activates gene expression of thromobospondin suggests that the

regulation of cell growth involves an interaction between autocrine/paracrine growth factors and matrix proteins.[57] Thus, matrix components produced by vascular cells can influence vascular structure by modulating cell phenotype and growth response to mitogens.

Vascular remodeling also entails changes in the mass and cell composition of the vessel wall. This process must involve a reconstruction of the matrix scaffolding and therefore a process of active proteolysis and resynthesis of these proteins. Similarly, the migration of VSMCs from the media to the subintimal space must involve a complex process of ligand-receptor binding, coupling, and proteolysis. The cytoskeletal scaffolding (e.g., actin) must change with cell movement, the points of contact with the extracellular matrix mediated by integrins and other membrane receptor proteins must change with movement, and the barrier created by the scaffolding and ground substance of the extracellular matrix must be destroyed by proteolytic action.[36,54,75]

As discussed above, vascular cells have the capacity to synthesize the collagens, glycoproteins, and proteoglycans that compose the extracellular matrix.[58,81,87] It is also apparent that these cells have the capacity to produce the proteases necessary for vascular remodeling. Endothelial cells synthesize the plasminogen activators urokinase and tissue plasminogen activator.[28,75] The inactive proenzyme plasminogen binds to the matrix and is abundant in the vasculature.[75] The plasmin produced by plasminogen activation is not only the critical protease in thrombolysis but is also capable of activating procollagenases and participating in the proteolysis of other matrix proteins. In addition to its effect on matrix proteins, plasmin also converts the latent transforming growth factor beta precursor into its active form.[77] Hence, the production of plasmin not only modifies the matrix as a result of its own proteolytic activity but also through its effect on other protease enzymes and matrix-modulating growth factors.

It is noteworthy that other agents such as FGF, thrombin, and phorbol esters also induce increased plasminogen activator synthesis by endothelial cells.[28,50,76] Indeed, it has recently been reported that shear stress stimulates the secretion of tissue plasminogen activator by endothelial cells.[18] These data suggest hemodynamic or humoral factors may modulate vascular remodeling by activating factors that regulate the proteolytic activity within the vessel wall.

The regulation of vessel wall proteolytic activity not only involves the plasminogen activator/plasmin system, but also interstitial and type IV collagenases, stromelysin, tissue inhibitor of metalloproteinases, as well as plasminogen activator inhibitor.[17,54,75,78] Vascular smooth muscle cells may modulate this proteolytic activity by secreting plasminogen activator inhibitor into the matrix.[46]

Thus, matrix proteins, cell-derived proteases, and cell-derived protease inhibitors provide a critically important element of the endothelial cell effector system modulating vascular structure. The interaction between vasoactive substances, hemodynamic stimuli, autocrine/paracrine growth factors, matrix proteins, and matrix-modulating proteases will be an area of fruitful research.

Models of Vascular Remodeling

In this section we will review several animal models in which vascular remodeling is a prominent feature and examine the potential role of the endothelium in these models.

The vasculature responds to changes in flow or shear stress. Changes in shear stress not only involve acute adaptive changes in vascular tone but also appear to modulate vascular structure. An artery exposed to increased blood flow on a chronic basis dilates over time. Given that shear stress is directly proportional to flow rate and inversely related to vessel radius, vessel dilation normalizes the wall shear stress.[43] Recently, Langille et al. provided confirmatory data by demonstrating that an artery exposed to a chronic decrease in shear stress undergoes an adaptive decrease in caliber. This response appears to be endothelium-dependent and involves alterations in the matrix and cell involution but not cell proliferation.[47] Hence, shear stress appears to be an important determinant of vascular remodeling mediated by the endothelium.

Structural alterations can be seen in the veins of patients with long-standing elevation in venous pressure or in the portal veins of patients with cirrhosis of the liver. Studies of animal models of venous hypertension such as partial portal vein ligation have described VSMC hypertrophy without hyperplasia.[83] Similarly, animal models of arterial hypertension demonstrate VSMC hypertrophy and increased matrix production within the conduit vessel walls.[39] These in vivo observations have been confirmed by in vitro models of mechanical stretch that demonstrate that VSMCs adapt to mechanical stretch by hypertrophy and increased matrix production.[49] Tozzi et al. have recently observed that in the pulmonary vasculature the induction of increased matrix production in response to mechanical stretch is an endothelium-dependent process.[82] These studies suggest that the vasculature remodels itself in response to increased intraluminal pressure transduced by the endothelium.

Another model of vascular remodeling of particular clinical relevance is the adaptation of vein grafts to the arterial circulation. Vein grafts in the arterial circulation are characterized by a process of myointimal hyperplasia which is most prominent at the site of anastomosis. The vein grafts with prominent myointimal hyperplasia also exhibit endothelial dysfunction as demonstrated by impaired EDRF release in response to acetylcholine, ADP, and thrombin.[60] Clinicians have observed that vein grafts exposed to high flow rates in the renal circulation have higher patency rates than those in other circulatory beds. In animal models, grafts that are established with a distal fistula and increased shear stress have minimal myointimal hyperplasia compared to grafts with distal stenosis and decreased flow.[20] These data suggest that the vascular remodeling of vein grafts is influenced by hemodynamic stimuli. The role of the endothelium in this process remains to be further elucidated.

Finally, the myointimal hyperplasia observed after balloon injury of an artery is another example of vascular remodeling secondary to endothelium denudation/dysfunction. In the absence of endothelium, platelets aggregate and release VSMC growth factors such as PDGF, serotonin, etc. In addition, the subintimal smooth muscle cells migrate, proliferate, and express PDGF even in the presence of a regenerated endothelium several weeks later.[82] Moreover, the regenerated endothelium is dysfunctional, as documented by impaired EDRF release.[13] We would speculate that the dysfunctional endothelium may produce less growth inhibitory mediators such as nitric oxide, prostaglandins, heparan sulfate, and TGF-beta and/or increased growth promoting factors such as FGF, PDGF, and IGF-1. The regenerated endothelium may also participate in the proteolysis and resynthesis of the matrix to promote VSMC invasion into the subintimal space. It is intriguing to note that three factors appear to inhibit myointimal hyperplasia in vivo: shear stress, heparin, and angiotensin converting enzyme inhibitors.[11,20,69,85] The importance of the endothelium in the remodeling process can be inferred from the fact that these three factors are either transduced or synthesized by the endothelium. These observations are consistent with the hypothesis that endothelial denudation/dysfunction results in an imbalance of inhibitory and stimulatory forces that promote VSMC proliferation and migration. We speculate that future developments in effective therapy of myointimal hyperplasia may involve the enhancement of growth-inhibitory mediators (e.g., heparin) or the blockade of growth-promoting mediators (e.g., angiotensin II).

In summary, the endothelium appears to play an important role in vascular remodeling by detecting changes in humoral or hemodynamic conditions within the circulation, by transducing the signals to the underlying blood vessel wall and by the production of mediators which modify vascular structure. An alteration in endothelial function may promote adaptive changes in vascular structure that may assume pathophysiological significance such as myointimal hyperplasia.

Acknowledgment: This work is supported by NIH grants HL35610, HL35792, HL19259, HL35252, HL43131, HL42663, and NIH Specialized Center of Research in Hypertension HL36568. Dr. Gary Gibbons is a recipient of a Robert Wood Johnson Foundation Minority Faculty Development Fellowship. The authors wish to thank Ms. Donna MacDonald for her expert secretarial assistance.

References

1. Ando J., Komatsuda T., Kamiya A.: Cytoplasmic calcium response to fluid shear stress in cultured vascular endothelial cells. In Vitro 24:871–877, 1988.
2. Antonelli-Orlidge A., Saunders K.B., Smith S., D'Amore P.A.: An activated form of transforming growth factor-beta is produced by cocultures of endothelial cells and pericytes. Proc. Natl. Acad. Sci. USA 86:4544–4548, 1989.
3. Berk B.C., Brock T.A., Webb R.C., Taubman M.B., Atkinson W.J., Gimbrone M.A.,

Alexander R.W.: Epidermal growth factor, a vascular smooth muscle mitogen, induces rat aortic contraction. J. Clin. Invest. 75:1083–1086, 1985.

4. Berk B.C., Brock T.A., Gimbrone M.A., Alexander R.W.: Early agonist-mediated ionic events in cultured vascular smooth muscle cells: calcium mobilization is associated with intracellular acidification. J. Biol. Chem. 262:5065–5072, 1987.

5. Block L.H., Emmans L.R., Vogt E., Sachinidis A., Vetter W., Hoppe J.: Ca^{2+} channel blockers inhibit the action of recombinant platelet-derived growth factor in vascular smooth muscle cells. Proc. Natl. Acad. Sci. USA 86:2388–2392, 1989.

6. Brock T.A., Capasso E.A.: Thrombin and histamine activate phospholipase C in human endothelial cells via a phorbol ester-sensitive pathway. J. Cell Physiol. 136:54–62, 1988.

7. Campbell J.H., Campbell G.R.: Endothelial cell influences on vascular smooth muscle phenotype. Annu. Rev. Physiol. 48:295–306, 1986.

8. Campbell-Boswell M., Robertson A.L.: Effects of angiotensin II and vasopressin on human smooth muscle cells in vitro. Exp. Mol. Pathol. 35:265–276, 1981.

9. Castellot J.J., Farreau L.T., Karnovsky M.J., Rosenberg R.D.: Inhibition of vascular smooth muscle cell growth by endothelial cell-derived heparin: possible role of a platelet endoglycosidase. J. Biol. Chem. 257:11256–11260, 1982.

10. Clemmons D.R.: Interaction of circulating cell-derived and plasma growth factors in stimulating cultured smooth muscle cell replication. J. Cell. Physiol. 121:425–430, 1984.

11. Clowes A.W., Clowes M.M. Kinetics of cellular proliferation after arterial injury. IV. Heparin inhibits rat smooth muscle mitogenesis and migration. Circ. Res. 58:839–845, 1986.

12. Colden-Stanfield M., Schilling W.P., Ritchie A.K., Eskin S.G., Navarro L.T., Kunze D.L.: Bradykinin-induced increases in cytosolic calcium and ionic currents in cultured bovine aortic endothelial cells. Circ. Res. 61:632–640, 1987.

13. Cooke J.P., Rossitch E. Jr., Andon N., Loscalzo J., Dzau V.J.: Flow activates a specific endothelial potassium channel to release an endogenous nitrovasodilator. J. Am. Coll. Cardiol. 15:1A. 1990.

14. Daniel T.O., Gibbs V.C., Milfay D.F., Williams L.T.: Agents that increase cAMP ac-cumulation block endothelial c-sis induction by thrombin and transforming growth factor-B. J. Biol. Chem. 262:11893–11896, 1987.

15. Danthuluri N.R., Cybulsky M.I., Brock T.A.: Ach-induced calcium transients in primary cultures of rabbit aortic endothelial cells. Am. J. Physiol. 255:H1549-H1553, 1988.

16. DeForrest J.M., Hollis T.M.: Shear stress and aortic histamine synthesis. Am. J. Physiol. 234:H701-H705, 1978.

17. Delvos V., Gajdusek C., Sage H., Harker L.A., Schwartz S.M.: Interactions of vascular wall cells with collagen gels. Lab. Invest. 46:61–72, 1982.

18. Diamond S.E., Eskin S.G., McIntire I.V.: Fluid flow stimulates tissue plasminogen activator secretion by cultured human endothelial cells. Science 243:1483–1485, 1989.

19. Dubin D., Pratt R.E., Cooke J.P., Dzau V.J.: Endothelin, a potent vasoconstrictor is a vascular smooth muscle mitogen. J. Vasc. Med. Biol. 1:150–154, 1989.

20. Faulkner S.L., Fisher R.D., Conkle D.M., Page D.L., Bender H.W. Effect of blood flow rate on subendothelial proliferation in venous autografts used as arterial substitutes. Circulation 51/52 (Suppl. I)I-163-I-172, 1975.

21. Fox P.L., DiCorleto P.E.: Regulation of production of a platelet-derived growth factor-like protein by cultured bovine aortic endothelial cells. J. Cell. Physiol. 121:298–308, 1984.

22. Frangos V.A., Eskin S.G., McIntire L.V., Ives C.L.: Flow effects on prostacyclin production by cultured human endothelial cells. Science 227:1477–1479, 1985.

23. Garg U.C., Hassid A.: Nitric oxide-generating vasodilators and 8-bromo-cyclic guanosine monophosphate inhibit mitogenesis and proliferation of cultured rat vascular smooth muscle cells. J. Clin. Invest. 83:1774–1777, 1989.

24. Geisterfer A.A.T., Peach M.J., Owens G.K.: Angiotensin II induces hypertrophy, not hyperplasia, of cultured rat aortic smooth muscle cells. Circ. Res. 62:749–756, 1988.

25. Gibbons G.H., Pratt R.E., Dzau V.J.: Angiotensin II is a bifunctional vascular smooth muscle cell growth factor. Hypertension 14:358, 1989.

26. Gibbons G.H., Pratt R.E., Dzau V.J.: Platelet-derived growth factor isoforms differ in mitogenic effect on adult vascular smooth muscle cells. Circulation 80(Suppl. II):II-93, 1989.

27. Gibbons G.H., Pratt R.E., Dzau V.J.: Transforming growth factor-beta expression modulates the bifunctional response of vascular smooth muscle cell to angiotensin. Clin. Res. 38:287, 1990.

28. Gross J.L., Moscatelli D., Jaffe E.A., Rifkin D.B.: Plasminogen activator and collagenase production by cultured capillary endothelial cells. J. Cell Biol. 95:974–981, 1982.

29. Hajjar K.A., Hajjar D.P., Silverstein R.L., Nachman R.L.: Tumor necrosis factor-mediated release of platelet-derived growth factor from cultured endothelial cells. J. Exp. Med. 166:235–245, 1987.

30. Hansson H.-A., Jennische E., Skottner A.: Regenerating endothelial cells express insulin like growth factor-1 immunoreactivity after arterial injury. Cell Tissue Res. 250:499–505, 1987.

31. Harder D.R.: Pressure-induced myogenic activation of cat cerebral arteries is dependent on intact endothelium. Circ. Res. 60:102–107, 1987.

32. Hart C.E., Forstrom J.W., Kelly J.D., Seifert R.A., Smith R.A., Ross R., Murray M.J., Bowen-Pope D.F.: Two classes of PDGF receptor recognize different isoforms of PDGF. Science 240:1529–1531, 1988.

33. Hedin U., Bottger B.A., Forsberg E., Johansson S., Thyberg J.: Diverse effects of fibronectin and laminin on phenotypic properties of cultured arterial smooth muscle cells. J. Cell Biol. 107:307–319, 1988.

34. Heimark R.L., Twardzik D.R., Schwartz S.M.: Inhibition of endothelial regeneration by type-beta transforming growth factor from platelets. Science 233:1078–1080, 1986.

35. Hoover R.L., Rosenberg R., Haering W., Karnovsky M.J.: Inhibition of rat arterial smooth muscle cell proliferation by heparin: II in vitro studies. Circ. Res. 47:578–583, 1980.

36. Hynes R.O.: Integrins: a family of cell surface receptors. Cell 48:549–554, 1987.

37. Ishimitsu T., Uehara Y., Ishii M., Ikeda T., Matsuoka H., Sugimoto T.: Thromboxane and vascular smooth muscle cell growth in genetically hypertensive rats. Hypertension 12:46–51, 1988.

38. Itoh H., Pratt R.E., Dzau V.J.: Growth inhibitory action of atrial natriuretic polypeptide on vascular smooth muscle cell: new antagonistic relationship to the renin-angiotensin system. Clin. Res. 38:239A, 1990.

39. Iwatsuki K., Cardinale G.J., Spector S., Udenfriend S.: Hypertension: increase of collagen biosynthesis in arteries but not in veins. Science 198:403–405, 1977.

40. Jaffe E.A., Grulich J., Weksler B.B., Hampel G., Watanabe K.: Correlation between thrombin-induced prostacyclin production and inositol-triphosphate and cytosolic free calcium level in cultured human endothelial cells. J. Biol. Chem. 262:8557–8565, 1987.

41. Johns A., Lategan T.W., Lodge N.J., Ryan U.S., Van Breeman C., Adams D.J.: Calcium entry through receptor-operated channels in bovine pulmonary artery endothelial cells. Tissue Cell 19:733–745, 1987.

42. Kaiser L., Hull S.S., Sparks H.V.: Methylene blue and ETYA block flow-dependent dilation in canine femoral artery. Am. J. Physiol. 250:H974-H987, 1986.

43. Kamiya A., Togawa T.: Adaptive regulation of wall shear stress to flow change in the canine carotid artery. Am. J. Physiol. 239:H14-H21, 1980.

44. Kifor I., Dzau V.J.: Endothelial renin-angiotensin pathway: evidence for intracellular synthesis and secretion of angiotensins. Circ. Res. 60:422–428, 1987.

45. King G.L., Goodman A.D., Buzney S., Moses A., Kahn C.R.: Receptors and growth-promoting effects of insulin and insulin-like growth factors on cells from bovine retinal capillaries and aorta. J. Clin. Invest. 75:1028–1036, 1985.

46. Knudsen B.S., Harpel P.C., Nachman R.L.: Plasminogen activator inhibitor is associated with the extracellular matrix of cultured bovine smooth muscle cells. J. Clin. Invest. 80:1082–1089, 1987.

47. Langille B.L., Bendeck M.P., Keeley F.W.: Adaptations of carotid arteries of young and mature rabbits to reduced carotid blood flow. Am. J. Physiol. 256:H931-H939, 1989.

48. Lansman J.B., Hallam TJ., Rink T.J.: Single stretch-activated ion channels in vascular endothelial cells as mechanotransducers? Nature 325:811–813, 1987.

49. Leung D.Y.M., Glagov S., Mathews M.B. Cyclic stretching stimulates synthesis of matrix components by arterial smooth muscle cells in vitro. Science 191:475–477, 1986.

50. Levin E.G., Marzec U., Anderson J., Harker L.A.: Thrombin stimulates tissue plasminogen activation release from cultured human endothelial cells. J. Clin. Invest. 74:1988–1995, 1984.

51. Libby P., O'Brien K.L.: Culture of quiescent arterial smooth muscle cells in a defined serum-free medium. J. Cell. Physiol. 115:217–223, 1983.

52. Libby P., Warner S.J.C., Friedman G.B.: In-

terleukin 1: a mitogen for human vascular smooth muscle cells that induces the release of growth inhibitory prostanoids. J. Clin. Invest. 81:487–498, 1988.

53. Lilly L.S., Pratt R.E., Alexander R.W., Larson D.M., Ellison K.E., Gimbrone M.A., Dzau V.J.: Renin expression by vascular endothelial cells in culture. Circ. Res. 57:312–218, 1985.

54. Liotta L.A., Rao C.N., Wewer U.M.: Biochemical interactions of tumor cells with the basement membrane. Annu. Rev. Biochem. 55:1037–1057, 1986.

55. Loesberg C., Wijk R.V., Zandbergen J., Van Aken W.G., Van Mourik J.A., DeGroot Ph.G.: Cell cycle-dependent inhibition of human vascular smooth muscle cell proliferation by prostaglandin E_1. Exp. Cell Res. 160:117–125, 1985.

56. Majack R.A.: Beta type transforming growth factor specifies organizational behavior in vascular smooth muscle cultures. J. Cell Biol. 105:465–471, 1987.

57. Majack R.A., Goodman L.V., Dixot V.M.: Cell surface thrombospondin is functionally essential for vascular smooth muscle cell proliferation. J. Cell Biol. 106:415–422, 1988.

58. Mayne R.: Collagenous proteins of blood vessels. Arteriosclerosis 6:585–593, 1986.

59. Mignatti P., Tsuboi R., Robbins E., Rifkin D.B.: In vitro angiogenesis on the human amniotic membrane: requirement for basic fibroblast growth factor-induced proteinases. J. Cell Biol. 108:671–682, 1989.

60. Miller V.M., Reigel M.M., Hollier L.H., Vanhoutte A.M.: Endothelium-dependent responses in autogenous femoral veins grafted into the arterial circulation of the dog. J. Clin. Invest. 80:1350–1357, 1987.

61. Naftilan A.I., Pratt R.E., Dzau V.J.: Induction of platelet-derived growth factor A-chain and c-myc gene expressions by angiotensin II in cultured rat vascular smooth muscle cells. J. Clin. Invest. 83:1419–1424, 1989.

62. Nemecek G.M., Coughlin S.R., Handley D.A., Moskowitz M.A.: Stimulation of aortic smooth muscle cell mitogenesis by serotonin. Proc. Natl. Acad. Sci. USA 83:674–678, 1986.

63. Nilsson J., von Euler A.M., Dalsgaard C.-J.: Stimulation of connective tissue cell growth by substance P and substance K. Nature 315:61–63, 1985.

64. Olesen S.-P., Davies P.F., Clapham D.E.: Muscarinic-activated K^+ current in bovine aortic endothelial cells. Circ. Res. 62:1059–1064, 1988.

65. Olesen S.-P., Clapham D.E., Davies P.F.: Hemodynamic shear stress activates a K+ current in vascular endothelial cells. Nature 331:168–170, 1988.

66. Owens G.K., Geisterfer A.A.T., Yang Y.W.-H., Komoriya A.: Transforming growth factor B-induced growth inhibition and cellular hypertrophy in cultured vascular smooth muscle cells. J. Cell Biol. 107:771–780, 1988.

67. Palmberg L., Claesson H.-E., Thyberg J.: Leukotrienes stimulate initiation of DNA synthesis in cultured arterial smooth muscle cells. J. Cell Sci. 88:151–159, 1987.

68. Pohl U., Holtz J., Busse R., Bassenge E.: Crucial role of endothelium in the vasodilator response to increased flow in vivo. Hypertension 8:37–44, 1986.

69. Powell J.S., Clozel J.-P., Muller R.K.M., Kuhn H., Hefti F., Hosang M., Baumgartner H.R.: Inhibitors of angiotensin-converting enzyme prevent myointimal proliferation after vascular injury. Science 245:186–188, 1989.

70. Raines E.W., Dower S.K, Ross R.: Interleukin-1 mitogenic activity for fibroblasts and smooth muscle cells is due to PDGF-AA. Science 243:393–395, 1989.

71. Roberts A.B., Sporn M.B., Assoian R.K., Smith J.M., Roche N.S., Wakefield L.M., Heine U.I., Liotta L.A., et al.: Transforming growth factor type beta: rapid induction of fibrosis and angiogenesis in vivo and stimulation of collagen formation in vitro. Proc. Natl. Acad. Sci. USA 83:4167–4171, 1986.

72. Rubanyi G.M.: Endothelium-dependent pressure-induced contraction of isolated carotid arteries. Am. J. Physiol. 255(Pt.2):H783-H788, 1988.

73. Rubanyi G.M., Romero J.C., Vanhoutte P.M.: Flow-induced release of endothelium-derived relaxing factor. Am. J. Physiol. 250 (Pt. 2):H1145-H1149, 1986.

74. Ryan U.S.: Endothelium as a transducing surface. J. Mol. Cell Cardiol. 2l(Suppl. 1):85–90, 1989.

75. Saksela O., Rifkin D.B.: Cell-associated plasminogen activation: regulation and physiological functions. Annu. Rev. Cell Biol. 4:93–126, 1988.

76. Sato Y., Rifkin D.B.: Autocrine activities of basic fibroblast growth factor: regulation of endothelial cell movement, plasminogen activator synthesis, and DNA synthesis. J. Cell Biol. 107:1199–205, 1988.

77. Sato Y., Rifkin D.B.: Inhibition of endothelial cell movement by pericytes and smooth muscle cells: activation of a latent trans-

forming growth factor-beta 1-like molecule by plasmin during co-culture. J. Cell Biol. 109:309–315, 1989.

78. Sawdey M., Podor T.J., Loskutoff D.J.: Regulation of type 1 plasminogen activator inhibitor gene expression in cultured bovine aortic endothelial cells. J. Biol. Chem. 264:10396–10401, 1989.

79. Vanhoutte P.M., Shimokawa H.: Endothelium-derived relaxing factor and coronary vasospasm. Circulation 80:1–9, 1989.

80. Starksen N.F., Harsh G.R., Gibbs V.C., Williams L.T.: Regulated expression of the platelet-derived growth factor A chain gene in microvascular endothelial cells. J. Biol. Chem. 262:14381–14384, 1987.

81. Stepp M.A., Kindy M.S., Franzblau C., Sonenshein G.E.: Complex regulation of collagen gene expression in cultured bovine aortic smooth muscle cells. J. Biol. Chem. 261:6542–6547, 1986.

82. Tozzi C.A., Poiani G.J., Harangozo A.M., Boyd C.D., Riley D.J. Pressure-induced connective tissue synthesis in pulmonary artery segments is dependent on intact endothelium. J. Clin. Invest. 84:1005–1012, 1989.

83. Uvelius B., Arner A., Johansson B.: Structural and mechanical alterations in hyper-trophic venous smooth muscle. Acta Physiol. Scand. 112:463–471, 1981.

84. Vlodavsky I., Folkman J., Sullivan R., Fridman R., Ishai-Michaeli R., Sasse J., Klagsbrun M.: Endothelial cell-derived basic fibroblast growth factor: synthesis and deposition into subendothelial extracellular matrix. Proc. Natl. Acad. Sci. 84:2292–2296, 1987.

85. Walker L.N., Bowen-Pope D.F., Reidy M.A.: Production of platelet-derived growth factor-like molecules by cultured arterial smooth muscle cells accompanies proliferation after arterial injury. Proc. Natl. Acad. Sci. USA 83:7311–7315, 1986.

86. Welch H.A., Iberg N., Klagsbrun M., Folkman J.: Transcriptional regulation of the gene of basic fibroblast growth factor in capillary endothelial cells. J. Cell Biochem. Suppl. 14E:205, 1990.

87. Wight T.N.: Proteoglycans in pathological conditions: atherosclerosis. Fed. Proc. 44:381–385, 1985.

88. Yoshizumi M., Korihara H., Sugiyama T., Takaku F., Yanagisawa M., Masaki T., Yazaki Y.: Hemodynamic shear stress stimulates endothelin production by cultured endothelial cells. Biochem. Biophys. Res. Commun. 161:859–864, 1989.

14

Platelets, Thrombosis, and the Endothelium

M.J. Lewis, J.A. Smith

Introduction

Endothelium, as well as having an important role in the regulation of vascular smooth muscle tone, also acts as an important modulator of interactions between platelets and the underlying vascular smooth muscle.[106] Endothelium also plays a crucial role in maintaining a balance between pro- and antiaggregatory influences on platelets to prevent inappropriate thrombotic events in the circulation. Some of the pro- and antiaggregatory properties of endothelium are summarized in Table 1.

Normally, the endothelium presents a nonthrombogenic surface to blood. The mechanisms responsible for this feature of endothelial function are, however, poorly understood. The anionic charge presented by the glycocalyx of the endothelium is thought to play a major role, though heparan sulphate; prostacyclin (PGI$_2$) and more recently endothelium-derived relaxing factor (EDRF) have also been implicated. The remainder of this chapter will concentrate on the antiplatelet properties of PGI$_2$ and in particular of EDRF.

Prostacyclin

The principal role of PGI$_2$ as an antithrombogenic agent is in the inhibition of platelet aggregation. The source of PGI$_2$ is mainly endothelial cells, though vascular smooth muscle can also synthesize it from prostaglandin endoperoxides released from platelets.[101] It is the most potent endogenous inhibitor of platelet aggregation yet discovered being 30–40 times more potent than PGE$_1$[72] and about 1000 times more potent than adenosine.[4] It also has two other properties that may contribute to its antithrombogenic role. It can disaggregate platelets that have already aggregated[43,72,98,104] and it can inhibit platelet adhesion to a variety of surfaces.[19,110]

It is unlikely that PGI$_2$ contributes significantly to the inhibition of platelet adhesion to endothelium (or subendothelium if exposed) in vivo. Compared with its antiaggregatory properties, PGI$_2$ is a relatively poor inhibitor of platelet adhesion.[51] Basal production of PGI$_2$ by endothelium is very low[111] and the presence of red blood

Rubanyi G.M.: Cardiovascular Significance of Endothelium-Derived Vasoactive Factors, Futura Publishing Co., Inc., Mount Kisco, NY, © 1991.

Table 1

Pro- and Anti-Aggregatory Properties of Endothelium

Antithrombotic Properties	Prothrombotic Properties
Heparan sulphate	Von-Willebrand
Thombomodulin	Factor
Antithrombin III	Factor VIII
Protein S	Factor V
Ectonucleotidases	Platelet-activating
Prostacyclin	factor
Endothelium-derived	Thromboplastin
relaxing factor	Thrombospondin
Activates Protein C	Fibronectin
with antithrombin	Binds factors IXa,
III, inactivates	VIIa, and high MW
thrombin	kinogen
	Activates Hageman
	factor

cells in vivo, which strongly bind PGI_2[118] make it unlikely that PGI_2 contributes significantly to the prevention of platelet adhesion to the vessel wall. Studies by several groups have confirmed this view.[1,20,23]

The most important functions of PGI_2 seem, therefore, to be inhibition of intravascular platelet aggregation and the disaggregation of already formed aggregates. Since the basal production of PGI_2 by endothelium is low and circulatory levels in rabbits[46] and man[9,49] are below those necessary to inhibit aggregation, it seems likely that the effect of PGI_2 becomes important only when platelets start to aggregate. Under these conditions, the endothelium is stimulated to release PGI_2 by several products of the platelet release-reaction, e.g., ATP, ADP, 5HT, and of course thrombin from the coagulation cascade. Each of these products (and many more derived from tissue damage) acting through PGI_2 thus limit further platelet aggregation and thrombus formation.

The mechanism of action of PGI_2 on platelets is through stimulation of adenylate cyclase via specific cell surface receptors, leading to an increase in cyclic AMP.[41,71,102,112] The mechanism of action of cyclic AMP in platelets has not been clearly identified, however. It has been known for several years that it inhibits the formation of diacylglycerol in platelets activated by thrombin[55,87] and more recently to decrease inositol trisphosphate formation.[109] These effects are thought to be attributable to an indirect inhibition of phospholipase C through the ability of cyclic AMP to sequester intracellular Ca^{++},[58] though a direct effect of cyclic AMP on the activation of phospholipase C has been suggested, but not confirmed.[8] More recently, an effect of cyclic AMP at the level of G-proteins has been suggested.[44] It is probable, therefore, that cyclic AMP exerts its inhibitory activity at more than one level in the platelet (Fig. 1B). These effects of cyclic AMP are almost certainly the result of phosphorylation of specific intracellular proteins through the action of protein kinase A, though the proteins involved have yet to be identified.

Endothelium-Derived Relaxing Factor

Since the first description of endothelium-dependent relaxation by Furchgott and Zawadski in 1980,[34] it has become apparent that as well as being a potent inhibitor of vascular smooth muscle contraction, EDRF also possesses platelet inhibitory properties.

With hindsight, it might have been expected that EDRF would act as an inhibitor of platelet aggregation since it was shown as long ago as 1972 that sodium nitroprusside (which like EDRF stimulates soluble guanylate cyclase and increases intracellular cyclic GMP) was a potent platelet disaggregatory agent.[80] This was followed in 1974 by the demonstration that nitroprusside inhibited platelet aggregation induced by a variety of agents.[38] These original observations were later confirmed by Saxon

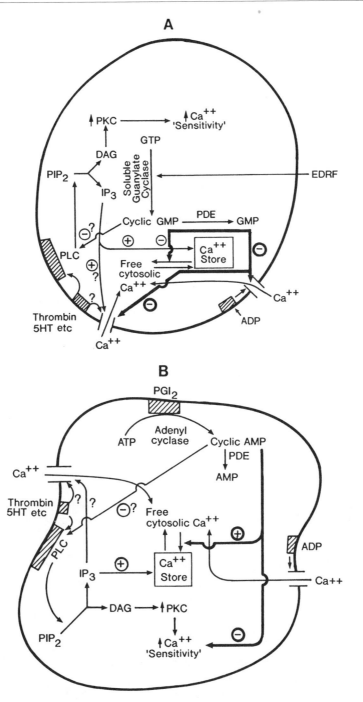

Figure 1: Proposed scheme for possible mechanisms of action of cyclic GMP (A) and cyclic AMP (B) in platelets. From the presently available data, it appears that the principal effect of cyclic GMP is inhibition of Ca^{++} influx and mobilization. The principal effects of cyclic AMP are probably reduction of intracellular Ca^{++} sequestration. Major effects of both cyclic nucleotides are shown by bold lines. PDE = phosphodiesterase; PKC = protein kinase C; PIP_2 = phosphatidylinositol 4,5-bisphosphate; PLC = phospholipase C; DAG = diacylglycerol; IP_3 = inositol 1,4,5-trisphosphate.

and Kattlove in 1976.[89] The involvement of cyclic GMP in the platelet response to sodium nitroprusside and other nitrovasodilators was demonstrated for the first time by Haslam and colleagues in 1978[45] and later by Mellion and co-workers.[70]

In 1986, Azuma and co-workers[5] reported that EDRF inhibited in vitro platelet aggregation. However, the published data do not exclude a contribution to inhibition of aggregation by PGI_2. In the study by Furlong and colleagues,[35] however, the effect of PGI_2 and other prostanoids was excluded by inclusion of a cyclooxygenase inhibitor in the experiments. These original observations have subsequently been confirmed by several other groups.[3,7,12,14,48,81]

That EDRF can act as an inhibitor of platelet aggregation when its release is stimulated in vivo was first demonstrated by Hogan and colleagues in 1988.[52] In this study, EDRF release was stimulated in vivo with carbachol, and platelet aggregation (whole blood) was induced by the ex vivo addition of ADP. More recently, EDRF has been shown to inhibit the ADP-induced accumulation of radiolabeled platelet aggregates in the pulmonary circulation of anesthetized rats.[7]

The antiaggregatory action of EDRF has now been attributed to nitric oxide. That EDRF is nitric oxide (or a nitric oxide-containing moiety) was first suggested by both Furchgott and Ignarro in 1986 at the fourth meeting of "Mechanisms of Vasodilatation" held in Rochester, Minnesota, in 1986. The proceedings of this meeting were subsequently published in 1988.[33,34] Final confirmation that the actions of EDRF were due to nitric oxide was provided by Palmer and co-workers in 1987.[78] The platelet antiaggregatory actions of nitric oxide were first demonstrated in 1981[70] and have subsequently been confirmed by several groups.[64,81,82]

Although EDRF (and therefore nitric oxide) has important antiaggregatory properties, its role in vivo as a platelet an-

tiadhesive agent may under normal physiological conditions be its more important action. The ability of EDRF to prevent platelets adhering to endothelial cells, collagen, and endothelial cell matrix was first shown by Radomski and co-workers[83,84] and later confirmed by Sneddon and colleagues.[97] PGI_2 also has antiadhesive properties, but as mentioned earlier, it is much less potent in this respect than as an antiaggregatory agent. EDRF (i.e., nitric oxide) on the other hand can completely inhibit adhesion of washed human platelets to collagen at a concentration of 10 μM, compared with PGI_2 which showed only about 25% inhibition at this concentration.[84] This action of EDRF may be important in vivo in the prevention of platelet adherence to vessel walls. The local concentration of EDRF is likely to be much higher at the vessel wall than in the lumen. This is because of the presence of the haptoglobin-hemoglobin complex and red blood cells, both of which act as "sinks" for EDRF; hence its concentration will be very low away from the vessel wall.[30,31] EDRF may therefore be viewed as acting as a "lubricant" in the circulation, preventing platelets adhering to vessel walls and the formation of platelet emboli with their consequences.

Synergism between sodium nitroprusside and PGI_2 to inhibit platelet aggregation was shown originally by Levin and colleagues in 1982.[61] Similarly, PGI_2 has been shown to potentiate the antiaggregating and disaggregating activity of both EDRF and nitric oxide.[4,82] Unexpectedly perhaps, the platelet antiadhesive properties of nitric oxide do not appear to be potentiated by PGI_2.[84]

The platelet inhibitory properties of nitric oxide (EDRF and nitrovasodilators) is now known to be due to activation of platelet-soluble guanylate cyclase and elevation of intracellular cyclic GMP. In this respect, its mechanism in platelets is identical to its mechanism of action in vascular smooth muscle. The association of the antiaggregatory properties of sodium nitro-prusside with an elevation of cyclic GMP was noticed as long ago as 1978.[45] That this was due to nitric oxide was not recognized, however, until much later in 1981.[70] These workers suggested that nitric oxide was the active species of several nitrovasodilators and was the agent responsible for the in-hibition of platelet aggregation through stimulation of soluble guanylate cyclase and elevation of cyclic GMP. That EDRF directly stimulates soluble guanylate cy-clase was first shown by Forstermann and colleagues.[32]

The mechanism(s) by which cyclic GMP exerts its antiaggregatory and an-tiadhesion effects on platelets is by no means clear. In contrast to the mechanism of cyclic GMP in vascular smooth muscle, few studies have addressed this question in platelets. In vascular smooth muscle, cyclic GMP has several actions (for review see ref. 62), including reduction of Ca^{++} sensitivity of the contractile proteins;[79] in-hibition of Ca^{++} influx and intracellular Ca^{++} release,[17] reduction of phosphati-dylinositol hydrolysis[85] and inositol tri-phosphate generation,[59] increased Ca^{++} extrusion by the sarcolemma,[86,108] and in-creased Ca^{++} sequestration by the sarco-plasmic reticulum.[103]

Takai and colleagues demonstrated an inhibitory action of cyclic GMP on throm-bin-induced phosphatidylinositol turnover and protein phosphorylation in platelets,[99] similar to that shown in vascular smooth muscle.[59,85] They later showed that in the presence of raised cyclic GMP levels, these thrombin-stimulated events were associ-ated with phosphorylation of a range of other cell proteins with molecular weights ranging from 22,000 to 240,000. They con-cluded that cyclic GMP acts as an indirect inhibitor of protein kinase C activation by inhibition of receptor-linked phosphati-dylinositol breakdown, probably through the actions of cyclic nucleotide-dependent protein kinases.[100] A more recent study by Nakashima and co-workers[75] showed sim-

ilar findings of reduced thrombin-stimu-lated phosphatidylinositol breakdown in the presence of 8-bromo cyclic GMP which was associated with reduced inositol tris-phosphate formation and reduced levels of intracellular Ca^{++}. This group concluded that cyclic GMP acted to reduce receptor-activated stimulation of phospholipase C. A similar inhibitory effect of EDRF on thrombin-induced increase in platelet in-tracellular Ca^{++} has recently been shown by Busse and colleagues,[14] confirming ear-lier studies with nitroprusside showing an inhibition of both Ca^{++} influx and mobi-lization in response to thrombin[56,75] and platelet-activating factor.[65]

The action of cyclic GMP on inhibi-tion of phospholipase C stimulation and protein kinase C activation has recently been suggested to be secondary to a reduction of Ca^{++} influx rather than a primary event. This conclusion comes from the studies of Marie-Françoise and colleagues[66] and Morgan and Newby[74] who showed that elevation of platelet cyclic GMP with nitroprusside or Sin-1, the active metabolite of molsidomine, resulted in a greater inhibition of Ca^{++} influx than of intracellular Ca^{++} mobilization. The study by Marie-Françoise and co-workers further showed that maximum inhibition of receptor-operated phospholipase C ac-tivation occurred only in the presence of extracellular Ca^{++}, indicating that the ef-fect of phospholipase C was secondary to inhibition of Ca^{++} influx.

It is unlikely that cyclic GMP affects the sensitivity of platelets to Ca^{++} since platelet responses to the calcium iono-phore, ionomycin, or phorbol ester are un-affected by elevation of cyclic GMP.[74] Fur-thermore, cyclic GMP has been shown not to decrease the sensitivity to Ca^{++} of stim-ulated permeabilized platelets.[58] There is also evidence that cyclic GMP has no part to play in the regulation of Ca^{++} extrusion or sequestration in platelets since it failed to affect ionomycin-induced rises in intra-cellular Ca^{++} concentration.[74]

Thus, from presently available data, it appears that the principal effect of cyclic GMP in platelets is inhibition of Ca^{++} influx and mobilization (Fig. 1A). It is possible, but by no means proven, that the marked antiadhesion effects of cyclic GMP in platelets can be related to its effect on Ca^{++} influx, whereas the potent antiaggregatory effects of cyclic AMP are related to its ability to increase Ca^{++} sequestration[114] and to reduce intracellular Ca^{++} sensitivity in platelets.[47]

Although EDRF is undoubtedly the major source of nitric oxide in the circulation, it is perhaps worthwhile mentioning that two other sources of nitric oxide are available in blood that may influence platelet activity, namely macrophages and neutrophils.[50,68] The role of macrophage-generated nitric oxide in influencing platelet responses remains unclear at present but recent work with neutrophils has clearly shown that platelet aggregation can be markedly inhibited by neutrophil-derived nitric oxide.[68] The exact biological role of neutrophil-derived nitric oxide remains unknown at present, however. Perhaps it plays a role in regulating the concentration of superoxide anion produced by neutrophils since nitric oxide and superoxide anions interact chemically. It is unlikely that nitric oxide has any direct effect in regulating neutrophil function, however, since 8-bromo cyclic GMP, nitric oxide, and nitrovasodilators have no effect on superoxide anion production by neutrophils [15] (Evans H.G., Lewis M.J. unpublished observations).

Pathophysiology

No review on platelets and endothelium would be complete without a brief mention of their role in the pathophysiological mechanisms of vascular diseases.

Under normal physiological conditions, both PGI_2 and EDRF will act to inhibit intravascular platelet aggregation and adhesion to vessel walls.

In experimental models and in some cases man, diseases like atheroma, diabetes, hypertension, and aging, and in situations where endothelium has been removed as in angioplasty, or where areas of damaged endothelium have regenerated, all result in reduced endothelium-dependent relaxations and in some instances release of EDRF.[16,24,37,63,77,91,92,95,105,107] In such situations, it is likely that intravascular platelet aggregates will develop and that platelets will adhere to the damaged endothelium or the underlying exposed collagen. Platelet activation will in turn release ADP, ATP, 5-hydroxytryptamine, and thromboxane A_2, each of which will promote further aggregation and constriction of the underlying vascular smooth muscle. At the edge of the endothelial damage or loss, however, these substances will promote the release of EDRF and PGI_2, which will result in local inhibition of further platelet adhesion, aggregation, and vasodilatation (for review, see reference 106). The endothelium thus acts to localize the platelet response to the damaged area, preventing intravascular coagulation and vasoconstriction downstream from the damaged are (Fig. 2).

Therapeutic Implications and Speculations

The beneficial use of drugs like aspirin, dipyridamole, and PGI_2 that suppress platelet aggregation has been proven in a variety of conditions where platelet aggregation is thought to play a major pathophysiological role, e.g., unstable angina, myocardial infarction, thrombotic complications of artificial heart valves, cardiopulmonary bypass, hemodialysis etc (for review, see reference 36). The possible therapeutic benefits resulting from manipulation of platelet cyclic GMP levels, how-

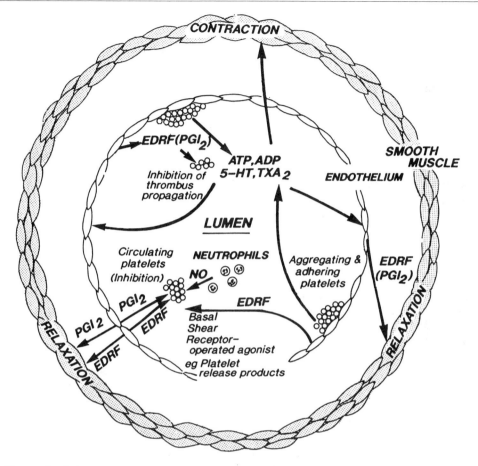

Figure 2: Schematic illustration showing sequence of events, following platelet activation, leading to relaxation (in presence of intact endothelium) or contraction (in presence of impaired endothelium) of vascular smooth muscle. Release of EDRF (and PGI_2) from endothelium and nitric oxide from neutrophils, inhibit intraluminal aggregation and thrombus propagation. EDRF is released in response to shear stress and products of the platelet release reaction (e.g., ATP, ADP, 5-HT, and possibly TXA_2) as well as having a basal release.

ever, have been less extensively investigated.

Nitrovasodilators

Of the currently available nitrovasodilator drugs, only nitroprusside has been shown to inhibit ex vivo platelet aggregation following in vivo administration in humans.[69,89] Glyceryl trinitrate is ineffective as an inhibitor of platelet aggregation when given in vivo, probably because unlike nitroprusside, it requires intracellular metabolism before releasing its nitric oxide, a metabolic step that platelets seem incapable of performing.[53,69] Isosorbide dinitrate has been shown to be a more potent inhibitor of platelet aggregation when given in vivo than when tested in vitro situations.[21,22] This difference between in vivo and in vitro effects has been variously attributed to release of PGI_2 by isosorbide dinitrate,[60,90] to the mononitrate metabolic breakdown products of isosorbide dinitrate being more potent inhibitors of platelet aggregation,[22] to the low potency of isosorbide dinitrate found in vitro being potentiated by PGI_2 in vivo[22] or to the stimulation by isosorbide dinitrate of the release of an as yet unidentified substance with platelet inhibitory properties.[6] Although there is some evidence that supports each of these possibilities, it may simply be that the metabolism of isosorbide dinitrate in vivo by vascular smooth muscle cells, endothelium, and perhaps liver cells, releases free nitric oxide which then acts as the platelet inhibitor.

An overview of the randomized trials studying the effect of intravenous nitrates on mortality in acute myocardial infarction certainly shows benefical effects of both glyceryl trinitrate and nitroprusside in this respect.[115] In view of the lack of effect of glyceryl trinitrate on platelet aggregation when given in vivo, however, it is unlikely that the effects of these drugs can be ascribed solely to their effects on aggregation.

Molsidomine, another nitrovasodilator and its active metabolite Sin-1 have been shown to possess potent platelet antiaggregatory properties in vitro.[76] In a recent unpublished study (Penny W.J., Hallet I., Lewis M.J.) Sin-1 also inhibited ex vivo platelet aggregation to ADP and elevated platelet cyclic GMP levels following in vivo infusion in the pig. Molsidomine has also been shown to inhibit experimentally induced coronary artery thrombosis in the dog, effects that were not demonstrable with either glyceryl trinitrate or isosorbide dinitrate.[67]

Dipyridamole

The beneficial therapeutic effects of dipyridamole as a platelet inhibitor drug are usually attributed to its effect on inhibition of adenosine uptake, the raised levels of adenosine elevating platelet cyclic AMP levels. Combined with its inhibition of cyclic AMP phosphodiesterase, these mechanisms are probably adequate to explain the effects of dipyridamole on aggregation.[18,42,57,73,88] Nevertheless, dipyridamole is also a potent inhibitor of cyclic GMP phosphodiesterase and potentiates the platelet inhibitory action of EDRF.[2,11] Could part of the platelet inhibitory action of dipyridamole in vivo be explained by its potentiating effect on EDRF? This is an interesting but as yet unproven possibility.

Omega-3 Fatty Acids

Dietary supplementation in man with fish oil, which contains the omega-3 fatty acids eicosapentaenoic acid and docosahexaenoic acid, has been shown to markedly inhibit platelet aggregation.[39,40,96] Interest in the use of these fatty acids, provided in the diet by fatty fish such as salmon or mackerel, as prophylaxis against the development of coronary artery disease has grown over the last 10 years since the original observations that Greenland Eskimos have a reduced incidence of coronary disease and atherosclerosis generally.[25–29] Until recently, firm recommendations regarding the beneficial dietary use of these fatty acids were lacking. A recently published report has shown for the first time clear evidence of a reduction in reinfarction and mortality from ischemic heart disease by the regular inclusion of fatty fish in the diet.[13] The mechanism of this effect is likely to be complex since the omega-3 fatty acids have many diverse actions on platelets, monocytes, red cells, and endothelium. One of their effects on endothelium is to increase endothelium-dependent relaxation in both large[94] and small[93] arteries. Thus, part of the platelet inhibitory action of the omega-3 fatty acids may be through augmentation of the effects of

EDRF on aggregation, and possibly adhesion.

It would seem, then, that to achieve maximum effects on inhibition of platelet aggregation and adhesion, the therapeutic combination of agents that elevate platelet cyclic AMP (such as PGI_2 or dipyridamole), cyclic GMP (such as nitroprusside or molsidomine or dipyridamole), together with agents that augment EDRF release or activity (such as omega-3 fatty acids) would prove to be the most effective way of inhibiting platelets with obvious therapeutic benefits.

Acknowledgment: We would like to thank Miss W. Simons for secretarial assistance during the preparation of this chapter.

References

1. Adelman B., Stemerman M.B., Mendell D., Handin R.I.: The interaction of platelets with aortic subendothelium: inhibition of adhesion and secretion by prostaglandin I_2. Blood 58:198–205, 1981.
2. Ahlner J., Andersson R.G.G., Axelsson K.L., Bunnfors I., Wallentin L.: Effects of dipyridamole on the glyceryl-trinitrate-induced inhibition of coronary artery muscle tone and platelet aggregation in relation to cyclic nucleotide metabolism. Acta Pharmacol. Toxicol. 57:88–95, 1985.
3. Alheid U., Frolich J.C., Forstermann U.: Endothelium-derived relaxing factor from cultured human endothelial cells inhibits aggregation of human platelets. Thromb. Res. 47:561–571, 1987.
4. Alheid Y., Reichwehr I., Forstermann U.: Human endothelial cells inhibit platelet aggregation by separately stimulating platelet cyclic AMP and cyclic GMP. Eur. J. Pharmacol. 164:103–110, 1989.
5. Azuma H., Masayuki I., Sekizaki S.: Endothelium-dependent inhibition of platelet aggregation. Br. J. Pharmacol. 88:411–415, 1986.
6. Berenger F.P., Friggi A., Bodard H., Rolland P.H.: Control of the antithrombogenic endothelial cell defense by short- and long-term exposure of cultured endothelial cells to isosorbide nitrates. Eur. Heart J. 9(Suppl. A):3–10, 1988.
7. Bhardwaj R., Page C.P., May G.R., Moore P.K.: Endothelium-derived relaxing factor inhibits platelet aggregation in human whole blood in vitro and in the rat in vivo. Eur. J. Pharmacol. 157:83–91, 1988.
8. Billah M.M., Lapetina E.G., Cuatrecasas P.: Phosphotidylinositol-specific phospholipase-C of platelets: association with 1,2-diacylglycerol-kinase and inhibition by cyclic-AMP. Biochem. Biophys. Res. Commun. 90:92–98, 1979.
9. Blair I.A., Barrow S.E., Waddell K.A., Lewis P.J., Dollery C.T.: Analysis of 6-oxo-prostaglandin $F_{1\alpha}$ in human plasma by gas chromatography negative chemical ionization mass spectrometry. Prostaglandins 23:579–589, 1982.
10. Born G.V.R.: Aggregation of blood platelets by adenosine diphosphate and its reversal. Nature (Lond.) 194:927–929, 1962.
11. Bult H., Fret H.R.L., Herman A.G., Jordaens F.H.: Blood platelet inhibition by endothelium-derived relaxing factor in the presence of dipyridamole. Pflügers Archiv Eur. J. Physiol. 412:S44, 1988.
12. Bult H., Fret H.R.L., Van de Bossche R.M., Herman A.G.: Platelet inhibition by endothelium-derived relaxing factor from the rabbit perfused aorta. Br. J. Pharmacol. 95:1308–1314, 1988.
13. Burr M.L., Gilbert J.F., Holliday R.M., Elwood P.C., Fehily A.M., Rogers S., Sweetnam P.M., Deadman N.M.: Effects of changes in fat, fish, and fibre intakes on death and myocardial infarction: diet and reinfarction trial (DART). Lancet ii:757–761, 1989.
14. Busse R.A., Luckhoff E., Bassenge E.: Endothelium-derived relaxant factor inhibits platelet activation. Naunyn-Schmied. Arch. Pharmacol. 336:566–571, 1987.
15. Cantor E.H., Ho E.H., Parker-Botelhs L.H., Lumma W.C., Rubanyi G.M.: Effect of nitric oxide and nitrovasodilators on human platelets and neutrophils. J. Vasc. Med. Biol. 1:80, 1989.
16. Chappell S.P., Lewis M.J., Henderson A.H.: Effect of lipid feeding on endothe-

lium-dependent relaxation in rabbit aortic preparations. Cardiovasc. Res. 21:34–38, 1986.

17. Collins P., Griffith T.M., Henderson A.H., Lewis M.J.: Endothelium-derived relaxing factor alters calcium fluxes in rabbit aorta: a cyclic guanosine monophosphate-mediated effect. J. Physiol. 381:427–437, 1986.

18. Crutchley D.J., Ryan U.S., Ryan W.J.: Effects of aspirin and dipyridamole on the degradation of adenosine diphosphate by cultured cells derived from bovine pulmonary artery. J. Clin. Invest. 66:29–35, 1980.

19. Curwen K.D., Gimbrone M.A., Jr., Handin R.I.: In vitro studies of thromboresistance. The role of prostacyclin (PGI$_2$) in platelet adhesion to cultured normal and virally transformed human vascular endothelial cells. Lab. Invest. 42:366–374, 1980.

20. Czervionke R.L., Smith J.D., Fry G.L., Hoak J.C., Haycraft D.L.: Inhibition of prostacyclin by treatment of endothelium with aspirin: correlation with platelet adherence. J. Clin. Invest. 63:1089–1092, 1979.

21. Decaterina R., Giannessi D., Crea F., Chierchia S., Bernini W., Gazzetti P., L'Abbate A.: Inhibition of platelet function by injectable isosorbide dinitrate. Am. J. Cardiol. 53:1683–1687, 1984.

22. Decaterina R., Giannessi D., Mazzone A., Bernini W.: Mechanisms for the in vivo anti-platelet effects of isosorbide dinitrate. Eur. Heart J. 9(Suppl.A):45–49, 1988.

23. Dejana E., Cazenava J.P., Groves H.M., Kinlough-Rathbone R.L., Richardson M., Packman M.A., Mustard J.F.: The effect of aspirin inhibition of prostacyclin production on platelet adherence to normal and damaged rabbit aorta. Thromb. Res. 17:453–464, 1979.

24. Dorros G., Cowley M.J., Simpson J., Bentivoglio L.G., Block P.C., Bourassa M., Detre K., Gosselin A.J., Gruenzig A.R., Helsey S.F., et al.: Percutaneous transluminal coronary angioplasty: report of complications for the National Heart, Lung and Blood Institute PTCA registry. Circulation 67:723–730, 1983.

25. Dyerberg J.: In: Nutritional Evaluation of Long Chain Fatty Acids in Fish Oil. Orlando, Florida, Academic Press, 1982, pp 245–261.

26. Dyerberg J., Bang H.O.: Haemostatic function and platelet polyunsaturated

fatty acids in Eskimos. Lancet ii:433–435, 1979.

27. Dyerberg J., Bang H.O., Stoffersen E., Moncada S., Vane J.R.: Eicosapentaenoic acid and prevention of thrombosis and atherosclerosis? Lancet ii:117–119, 1978.

28. Dyerberg J., Bjerregaard P.: Proceedings of the AOCS short course on polyunsaturated fatty acids and eicosanoids. Biloxi, Mississippi. American Oil Chemists Society, 1987, pp 2–8.

29. Dyerberg J., Jorgensen K.A.: Marine oils and thrombogenesis. Prog. Lipid Res. 21:255–269, 1982.

30. Edwards D.H., Griffith T.M., Ryley H.C., Henderson A.H.: Haptoglobin-haemoglobin complex in human plasma inhibits endothelium-dependent relaxation: evidence that endothelium-derived relaxing factor acts as a local autocoid. Cardiovasc. Res. 20:549–556, 1986.

31. Evans H.G., Ryley H.C., Hallet I., Lewis M.J.: Human red blood cells inhibit endothelium-derived relaxing factor (EDRF) activity. Eur. J. Pharmacol. 163:361–364, 1989.

32. Forstermann U., Mulach A., Bohme E., Busse R.: Stimulation of soluble guanylate cyclase by an acetylcholine-induced endothelium-derived factor from rabbit and canine arteries. Circ. Res. 58:531–538, 1986.

33. Furchgott R.F.: In: Vasodilatation: Vascular Smooth Muscle, Peptides, Autonomic Nerves, and Endothelium. New York, Raven Press, pp 401–414, 1988.

34. Furchgott R.F., Zawadzki J.V.: The obligatory role of endothelial cells in the relaxation of arterial smooth muscle by acetylcholine. Nature (Lond.) 288:373–376, 1980.

35. Furlong B., Henderson A.H., Lewis M.J., Smith J.A.: Endothelium-derived relaxing factor inhibits in vitro platelet aggregation. Br. J. Pharmacol. 90:687–692, 1987.

36. Fuster V., Badimon L., Badimon J., Adams P.C., Turitto V., Chesebro J.H.: Drugs interfering with platelet functions: mechanisms and clinical relevance. Thrombosis and Haemostasis, Leuven University Press, Leuven, pp 349–418, 1987.

37. Ginsburg R., Bristow M.R., Davis K., Dibiase A., Billingham M.E.: Quantitative pharmacologic responses of normal and atherosclerotic isolated human epicardial coronary arteries. Circulation 69:430–440, 1984.

38. Glusa E., Markwadt F., Sturzebecher J.: Effects of sodium nitroprusside and other pentacyanonitrosyl complexes on platelet aggregation. Haemostasis 3:249–256, 1974.

39. Goodnight S.H., Harris W.S., Connor W.E.: The effects of dietary omega-3 fatty acids on platelet composition and function in man: a prospective, controlled study. Blood 58:880–885, 1981.

40. Goodnight Jr. S.H., Harris W.S., Connor W.E., Illingworth D.R.: Polyunsaturated fatty acids, hyperlipidaemia, and thrombosis. Arteriosclerosis 2:87–113, 1982.

41. Gorman R.R., Bunting S., Miller O.V.: Modulation of human platelet adenylate cyclase by prostacyclin (PGX). Prostaglandins 13:377–388, 1977.

42. Gresele P., Zoja C., Deckmyn H., Arnout J., Vermylen J., Verstraete M.: Dipyridamole inhibits platelet aggregation in whole blood. Thromb. Haemost. 50:852–856, 1983.

43. Gryglewski R.J., Korbut R., Ocetkiewicz A.C.: Generation of prostacyclin by lungs in vivo and its release into the arterial circulation. Nature (Lond.) 273:765–767, 1978.

44. Halenda S.P., Volpi M., Zavoko G.B., Sh'afri R.I., Feinstein M.B.: Effects of thrombin, phorbol myristate acetate and prostaglandin D_2 on 40-41 kDa protein that is ADP-ribosylated by pertussis toxin in platelets. FEBS Lett. 204:341–346, 1986.

45. Haslam R.J., Davidson M.M.L., Davies T., Lynham J.A., McClenaghan M.D.: Regulation of blood platelet function by cyclic nucleotides. Adv. Cycl. Nucl. Res. 9:533–552, 1978.

46. Haslam R.J., McClenaghan M.D.: Measurement of circulating prostacyclin. Nature 292:364–366, 1981.

47. Hathaway D.R., Konicki M.V., Coolican S.A.: Phosphorylation of myosin light chain kinase from vascular smooth muscle by cAMP- and cGMP-dependent protein kinases. J. Mol. Cell. Cardiol. 17:841–850, 1985.

48. Hawkins D.J., Meyrick B.O., Murray J.J.: Activation of guanylate cyclase and inhibition of platelet aggregation by endothelium-derived relaxing factor released from cultured cells. Biochim. Biophys. Acta 969:289–296, 1988.

49. Heavey D.J., Barrow S.E., Hickling N.E., Ritter J.M.: Aspirin causes short-lived inhibition of bradykinin-stimulated prostacyclin production in man. Nature (Lond.) 318:186–188, 1985.

50. Hibbs J.B., Taintor R.R., Vavrin Z.: Macrophage cytotoxicity: role for L-arginine deiminase and imino nitrogen oxidation to nitrite. Science 235:473–476, 1987.

51. Higgs E.A., Moncada S., Vane J.R., Caen J.P., Michel H., Tobelem G.: Effect of prostacyclin (PGI_2) on platelet adhesion to rabbit arterial subendothelium. Prostaglandins 16:17–22, 1978.

52. Hogan J.C., Lewis M.J., Henderson A.H.: In vivo EDRF activity influences platelet function. Br. J. Pharmacol. 94:1020–1022, 1988.

53. Hogan J.C., Lewis M.J., Henderson A.H., Glyceryl trinitrate and platelet aggregation: effects of N-acetyl-cysteine. Br. J. Clin. Pharmacol. 27:617–619, 1989.

54. Ignarro L.J., Byrns R.E., Wood K.S.: In: Vasodilatation: Vascular Smooth Muscle, Peptides, Autonomic Nerves, and Endothelium. New York, Raven Press, pp 427–435, 1988.

55. Imai A., Nakashima S., Nozawa Y.: The rapid polyphosphoinositide metabolism may be a triggering event for thrombin-mediated stimulation of human platelets. Biochem. Biophys. Res. Comm. 110:108–115, 1983.

56. Kawahara Y., Yamanishi J., Fukuzaki H.: Inhibitory action of guanosine 3′,5′-monophosphate on thrombin-induced calcium mobilization in human platelets. Thromb. Res. 33:203–209, 1984.

57. Klabunde R.E.: Dipyridamole inhibition of adenosine metabolism in human blood. Eur. J. Pharmacol. 93:21–26, 1983.

58. Knight D.E., Scrutton M.C.: Cyclic nucleotides control a system which regulates Ca^{2+} sensitivity of platelet secretion. Nature (Lond.) 309:66–68, 1984.

59. Lang D., Lewis M.J.: Endothelium-derived relaxing factor inhibits the formation of inositol trisphosphate by rabbit aorta. J. Physiol. 411:45–52, 1989.

60. Levin R.I., Jaffe E.A., Weksler B.B., Tack-Goldman K.: Nitroglycerin stimulates synthesis of prostacyclin by human endothelial cells. J. Clin. Invest. 67:762–769, 1981.

61. Levin R.I., Weksler B.B., Jaffe E.A.: The interaction of sodium nitroprusside with human endothelial cells and platelets: nitroprusside and prostacyclin synergistically inhibit platelet function. Circulation 66:1299–1309, 1982.

62. Lincoln T.M.: Cyclic GMP and mechanisms of vasodilatation. Pharmacol. Ther. 41:479–502, 1989.

63. Ludmer P.L., Selwyn A.P., Shook T.L.,

Wayne R.R., Mudge G.H., Alexander R.W., Ganz P.: Paradoxical vasoconstriction induced by acetylcholine in atherosclerotic coronary arteries. N. Engl. J. Med. 315:1046–1051, 1986.

64. Macdonald P.S., Read M.A., Dusting G.J.: Synergistic inhibition of platelet aggregation by endothelium-derived relaxing factor and prostacyclin. Thromb. Res. 49:437–449, 1988.

65. MacIntyre D.E., Bushfield M., Shaw A.M.: Regulation of platelet cytosolic free calcium by cyclic nucleotides and protein kinase C. FEBS Lett. 188:383–388, 1985.

66. Marie-Francoise S., Chap H., Douste-Blazy L.: Effect of a stimulant of guanylate cyclase, SIN 1, on calcium movements and phospholipase C activation in thrombin-stimulated human platelets. Biochem. Pharmacol. 37:1263–1269, 1988.

67. Martorana P.A., Kettenback B., Gobel H., Nitz R.E.: Comparison of the effects of molsidomine, nitroglycerin and isosorbide dinitrate on experimentally induced coronary artery thrombosis in the dog. Basic Res. Cardiol. 79:503–512, 1984.

68. McCall T.B., Boughton-Smith N.K., Palmer R.M.J., Whittle B.J.R., Moncada S.: Synthesis of nitric oxide from L-arginine by neutrophils. Biochem. J. 261:293–296, 1989.

69. Mehta J., Mehta P.: Comparative effects of nitroprusside and nitroglycerin on platelet aggregation in patients with heart failure. J. Cardiovasc. Pharmacol. 2:25–33, 1980.

70. Mellion B.T., Ignarro L.J., Ohlstein E.H., Pontecorvo E.G., Hyman A.L., Kadowitz P.J.: Evidence for the inhibitory role of guanosine 3′,5′-monophosphate in ADP-induced human platelet aggregation in the presence of nitric oxide and related vasodilation. Blood 57:946–955, 1981.

71. Miller O.V., Gorman R.R.: Evidence for distinct PGI_2 and PGD_2 receptors in human platelets. J. Pharmacol. Exp. Ther. 210:134–140, 1979.

72. Moncada S., Gryglewski R.J., Bunting S., Vane J.R.: An enzyme isolated from arteries transforms prostaglandin endoperoxides to an unstable substance that inhibits platelet aggregation. Nature (Lond.) 263:663–665, 1976.

73. Moncada S., Korbut R.: Dipyridamole and other phosphodiesterase inhibitors act as antithrombotic agents by potentiating endogenous prostacyclin. Lancet i:1286–1289, 1978.

74. Morgan R.O., Newby A.C.: Nitroprusside differentially inhibits ADP-stimulated calcium influx and mobilization in human platelets. Biochem. J. 258:447–454, 1989.

75. Nakashima S., Tomatsu T., Hattori H., Okano Y., Nozawa Y.: Inhibitory action of cyclic GMP on secretion polyphosphoinositide hydrolysis and calcium mobilization in thrombin-stimulated platelets. Biochem. Biophys. Res. Comm. 135:1099–1104, 1986.

76. Nishikawa M., Kanamori M., Hidaka H.: Inhibition of platelet aggregation and stimulation of guanylate cyclase by an antianginal agent molsidomine and its metabolites. J. Pharmacol. Exp. Ther. 220:183–190, 1982.

77. Oyama K., Kawasaki H., Hattori Y., Kanno M.: Attenuation of endothelium-dependent relaxation in aorta from diabetic rats. Eur. J. Pharmacol. 131:75–78, 1986.

78. Palmer R.M.J., Ferrige A.G., Moncada S.: Nitric oxide release accounts for the biological activity of endothelium-derived relaxing factor. Nature (Lond.) 327:524–526, 1987.

79. Pfitzer G., Hoffman F., Disalvo J., Ruegg J.C.: cGMP and cAMP inhibit tension development in skinned coronary arteries. Pflügers Arch. 401:277–280, 1984.

80. Pleiderer T.: Na-nitroprusside, a very potent platelet disaggregating substance. Acta Univ. Carol. Med. (Praha) 53:247–250, 1972.

81. Radomski M.W., Palmer R.M.J., Moncada S.: Comparative pharmacology of endothelium-derived relaxing factor, nitric oxide and prostacyclin in platelets. Br. J. Pharmacol. 92:181–187, 1987a.

82. Radomski M.W., Palmer R.M.J., Moncada S.: The anti-aggregating properties of vascular endothelium: interactions between prostacyclin and nitric oxide. Br. J. Pharmacol. 92:639–646, 1987b.

83. Radomski M.W., Palmer R.M.J., Moncada S.: Endogenous nitric oxide inhibits human platelet adhesion to vascular endothelium. Lancet ii:1057–1058, 1987c.

84. Radomski M.W., Palmer R.M.J., Moncada S.: The role of nitric oxide and cGMP in platelet adhesion to vascular endothelium. Biochem. Biophys. Res. Comm. 148:1482–1489, 1987d.

85. Rapoport R.M.: Cyclic guanosine monophosphate inhibition of contraction may be mediated through inhibition of phosphatidylinositol hydrolysis in rat aorta. Circ. Res. 58:407–410, 1986.

86. Rashatwar S.S., Cornwell T.L., Lincoln T.M.: Effects of 8-bromo-cGMP on Ca^{2+} levels in vascular smooth muscle cells: possible regulation of Ca^{2+}-ATPase by cGMP-dependent protein kinase. Proc. Natl. Acad. Sci. USA 84:5685–5689, 1987.

87. Rittenhouse-Simmons S.: Production of diglyceride from phosphatidyl inositol in activated human platelets. J. Clin. Invest. 63:580–587, 1979.

88. Sattini A., Rall T.: The effect of adenosine and adenine nucleotides on the cyclic adenosine 3'-5'-phosphate content of guinea pig central cortex slices. Mol. Pharmacol. 6:13–23, 1970.

89. Saxon A., Kattlove H.E.: Platelet inhibition by sodium nitroprusside, a smooth muscle inhibitor. Blood 47:957–961, 1976.

90. Schror K., Ahland B., Weiss P., Konig E.: Stimulation of coronary vascular PGI_2 by organic nitrates. Eur. Heart J. 9 (Suppl. A):25–32, 1988.

91. Screeharan N., Jayacody R.L., Senaratne P.J., Thomson A.B.R., Kappagoda C.T.: Endothelium-dependent relaxation and experimental atherosclerosis in the rabbit aorta. Can. J. Pharmacol. 64:1451–1453, 1986.

92. Shimokawa H., Aarhus L.L., Vanhoutte P.M.: Porcine coronary arteries with regenerated endothelium have a reduced endothelium-dependent responsiveness to aggregating platelets and serotonin. Circ. Res. 61:256–270, 1987.

93. Shimokawa H., Aarhus L.L., Vanhoutte P.M.: Dietary ω3 polyunsaturated fatty acids augment endothelium-dependent relaxation to bradykinin in coronary microvessels of the pig. Br. J. Pharmacol. 95:1191–1196, 1988.

94. Shimokawa H., Lam T.Y.T., Chesebro J.H., Bowie E.J.W., Vanhoutte P.M.: Effects of dietary supplementation with cod-liver oil on endothelium-dependent responses in porcine coronary arteries. Circulation 76:898–905, 1987.

95. Shirasaki Y., Su C., Lee T.J.-F., Kolm P., Cline W.H., Nickols G.A.: Endothelial modulation of vascular relaxation to nitrovasodilators in aging and hypertension. J. Pharmacol. Exp. Ther. 239:861–866, 1986.

96. Siess W., Scherer B., Bohlig B., Roth P., Kurzmann I., Weber P.C.: Platelet-membrane fatty acids, platelet aggregation, and thromboxane formation during a mackerel diet. Lancet i:441–444, 1980.

97. Sneddon J.M., Bearpark T., Vane J.R.: Endothelial derived relaxing factor (EDRF)

inhibits platelet adhesion to bovine endothelial cells. Br. J. Pharmac. 93:100P, 1988.

98. Szczeklik A., Gryglewski R.J., Nizankowski R., Musial J., Pieton R., Mruk J.: Circulatory and antiplatelet effects of intravenous prostacyclin in healthy man. Pharmacol. Res. Commun. 10:545–556, 1978.

99. Takai Y., Kaibuchi K., Matsubara T., Mishizuka Y.: Inhibitory action of guanosine-3'-5'-monophosphate on thormbin-induced phosphatidylinositol turnover and protein phosphorylation in human platelets. Biochem. Biophys. Res. Comm. 101:61–67, 1981.

100. Takai K., Kaibuchi K., Sano K., Nishizuka Y.: Counteraction of calcium-activated phospholipid dependent protein kinase activation by adenosine-3'5'-monophosphate and guanosine-3'5'-monophosphate in platelets. J. Biochem. 91:403–406, 1982.

101. Tansik R.L., Namm D.H., White H.L.: Synthesis of prostaglandin 6-keto-$F_{1\alpha}$ by cultured aortic smooth muscle cells and stimulation of its formation in a coupled system with platelet lysates. Prostaglandins 15:399–408, 1978.

102. Tateson J.E., Moncada S., Vane J.R.: Effects of prostacyclin (PGX) on cyclic AMP concentrations in human platelets. Prostaglandins 13:389–399, 1977.

103. Twort C.H.C., van Breemen C.: Cyclic guanosine monophosphate-enhanced sequestration of Ca^{2+} by sarcoplasmic reticulum in vascular smooth muscle. Circ. Res. 62:961–964, 1988.

104. Ubatuba F.B., Moncada S., Vane J.R.: The effect of prostacyclin (PGI_2) on platelet behaviour, thrombus formation in vivo and bleeding time. Thromb. Diath. Haemorrh. 41:425–434, 1979.

105. Van de Voorde J., Leusen I.: Endothelium-dependent and independent relaxation of aortic rings from hypertensive rats. Am. J. Physiol. 250:H711–H717, 1986.

106. Vanhoutte P.M., Shimokawa H.: Endothelium-derived relaxing factor and coronary vasospasm. Circulation 80:1–9, 1989.

107. Verbeuren T.J., Jordaens F.H., Zonnekeyn L.L., Van Hove C.E., Coene M.C., Herman A.G.: Effect of hypercholesterolaemia on the vascular reactivity in the rabbit. Circ. Res. 58:552–564, 1986.

108. Vrolix M., Raeymaekers L., Wuytack F., Hofmann F., Casteels R.: Cyclic GMP-dependent protein kinase stimulates the

plasmalemmal Ca^{2+} pump of smooth muscle via phosphorylation of phosphatidylinositol. Biochem. J. 255:855–863, 1988.

109. Watson S.P., McConnell R.T., Lapetina E.G.: The rapid formation of inositol phosphates in human platelets by thrombin is inhibited by prostacyclin. J. Biol. Chem. 259:13199–13203, 1984.

110. Weiss H.J., Turitto V.T.: Prostacyclin (prostaglandin I_2, PGI_2) inhibits platelet adhesion and thrombus formation on subendothelium. Blood 53:244–250, 1979.

111. Weksler B.B., Ley C.W., Jaffe E.A.: Stimulation of endothelial prostacyclin production by thrombin, trypsin and the ionophore A23187. J. Clin. Invest. 62:923–930, 1978.

112. Whittle B.J.R., Moncada S., Vane J.R.: Comparison of the effects of prostacyclin (PGI_2), prostaglandin E_1 and D_2 on platelet aggregation in different species. Prostaglandins 16:373–388, 1978.

113. Willems C., Stel H.V., van Aken W.G., van Mourik J.A.: Binding and inactivation of prostacyclin by human erythrocytes. Br. J. Haemat. 54:43–52, 1983.

114. Yoshida K., Stark F., Nachmias V.T.: Comparison of the effects of phorbol 12-myristate 13-acetate and prostaglandin E_1 on calcium regulation in human platelets. Biochem. J. 249:487–493, 1988.

115. Yusuf S., Collins R., Macmahon S., Petro P.: Effect of intravenous nitrates on mortality in acute myocardial infarction: an overview of the randomised trials. Lancet ii:1088–1092, 1988.

Part IV
Therapeutic Considerations

15

Iloprost: Stable Prostacyclin Analogue

B. Müller, W. Witt, F.M. McDonald

Introduction

In 1976 when Moncada, Gryglewski, Bunting, and Vane[90] described the biological profile of prostacyclin (PGI$_2$), its potent inhibition of platelet aggregation and pronounced vasodilator effects raised the hope of broad therapeutic utility. Among other clinical indications, myocardial infarction, stroke, peripheral vascular disease, and replacement of heparin in extracorporeal circulations were discussed. However, though PGI$_2$ has been used therapeutically to a certain extent, it soon became obvious that the chemical instability of this molecule would severely limit its clinical use.

Considerable efforts were made by several groups to develop stable PGI$_2$ derivatives, and studies on the structure-activity relationship of carbacyclin PGI$_2$ mimetics resulted in the synthesis of iloprost, a very close image of PGI$_2$ with respect to its biological profile and PGI$_2$ mimetic potency.[134]

Besides being the first PGI$_2$ analogue in the process of registration in Europe as a drug for treatment of arterial occlusive diseases, the close similarity to PGI$_2$ and the convenience of its stability triggered a widespread interest in iloprost in different areas of experimental research. Iloprost rapidly became the most widely used substitute for PGI$_2$, and the literature on this compound comprises already more than 700 references.

The main pharmacological properties of iloprost, like those of PGI$_2$, are inhibition of platelet aggregation, vasodilatation, and still poorly defined cytoprotective properties. Reviews on iloprost's chemistry[103] and on pharmacodynamic, toxicological, and pharmacokinetic properties[121] as well as an overview of clinical results[104] are available. This review summarizes the current state of knowledge on the pharmacology of iloprost with regard

Rubanyi G.M.: Cardiovascular Significance of Endothelium-Derived Vasoactive Factors, Futura Publishing Co., Inc., Mount Kisco, NY, © 1991.

to established or hypothetical clinical indications.

Effects on Hemostasis and Experimental Thrombosis

Binding to the Platelet Receptor and Signal Transduction

Inhibition of platelet function represents one of the major pharmacological properties of iloprost. Many effects of the drug not obviously related to platelets at first glance may eventually turn out to be due to the potent inhibition of various platelet functions by iloprost (see below). Binding to specific PGI_2 receptors is the prerequisite for iloprost's action on platelets. The very first published results on iloprost describe that [^{3}H]-iloprost competes with [^{3}H]-PGI_2 for the same specific binding sites on particulate fractions of human and bovine platelets.[122] Since then, [^{3}H]-iloprost has become the standard ligand for PGI_2-receptor tests in most laboratories. PGI_2 and iloprost bind to a common site, termed IP-receptor,[69] which was only recently solubilized from human platelet membranes.[148] Binding is saturable and reversible and both compounds have similar receptor affinities, i.e., dissociation constants. The number of binding sites has been estimated to be in the range of 4000 sites/platelet.[130] Binding of PGI_2 and iloprost leads to similar degrees of activation of platelet adenylate cyclase, i.e., increases in intracellular cAMP levels.[141] The activity of cAMP-dependent protein kinases, which are known to phosphorylate a variety of platelet proteins, is then believed to mediate the inhibitory effects on different biochemical pathways involved in the activation of platelets by stimuli such as thrombin, collagen, ADP, PAF, etc.[86] (See also Chapter 14.)

Prolonged exposure to iloprost leads to heterologous desensitization of platelets,[64,82] i.e., platelets are also desensitized to PGD_2, which binds to a distinct DP-type receptor, and adenosine. Platelets desensitized to iloprost show a decrease in iloprost binding as well as cAMP production. Desensitization is time- and dose-dependent. It might involve a change in the regulatory Gs subunit of the adenylate cyclase[40] and an increase in phosphodiesterase activity possibly linked to cAMP-dependent phosphorylation of the enzyme,[55] which may explain the heterologous desensitization. It was also hypothesized that iloprost binds to a putative low affinity receptor which inhibits adenylate cyclase.[9] In clinical therapy with intermittent infusions of iloprost up to 6 hours per day, platelet inhibition is maintained throughout the infusion period.[33]

Inhibition of Platelet Function

In hemostasis and thrombosis, circulating discoid platelets become activated by stimuli such as thrombin, collagen, ADP, PAF, or epinephrine. Upon activation, these platelets change shape, adhere to the damaged vessel wall, aggregate, express procoagulant activity, and release many biologically active compounds.

Iloprost has been shown to equally inhibit aggregation induced by all commonly used physiological activators in platelet-rich plasma of various mammalian species,[141] a unique property of agents that act through stimulation of platelet adenylate cyclase resulting in common pathway inhibition, i.e., an inhibition of all (or a common step of all) different biochemical activation pathways of platelets. This type of platelet inhibition markedly differs from the effect of antiplatelet agents such as aspirin, which selectively inhibit only one pathway of platelet activation, explaining the dependence of their efficacy on the respective stimulus used: blocking the formation of thromboxane (aspirin) or its receptors (TXA$_2$ angatonists) results in a good inhibition of aggregation induced by low concentrations of collagen, with no effect against ADP (at physiological conditions)[164] or high concentrations of collagen.[35,56]

Inhibition of platelet aggregation by iloprost was observed in human platelets in vitro[49,124] or ex vivo in volunteers and patients treated with iloprost[16,33] and various animal species[2,25,141] in platelet-rich plasma as well as in whole blood.[83,120] Besides aggregation, iloprost also inhibits shape change,[109] thromboxane formation and release,[141] as well as the secretion of biological mediators stored in different platelet vesicles, like the dense body contents serotonin[30] and ATP[141] or the alpha granule proteins PDGF[142] and PAI-1 (Baldus et al., unpublished observations) (see Table 1). In contrast to aspirin, it has been shown for PGI$_2$ and PGI$_2$ derivatives that they can also inhibit the expression of procoagulant activity on the surface of activated platelets.[133,166] All these effects of iloprost hold true when the drug is added to platelet suspensions prior to addition of platelet activators. Interestingly, iloprost added to preactivated platelets also shows some ability to disaggregate freshly formed platelet aggregates.[124,141]

In summary, iloprost, is a very potent and efficacious inhibitor of platelet function in vitro. Due to common pathway inhibition, it is effective against all types of physiological platelet activators. The extent of inhibition of platelet function that can be achieved in vivo by iloprost therapy in patients is, on the other hand, limited by the maximum tolerable dose, determined by increasing hemodynamic effects with higher doses (see below). In this respect, iloprost may show some favorable dissociation towards a more pronounced platelet inhibition when compared to natural prostaglandins such as PGI$_2$[17,124] or PGE$_1$.[1,163]

Effects on Coagulation

No direct effects of iloprost or other PGI$_2$ derivatives on fibrin formation in plasma systems are known. The role of platelets, on the other hand, in coagulation in vivo has probably been underestimated for a long time. Activated platelets release factors that can enhance coagulation, such as protein S and platelet factor 4, as well as coagulation factors V and VII. Iloprost was shown to inhibit their release.[11] The assembly of coagulation factor complexes on the platelet surface, such as that of the so-called prothrombinase complex (factors Va, Xa, and Ca^{2+}), strongly enhances the rate of thrombin formation. It was demonstrated that this procoagulant activity of activated platelets can be inhibited by PGI$_2$ and PGI$_2$ derivatives (see above). Iloprost prolongs the time as well as reduces the maximum amount of thrombin generation in platelet-rich plasma (Baldus et al., unpublished observations). These results suggest that common pathway inhibitors of platelet function such as iloprost may

Table 1
Inhibition of Collagen-Induced Platelet Aggregation and Release of PAI-1 Measured by ELISA in Human PRP (means ± SEM, n = 6)

		% Inhibition	
		Aggregation	PAI-1
Iloprost	3 × 10^{-10} M	3 ± 2	7 ± 5
	10^{-9} M	7 ± 5	2 ± 1
	3 × 10^{-9} M	53 ± 14	39 ± 5
	10^{-8} M	92 ± 2	68 ± 7
	3 × 10^{-8} M	98 ± 1	80 ± 8
	3 × 10^{-7} M	97 ± 1	74 ± 6
ASA	10^{-4} M	9 ± 3	10 ± 8
	10^{-3} M	46 ± 6	27 ± 10

Data are shown as percent of control (= 100%) ASA = acetylsalicylic acid (Baldus et al., submitted for publication).

actually possess anticoagulant activity in vivo in platelet-dependent thrombosis.

Profibrinolytic Effects

The first evidence for a profibrinolytic effect of iloprost was provided by studies in rabbits where a shortening of euglobulin clot lysis time was demonstrated after iloprost injection.[73] This effect has been verified in rats[163] and also in humans.[18,99] It is interesting that aspirin has an inhibitory influence on the fibrinolytic system[79] and that this inhibition can be reversed by concomitant infusion of iloprost in human volunteers,[19] suggesting that the effect of aspirin might be related to inhibition of endogenous PGI_2 formation. There is some controversy on the underlying mechanism(s) of profibrinolytic effects of iloprost and other prostaglandins. There has been one case described where PGI_2 infusion led to an elevation of tissue-type plasminogen activator (t-PA) levels in plasma of a woman suffering from peripheral vascular disease.[160] The ineffectiveness of iloprost and related compounds in releasing plasminogen activator activity in the buffer-perfused rat hindlimb system,[147] however, argues against an induction of t-PA release from endothelial stores. Adenylate cyclase stimulators such as iloprost may actually cause inhibition of t-PA liberation from human umbilical vein endothelial cells.[51] One possible mechanism explaining a profibrinolytic effect of iloprost may be the observed (see above) inhibition of the release of plasminogen activator inhibitor-1 (PAI-1) from activated platelets. PAI-1 stored in platelets constitutes the major pool of total blood PAI-1 and there is recent evidence that platelet PAI-1 may actively impair fibrinolytic activity.

Hemostasis In Vivo and Experimental Thrombosis

Inhibition of platelet aggregate formation and embolization by iloprost was also shown in vivo in different animal species where platelet activators were injected directly into the circulation.[161,162] The potent antiplatelet effects of iloprost will explain the prolongation of bleeding times obtained in rats and mice.[25,161] There is no indication that iloprost or related agents induce spontaneous bleeding such as gastrointestinal bleeding in the same manner as aspirin. This might be related to the protective effect of iloprost on the endothelium (see below). Also, platelet adhesion, i.e., the primary interaction of platelets with exposed subendothelial layers, has been shown to be partially independent of PGI_2,[78] or only affected by high doses.[63]

Iloprost has shown antithrombotic efficacy in various animal models of thrombosis. In electrically damaged mesenteric arterioles of rats and guinea pigs, superfusion of ADP at concentrations specific for an individual vessel induces reversible thrombus formation at the lesion site. Iloprost infusion led to increases of the ADP concentration needed to induce thrombus formation in this model of microvascular thrombosis, i.e., an elevation of the thrombogenetic threshold.[161] Large vessel thrombosis was produced by damaging carotid arteries or jugular veins of rats through a combination of crushing and cooling. Several hours later, thrombus size was evaluated by measuring thrombus hemoglobin content. Iloprost not only potently inhibited arterial and venous thrombus formation but also led to a significant decrease of the size of preformed thrombi.[161] This thrombolytic effect on fresh thrombi may be related to the profibrinolytic as well as disaggregatory properties of iloprost described above. In the same rat model of thrombosis, iloprost showed cooperative antithrombotic effects in combination with a TXA_2 receptor blocker.[162] In another rat model, where thrombosis was induced by applying electrical current to carotid arteries, iloprost effectively antagonized the incidence of loss of righting reflexes which developed as a consequence of carotid thrombosis.[112]

Coronary thrombosis is probably of major importance in the pathogenesis of myocardial infarction. In a coronary thrombosis model in pigs, iloprost was found to have antithrombotic effects, in that the time to occlusion after electrical damage to the coronary artery was significantly delayed.[154] One of the main problems of thrombolytic therapy in myocardial infarction is reocclusion. In experimental coronary thrombosis in dogs, iloprost at 100 ng/kg/min IV completely prevented reocclusion after successful thrombolysis with tissue-type plasminogen activator (t-PA).[54] Iloprost infusion was started together with t-PA, 30 minutes after total occlusion of the arteries and it was actually shown that the time to reperfusion was also significantly shortened in the iloprost group. We have recently obtained similar results (see Table 2) with an intracoronary infusion of 30 ng/kg/min iloprost + t-PA in a model of canine coronary thrombosis.

We also included a subgroup with iloprost alone without t-PA. Intracoronary infusion of iloprost completely prevented reocclusion after reperfusion with t-PA, and iloprost alone seemed to enhance spontaneous clot lysis.

An interesting application of iloprost as an antithrombotic agent is suggested by several experiments using bound iloprost rather than free drug. Surgical suture containing iloprost completely prevented occlusion of femoral vein anastomosis in rats.[39] Iloprost can also be bound to dacron grafts which then slowly delivers the drug in a biologically active form resulting in inhibition of platelet aggregation.[71] We have used iloprost bound to charcoal in an experimental in vitro hemoperfusion circuit where iloprost completely antagonized the loss of platelets during perfusion (Fig. 1).

Effects on the Vessel Wall

Binding to Prostanoid Receptors and Mechanisms of Vasodilation

In isolated strips of bovine coronary artery, a bioassay commonly used to demonstrate PGI_2-like effects, iloprost is a slightly more active relaxant compound than PGI_2.[32] In the same preparation, iloprost, with a dissociation constant of 21 nM, was shown to bind to specific membrane PGI_2 receptors.[146] This was demonstrated also in preparations from pig aorta, where the dissociation constant was 8 nM,[119] and from dog femoral arteries.[122] Further experiments in various prostanoid receptor-containing smooth muscle preparations, using the prostanoid receptor classification proposed by Coleman et al.,[28] classified iloprost to be a potent agonist at IP (PGI_2) receptors with no affinity towards FP ($PGF_{2\alpha}$), TP (TXA_2), and DP (PGD_2) receptors and weak agonist activity at EP_1

Table 2

Effects of 30 ng/kg/min IC Iloprost on Spontaneous as well as t-PA-Induced Thrombolysis (Reperfusion Rate) and Reocclusion Rate in a Coronary Thrombosis Model in Dogs

	Control	Iloprost	t-PA	Ilo + t-PA
Reperfusion rate	2/6	3/6	6/6	6/6
Reocclusion rate	2/2	1/3	6/6	0/6
Persisting reperfusion rate	—	2/3	—	6/6
% of total	0%	33%	0%	100%

(Own results, submitted for publication.) Thrombotic occlusion was produced by introduction of a copper coil into the coronary artery. Reperfusion occurred within 50 minutes after beginning of treatment. Patency of the vessel was then angiographically monitored for a further 180 minutes.

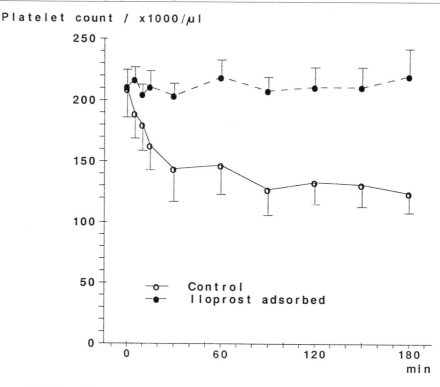

Platelet count / x1000/µl

Figure 1: Effect of iloprost adsorbed onto charcoal on thrombocytopenia in simulated hemoperfusion in vitro with human whole blood. The charcoal was incubated with iloprost at 10 µg/ml for 30 minutes and then washed with saline before it was used in the perfusion circuit.

(exitatory PGE) but not EP_2 (inhibitory PGE) receptors.[28,38]

As in platelets, binding of iloprost to smooth muscle PGI_2 receptors is followed by stimulation of adenylate cyclase and by an increase in cyclic AMP, as shown in cultured smooth muscle cells[105] and in preparations from dog femoral artery[122] and rabbit mesenteric artery.[123] Smooth muscle cGMP in rabbit femoral arteries was not changed by vasodilator concentrations of iloprost.[123]

Besides binding to PGI_2 receptors and increasing cAMP, iloprost-induced vascular relaxation in canine carotid artery and rat portal vein is accompanied by a concentration-dependent increase in smooth muscle resting membrane potential, and this hyperpolarization can be attributed to

a selectively increased membrane conductivity for potassium ions.[128,129]

Relaxant Effects in Isolated Arteries and Veins

Iloprost, like PGI_2, at nanomolar concentrations relaxes isolated arteries and veins, either precontracted by different agonists or displaying spontaneous tone, from different vascular beds of animals and man (Table 3). A direct comparison of vasorelaxant potencies between iloprost and PGI_2 is available only from bovine coronary artery strips, where the relaxant EC_{50} was 45 nM for iloprost and 65 nM for PGI_2.[140]

Iloprost does not relax the rabbit aortic

Table 3
Relaxation of Vascular Preparations In Vitro by Iloprost

Preparation	Precontraction	EC_{50} (nM)	Reference Number
Bovine coronary artery strip	none	45	140
Bovine coronary vein strip	none	inactive	124
Rabbit femoral artery strip	$PGF_{2\alpha}$	180	123
Rabbit mesenteric artery strip	$PGF_{2\alpha}$	42	123
Rabbit pulmonary artery strip	$PGF_{2\alpha}$	5200	123
Rabbit aortic strip	$PGF_{2\alpha}$	inactive	123
Rabbit ear artery perfused segment	phenylephrine	170	13
Rabbit saphenous vein strip	$PGF_{2\alpha}$	220	123
Dog carotid artery strip	none	6.7	128
Cat cerebral artery rings	5-HT	≈50	158
Human intrapulmonary artery strip	histamine	38	61

strip[123], which, presumably due to a lack of PGI_2 receptors, is considered as a PGI_2-insensitive preparation.[106]

At concentrations exceeding 10^{-6}M, iloprost increased the tone of dog coronary artery strips[128] and, like PGI_2, of human cerebral arteries.[81] Since cicaprost, a PGI_2 analogue with only negligible affinity towards PGE receptors, did not show this effect (Siegel, personal communication), vasoconstriction at high concentrations of iloprost may be mediated by its agonist activity at EP_1 receptors. Though the concentrations necessary to elicit EP_1 receptor agonist activity cannot be reached in vivo, in vitro results using PGE-sensitive preparations and high concentrations of iloprost should be interpreted with caution, since PGI_2 mimetic properties could be overridden by EP_1 agonistic activity.

Although in rings from rabbit mesenteric artery the relaxing potency was slightly less after removal of the endothelium, iloprost-induced vasorelaxation can be considered to be basically independent of endothelium.[123] Endogenous cyclooxygenase products seem not to modify iloprost's vasorelaxant effects, since indomethacin pretreatment of rabbit mesenteric artery was without influence.[123] As could be expected from the lack of effect on smooth muscle cGMP (see above), inhibition of guanylate cyclase with methylene blue did not modify vasorelaxation by iloprost,[123] and no potentiation of relaxation by sodium nitroprusside, a vasodilator stimulating smooth muscle cGMP, was noted in rabbit arteries.[5]

As neither iloprost perfusion through isolated rat blood vessels nor ex vivo assay of vascular PGI_2 synthesis after chronic iloprost infusion showed effects on PGI_2 synthesis, iloprost seemingly does not interfere with endogenous vascular PGI_2 formation.[84]

Inhibition of vascular sympathetic neurotransmission, in contrast to prostaglandins of the E-type, does not contribute to iloprost's vasorelaxant effect, as investigated in perfused rabbit ear arteries using transmural nerve stimulation to elicit contractions.[13]

Summarizing these data, iloprost, with a potency similar to PGI_2, relaxes PGI_2-sensitive isolated blood vessels in an endothelium-independent way, its vasodilator mechanisms involving binding to smooth muscle PGI_2 receptors, stimulation of adenylate cyclase, increase in cAMP, hyperpolarization of smooth muscle, and selective increase of membrane potassium conductivity.

Hemodynamic Action

Like PGI$_2$, iloprost dose-dependently lowers arterial vascular resistance and systemic blood pressure.[59] Its half-life being short (5 and 14 minutes in rat and dog, respectively),[121] steady-state hemodynamic effects are reached within 15 to 40 minutes of continuous intravascular infusion and are readily reversible after ceasing infusion.

At hypotensive doses, iloprost, like other vasodilators, activates baroreceptor reflex mechanisms increasing heart rate, cardiac output, splanchnic nerve activity, and plasma renin activity.[59,138]

As investigated in anesthetized dogs where both venous and arterial compliance were measured, the overall hemodynamic profile of iloprost is that of a preferential arterial vasodilator.[76]

The blood pressure lowering potency of iloprost is similar to PGI$_2$ (Fig. 2) and varies considerably according to animal species and experimental conditions, such as anesthesia, surgery, etc. (for review, see references 105, 121).

Although in vitro experiments in isolated rat atria showed a weak positive inotropic and chronotropic effect,[44] there is no evidence for direct effects of iloprost on cardiac performance in vivo.

Since clinically iloprost is applied at vasoactive, but nonhypotensive doses, systemic vasodilator effects at this dose level are of considerable interest and have been investigated in conscious rats instrumented with Doppler flow probes,[138] and in anesthetized rats using radioactive tracer microspheres.[95] Iloprost at subhypotensive doses decreased vascular resistance in the hind limbs and in the mesenteric vascular bed and, like PGI$_2$, significantly increased blood flow to the distal (nonmuscular) parts of the limbs. This dissociation between vasodilator and hypotensive effects clearly could be relevant to

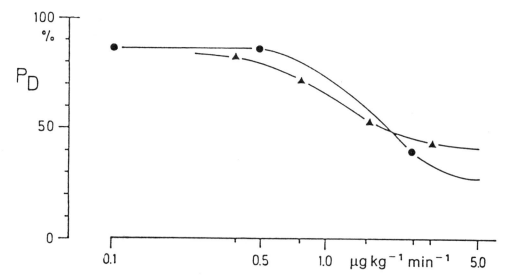

Figure 2: Lowering of diastolic arterial blood pressure (P$_D$) by iloprost (▲—▲) and PGI$_2$ (●—●) infused intravenously in conscious, spontaneously hypertensive rats.

iloprost's therapeutic effects in peripheral ischemic disease.[138] (See Chapter 16.)

At hypotensive doses, iloprost increases blood flow towards other vascular beds, such as mesentery, kidney, and skeletal muscle and causes redistribution of cardiac output towards gastrointestinal and skeletal muscle.[95] It is noteworthy that even in the presence of marked hypotension due to iloprost, a concomitant decrease of coronary vascular resistance maintains an increased coronary blood flow,[95] presumably due to the potent PGI_2-like coronary vasodilator action of iloprost shown also in isolated perfused hearts.[124] An effect of potential therapeutic relevance might be iloprost's potent dilatation of pulmonary arteries: in anesthetized dogs, iloprost effectively prevented hypoxia- and $PGF_{2\alpha}$-induced increases in pulmonary arterial pressure and resistance without lowering arterial blood pressure or affecting blood gases.[7]

Effects on the Microcirculation and on Vascular Endothelium

Since trophic lesions in advanced stages of peripheral arterial occlusive disease represent a breakdown of skin microcirculation, and iloprost has convincingly been shown to improve ischemic ulcer healing,[104] the effects on microvasculature represent an important facet of iloprost's pharmacology.

In the hamster cheek pouch preparation, iloprost, at a nonhypotensive dose, significantly dilated arterioles and venules, and markedly increased the number of blood-perfused capillaries.[96]

Microvascular vasospasm in the hamster cheek pouch induced by leukotriene D_4 (LTD_4) was functionally antagonized by iloprost,[96] as was LTD_4-induced coronary vasocontriction in isolated, perfused guinea pig hearts.[20] Recently, we could

demonstrate that arteriolar spasm in the hamster cheek pouch induced by the endothelium-derived vasoconstrictor peptide endothelin is totally reversed by IV infusion of a nonhypotensive dose of iloprost (Fig. 3) (unpublished observation).

Increases in microvascular macromolecular permeability as induced by inflammatory mediators (histamine, 5-HT, bradykinin) or by reperfusion after ischemia were effectively prevented by iloprost infusion at subhypotensive doses.[45,96]

Antiedematous effects of iloprost were also demonstrated in inflamed rat skin[41] and in isolated, perfused, angiotensin II-challenged rat lungs.[149] Furthermore, a distinct increase in rabbit cutaneous blood flow without increase in microvascular permeability was shown after topical application of iloprost.[42] The mechanism of iloprost's microvascular antiedematous effect (which, considering the regular finding of pericapillary protein-rich edema in peripheral ischemic disease, might be therapeutically relevant) has not been elucidated yet.

However, iloprost, like PGI_2, increases cAMP in cultured bovine endothelial cells,[36] and PGI_2 and carbacyclic PGI_2 analogues, in parallel with increasing cAMP-level, inhibit the passage of high molecular weight dextran through endothelial monolayers.[89] While it is not yet clear whether PGI_2/iloprost inhibits intercellular and/or transcellular endothelial passage of macromolecules, an increase of endothelial cAMP seems to be involved.

Supporting evidence for a role of iloprost in directly modulating endothelial cell function comes from experiments in isolated rabbit aorta, where iloprost preserved non-PGI_2-like, endothelium-dependent vasodilatation under the influence of hypoxia[151] and in perfused rat lung where iloprost, under hypoxic conditions, preserved the activity of an endothelial ectoenzyme, angiotensin converting enzyme.[3]

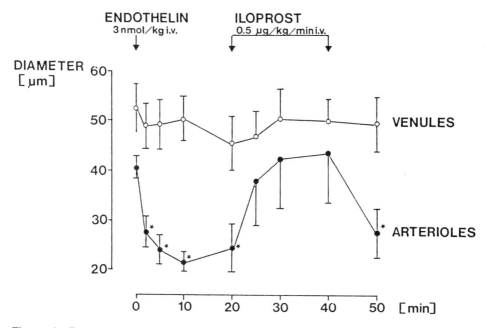

Figure 3: Reversal of endothelin-induced vasospasm by iloprost in the microcirculation of the exteriorized hamster cheek pouch. Data are means ± SD from five experiments/group. Asterisks indicate significant differences from control (p ≤ 0.05; rank sum test).

Effects on Leukocytes and on Leukocyte-Vessel Wall Interaction

Considerable evidence suggests that leukocyte-vessel wall interactions represent an important pathomechanism in ischemic diseases.[60] In pure in vitro preparations of human polymorphonuclear leukocytes (PMN), iloprost only weakly inhibited fMLP-induced aggregation at a concentration of 28 nM,[15] did not inhibit fMLP- and zymosan-induced superoxide anion formation up to a concentration of 30 μM[58] and only weakly inhibited aggregation of PMN induced by supernatant from aggregating platelets.[108] Superoxide anion formation by canine leukocytes stimulated by zymosan-activated plasma was partly inhibited by 50 μM iloprost or 100 μM PGI$_2$.[131] No effect was noted on zymosan-stimulated chemoluminescence of murine peritoneal macrophages up to 1 μM iloprost.[107]

According to these findings, iloprost is not a direct inhibitor of leukocyte activation. The effects shown in some preparations at high concentrations may well be attributed to iloprost's weak PGE-like agonist activity, since E-prostaglandins generally are potent direct inhibitors of leukocyte activation.[58]

On the other hand, iloprost already at 0.1 nM half-maximally inhibited human PMN-aggregation induced by collagen- and ADP-stimulated platelets,[108] and at 4 nM completely prevented fMLP- and Ca^{2+}-ionophore-induced leukocyte aggregation in human whole blood.[15] In vitro, inhibition of PMN adhesion to human umbilical vessels preincubated with iloprost,[15] and dose-dependent inhibition of spontaneous and complement peptide-stimulated guinea pig leukocyte adhesion to autologous aortic strips[52] have been described. In vivo, iloprost, at a non-hypotensive dose of 100 ng/kg/min IV, in rats completely inhibited increased leukocyte adherence to damaged mesenteric venules[97] and, in parallel to limiting infarct size, prevented leukocyte accumulation in feline and canine myocardium reperfused after ischemia.[8,131]

According to these data, iloprost is not a direct inhibitor of leukocyte activation but a potent inhibitor of platelet-induced leukocyte activation and stimulated adhesion of leukocytes to the vessel wall. The mechanism of iloprost's effect on leukocyte adhesion is not yet clear. However, inhibition of leukocyte adhesion after selective exposure of the blood vessel only to iloprost[15] suggests a role for direct effects on the vessel wall, besides inhibition of platelet-mediated leukocyte activation.

Cytoprotective and Tissue Protective Effects

The term *cytoprotection by prostaglandins* was first used by Robert[115] to describe protection by several prostaglandins and, later, also by PGI_2[72] of the gastric mucosa against various noxious stimuli. Subsequently, this term has been used frequently to describe protective effects of eicosanoids on tissues other than the stomach including the heart, liver, pancreas, and kidneys, and "cytoprotection," besides inhibition of platelet aggregation and vasodilator effects, is considered to represent one of the basic pharmacological properties of PGI_2 and iloprost.[57]

Cytoprotection, however, by no means refers to a defined pharmacological mechanism but rather is used with respect to tissue- and organ-protective effects in vitro and in vivo, where multiple PGI_2 effects, such as platelet inhibition, interference with leukocyte-vessel wall interactions, improved microcirculatory functions, etc., might be involved.

Cardioprotective Effects

In recent years, several studies have been published showing beneficial effects of iloprost (as well as, in some cases, prostacyclin itself and some other PGI_2 mimetics) in a variety of experimental models of myocardial injury. The diversity of pathophysiological models employed and the high number of parameters used to assess both myocardial damage and, consequently, the effectiveness of therapeutic intervention have resulted in a wide spectrum of "cardioprotective" effects being attributed to iloprost, some of which are summarized in Tables 4 and 5.

Cardioprotection in Ischemia-Reperfusion Situations

Much of the experimental evidence for cardioprotective effects of iloprost has been obtained in models of injury caused by myocardial ischemia with or without subsequent reperfusion (Tables 4 and 5). This probably reflects the general clinical situations in which cardioprotective therapy can be useful, e.g., acute myocardial infarction and angina pectoris.

During myocardial ischemia, cardiomyocytes in the underperfused region undergo a progressive change from the normal state to a state of irreversible injury. The rate at which this progression proceeds is primarily dependent on the extent of coronary collateral blood flow in the ischemic zone. Coronary collateral development and rate of infarction varies greatly in different species,[85] and is also dependent on clinical history, e.g., the normal human heart has only poorly developed collateral vessels, however, coronary stenosis (e.g., atherosclerotic) may result in the development of an extensive collateral network. The temporal progression of injury during ischemia means that there is a

Table 4
Cardioprotective Effects of Iloprost In Vitro

	Reference Numbers
Improved functional recovery during reperfusion after prolonged cold or short-term warm cardioplegia, or global ischemia	47, 125, 135, 155
Preservation of nerve stimulation-induced noradrenaline release following ischemia and reperfusion	125
Reduced oxidative stress during ischemia and reperfusion	47
Increased $CP:P_i$ ratio during reperfusion after global ishemia	110
Protection against arrhythmias induced by hypoxia and reoxygenation, aconitine, or cardiac glycosides	4, 87

"time window" during which therapeutic intervention should result in increased tissue salvage. The primary therapy for myocardial ischemia which has not yet progressed to irreversible injury must remain reperfusion—either pharmacological, physical, or surgical—as long-term viability is not feasible in the absence of restoration of blood flow. However, reperfusion may, in some situations, represent a "double-edged sword" as there is considerable experimental evidence to support the concept of reperfusion injury, i.e., reperfusion may lead to the death of some cardiomyocytes, which, at the time of reperfusion, were not yet irreversibly injured. Cardioprotective effects might therefore be expected with substances which can increase the "time window" for reperfusion (by reducing the severity of ischemia or increas-

Table 5
Cardioprotective Effects of Iloprost In Vivo

	Reference Numbers
Infarct size reduction following ischemia and reperfusion or coronary embolization	26, 34, 131
Enhanced recovery of regional myocardial function during reperfusion following ischemia	46, 153
Preservation of high-energy phosphates in ischemic myocardium	111
Preservation of myocardial CK and SOD activity following ischemia and reperfusion	31, 136, 145
Amelioration of ischemia-induced reductions in membrane phospholipids and intraneuronal catecholamines	31, 126
Reduction in ishemia-induced increases in cAMP and free lysosomal enzymes	111, 136
Inhibition of coronary thrombus formation induced by electrical stimulation	154
Prevention of cyclic reductions in coronary flow in the presence of a coronary stenosis	152
Antiarrhythmic effects against ischemia/reperfusion-induced and digoxin-induced arrhythmias	27, 34, 87, 94
Reduction of ischemia-induced ST elevation	34, 126

ing the ischemia tolerance of the cardiomyocytes) and/or reduce the extent of reperfusion injury.

Clinical myocardial infarction is usually initiated by thrombus formation in a coronary artery, often at the site of a ruptured atherosclerotic plaque, possibly accompanied by coronary vasoconstriction. Figure 4 shows a simplified schematic representation of this situation, and illustrates the self-amplifying nature of these events.

In such situations, iloprost, by virtue of its vasodilator and platelet antiaggregatory effects, should interrupt this vicious cycle and might therefore be expected to show beneficial effects. However, these effects alone do not provide sufficient explanation for the cardioprotective effects of iloprost seen in a number of ischemia-reperfusion situations. Improved functional recovery after ischemia is seen using doses of iloprost which cause only minor reductions in afterload and no increase in collateral blood flow during ischemia;[46] such beneficial effects were not seen with equi-

hypotensive doses of sodium nitroprusside. Iloprost has also been shown to improve functional recovery and/or reduce infarct size in rat, rabbit, and pig hearts, species in which coronary collateral development is minimal.[26,31,34,153,155] A primary role for platelets in the development of myocardial infarction in models of nonthrombotic coronary occlusion also seems doubtful, as infarct size is not reduced in dogs made acutely thrombocytopenic prior to the ischemic insult.[66,91]

In addition to vasodilation and inhibition of platelet activation, a number of other effects have been described for iloprost which may contribute to its cardioprotective actions. It has been reported to induce "membrane stabilization," assessed from washout profiles of labeled lipids,[135] though this effect differs from that of local anesthetics, as iloprost does not reduce the maximum rate of depolarization in arterial or ventricular muscle[68] The lysosomal stabilization[136] and preservation of intraneuronal catecholamines[126] ob-

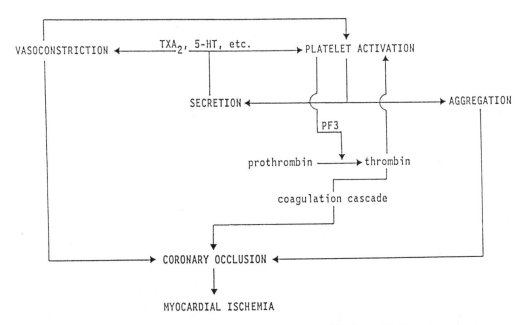

Figure 4: Schematic representation of events involved in the initiation of acute myocardial infarction.

served with iloprost in myocardial ischemia may also reflect some form of membrane stabilization.

A principal mechanism for the cardioprotective actions of iloprost in ischemia-reperfusion situations appears to be its ability to attenuate neutrophil-mediated cell injury (the effects of iloprost on leukocyte function have been dealt with in detail above). Reperfusion results in rapid accumulation of neutrophils in previously ischemic myocardium.[92] Activated neutrophils seem to play a central role in many models of ischemia-reperfusion damage, especially in those in which reperfusion injury is likely to occur. The deleterious effects of neutrophils are probably due mainly to release of reactive oxygen-derived free radicals, though proteolytic enzymes and myeloperoxidase-derived hypochlorous acid may also be involved. Neutrophils may also contribute to the "no reflow" phenomenon, by mechanical blockage of vessels in the microcirculation. The initial stimulus for neutrophil chemotaxis and diapedesis seems to be complement activation in the ischemic myocardium.[117] Leukotriene release from activated neutrophils will then increase leukocyte chemotaxis, as well as causing vasoconstriction and leakage of plasma proteins.[48] Support for the role of neutrophils in such situations comes from the apparent therapeutic efficacy of "antineutrophil" interventions, such as neutropenia,[43,67,116] treatment with antibodies inhibiting neutrophil adhesion[132] or treatment with oxygen radical scavengers,[6,88,100,113] in reducing infarct size and improving functional recovery following ischemia and reperfusion. Iloprost has been shown to reduce neutrophil accumulation in ischemic-reperfused myocardium, and this effect was associated with a reduction in infarct size of similar magnitude to. that seen in neutropenic animals.[131] It is likely that the most important "antineutrophil" effect of iloprost in this situation is its ability to inhibit neutrophil adhesion to the endothelial cell surface, which has been observed both in vitro[52] and in vivo.[97]

There is, therefore, considerable experimental evidence demonstrating cardioprotection of some form or another with iloprost. It also seems that no single mechanism of action can be proposed that would account for this beneficial effect in all the systems studied, for example, the effects on neutrophils, which seem to be of major importance in situations in vivo in which reperfusion damage occurs, cannot account for the improved functional recovery seen in buffer-perfused hearts in vitro. It seems more plausible that, of the broad spectrum of effects which have been demonstrated for iloprost, many may contribute to an overall "cardioprotective" action. The relative contribution of each of these effects will be intimately dependent on the pathophysiological changes that occur in the model or disease state under consideration.

Protective Effects on the Liver

Experimental evidence for cytoprotective effects in the strict sense—direct protection of mammalian cells against noxious stimuli—comes from experiments in isolated hepatocytes. In freshly isolated rat hepatocytes, iloprost at low concentrations (10^{-12} to 10^{-9}M) prevented cell death and sublethal morphological cell damage induced by carbon tetrachloride or bromobenzene and markedly attenuated bromobenzene-induced release of lactate dehydrogenase from the cells.[23] Similar protection of isolated hepatocytes by iloprost was shown against paracetamol toxicity.[101] No information is available, however, about the potential cytoprotective mechanisms of iloprost in these experiments.

Liver protective effects of iloprost were also described in vivo; IV infusion of

100 ng/kg/min in mice preserved liver cell morphology and attenuated enzyme release after sublethal doses of carbon tetrachloride.[23] Pretreatment of mice with iloprost protected against galactosamine/endotoxin-induced hepatitis.[157] This effect, however, rather than representing cytoprotection, was interpreted as functional antagonism by iloprost of a presumably leukotriene-mediated liver ischemia-reperfusion damage syndrome in this model.[157]

A potential therapeutic usefulness in liver transplantation is suggested by experiments in pig liver, demonstrating improved functional organ preservation with iloprost after 2 hours of warm ischemia.[139]

Protective Effects on the Kidney

The positive outcome of several studies investigating protective effects on the kidney suggest therapeutic potential of iloprost in kidney transplantation. Previous perfusion of isolated rabbit kidneys with 1–100 nM iloprost resulted in preservation of excretory function at reperfusion after 24 hours of cold storage.[150]

Reperfusion of dog kidneys in vivo following 180 minutes of renal artery occlusion after previous intraortic infusion of 50 ng/kg/min iloprost resulted in improved postischemic kidney perfusion and normal kidney function.[102] In pigs, reimplantation of in situ iloprost-preperfused kidneys after 45 minutes of warm ischemia or after 72 hours of hypothermic storage showed normal kidney perfusion, normal kidney function and no release of structural enzymes indicating cell damage.[62,114]

The precise mechanisms of iloprost's protective effects on the kidney are unknown, although improved blood flow at reperfusion seems to be involved.[102]

Protective Effects on Gastric Mucosa

Like PGI_2, iloprost protects gastric mucosa; in rats iloprost prevented indomethacin-induced gastric ulcers with an ED_{50} of 50 µg/kg p.o., thereby showing a potency approximately five times less than prostaglandin E_2.[156,165]

In rat stomach mucosal cells, iloprost at concentrations above 10 nM reduced ethanol-induced cell damage,[10] and also in dog gastric mucosa protective effects have been described.[72] In rat mucosal cells, specific binding of iloprost, but no correlation between mucosal cell cAMP and cell protection, was found.[10] Specific binding of iloprost to high affinity binding sites of gastric mucosa, not identical to PGI_2-binding sites, was shown in rats[144] but not in fundic mucosa from pigs, where iloprost at high concentrations bound to PGE_2-binding sites.[14]

In dog gastric mucosa, increased mucosal blood flow was proposed as the mechanism of iloprost's protective effect.[72]

Retardation of Allograft Rejection

Tissue protective effects may also be involved in effects of iloprost on rejection of organ or tissue transplants. In rats, iloprost infusion significantly prolonged rejection time of heterotopic cardiac allografts and, with respect to rejection time, showed synergistic effects with the immunosuppressive agent cyclosporine A.[50,118] Improvement of allograft blood flow was suggested as a potential mechanism of iloprost in this study.[118] Pretreatment with subcutaneous injections of iloprost significantly prolonged rejection time of murine skin allografts, and a concomitant reduction of thromboxane A_2 content in the ambient skin suggested inhibition of local platelet activation to play a role.[12]

Tissue Protective Effects in a Model of Skin Ischemia

Iloprost in patients with critical limb ischemia, which is not amenable to vascular reopening procedure, clearly promotes ischemic ulcer healing.[37,104] Pathomechanisms of critical ischemia comprise platelet activation, microvascular maldistribution of nutritive blood flow, increased microvascular permeability, and vasotoxic leukocyte vessel wall interactions; beneficial effects of iloprost on these mechanisms have been discussed above. Whether the effects of iloprost on microvessels, platelets, and leukocytes really would lead to a protective effect on critical ischemia was investigated in a model in which the ears of hairless mice were made critically ischemic by permanently interrupting two of the three neurovascular trunks supplying the ears.[98] In this model, continuous IV infusion of iloprost (100 ng/kg/min) limited the resulting final ischemic necrosis of the ears to approximately 50% of control values. Interestingly, in controls, functional vessel density decreased and total capillary flow increased, while with iloprost, functional vessel density increased and capillary flow remained unchanged. This indicates maldistribution of microvascular blood flow rather than critically low total flow in ischemic necrosis, and iloprost prevents ischemic necrosis by correcting microvascular flow maldistribution rather than by increasing total microvascular blood flow.

Effects in Cerebral Ischemia

In rats subjected to 60 minutes of cerebral ischemia by clamping of both carotid arteries and concomitant lowering of blood pressure with IV infusion of sodium nitroprusside, a neurological deficit, impaired learning behavior, and brain accumulation of Ca^{2+} as well as potassium loss and brain edema developed within the subsequent days. Iloprost infusion, at 0.16 μg/kg/min starting after ischemia, largely prevented potassium loss, Ca^{2+} accumulation and brain edema, improved postischemic learning capability, and attenuated the neurological deficit.[21,24]

In anesthetized dogs after 10 minutes of occlusion of both carotid and vertebral arteries, iloprost (12.5 ng/kg/min IV) prevented the postischemic decline of cerebral blood flow and cerebral oxygen extraction and maintained tissue PO_2 above hypoxia threshold levels.[24]

As potential mechanisms of these protective effects in cerebral ischemia, the authors suggested maintenance of cerebral microcirculatory viability by an effect of iloprost on microvascular tone and on platelet aggregation.

Antiatherosclerotic Effects

Considerable interest in the potential antiatherosclerotic properties of PGI_2 and PGI_2 analogues was raised by the finding that these substances inhibit basic mechanisms of early atherosclerosis, such as liberation of mitogens from platelets, leukocytes, and vascular endothelium and accumulation of cholesteryl esters in mononuclear leukocytes.[159]

In vitro, iloprost at nanomolar concentrations inhibits the release of mitogenic activity from cultured human umbilical endothelium.[159] Some controversy exists with respect to the inhibitory effect of iloprost and other prostanoids on growth factor release from platelets. Willis et al.,[159] using cultured 3T3 fibroblasts as a rather crude bioassay system for platelet-derived mitogenic activity, suggested that some PGI_2 mimetics could inhibit platelet-derived growth factor (PDGF) release at concentrations even below those inhibiting platelet activation. Subsequent studies, however, using a sensitive radioimmunoassay against human PDGF, showed for iloprost, as well as for a series of prostanoid platelet inhibitors, strict parallels between inhibition of PDGF release and inhibition of aggregation in thrombin-challenged human platelets.[142]

In freshly isolated human mononuclear leukocytes in lipid-depleted medium, iloprost (at concentrations of 1 nM and above) dependently inhibited cholesterol synthesis and LDL-receptor activity.[74,75]

In vivo, Jellinek et al.[65] showed that continuous infusion of iloprost prevented early atherosclerotic changes (deposition of basal membrane-like material in the subendothelial space, mitosis and subendothelial migration of smooth muscle cells) in the aorta of rats challenged with high doses of a soya-bean lipid emulsion.

In rats, where the endothelium in the abdominal aorta was denuded with a balloon catheter, iloprost diminished platelet adhesion to the denuded area and limited the intimal vascular proliferation, as assessed morphometrically 14 days after balloon catheter damage, to approximately 50% of control values.[70] Also in balloon catheter-denuded rat carotid arteries, iloprost significantly limited intimal proliferation after 14 days.[22]

According to these data, iloprost, like PGI_2, shows antiatherosclerotic properties by inhibiting mitogen release from platelets and endothelial cells, beneficially influencing mechanisms of cholesterol deposition in macrophages, and attenuating proliferative vascular changes following challenge by lipids or endothelial denudation.

Effects in Circulatory Shock

In rats injected with a 90% lethal dose of gram-negative bacterial endotoxin, iloprost (0.5 μg/kg/min IV) failed to correct endotoxic hypotension, leukopenia, and thrombocytopenia.[137] Survival time of endotoxemic rats, however, was significantly prolonged by iloprost.[127]

In lethal traumatic shock in anesthetized rats, iloprost significantly prolonged survival time and attenuated increases in plasma cathepsin D and plasma myocardial depressant factor-activity.[80] As a

mechanism of these protective effects, stabilizing of lysosomal membranes and preservation of splanchic circulation were proposed.[80]

In anesthetized cats, iloprost (0.2 and 1.0 μg/kg/min IV) dose-dependently attenuated hypotension and depression of cardiac function, and improved recovery from thrombocytopenia in systemic passive anaphylaxis.[93]

Negative results were obtained in porcine septic shock, where iloprost, like other antiplatelet drugs, did not markedly influence thrombocytopenia, leukopenia, decreases of antithrombin II and α_2-macroglobulin, and stimulation of coagulation system following injection of live *Escherichia coli*.[143]

Outlook

As discussed in Chapter 16 of this volume, the therapeutic potential of iloprost so far has been established clinically in the indications of severe peripheral arterial occlusive diseases, such as arteriosclerosis obliterans stage III and stage IV (according to Fontaine), thrombangiitis obliterans, and Raynaud's syndrome.

Its use as an adjunct to surgical recanalization therapy in vascular disease, as an adjunct to enzymatic thrombolysis in myocardial infarction, for preservation of transplant kidneys, and as an adjunct in heparin-induced thrombocytopenia is currently being investigated in prospective clinical trials.

Further investigations with iloprost and other PGI_2 mimetics, such as the metabolically stable compound cicaprost,[140] will show whether some of the potential therapeutic uses suggested by experimental data, such as ischemic stroke, platelet preservation in extracorporeal circulation systems, and prevention of vascular proliferative reocclusion in coronary and peripheral bypass surgery, can be established in clinical practice.

An exciting new field of experimental research is opened up by the question of how long-term therapeutic effects, as demonstrated in peripheral vascular disease,[37] can result from limited infusion cycles with a short-lived compound such as iloprost. At the level of platelets, Cottrell et al.[29] demonstrated that a short infusion of iloprost preserved normal platelet function throughout a 3-hour extracorporeal membrane oxygenation.

Recently, Lapetina[77] showed in human platelets that following incubation with iloprost a ras-related 22 kDa membrane protein is phosphorylated and translocated from the cell membrane to the cytosol. However, the relevance of this finding for platelet function is not known. Generally, our current understanding is incomplete with regard to long-term consequences of PGI_2- and iloprost-induced transient increases in cAMP in target cells, such as endothelium, vascular smooth muscle, and platelets, and further research on this subject is required.

References

1. Adaikan P.G., Kottegoda S.R.: Prostacyclin Analogs. Drugs Future 10:765–774, 1985.
2. Adaikan P.G., Karim S.M., Lau L.C., Tai M.Y., Kottegoda S.R.: Inhibition of platelet aggregation and antagonism of vasopressin-induced ECG changes in primates by a carboprostacyclin analogue, ZK 36374. Thromb. Res. 33:333–340, 1984.
3. Aksulu H.E., Türker R.K.: Iloprost preserves angiotensin-I conversion in the isolated perfused rat lung against anoxia. Eur. J. Pharmacol. 128:67–72, 1986.
4. Aksulu H.E., Ercan Z.S., Türker R.K.: Further studies on the antiarrhythmic effect of iloprost. Arch. Int. Pharmacodyn. Ther. 277:223–234, 1985.
5. Antunes E., Lidbury P.S., de Nucci G., Vane J.R.: Lack of synergism of iloprost and sodium nitroprusside on rabbit vascular smooth muscle. Br. J. Pharmacol. 95(Suppl.):516P, 1988.
6. Ambrosio G., Becker L.C., Hutchins G.M., Weisman H.F., Weisfeldt M.L.: Reduction in experimental infarct size by recombinant human superoxide dismutase: insights into the pathophysiology of reperfusion injury. Circulation 74:1424–1433, 1986.
7. Archer S.L., Chesler E., Cohn J.N., Weir E.K.: ZK 36.374, a stable analog of prostacyclin, prevents acute hypoxic pulmonary hypertension in the dog. J. Am. Coll Cardiol. 8:1189–1194, 1986.
8. Arnold G., Thiemermann C., Heymans L., Schroer K.: Morphological analysis of the iloprost effects on reperfused ischaemic myocardium. In: Prostaglandins and Other Eicosanoids in the Cardiovascular System, K. Schorr (ed.). Karger, Basel, 1985, pp 254–258.
9. Ashby B.: Kinetic evidence indicating separate stimulatory and inhibitory prostaglandin receptors on human platelet membranes. J. Cyc. Nucl. Prot. Phosph. Res. 11:291–300, 1986.
10. Barr D.B., Duncan J.A., Kiernan J.A., Soper B.D., Teppermann B.L.: Binding and biological actions of prostaglandin E_2 and I_2 in cells isolated from rabbit gastric mucosa. J. Physiol. 405:39–55, 1988.
11. Baruch D., Hemker H.C., Lindhout T.: Kinetics of thrombin-induced release and activation of platelet factor V. Eur. J. Biochem. 154:213–218, 1986.
12. Becker K.G., Lueddeckens R., Von Baehr W., Forster W.: Influence of the PG analogues iloprost, nalador and nileprost on rejection time and TXB2 content of murine tail skin allografts. Biomed. Biochim. Acta 47:117–120, 1988.
13. Beckmann R., Müller B.: Pre- and postsynaptic vascular effects of the PGI_2-analogues iloprost and ZK96.480, PGE_2 and PGE^1 in isolated rabbit ear arteries. In: Proc. 4th Con. Hung. Pharmacol. Soc. Vol. 3, U. Kecskemiti, K. Gyires, G. Kovacs (eds.). Budapest, 1985, pp 373–376.

14. Beinborn M., Netz S., Staar U., Sewing K.F.: Enrichment and characterization of specific (^{3}H) PGE$_2$ binding sites in the porcine gastric mucosa. Eur. J. Pharmacol. 147:217–226, 1988.

15. Belch J.J.F., Saniabadi A., Dickson R., Sturrock R.D., Forbes C.D.: Effect of iloprost on white cell behaviour. In: Prostacyclin and its Stable Analogue Iloprost, R.J. Gryglewsky, G. Stock (eds.). Springer, Berlin, 1987, pp 97–102.

16. Belch J.J., Greer I., McLaren M., Saniabadi A.R., Miller S., et al.: The effects of intravenous ZK 36374, a stable prostacyclin analogue, on normal volunteers. Prostaglandins 28:67–77, 1984.

17. Bergmann G., Kiff P.S., Atkinson L.,. Kerkez S., Jewitt. D.E.: Dissociation of platelet aggregation and vasodilatation with iloprost: a stable orally active, prostacyclin derivative. Circulation 68:398, 1983.

18. Bertele V.L., Mussoni G., Del Rosso G., Pintucci M.R., Carriero M.R., Merati G., et al.: Defective fibrinolytic response in atherosclerotic patients: effect of iloprost and its possible mechanism of action. Thromb. Haemostas. 60:141–144, 1988.

19. Bertele V., Mussoni L., Pintucci G., DelRosso G., Romano G., De Gaetano G., Libretti A.: The inhibitory effect of aspirin on fibrinolysis is reversed by iloprost, a prostacyclin analogue. Thromb. Haemostas. 61:286–288, 1989.

20. Bjornsson O.G., Kobayashi K., Williamson J.R.: Inducers of adenylate cyclase reverse the effect of leukotriene D4 in isolated working guinea pig heart. Am. J. Physiol. 252:H1235–H1242, 1987.

21. Borzeix M.G., Cahn R., Cahn J.: Effects of new chemically and metabolically stable prostacyclin analogues (iloprost and ZK96.480) on early consequences of a transient oligemia in the rat. Prostaglandins 35:653–664 1988.

22. Broszey T., Wülfroth P., Grünwald J.: Effects of the prostacyclin analogue iloprost and of heparin on experimentally induced lesion after ballooning of the rat carotid artery. In: 8th Int. Sympos. Atherosclerosis, Rome Abstr. 106, 1988.

23. Bursch W., Schutle-Hermann R.: Cytoprotective effect of the prostacyclin derivative iloprost against liver cell death induced by the hepatotoxins carbon tetrachloride and bromobenzene. Klin. Wochenschr. 64(Suppl.):47–50, 1986.

24. Cahn J., Borzeix M.G.: Iloprost in experimental cerebral ischaemia. In: Prostacyclin and its Stable Analogue Iloprost, R.J. Gryglewski, G. Stock (eds.). Springer, Berlin, 1987, pp 247–255.

25. Casals-Stenzel J., Buse M., Losert W.: Comparison of the vasodepressor action of ZK 36 374, a stable prostacyclin derivative, PGI$_2$ and PGE^1 with their effect on platelet aggregation and bleeding time in rats. Prostagl. Leukotr. Med. 10:197–212, 1983.

26. Chiariello M., Golino P., Cappelli-Bigazzi M., Ambrosio G., Tritto I., Salvatore M.: Reduction in infarct size by the prostacyclin analogue iloprost (ZK 36.374) after experimental coronary artery occlusion-reperfusion. Am. Heart J. 115:499–504, 1988.

27. Coker S.J., Parratt J.R.:. Prostacyclin: antiarrhythmic or arrhythmogenic? Comparison of the effects of intravenous and intracoronary prostacyclin and ZK36374 during coronary artery occlusion and reperfusion in anaesthetised greyhounds. J. Cardiovasc. Pharmacol. 5:557–567, 1983.

28. Coleman R.A., Humphrey P., Kennedy I.: Prostanoid receptors in smooth muscle: further evidence for a proposed classification. In: Trends in Autonomic Pharmacology, S. Kalsner (ed.). Taylor and Francies, London/Philadelphia, pp 35–49, 1985.

29. Cottrell E.D., Kappa J.R., Stenach N., et al.: Temporary inhibition of platelet function with iloprost (ZK 36.374) preserves canine platelets during extracorporeal membrane oxygenation. J. Thorac. Cardiovasc. Surg. 96:535–541, 1988.

30. Cowley A.J., Heptinstall S., Hampton J.R.: Effects of prostacyclin and of the stable prostacyclin analogue ZK 36374 on forearm blood flow and blood platelet behaviour in man. Thromb. Haemostas. 53:90–94, 1985.

31. Darius H., Osborne J.A., Reibel D.K., Lefer A.M.: Protective actions of a stable prostacyclin analog in ischemia induced membrane damage in rat myocardium. J. Mol. Cell. Cardiol. 19:243–250, 1987.

32. Darius H., Matzky R.: The actions of ZK36.374, a chemically stable carbacycline derivative, on platelet aggregation and vascular tone in vitro. Naunyn-Schmiedebergs Arch. Pharmacol. 316:R29, 1981.

33. Darius H., Hossmann V., Schorr K.: Antiplatelet effects of intravenous iloprost in patients with peripheral arterial obliterative disease. Klin. Wochenschr. 64:545–551, 1986.

34. De Langen C.D.J., van Gilst W.H., Wes-

seling H.: Sustained protection by iloprost of the porcine heart in the acute and chronic phases of myocardial infarction. J. Cardiovasc. Pharmacol. 7:924–928, 1985.

35. De Caterina R., Giannessi D., Gazzetti P., Bernini W.: Inhibition of platelet aggregation and thromboxane B2 production during aspirin treatment: dependence on the dose of the aggregating agent. Thromb. Res. 37:337–342, 1985.

36. Dembinska-Kiec A., Rücker W., Schonhofer P.S.: Effects of PGI$_2$ and PGI$_2$ analogues on c-AMP levels in cultured endothelial and smooth muscle cells derived from bovine arteries. Naunyn-Schmiedebergs Arch. Pharmacol. 311:R67, 1980.

37. Diehm C., Abri O., Baitsch G., Bechara G., Beck K., et al.: Iloprost, ein stabiles Prostacyclinderivat bei arterieller Verschluakrankheit im Stadium IV. Dtsch. Med. Wochenschr. 114:783–788, 1989.

38. Dong Y.J., Jones R.L., Wilson N.H.: Prostaglandin E-receptor subtypes in smooth muscle: agonist activities of stable prostacyclin analogues. Br. J. Pharmacol. 87:97–107, 1986.

39. Eddy C.A., Laufe L.E., Dunn R.L., Gibson J.W.: The use of prostacyclin analogue containing suture for the prevention of postoperative venous thrombosis in the rat. Plast. Reconstr. Surg. 78:504–512, 1986.

40. Edwards R.J., MacDermot J., Wilkins J.: Prostacyclin analogues reduce ADP-ribosylation of the alpha subunit of the regulatory G-S-protein and diminish adenosine A2 responsiveness of platelets. Br. J. Pharmacol. 90:501–510, 1987.

41. Ekerdt R., Luhm H.D., Opitz D.: Local effects of the prostacyclin analogue iloprost on cutaneous blood supply and oedema formation. Biomed. Biochim. Acta 47:S52-S55, 1988.

42. Ekerdt R., Luhm H., Toepert M.: Blood supply can be increased in rabbit skin by a stable prostacyclin derivative without potentiation of plasma extravasation. Br. J. Dermatol. 111 (Suppl.):144–146, 1984.

43. Engler R., Covell J.W.: Granulocytes cause reperfusion ventricular dysfunction after 15 minute ischemia in the dog. Circ. Res. 61:20–28, 1987.

44. Ercan Z.S., Turker R.K.: Possible beta adrenoceptor modulating effect of ZK36.374, a stable analogue of carbacyclin. Prostagl. Leukotrienes Med. 15:45–52, 1984.

45. Erlansson M., Bergqvist D., Persson D.H., Svensjoe E: Modulation of ischemia and histamine-induced macromolecular permeability increase in the hamster by a stable prostacyclin analogue (iloprost). Int. J. Microcir. Clin. Exp 6:183, 1987.

46. Farber N.E., Pieper G.M., Thomas J.P., Gross G.: Beneficial effects of iloprost in the stunned canine myocardium. Circ. Res. 62:204–215, 1988.

47. Ferrari R., Cargnoni A., Ceconi C., Curello S., Belloli S., et al.: Protective effect of a prostacyclin-mimetic on the ischaemic-reperfused rabbit myocardium. J. Mol. Cell. Cardiol. 20:1095–1106, 1988.

48. Feuerstein G.T., Hallenbeck J.M.: Leukotrienes in health and disease. FASEB J. 1:186–192, 1987.

49. Fisher C.A., Kappa J.R., Sinha A.K., Cottrell E.D., et al.: Comparison of equimolar concentrations of iloprost, prostacyclin, and prostaglandin E1 on human platelet function. J. Lab. Clin. Med. 109:184–90, 1987.

50. Foegh M.L., Rowles J., Khirabadi B.S., Ramwell P.W.: Allograft survival with iloprost. In: Prostaglandins and Other Eicosanoids in the Cardiovascular System, K. Schorr (ed). Karger, Basel, 1985, pp 243–246.

51. Frances R.B., Neely S.: Regulation by cyclic AMP of endothelial secretion of tissue-type plasminogen activator and its rapid inhibitor. Blood 72 (Suppl.1):296a (Abstr.1093), 1988.

52. Fricke D., Damerau B., Vogt W.: Adhesion of guinea pig poly morphonuclear leucocytes to autologous aortic strips: Influence of chemotactic factors and of pharmacological agents with affect arachidonic acid metabolism. Int. Arch. Allergy appl. Immunol. 78:429–437, 1985.

53. Giessen W.J., Van Mooi W.J., Rutteman A.M., Berk L., Verdouw P.D.: The effect of the stable prostacyclin analogue ZK 36374 on experimental coronary thrombosis in the pig. Thromb. Res. 36:45–51, 1984.

54. Golino P., Focaccio A., Eidt J., Buja L.M., Willerson J.T.: Iloprost reduces the time to thrombolysis and alters reocclusion after tDA in a canine model of coronary thrombosis. Circulation 78(Suppl.II):16(Abstr. 61), 1988.

55. Grant P.G., Mannarino A.F., Colman A.W.: cAMP mediated phosphorylation of the low K(m)cAMP phosphodiesterase markedly stimulates its catalytic activity. Proc. Natl. Acad. Sci. USA 85:9071–9075, 1988.

56. Gresele P., Arnout J., Deckmyn H., Huybrechts E., Pieters G., Vermylen J.: Role of proaggregatory and antiaggregatory prostaglandins in hemostasis. J. Clin. Invest. 80:267–271, 1987.

57. Gryglewski R.J.: The impact of prostacyclin studies on the development of its stable analogs. In: Prostacyclin and its Stable Analogue Iloprost, R.J. Gryglewski, G. Stock (eds.). Springer, Berlin, 1987, pp 3–15.

58. Gryglewski R.J., Szceklik A., Wandzilak M.: The effect of six prostaglandins, prostacyclin and iloprost on generation of superoxide anions by human polymorphonuclear leukocytes stimulated by zymosan or formyl methionyl leucyl phenylalanine. Biochem. Pharmacol. 36:4209–4213, 1987.

59. Haberey M., Loge O., Maass B., Ohme G.: Haemodynamic profile of iloprost in rats, rabbits and cats. In: Prostacyclin and its Stable Analogue Iloprost, R.J. Gryglewski, G. Stock (eds.). Springer, Berlin, 1987, pp 151–158

60. Harlan J.M.: Neutrophil-mediated vascular injury. Acta Med. Scan. 715(Suppl.):123–129, 1988.

61. Haye-Legrand I., Brink C., Bourdillat B., Labat C., Cerrina J., et al.: Relaxation of human pulmonary muscle preparations with PGI_2 and its analog. Prostaglandins 33:845–867, 1987.

62. Heynemann H.U., Rebmann J., Schabel B., Langkopf H., Pauer D., et al.: Hemodynamic studies of iloprost: conditioned ischemically stressed kidneys in animal experiments. Z. Urol. Nephrol. 79:329–334, 1986.

63. Higgs E.A., Moncada S., Vane J.R., Caen J.P., Michel H., Tobelem B.: Effect of prostacyclin (PGI_2) on platelet adhesion to rabbit arterial subendothelium. Prostaglandins 16:17–22, 1978.

64. Jaschonek K., Faul C., Schmidt H., Renn W.: Desensitization of platelets to iloprost. Loss of specific binding sites and heterologous desensitization of adenylate cyclase. Eur. J. Pharmacol. 147:187–196, 1988.

65. Jellinek H., Stock G., Takacs E.: Lipofundin arteriosclerosis and iloprost treatment. In: Prostacyclin and its Stable Analogue Iloprost, R.J. Gryglewski, G. Stock (eds.). Springer, Berlin, 1987, pp 269–278.

66. Jolly S.R., Schumacher W.A., Kunkel S.L., Abrams G.D., Liddicoat J., Lucchesi B.R.: Platelet depletion in experimental myocardial infarction. Basic Res. Cardiol. 80:269–279, 1985.

67. Jolly S., Kane W.J., Hoiok B.G., Abrams G.D., Kunkel S.L., Lucchesi B.R.: Reduction of myocardial infarct size by neutrophil depletion: effect of duration of occlusion. Am. Heart J. 112:682–690, 1986.

68. Kecskemeti V.: Cardiac electrophysiological effects of prostacyclin analogues, 7-oxo-PGI_2 and iloprost. Biomed. Biochim. Acta 46:S460-S464, 1987.

69. Kennedy I., Coleman R.A., Humphrey P.P.A., Lumley P.: Studies on the characterization of prostanoid receptors. In: Advances in Prostaglandin, Thromboxane, and Leukotriene Research, B. Samuelsson, R. Paoletti, P. Ramwell (eds). Raven Press, New York, 1983, pp 327–331.

70. Kerenyi A., Pustbai P., Takacs E., Kerenyi T., Schonfeld T., et al.: Reendothelialisations and prostacyclin therapy. In: Int. Congr. Atheroscl. Vienna, Abstr. No. 154, 1989.

71. Kim H.C., Harvey R., Kim E.J., Dole W., Saidi P., Trooskin S., Greco R.: Binding of a prostacyclin analogue (iloprost) to vascular prosthetic graft. Blood 72 (Suppl.1):369a, 1988.

72. Konturek S.J., Robert A.: Cytoprotection of canine gastric mucosa by prostacyclin: possible mediation by increased mucosal blood flow. Digestion 25:155–163, 1982.

73. Korbut R., Byrska Danek A., Gryglewski R.J.: Fibrinolytic activity of 6 keto prostaglandin E1. Thromb. Haemostas. 50:893, 1983.

74. Krone W., Klass A., Naegele H., Behnke B., Greten H.: Influence of prostaglandins on LDL receptor activity and cholesterol biosynthesis in human mononuclear leukocytes. Klin. Wochenschr. 65 (Suppl.):198, 1987.

75. Krone W., Kaczmarczyk P., Müller-Wieland D., Greten H.: The prostacyclin analogue iloprost and PGE_1 suppress sterol synthesis in freshly isolated human mononuclear leucocytes. Biochim. Biophys. Acta 835:154–157, 1985.

76. Krug B., Küpper J., Arnold G.: Effects of a prostacyclin analogue (ZK 36.374) on the arterial vascular system and on integrated systemic venous bed in anaesthetized dogs. In: Prostaglandins and Other Eicosanoids in the Cardiovascular System, K. Schorr (ed.). Karger, Basel, 1985, pp 292–297.

77. Lapetina E.G.: Iloprost causes the phosphorylation and translocation of a ras-related protein. J. Vasc. Med. Biol. 1:98, 1989.

78. Lapetina E.G., Reep B., Read N.G., Moncada S.: Adhesion of human platelets to collagen in the presence of prostacyclin, indo methacin and compound BW 755C. Thromb. Res. 41:325–335, 1986.

79. Levin R.I., Harpel P.C., Weil D., Chang T.S., Rifkin D.B.: Aspirin inhibits vascular plasminogen activator activity in vivo. J. Clin. Invest. 74:571–580, 1984.

80. Levitt M., Lefer A.M.: Anti-shock properties of the prostacyclin analog iloprost in traumatic shock. Prostaglandins Leukotr. Med. 25:175–185, 1986.

81. Lye R.H., Parsons A.A., Whalley E.T.: Effect of iloprost and PGI_2 on in vitro human cerebral arteries. Br. J. Pharmacol. 89 (Suppl.):691P, 1986.

82. MacDermot J., Wilkins A.J., Edwards R.J.: Heterologous desensitization of platelet adenosine (A2) responses by iloprost. Adv. Prostagl. Thrombox. Leukotriene Res. 17A:479–481, 1987.

83. Mackie I.J., Jones R., Machin S.L.: Platelet impedance aggregation in whole blood and its inhibition by antiplatelet drugs. J. Clin. Pathol. 37:874–878, 1984.

84. Masi I., Giani E., Mosconi C., Galli C.: Effects of iloprost treatment in the rat on prostacyclin release from isolated aortas. In: Prostacyclin and its Stable Analogue Iloprost, R.J. Gryglewski, G. Stock (eds.). Springer, Berlin, 1987, pp 139–142.

85. Maxwell M.P., Hearse D.J., Yellon D.M.: Species variation in the coronary collateral circulation during regional myocardial ischaemia: a critical determinant of the rate of evolution and extent of myocardial infarction. Cardiovasc. Res. 21:737–746, 1987.

86. McIntyre D.E., Bushfield M., McMillan M.J., Moffat K.J., et al.: Receptors and receptor mechanisms of endogenous platelet stimulatory and inhibitory mediators. Agents Actions 20(Suppl.):45–62, 1986.

87. Metin M., Dörtlemez O., Dörtlemez H., Akar F., Ercan Z.S., et al.: Prevention by a carbacyclin analogue (ZK36374) of digoxin-induced ventricular extrasystoles in guinea-pig myocardium. Eur. J. Pharmacol. 98:125–128, 1984.

88. Mitsos S.E., Fantone J.C., Gallgher K.P., Walden K.M., Simpson P.J., et al.: Canine myocardial reperfusion injury: protection by a free radical scavenger, N-2-mercaptopropionyl glycine. J. Cardiovasc. Pharmacol. 8:978–988, 1986.

89. Mizuno-Yagyo Y., Hashida R., Mineo C., Ikegami S., Oshuma S., Takano T.: Effect of PGI_2 on transcellular transport of fluorescein dextran through on arterial endothelial monolayer. Biochem. Pharmacol. 36:3809–3813, 1987.

90. Moncada S.R., Gryglewski J., Bunting S., Vane J.R.: An enzyme transforms prostaglandin endoperoxides to an unstable substance that inhibits platelet aggregation. Nature 263:663–665, 1976.

91. Mullane K.M., McGiff J.C.: Platelet depletion and infarct size in an occlusion-reperfusion model of myocardial ischemia in anesthetized dogs. J. Cardiovasc. Pharmacol. 7:733–738, 1985.

92. Mullane K.M., Kraemer R., Smith B.: Myeloperoxidase activity as a quantitative assessment of neutrophil infiltration into ischemic myocardium. J. Pharmacol. Methods 14:157–167, 1985.

93. Müller B., Maass B., Haberey M.: The stable prostacyclin analogue iloprost alleviates cardiovascular symptoms of systemic anaphylaxis in anaesthetized cats. Prostagl. Leukotr. Med. 17:147–148, 1985.

94. Müller B., Maass B., Stürzebecher S., Skuballa W.: Antifibrillatory action of the stable orally active prostacyclin analogues iloprost and ZK96480 in rats after coronary artery ligation. Biomed. Biochim. Acta 43:S175-S178, 1984.

95. Müller B., Maass B., Kuhles T.: Effect of PGI_2 and iloprost on regional blood flow in rats. Naunyn-Schmiedebergs Arch. Pharmacol. 332(Suppl.):36, 1986.

96. Müller B., Schmidtke M., Witt W.: Action of the stable prostacyclin analogue iloprost on microvascular tone and perme ability in the hamster cheek pouch. Prostagl. Leukotr. Med. 29:187–198, 1987.

97. Müller B., Schmidtke M., Witt W.: Adherence of leucocytes to electrically damaged venules in vivo. Effects of iloprost, PGE_1-indomethacin, forskolin, BW 755C, sulotroban, hirudin and throbocytopenia. Eicosanoids 1:13–17, 1988.

98. Müller B., Schmidtke M.: Effect of iloprost on spreading of ischaemic necrosis in the hairless mouse ear. Prostagl. Leukotr. Essent. Fatty Acids 39(1):63–64, 1990.

99. Musial J., Wilczynska M., Sladek K., Cierniewski C.S., Nizankowski R., Szczeklik A.: Fibrinolytic activity of prostacyclin and iloprost in patients with peripheral arterial disease. Prostaglandins 31:61–70, 1986.

100. Myers M.L., Bolli R., Lekich R.F., Hartley C.J., Roberts R.: N-2-mercaptopropionylglycine improves recovery of myocardial function after reversible regional ischemia. J. Am. Coll. Cardiol. 8:1161–1168, 1986.

101. Nasseri Sina P., Boobis A.R., Davies D.S.: Cytoprotection against paracetamol induced toxicity in isolated hepatocytes with iloprost a stable analogue of prostacyclin. Hum. Toxicol. 6:429–430, 1987.

102. Neumayer H.H., Wagner K., Preuschof L., Stanke H., Schultze G., et al.: Amelioration of postischemic acute renal failure by prostacyclin analogue (Iloprost): long-term studies with chronically instrumented conscious dogs. J. Cardiovasc. Pharmacol. 8:785–790, 1986.

103. Nickolson R.C., Town M.H., Vorbrüggen H.: Prostacyclin analogs. Med. Res. Rev. 5:1–53, 1985.

104. Oberender H., Krais T., Schäfer M., Belcher G.: Clinical benefits of iloprost, a stable prostacyclin (PGI_2) analog, in severe peripheral arterial disease (PAD). Adv. Prostaglandins, Thromboxane Leukotriene Res. 19:311–316, 1989.

105. Oliva D., Nicosia S.: PGI_2 receptors and molecular mechanisms in platelets and vasculature. Pharmacol. Res. Commun. 19:735–765, 1987.

106. Omini C., Moncada S., Vane J.R.: The effects of PGI_2 on tissues which detect prostaglandins. Prostaglandins 14:625–632, 1977.

107. Parnham M.J., Bittner C.: Pharmacological analysis of guinea pig macrophage chemiluminescence responses to platelet activating factor and opsonized zymosan. Int. J. Immunopharmacol. 8:951–959, 1986.

108. Pecsvarady Z., Nash G., Thomas P., Dormandy J.: Protective effect of a prostacyclin analogue (iloprost) against platelet-induced granulocyte aggregation. Thromb. Haemostas., in press, 1989.

109. Pedvis L.G., Wong T., Frojmovic M.M.: Differential inhibition of the platelet activation sequence: shape change, micro and macro aggregation, by a stable prostacyclin analogue (iloprost). Thromb. Haemostas. 59:323–328, 1988.

110. Pissarek M., Gründer W., Keller T.: 31-P.NMR-spectroscopy on ischemic and reperfused rat hearts: effects of iloprost. Biomed. Biochim. Acta 46:S564-S567, 1987.

111. Pissarek M., Goos H., Nöhring J., Graff J., Buller G., et al.: Prostacyclin and iloprost: Equal efficiency in preserving high energy phosphates in the dog heart following coronary artery ligation. Basic Res. Cardiol. 82:566–575, 1987a.

112. Plotkine M., Massad L., Allix M., Boulu R.G.: A new arterial thrombosis model to study antithrombotic agents: efficacy of naftidrofuryl. Clin. Hemorheol. 9:339–349, 1989.

113. Przyklenk K., Kloner R.A.: Superoxide dismutase plus catalase improve contractile function in the canine model of the "stunned myocardium." Circ. Res. 58:148–156, 1986.

114. Rebmann U., Langkopf B., Schabel I., Pauer H.D., Heynemann H., Forster W.: Extended storage preservation of swine kidneys to 72 hours using iloprost. Z. Urol. Nephrol. 78:611–617, 1985.

115. Robert A.: Antisecretory, antiulcer, cytoprotective and diarrheogenic properties of prostaglandins. Adv. Prostaglandin Thromboxane Res. 2:507–520, 1976.

116. Romson J.L., Hook B.G., Kunkel S.L., Abrams G.D., et al.: Reduction of the extent of ischemic myocardial injury by neutrophil depletion in the dog. Circulation 67:1016–1023, 1983.

117. Rossen R.D., Swain J.L., Michael L.H., Weakley S., Giannini E., Entman M.L.: Selective accumulation of the first component of complement and leucocytes in ischemic canine heart muscle. A possible initiator of an extra myocardial mechanism of ischemic injury. Cir. Res. 57:119–130, 1985.

118. Rowles J.R., Foegh M.L., Khirabadi B.S., Ramwell P.W.: The synergistic effect of cyclosporine and iloprost on survival of rat cardiac allografts. Transplantation 42:94–96, 1986.

119. Rücker W., Schrör K.: Evidence for high affinity prostacyclin binding sites in vascular tissue: radioligand studies with a chemically stable analogue. Biochem. Pharmacol. 32:2405–2410, 1983.

120. Saniabadi A.R., Lowe G.D.O., Belch J.J.F.: The novel effect of a new prostacyclin analogue ZK36374 on the aggregation of human platelets in whole blood. Thromb. Haemostas. 50:718–721, 1983.

121. Schillinger E., Krais T., Lehmann M., Stock G.: Iloprost. In: New Cardiovascular Drugs, A. Scriabine (ed.). Raven Press, New York, 1986, pp 209–231.

122. Schillinger E., Losert W.F.: Identification of PGI_2-receptors and cAMP levels in platelets and femoral arteries. Acta Therapeutica 6 (Suppl.):37, 1980.

123. Schröder G., Beckmann R., Schillinger E.: Studies on vasorelaxant effects and mechanisms of iloprost in isolated preparations. In: Prostacyclin and its Stable Analogue Iloprost, R.J. Gryglewski, G. Stock (eds.). Springer, Berlin, 1987, pp 129–137.

124. Schrör K., Darius H., Matzky R., Ohlendorf R.: The antiplatelet and cardiovascular actions of a new carbacyclin derivative (ZK 36.374) equipotent to PGI₂ in vitro. Naunyn-Schmiedebergs Arch. Pharmacol. 316:252–256, 1981.

125. Schrör K., Funke K.: Prostaglandins and myocardial noradrenaline overflow after sympathetic nerve stimulation during ischemia and reperfusion. J. Cardiovasc. Pharmacol. 7(Suppl. 5):S50-S54, 1985.

126. Schrör K., Ohlendorf R., Darius H.: Beneficial effects of a new carbacyclin derivative, ZK36374, in acute myocardial ischemia. J. Pharmacol. Exp Ther. 219:243–249, 1981.

127. Schutt W.A., Hom G.J.: Iloprost a stable prostacyclin analogue increases survival time in conscious rats treated with lipopolysaccharide endotoxin LPS. FASEB J. 2:Abstr. 7406, 1988.

128. Siegel G., Stock G., Schnalke F., Litza B.: Electrical and mechanical effects of prostacyclin in the canine carotid artery. In: Prostacyclin and its Stable Analogue Iloprost, R.J. Gryglewski, G. Stock (eds.). Springer, Berlin, 1987, pp 143–149.

129. Siegel G., Mironneau J., Schnalke F., Loirand G., Stock G.: Potassium channel opening and vasorelaxation. J. Vasc. Med. Biol. 1:116, 1989.

130. Siegl A.M.: Receptors for PGI₂ and PGD₂ on human platelets. Methods. Enzymol. 86:179–192, 1982.

131. Simpson P.J., Mickelson J., Fantone J.C., Gallagher K.P., Lucchesi B.R.: Iloprost inhibits neutrophil function in vitro and in vivo and limits experimental infarct size in canine heart. Circ. Res. 60:666–673, 1987.

132. Simpson P.J., Todd R.F. III, Fantone J.C., Fantone J.K., et al.: Reduction of experimental canine myocardial reperfusion injury by a monoclonal antibody (Anti-Mol, Anti-CD11b) that inhibits leucocyte adhesion. J. Clin. Invest. 81:624–629, 1988.

133. Skopal J., Kovacs M., Stadler I., Galambos G., Kovacs G.: Effect of prostacyclin derivatives on platelet factor 3 availability. Thromb. Res. 47:117–121, 1987.

134. Skuballa W., Vorbrüggen H.: A new route to 6a-carbacyclins. Synthesis of a stable biologically potent prostacyclin analogue. Angew. Chem. Int. Ed. Engl. 20:1046–1048, 1981.

135. Smith E.F. III, Kloster G., Stocklin G., Schrör K.: Effect of iloprost (ZK 37.374) on membrane integrity in ischemic rabbit hearts. Biomed. Biochim. Acta 43:S155-S158, 1984.

136. Smith E.F. III, Gallenkämper W., Beckmann R., Thomsen T., Mannesmann G., et al.: Early and late administration of a PGI₂-analogue, ZK36374 (iloprost): effects on myocardial preservation, collateral blood flow and infarct size. Cardiovasc. Res. 18:163–173, 1984.

137. Smith E.F., Tempel G.E., Wise W.C., Halushka P.V., Cook J.A.: The effect of PGI₂ or iloprost on eicosanoid formation and the leukopenia of endotoxin shock. In: Prostaglandins and Other Eicosanoids in the Cardiovascular System, K. Schrör (ed.). Karger, Basel, 1985, pp 202–206.

138. Steinberg H., Medvedev O.S., Luft F.C., Unger T.: Effect of a prostacyclin derivative (iloprost) on regional blood flow, sympathetic nerve activity, and baroreceptor reflex in the conscious rat. J. Cardiovasc. Pharmacol. 11:84–89, 1988.

139. Steininger R., Mühlbacher F., Rauhs R., Roth E., Bursch W.: Protective effect of PGI₂ and diltiazem on liver ischaemia and reperfusion in pigs. Transplant Proc. 20:999–1002, 1988.

140. Stürzebecher C.S., Haberey M., Müller B., Schillinger E., Schroder G., et al.: Pharmacological profile of ZK96.480, a new chemically and metabolically stable prostacyclin analogue with oral availability and high PGI₂ intrinsic activity. In: Prostaglandins and Other Eicosanoids in the Cardiovascular System, K. Schrör (ed.). Karger, Basel, 1985, pp 485–491.

141. Stürzebecher C.S., Losert W.: Effects of iloprost on platelet activation in vitro. In: Prostacyclin and its Stable Analogue Iloprost, R.J. Gryglewski, G. Stock (eds.). Springer, Berlin, 1987, pp 39–46.

142. Stürzebecher S., Nieuweboer B., Matthes S., Schillinger E.: Effects of PGD₂, PGE₁, and PGI₂-analogues on PDGF-release and aggregation of human gel-filtered platelets. In: Prostaglandins in Clinical Research: Cardiovascular system, K. Schrör, H. Sinzinger (eds.). Alan R. Liss, New York, 1989, pp 365–369.

143. Svartholm E., Bergquist D., Haglund U., Ljungberg J., Hedner U.: Coagulation and fibrinolytic reactions in experimental porcine septic shock: pretreatment with different antiplatelet factors. Circ. Shock 22:291–301, 1987.

144. Teppermann B.L., Soper B.D., Emery S.K.: Specific binding of a stable prostacyclin analogue (iloprost) to rat oxyntic mucosa. Prostaglandins 28:477–484, 1984.

145. Thiemermann C., Steinhagen-Thiessen

E., Schrör K.: Inhibition of oxygen centered free radical formation by the stable prostacyclin-mimetic iloprost (ZK 36.374) in acute myocardial ischemia. J. Cardiovasc. Pharmacol. 6:365–366, 1984.

146. Town M.H., Schillinger E., Speckenbach A., Prior G.: Idenfication and characterisation of a prostacyclin-like receptor in bovine coronary arteries using a specific and stable prostacyclin analogue, iloprost as radioactive ligand. Prostaglandins 24:61D72, 1982.

147. Tranquille N., Emeis J.J.: Release of tissue type plasminogen activator is induced in rats by leukotrienes C4 and D4, but not by prostaglandins E1, E2 and I2. Br. J. Pharmacol. 93:156–164, 1988.

148. Tsai A., Hsu M.J., Vijjeswarapu H., Wu K.K.: Solubilization of prostacyclin membrane receptors from human platelets. J. Biol. Chem. 264:61–67, 1989.

149. Türker R.K., Aksulu H.E., Ercan Z.S., Aslan S.: Thromboxane A_2-inhibitors and iloprost prevent angiotensin-II-induced edema in the isolated perfused rat lung. Arch. Int. Pharmacodyn. Ther. 287:323–329, 1987.

150. Türker R.K., Demirel E., Ercan Z.S.: Iloprost preserves kidney function against anoxia. Prostagl. Leukotr. Med. 31:45–52, 1988.

151. Türker R.K., Demirel E.: Iloprost maintains acetylcholine relaxations of isolated rabbit aortic strips submitted to hypoxia. Pharmacology 36:151–155, 1988.

152. Uchida Y., Murao S.: Effects of a prostaglandin I_2-analogue, ZK 36.374, on recurring reduction of coronary blood flow. Jpn. Heart J. 24:641–647, 1983.

153. Van der Giessen W.J., Schoutsen B., Tijssen J.G.P., Verdouw P.D.: Iloprost (ZK36374) enhances recovery of regional myocardial function during reperfusion after coronary artery occlusion in the pig. Br. J. Pharmacol. 87:23–27, 1986.

154. Van der Giessen W.J., Mooi W.J., Rutteman A.M., Berk L., et al.: The effects of the stable prostacyclin analogue ZK 36.374 on experimental coronary thrombosis in the pig. Thromb. Res. 36:45–51, 1984.

155. Van Gilst W.H., Boonstra P.W., Terpstra J.A., Wildevuur C.R.H., et al.: Improved recovery of cardiac function after 24 h of hypothermic arrest in the isolated rat heart: comparison of a prostacyclin analogue (ZK36374) and a calcium entry

156. Vischer P., Casals-Stenzel J.: Pharmacological properties of ciloprost, a stable prostacyclin analogue, on the gastrointestinal tract. Prostagl. Leukotr. Med. 9:517–529, 1982.

157. Wendel A., Tiegs G., Werner C.: Evidence for the involvement of a reperfusion injury in galactosamine/endotoxin induced hepatitis in mice. Biochem. Pharmacol. 36:2637–2639, 1987.

158. Whalley E.T., Schilling L., Wahl M.: Effects of various prostanoids on feline cerebral arteries in vivo and in vitro. Eur. J. Physiol. 411(Suppl.):R48, 1988.

159. Willis A.L., Smith D.L., Vigo L.: Suppression of principal atherosclerotic mechanisms by prostacyclin and other eicosanoids. Progr. Lipid Res. 25:645–666, 1986.

160. Winther K., Snorrason K., Knudsen L., Medgyesi S.: The effect of prostacyclin infusion on tissue plasminogen activator. Thromb. Res. 46:741–745, 1987.

161. Witt W., Müller B.: Antithrombotic profile of iloprost in experimental models of in vivo platelet aggregation and thrombosis. In: Advances in Prostaglandin, Thromboxane, and Leukotriene Research, B. Samuelsson, R. Paoletti, P. Ramwell (eds.). Raven Press, New York, 1983, pp 327–331.

162. Witt W., Stürzebecher S., Müller B.: Synergistic antiplatelet and antithrombotic effects of a prostacyclin analogue (iloprost) combined with a thromboxane antagonist (sulotroban) in guinea pigs and rats. Thromb. Res. 51:607–616, 1987.

163. Witt W., Baldus B.: Divergent effects of iloprost and alprostadil on platelets, blood pressure and fibrinolysis. In: Prostaglandins in Clinical Research: Cardiovascular System, K. Schrör, H. Sinzinger (eds.). Alan R. Liss, New York, 1989, p 347.

164. Witt W.: Differential efficacy in vivo of common versus specific pathway inhibitors of platelet aggregation. Blood 58:109 (Abstr. 62), 1989.

165. Zengil H., Onuk E., Ercan Z.S., Türker R.K.: Protective effect of iloprost and UK 38 485 against gastric mucosal damage induced by various stimuli. Prostagl. Leukotr. Med. 30:61–67, 1987.

166. Zwaal R.F.A., Comfurius P., Hemker H.C., Bevers E.M.: The inhibition of platelet prothrombinase activity by prostacyclin. Haemostasis 14:320–324, 1984.

16

Clinical Experience with Iloprost in the Treatment of Critical Leg Ischemia

John A. Dormandy

The Clinical Problem of Critical Leg Ischemia

It has been estimated that 1% of men under 50 years of age and 5% over that age have symptomatic arterial disease affecting the legs. In the early stages this may only manifest itself as intermittent claudication, that is, limitation of walking, but a proportion will progress until they can hardly move without pain, even indoors.[5] Finally, the blood supply to the legs may become so restricted that they have pain even at rest or frankly nonviable skin with ulceration or gangrene. The term critical limb ischemia (CLI) is applied to these final stages where the imminent prospect facing the patient is a major amputation. Neither the prevalence nor the incidence of critical leg ischemia has ever been directly documented in an adequate epidemiological study. However, from small population studies and national figures for amputations, it has been estimated that the incidence of critical leg ischemia is approxi-

mately 1000 per million population per year.[3] The fear of reaching this stage is something that is at the forefront of all patients' minds when told they have significant ischemic disease of their legs.

The pathophysiology and management of CLI has been a relatively neglected area of medicine until in 1988 there began in Europe a Consensus Process on Critical Limb Ischemia.[3] This brought together a number of specialists in the basic sciences and clinicians in the various disciplines involved with managing these patients. Because the underlying cause in the majority of CLI is atherosclerotic narrowing of the major arteries, traditionally its treatment has been the province of the vascular surgeon, who could possibly remove or bypass the obstruction. But unfortunately, reconstructive arterial surgery is only technically possible in a minority and major surgical intervention carries considerable risk in these patients. In the last decade, the increasing use of ingenious percutaneous catheter reopening procedures devised by radiologists has opened up an-

Rubanyi G.M.: Cardiovascular Significance of Endothelium-Derived Vasoactive Factors, Futura Publishing Co., Inc., Mount Kisco, NY, © 1991.

other possibility for correcting the basic arterial narrowing.[9] Nevertheless, even in centers where such specialized surgical and interventional radiological techniques are available, the fate of the patient with critical leg ischemia is dire. A recent survey has shown that even in centers of excellence, 19% of such patients have to undergo primary major amputation, 61% have an attempt at primary surgical or radiological treatment of the arterial occlusion, and the remaining 20% receive some type of temporary nonsurgical management. A year after developing CLI, only 56% will be alive with two legs, 26% will have had a major amputation and the other 18% will be dead.[17] The current prognosis for patients with critical leg ischemia is indeed very bleak.

Current Role of Pharmacotherapy in the Management of Critical Leg Ischemia

The consensus process on CLI brought together vascular surgeons and interventional radiologists, who in most countries provide treatment to the majority of these patients, with internists such as angiologists, cardiologists, and diabetologists, to determine the proper contribution from the respective specialties. Too frequently, angiology is still only practiced as a specialty in a few centers, although the pairing of angiologists and vascular surgeons should be as natural as that of cardiologists and cardiac surgeons. Figure 1

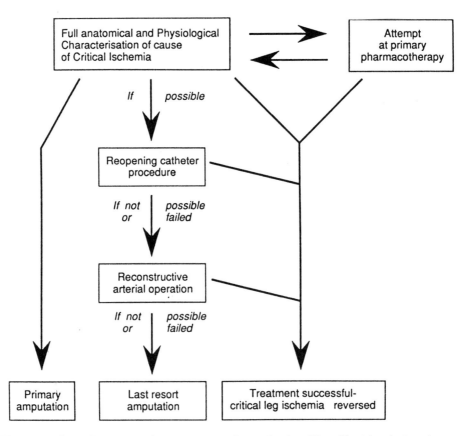

Figure 1: Overall pattern of management for patients with critical leg ischemia.

summarizes the current pattern of management of CLI, showing the possible place of pharmacotherapy. At least theoretically, pharmacotherapy may be a primary treatment, ideally avoiding the need for any form of mechanical procedure. A totally different and additional role of pharmacotherapy is as an adjuvant to arterial reconstructions, angioplasty, thrombolysis, or to improve healing in more distal amputations.

Unfortunately, there is little solid evidence that any of the older medications that are widely established in the management of patients with milder manifestations of leg ischemia, in particular intermittent claudication, are really effective in the treatment of CLI. Indeed, even their value in the treatment of claudication is still sometimes questioned.[8,14] The same has to be said for such maneuvers as isovolemic hemodilution. Recommendation 30 of the Consensus Document[3] summarizes the present situation regarding nonprostanoids in the primary treatment of critical ischemia as follows:

There is little evidence available for the efficacy of oral anticoagulants, other forms of anticoagulation, antiplatelet drugs, vasoactive drugs or fibrinogen-lowering drugs in the treatment of chronic critical limb ischemia. It is possible, but not formally proven, that oral and nonoral anticoagulant drugs may prevent macro- or micro-thromboembolic events in these patients. Similarly these drugs may also prevent the progression of peripheral arterial occlusive disease.

The background to this has been amplified in a subsequent book.[16] The use of drugs as adjuvant therapy during and following mechanical forms of therapy is much better established. But the amazing ingenuity of new percutaneous reboring techniques has not been matched by the necessary corollary of maintaining patency in the reopened arteries. There have been surprisingly few prospective controlled studies of adjuvant pharmacotherapy following peripheral angioplasty. The role of adjuvant pharmacotherapy is summarized in the following four recommendations of the Consensus Document on CLI:

Recommendation 19

On theoretical and clinical grounds, salicylate is recommended after PTA of stenoses and short occlusions. Treatment should be continued for at least one year, and longer in the absence of side effects if there are any residual lesions.

Recommendation 20

Heparin and overlapping oral anticoagulant therapy is recommended following local thrombolysis alone or in combination with PTA. The same regimen should be followed after PTA of long occlusions. Treatment should be continued for at least one year, or longer in the presence of any residual lesions.

Recommendation 28

No pharmacological therapy is required following reconstructive surgery above the inguinal ligament.

Recommendation 29

Following reconstructions below the inguinal ligament, some form of drug therapy may be useful to reduce graft failure, but its effectiveness still remains to be proven.

The place and usefulness of primary pharmacotherapy as an alternative and preferred treatment to surgery or interventional radiology has recently been altered by the advent of prostacyclin and its analogues. Although some prostaglandins have been used clinically, their role was difficult to establish because of the instability of the compounds and the need to administer some intra-arterially. Iloprost, however, is stable, can be administered intravenously, and has been evaluated clinically in a number of large multicenter studies of patients with CLI. The availability of iloprost as an effective form of pharmacotherapy for such patients with severe ischemia is likely to significantly improve the fate of patients with CLI. In the following sections, the probable mechanism of action of iloprost will be summarized and its clinical use will be described and discussed in more detail.

Pathophysiology of Critical Ischemia and Possible Mechanism of Action of Iloprost

The detailed pharmacological actions of iloprost are described in Chapter 15. How these varied properties of a prostacyclin-like drug may reverse the pathological changes seen in severe critical ischemia has been discussed in detail and published elsewhere.[4] While much is known of the actions of iloprost in vitro and in animal models, there is still much doubt about the basic pathophysiology of critical ischemia.

Critical ischemic changes in the distal part of the limb are almost always secondary to long-standing proximal arterial blocks and stenoses. These had been developing gradually over the decades, the distal blood supply being maintained by the development of collateral channels. In patients with CLI, the development of collateral channels has failed to compensate adequately for the progressive arterial occlusions. In diabetics, the proximal atherosclerosis may be accompanied or even largely replaced by a more localized distal angiopathy. The final changes in the mi-

crocirculation are the result of a decreased perfusion pressure. Iloprost acts largely at this microcirculatory level, reversing the changes resulting from a decreased perfusion pressure.

It has been suggested that the pathophysiology of CLI is essentially made up of two components: a deregulation of the microvascular flow regulating system (MFRS) and an inappropriate activation of the microvascular defense system (MDS). The MFRS regulates and distributes blood flow in the normal microcirculation. It is characterized by the phenomenon of normal vasomotion, which allows regular periodic perfusion of different capillary networks. Endothelium-derived relaxing factor (EDRF) and one or more endothelium-derived constricting factors (EDCF) also play a role in controlling normal microcirculatory flow. The MDS is primarily a property of the leukocytes and platelets in the circulating blood and also of the endothelium (Fig. 2a). In health, activation of platelets and leukocytes occurs and there are interactions between them and the endothelium, which is an entirely appropriate defensive response to injury and infection. It is suggested that in critical ischemia, there is a breakdown of both of these normal regulatory and defense systems. The components of the inappropriate activation of the MDS are shown in Figure 2b, which also illustrates the positive feedback vicious cycles that can be set up. The trigger for this is a marked decrease in the arterial perfusion pressure following occlusion of the larger proximal arteries by atherosclerosis. In addition, rheological changes occur in the distal microcirculation. The low shear stress and raised plasma fibrinogen allow erythrocyte aggregation. Similarly, the platelet and leukocyte aggregates also tend to cause microcirculatory occlusion. Leukocyte plugging is believed to be the principal effect of the low perfusion pressure at the level of individual capillaries. The overall changes in the arteries, arterioles, and cap-

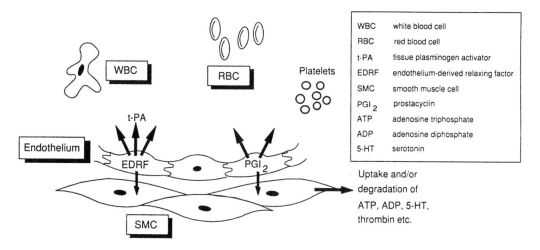

The blood cells (WBC, RBC, platelets) are under physiological conditions in a non-adhering, non-secretory state.

Figure 2a: Hypothesis of inappropriately activated microvascular defense system in critical ischemia: components of the microvascular defense system.

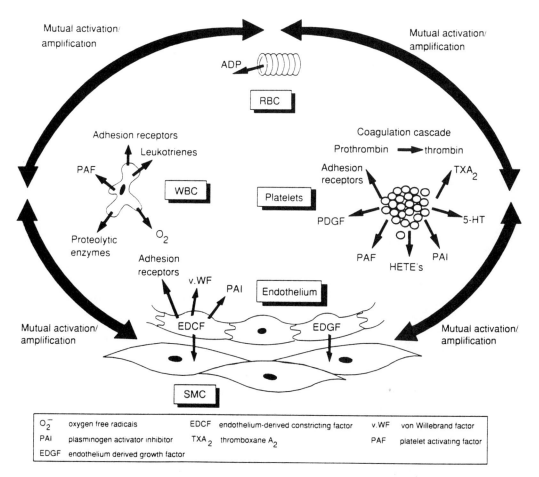

Figure 2b: Factors contributing to inappropriate activation of the microvascular defense system—alterations that may occur in critical ischemia.

illaries that may occur in critical ischemia are shown in greater detail in Figure 3.

The clinical benefit of iloprost is then due to a re- establishment of the MFRS and deactivation of the MDS. This is illustrated diagrammatically in the sequence of panels in Figure 4. Iloprost can have no immediate effect on the fixed arterial block and it is still uncertain whether it can substantially increase collateral blood flow. Clinical studies certainly do not suggest that it substantially improves the arterial perfusion pressure distal to the arterial block. Iloprost, however, improves the distribution of what blood flow there is by reversing many of the local microcirculatory changes

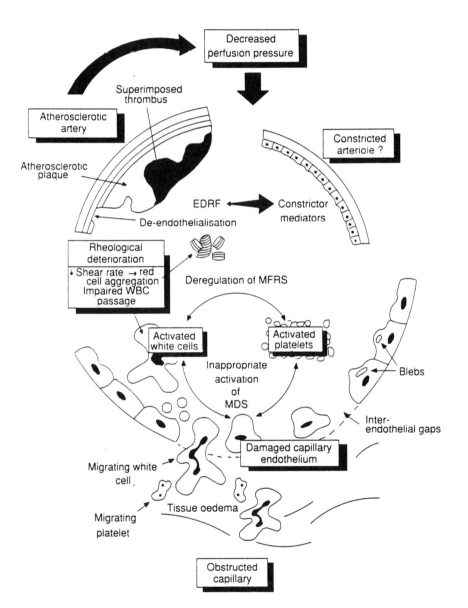

Figure 3: Summary of suggested pathophysiological changes in critical ischemia at different levels of the circulation.

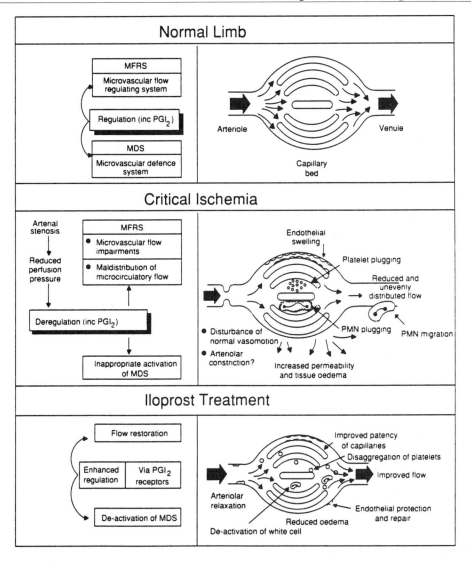

after Lowe

Figure 4: Microcirculatory response in critical ischemia and the effect of iloprost.

which had caused occlusion of the capillaries and by re-establishing normal vasomotion. The crucial, and ultimately the only, important question is whether iloprost works in practice. Most of the clinical experience so far has been in atherosclerotic critical leg ischemia and that experience will be reviewed first.

Clinical Efficacy of Iloprost in Patients with Critical Leg Ischemia Due to Atherosclerosis

In a disease such as CLI, where every patient's condition is different in terms of concurrent diseases, duration of disease, and many other risk factors, it is impossible to predict the outcome for individual patients. For this and many other reasons, it is essential that the efficacy of a new treatment should be assessed in a sufficiently large prospective study of patients randomly allocated to the test treatment and a placebo group. Double-blind assessment is also desirable, but cannot be fully achieved in practice with such a potent prostacyclin-like drug. It is therefore particularly important that the end-points used to measure efficacy are as hard and free of subjective judgment as possible.

Five large, prospective multicenter trials have been completed in four European countries, involving a total of 697 patients with CLI.[1,2,12,13] The outline of these studies is shown in Table 1. The dosage regime of iloprost was identical in all the studies; the maximum tolerated dose up to 2 ng/kg/minute was determined during the first 3 days and then continued as a 6-hour intravenous infusion every day for the duration of the study. This varied from 2 weeks in the Scandinavian study to 4 weeks in both the German (IV) and UK studies. Table 1 also shows two types of

patients with CLI who were studied, fitting into Fontaine's classification groups III and IV. In group III, patients had rest pain requiring continuous analgesia and hospitalization, but did not have any ulcers or gangrene. In stage IV, all the patients had such skin tissue loss and most also had pain. It is now increasingly appreciated that these two groups of patients should be considered separately, although both have CLI with a high amputation rate. Stages II, III, and IV do not necessarily form a continuum. Patients with severe claudication (stage II) frequently develop gangrene (stage IV) without passing through the stage of rest pain (stage III).

The characteristics of the patients entered in the five studies emphasize their severe local and generalized cardiovascular disease. The low ankle systolic Doppler pressure quantifies the extensive large vessel disease and the low perfusion pressure available to the microcirculation of the foot. Overall, approximately one-third of the patients already had attempts at arterial reconstructive operations or catheter opening procedures. Indeed, an entry criterion common to all the trials was the failure or impracticability of any revascularization

Table 1
Summary of Large, Prospective Placebo-Controlled Studies of Iloprost in CLI

Stage of CLI (Stage III: rest pain Stage IV: ulcers or gangrene)	German Study III	German Study IV	Scandinavian Study IV	U.K. Study III/IV	French Study IV
Number of patients	136	210	103	151	128
Period of treatment (weeks)	2	4	2	4	3
Age: years (mean)	70	66	70	73	68
Previous revascularization procedure	35%	n.a.	26%	44%	n.a.
Ankle Doppler pressure	87% <70 mm	52% <70 mm	64% <60 mm	59% <70 mm	n.a.
Diabetes	37%	52%	32%	40%	42
Hypertension	42%	42%	40%	n.a.	n.a.
Congestive heart failure	n.a.	29%	13%	n.a.	n.a.

Stage of CLI (Stage III: rest pain Stage IV: ulcers or gangrene)
n.a. = not available

procedure and, in this sense, the patients tended to have more advanced disease than a totally random selection of patients with CLI. The serious generalized cardiovascular disease is evidenced by the prevalence of hypertension and diabetes. Approximately three-quarters of the patients were already receiving medication for heart disease.

In all these trials, iloprost infusion was compared to a placebo infusion, but after the end of the treatment period, it was clearly impossible with such a severely ill group of patients to standardize the therapy after the infusion and individual investigators used whatever treatment they thought appropriate. At the end of the infusion period, patients were judged to be responders or nonresponders on the basis of pain relief in group III patients and signs of ulcer healing in group IV patients.

Figure 5 summarizes the responder rates in all the trials of patients with CLI. In all the studies, there was a greater response with iloprost than placebo. The fact that there was any response with a placebo infusion is not surprising since all the patients also received standard medical therapy for co-existing disease, such as heart failure or infection. The two German studies and the results in the two types of patients within the UK study suggest that iloprost was more effective in stage IV patients with ulcers than in stage III patients, who only had rest pain. Combining all the trials, 29.1% of the placebo-treated patients were responders compared to 51.5% of the patients receiving iloprost infusion. This difference in responder rate is impressive, but a formal statistical meta-analysis is also required, taking into account all patients who started treatment, even if they did not finish the full course. Patients who discontinued treatment because of treatment fail-

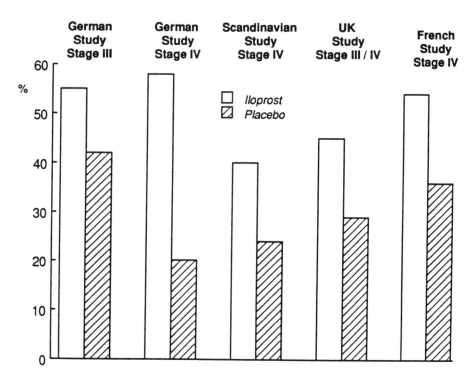

Figure 5: Response rate (%) at end of treatment with iloprost or placebo in the five CLI studies.

ure or early efficacy have to be considered as nonresponders and responders, respectively. Such a formal meta-analysis of the five studies, on an intention-to-treat basis, was carried out by the Technology Assessment Group of the Harvard School of Public Health[15] using the Yusuf-Peto modification[19] of the classic Mantel-Haenszel method.[10] The result shows that pain relief at end of treatment was significantly greater in the iloprost than in the placebo group (p<0.05), with an odds ratio of 1.58 (95% confidence limits 1.01 to 2.45). The difference between the two groups in terms of ulcer healing was even more impressive (p<0.0001), with an odds ratio of 2.48 (95% confidence limits 1.68 to 3.66).

The above analysis refers to results at the end of the infusion period and, while this gives us information about the pharmacological usefulness of the drug, real clinical efficacy needs to be judged in the longer term, even though the patients received an uncontrolled variety of treatments after their placebo or iloprost infusion. The end of treatment assessment may also be criticized because the rather subjective or soft end-points of pain relief and decrease in the ulcer size were used. There was, however, a formalized 6-month follow-up period of observation in the three most recent studies (Scandinavian, French, and UK) and in these studies, it is possible to look at the harder end-point of major (above the ankle) amputation in the two groups who had originally received iloprost or placebo infusion. These results are shown in Figure 6. In each study, fewer patients who had received iloprost required a major amputation in the subsequent 6 months than patients who had received placebo. A formal meta-analysis, as described above, on an intention-to-treat basis and, assuming that none of the lost

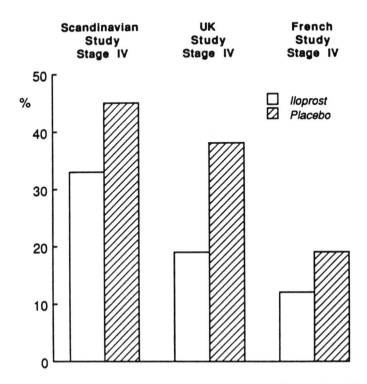

Figure 6: Major amputation rate during a 6-month observation period following iloprost and placebo infusions.

patients had an amputation, the improvement with iloprost therapy is significant (p = 0.01) with an odds ratio of 0.52 (95% confidence limits 0.31 to 0.89). (If all the patients lost to follow-up are assumed to have had an amputation, a significant difference persists at p<0.01.) These findings suggest the hypothesis that iloprost infusion reverses some of the microcirculatory changes associated with CLI and that the consequent benefit persists for at least some months.

The evidence from prospective placebo-controlled studies in nearly 700 patients with CLI unsuitable for any other forms of treatment strongly suggests that iloprost infusion for 2 to 4 weeks improves healing of ulcers, reduces rest pain, and decreases the incidence of major amputation within the subsequent 6 months.

Efficacy of Iloprost in Other Clinical Indications

There are two other, rarer, manifestations of severe ischemia where there is clinical evidence that iloprost is effective. The first is the rather intriguing condition of thromboangiitis obliterans (TAO), also known as Buerger's disease. The etiology of the characteristic narrowing of the distal arteries in this condition is uncertain, but it is definitely not atherosclerosis. In natives of Europe and North America, the condition is rare, but in many parts of Asia, it is almost as common a cause of leg ulcers and gangrene as atherosclerosis, often requiring amputation. Iloprost infusion for 4 weeks has been tested in 133 patients with ulcers due to TAO in what is probably the largest reported prospective controlled double-blind trial in such patients.[7] There has been a suggestion that low dose aspirin may be beneficial in TAO and therefore it was used in preference to placebo as the comparator drug. The beneficial effect of iloprost was even more striking than in patients with atherosclerotic leg ulceration. The overall response rate was 87% in the iloprost group, but only 17% in the aspirin-treated patients. In the iloprost group, 63% of the patients had complete pain relief, compared with 28% in the aspirin group; complete healing of ulcers was achieved in 35% of the iloprost group, compared with 13% in the aspirin group.

The particularly marked efficacy of iloprost in TAO is an interesting clue to a possible aspect of its mechanism of action. TAO is believed to be primarily an inflammatory response to an unknown stimulus. The protective effect of iloprost against inappropriate activation of leukocytes may therefore be an especially important mechanism.

The other clinical condition of severe ischemia, somewhat more common than TAO in the Western world, is Raynaud's phenomenon secondary to a connective tissue disease. These constitute a particularly malignant form of Raynaud's of the fingers, where there is usually severe pain and ulceration, not infrequently requiring amputation of one or more fingers. There is no established medical or surgical treatment for these cases. There have been several controlled, prospective studies of short-term (3 days) infusion of iloprost in a cross-over design.[11,18] Symptomatology was statistically significantly improved by iloprost, with substantial reduction in the frequency of the attacks, the benefit lasting for 4 to 6 weeks after infusion.

Future Perspectives

Iloprost and prostacyclin analogues are undoubtedly the most promising form of pharmacological therapy for severe peripheral ischemia to be introduced in the last decade. This is a clinical area that has been somewhat neglected in the past and has been particularly bereft of any established drug therapy with really significant and widely accepted clinical efficacy. Intravenous iloprost infusion for 2 to 4 weeks has been shown to relieve rest pain significantly, promote ulcer healing, and decrease the need for a major amputation for up to 6 months. There are several existing areas for the future clinical application of prostacyclin analogues and iloprost. Only patients with CLI who were unsuitable for surgical reconstruction and catheter reopening procedures, or where their attempt had failed, were entered in the current trials of iloprost. Given the excellent results in these patients, it may now be appropriate to compare an iloprost infusion with reconstructive arterial surgery as primary treatment of CLI. Limb salvage surgery carries a definite mortality and is frequently unsuccessful, leading directly to a major amputation. It may well be that for high risk patients, as many of these patients are, a course of iloprost will be preferred to a precarious arterial operation. At the same time, the use of iloprost as an adjunct to limb salvage surgery needs to be tested. It may well be that iloprost infusion during and after reconstructive surgery may improve patency and decrease mortality. Similarly, the combination of iloprost and percutaneous catheter procedures is an important study that needs to be carried out in the near future. With the present pharmacotherapy following angioplasty, there is still a high incidence of early reocclusion in distal lesions.

Finally, there is the completely unexplored area of adjuvant pharmacotherapy for major amputations. Even when a major amputation is inevitable, there is much advantage to be gained in terms of rehabilitation and mobility, if the amputation can be carried out below rather than above the knee. For this reason, a below-knee amputation is often attempted even when the chances of proper healing below the knee are uncertain. A review of the literature shows that 15% of below-knee amputations have to be revised above the knee, and in a further 15%[6] healing is very delayed. It seems logical to try and improve the success of below-knee amputations by an infusion of iloprost immediately after surgery, when increased skin blood flow is essential for proper healing. A trial of 700 below-knee amputations, looking at the possible benefit of an iloprost infusion immediately after surgery, has just been completed.

All of these areas remain to be fully explored with the present intravenous preparation. But orally effective prostacyclin analogues are not far away and they will open completely new areas of therapy, as well as possibly increasing the efficacy of the intravenous preparation by continuing with long-term oral medication. If intravenous iloprost significantly decreases the amputation rate within 6 months after cessation of the infusion, how much more effective would it be if during those 6 months the patients had been taking an oral prostacyclin analogue?

References

1. Balzer K., Bechara G., Bisler H., et al.: Placebo-kontrollierte, doppelblinde Multizenterstudie zur Wirksamkeit von iloprost bei der Behandlung ischamischer Ruheschmerzen von Patienten mit peripheren arteriellen Durchblutungsstorungen. Vasa (Suppl.) 20:379–381, 1987.
2. Diehm C., Abri O., Baitsch G., et al.: Iloprost, ein stabiles Prostacyclinderivat, bei arterieller Verschlusskrankheit im Stadium IV: eine placebo-Kontrollierte Multizenterstudie. Dtsch. Med. Wochenschr. 114:783–788, 1989.
3. Dormandy J.A. (Ed.): European Consensus Document on Critical Limb Ischaemia, Springer-Verlag, New York, 1989.
4. Dormandy J.A. (Ed.): The Pathophysiology of Critical Limb Ischaemia and Pharmaco-

logical Intervention with a Stable Prostacyclin Analogue, Iloprost. International Congress and Symposium Series, Royal Society of Medicine, 1989.

5. Dormandy J., Mahir M., Ascady G., et al.: Fate of the patient with chronic leg ischemia. J. Cardiovasc. Surg. 30:50–58, 1989.

6. Dormandy J.A., Thomas P.R.S.: What is the natural history of a critically ischaemic patient with and without his leg? In: Limb Salvage and Amputation for Vascular Disease, Greenhalgh R.M., Jamieson C.W., Nicolaides A.N., (eds.). W.B. Saunders Co., Philadelphia, 1988.

7. Fiessinger J.N.: A randomised double-blind study comparing iloprost and aspirin for the treatment of critical limb ischemia due to thromboangitis obliterans. Submitted for publication 1989.

8. Housley E.: Treating claudication in five words. Br. Med. J. 296:1483–1484, 1988.

9. Krings W., Peters P.E.: Percutaneous Procedures. In: Critical Leg Ischaemia: Its Pathophysiology and Management. Dormandy J., Stock G. (eds.). Springer-Verlag, New York, 1989.

10. Mantel N., Haenszel W.: Statistical aspects of the analysis of data from retrospective studies of disease. JNCI 22:719–748, 1959.

11. McHugh N.J., Csuka M., Watson H., et al.: Infusion of iloprost, a prostacyclin analogue, for treatment of Raynaud's phenomenon in systemic sclerosis. Ann. Rheum. Dis. 47:43–47, 1988.

12. Norgren L., Angqvist K.A., Bergqvist D., et al.: A stable prostacyclin analog (iloprost) in patients with ischemic ulcers of the lower limb. Eur. J. Vasc. Surg. (submitted).

13. Oberender H., Krais T., Schafer M., Belcher G.: Clinical benefits of iloprost, a stable prostacyclin (PGI_2 analog, in severe peripheral arterial disease (PAD). Adv. Prostaglandin, Thromboxane, Leukotriene Res. 19:311–316, 1989.

14. Ruckley C.V.: Claudication. Br. Med. J. 292:970–971, 1986.

15. Sacks H.S., Berrier J., Reitman D., et al.: Meta-analysis of randomized controlled trials. N. Engl. J. Med. 316:450–455, 1987.

16. Verstraete M., Verhaege R.: Primary pharmacotherapy other than prostanoids. In: Critical Leg Ischaemia: Its Pathophysiology and Management. Dormandy J., Stock G. (eds.). Springer-Verlag, New York, 1990.

17. Wolfe J.H.N.: The definition of critical ischaemia: is this a concept of value? In: Limb Salvage and Amputation for Vascular Disease, Greenhalgh R.M., Jamieson C.W., Nicolaides A.N. (eds.). W.B. Saunders Company, Philadelphia, 1988.

18. Yardumian D.A., Isenberg D.A., Rustin M., et al.: Successful treatment of Raynaud's syndrome with iloprost, a chemically stable prostacyclin analogue. Br. J. Rheumatol. 27:220–226, 1988.

19. Yusuf S., Peto R., Lewis J., et al.: Beta blockade during and after myocardial infarction: an overview of the randomised trials. Prog. Cardiovasc. Dis. 27:335–371, 1985.

Index